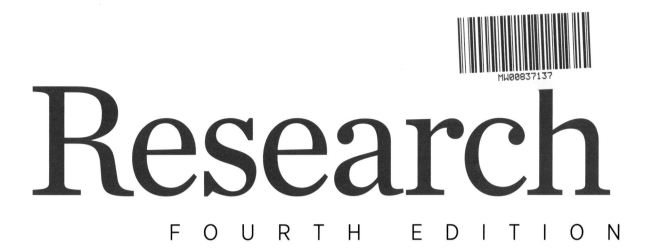

Research

FOURTH EDITION

Successful Approaches in Nutrition and Dietetics

Linda Van Horn, PhD, RDN,
and Judith Beto, PhD, RDN

EDITORS

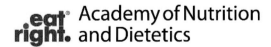

Academy of Nutrition and Dietetics

CHICAGO, IL

eat right. Academy of Nutrition and Dietetics

Academy of Nutrition and Dietetics
120 S. Riverside Plaza, Suite 2190
Chicago, IL 60606-6995

Research: Successful Approaches in Nutrition and Dietetics, Fourth Edition
ISBN 978-0-88091-946-3 (print)
ISBN 978-0-88091-947-0 (eBook)
Catalog Number 199919 (print)
Catalog Number 199919e (eBook)

10   9   8   7   6   5   4   3   2   1

For more information on the Academy of Nutrition and Dietetics, visit www.eatright.org.

Library of Congress Cataloging-in-Publication Data
Names: Van Horn, Linda, editor. | Beto, Judith A., editor. | Academy of
  Nutrition and Dietetics, issuing body.
Title: Research : successful approaches in nutrition and dietetics / [edited
  by] Linda Van Horn and Judith Beto.
Other titles: Research (Van Horn)
Description: 4th edition. | Chicago, IL : Academy of Nutrition and Dietetics,
  [2019] | Includes bibliographical references and index.
Identifiers: LCCN 2018060019 (print) | LCCN 2018061669 (ebook) | ISBN
  9780880919470 (eBook) | ISBN 9780880919463 (print : alk. paper)
Subjects: | MESH: Nutritional Physiological Phenomena | Research Design |
  Data Collection | Dietetics--methods | Epidemiologic Methods
Classification: LCC TX367 (ebook) | LCC TX367 (print) | NLM QU 145 | DDC
  613.2072--dc23
LC record available at https://lccn.loc.gov/2018060019

Contents

Section 1: An Introduction to Discovery Through Research in Nutrition and Dietetics

Section 2: Establishing and Maintaining a Research Environment

Section 3: Descriptive Research

Section 7: Key Aspects of Research in Food, Nutrition, and Dietetics

Section 8: Application of Statistical Analysis in Nutrition and Dietetics Research

Section 9: **Presentation of Research Data**

Section 10: **Applications of Research to Practice**

List of Boxes, Tables, and Figures

Boxes

Tables

Figures

Editors

Linda Van Horn, PhD, RDN, earned her bachelor's degree from Purdue University in Nutrition and Dietetics, her master's degree from the University of Pittsburgh in Exercise Physiology, and her doctorate from the University of Illinois at Chicago in Public Health. She completed her dietetic internship at Indiana University in Indianapolis. She began her career as a hospital dietitian I at the University of Illinois Hospitals and Clinics and eventually joined the faculty at Northwestern University Feinberg School of Medicine, where she is currently a tenured professor in the Department of Preventive Medicine and Associate Dean for Faculty Development. She served as Editor-in-Chief of the *Journal of the Academy of Nutrition and Dietetics* for the ten-year term limit and chaired the 2010 US Dietary Guidelines Advisory Committee.

Judith Beto, PhD, RDN, earned her bachelor's degree from Dominican University in Nutrition and Dietetics, her master's degree in Health Professions Education from the University of Illinois at Chicago, and her doctorate from the University of Chicago in Measurement, Evaluation, and Statistical Analysis. She completed her dietetic internship at the Hines Veterans Administration Hospital where she continued as a renal dietitian. She was the department chair and tenured professor of Nutrition Sciences at Dominican University until 2012. She still collaborates as a Research Associate in Nephrology and Hypertension at Loyola University Chicago, Health Sciences Division. She serves as a Research Editor for the *Journal of the Academy of Nutrition and Dietetics* and as an elected public member of the National Board of Podiatric Medical Examiners.

Contributors

Regan L. Bailey, PhD, MPH, RD
Associate Professor, Purdue University
West Lafayette, IN

Judith Beto, PhD, RDN
Research Associate, Loyola University Healthcare System
Maywood, IL

Carol J. Boushey, PhD, MPH, RDN
Associate Research Professor, Epidemiology Program, University of Hawaii Cancer Center
Honolulu, HI

Maureen Brady Moran, MPH
Assistant Professor of Preventive Medicine, Northwestern University, Feinberg School of Medicine,
Chicago, IL

Laura D. Byham-Gray, PhD, RDN, FNKF
Professor and Vice Chair of Research, Rutgers University, Department of Clinical and Preventive Nutrition Sciences
New Brunswick, NJ

Catherine M. Champagne PhD, RDN, LDN, FTOS, FAHA, FADA, FAND
Professor and Chief, Nutritional Epidemiology/Dietary Assessment & Nutrition Counseling, Pennington Biomedical Research Center, Part of Louisiana State University
Baton Rouge, LA

Feon Cheng, PhD, MPH, RDN, CHTS-CP
Nutrition Researcher, Academy of Nutrition and Dietetics
Los Angeles, CA

Marilyn C. Cornelis, PhD
Assistant Professor, Northwestern University Feinberg School of Medicine
Chicago, IL

Sharon M. Donovan, PhD, RD
Professor and Melissa M. Noel Endowed Chair in Diet and Health, University of Illinois at Urbana-Champaign
Urbana, IL

Judith A. Gilbride, PhD, RDN, FAND
Professor Emerita, Department of Nutrition and Food Studies, New York University Steinhardt
New York, NY

Philip Gleason, PhD
Senior Fellow, Mathematica Policy Research
Geneva, NY

Geoffrey W. Greene, PhD, RD, LDN
Professor and Dietetic Internship Director, University of Rhode Island
Kingston, RI

Mary B. Gregoire, PhD, RD, FADA, FAND
Executive Director, Accreditation Council for Education in Nutrition and Dietetics
Chicago, IL

Rosa K. Hand, PhD, RDN, LD, FAND
Instructor and Director, Combined Dietetic Internship/Master's Degree Program, Case Western Reserve University
Cleveland, OH

Deepa Handu, PhD, RDN
Senior Scientific Director, Evidence Analysis Center, Academy of Nutrition and Dietetics
Chicago, IL

Jeffrey Harris, DrPH, MPH, RDN, LDN, FAND
Professor, Department of Nutrition, West Chester University of Pennsylvania
West Chester, PA

David Haytowitz, MSc
Nutritionist, USDA-ARS-BHNRC Nutrient Data Laboratory
Beltsville, MD

James H. Hollis, PhD, BSc(Hons),
Associate Professor Food Science and Human Nutrition, Iowa State University
Ames, IA

Sharon I. Kirkpatrick, PhD, RD
Associate Professor, University of Waterloo
Waterloo, ON, Canada

Carol Koprowski, PhD, RDN
Clinical Assistant Professor of Preventative Medicine, Keck School of Medicine at the University of Southern California
Los Angeles, CA

Joanne Kouba, PhD, RDN
Associate Professor, Loyola University of Chicago, Health Science Campus
Maywood, IL

Nicole Larson, PhD, MPH, RDN
Senior Research Associate, University of Minnesota School of Public Health
Minneapolis, MN

JoAnn E. Manson, MD, DrPH
Chief, Division of Preventive Medicine, Brigham and Women's Hospital, and Professor of Medicine and the Michael and Lee Bell Professor of Women's Health, Harvard Medical School
Boston, MA

Kelsey Mangano, PhD, RD
Assistant Professor, Zuckerberg College of Health Sciences, University of Massachusetts Lowell
Lowell, MA

Shortie McKinney, PhD, RD, FADA
Dean, Zuckerberg College of Health Sciences, University of Massachusetts Lowell
Lowell, MA

Veronica McLymont, PhD, RD, CDN
Director, Food and Nutrition Services, Memorial Sloan Kettering Cancer Center
New York, NY

Jade McNamara, PhD
Assistant Professor of Human Nutrition, University of Maine
Orono, ME

Barbara Millen, DrPH, RD, FADA
President of Millennium Prevention, Inc. and Chairman of Boston Nutrition Foundation, Inc
Boston, MA

Lisa Moloney, MS, RDN
Nutrition Researcher, Academy of Nutrition and Dietetics
Chicago, IL

Yasmin Mossavar-Rahmani, PhD, RD
Associate Professor, Department of Epidemiology and Population Health, Albert Einstein College of Medicine,
Bronx, NY

Suzanne P. Murphy, PhD
Professor Emeritus, University of Hawaii Cancer Center
Honolulu, HI

William Murphy, MS, RDN
Chief Technology Officer, 3 Data, Inc
Austin, TX

Mary C. Naglak, PhD, RD
Clinical Research Director, Abington-Jefferson Health Memorial Hospital
Abington, PA

Dianne Neumark-Sztainer, PhD, MPH, RD
Mayo Professor and Division Head, Division of Epidemiology and Community Health, School of Public Health, University of Minnesota
Minneapolis, MN

Angela Odoms-Young, PhD
Associate Professor, University of Illinois at Chicago
Chicago, IL

Constantina Papoutsakis, PhD, RDN
Senior Director, Nutrition and Dietetics Data Science Center, Academy of Nutrition and Dietetics
Chicago, IL

Pamela R. Pehrsson, PhD
Research Leader, USDA-ARS-BHNRC Nutrient Data Laboratory
Beltsville, MD

Colleen A. Redding, PhD
Research Professor, University of Rhode Island
Kingston, RI

Mary Rozga, PhD, RDN
Nutrition Researcher, Academy of Nutrition and Dietetics
Chicago, IL

Lianne Russo, MS, RDN, CDN
Clinical Dietician and Nutritionist, Memorial Sloan Kettering Cancer Center
New York, NY

Kevin Sauer, PhD, RDN, LD, FAND
Associate Professor, Kansas State University
Manhattan, KS

Maria O. Scott, MPH
Academic/Scientific Editorial Manager, University of Iowa College of Public Health
Iowa City, IA

Madeleine Sigman-Grant, PhD, RD
Professor Emerita, University of Nevada, Reno
Las Vegas, NV

Linda Snetselaar, PhD, RDN, LD, FAND
Professor in Epidemiology, College of Public Health, University of Iowa
Iowa City, IA

Lyn M. Steffen, PhD, MPH, RDN, FAHA
Associate Professor of Epidemiology, University of Minnesota School of Public Health
Minneapolis, MN

Alison L. Steiber, PhD, RDN
Chief Scientific Officer, Research, International, and Scientific Affairs, Academy of Nutrition and Dietetics
Chicago, IL

Cynthia Thomson, PhD, RDN
Professor, Health Promotion Sciences, and Director, Canyon Ranch Center for Prevention & Health Promotion, Mel & Enid Zuckerman College of Public Health, University of Arizona
Tuscon, AZ

Linda Van Horn, PhD, RDN
Professor, Preventive Medicine and Chief, Nutrition Division, Northwestern University
Chicago, IL

Jacqueline A. Vernarelli, PhD
Assistant Professor of Public Health, Sacred Heart University
Fairfield, CT

Connie Weaver, PhD
Distinguished Professor, Nutrition Science, Purdue University
West Lafayette, IN

Miryam Yusufov, PhD
Research Fellow, Dana-Farber Cancer Institute, Harvard Medical School
Boston, MA

Reviewers

Melinda Anderson, PhD, RDN, LDN
DPD Director, School of Human Ecology, Tennessee
Technological University
Cookeville, TN

Shanna Beth Bernstein, MPH, RD, CDE
Metabolic Research Dietitian, National Institutes
of Health, Clinical Center
Bethesda, MD

Catherine M. Champagne, PhD, RDN, LDN, FTOS, FAHA, FADA,
FAND
Professor and Chief, Nutritional Epidemiology/Dietary
Assessment & Nutrition Counseling Pennington Biomedical
Research Center, Louisiana State University
Baton Rouge, LA

Natasha Chong Cole, PhD, MPH, RD
Postdoctoral Research Fellow
Baylor College of Medicine/Children's Nutrition
Research Center
Houston, TX

Brenda M. Davy, PhD, RD
Professor, Department of Human Nutrition, Foods and Exercise,
Virginia Polytechnic Institute and State University
Blacksburg, VA

Phillip Gleason, PhD
Senior Fellow, Mathematica Policy Research
Geneva, NY

Amanda Goldman, MS, RD, LD, FAND
System Director of Quality and Wellness; Director of Diabetes
and Nutrition Care, Catholic Health Initiatives
Lexington, KY

Rosa K. Hand, PhD, RDN, LD, FAND
Instructor and Director, Combined Dietetic Internship/Master's
Degree Program, Case Western Reserve University
Cleveland, OH

Kristen Heitman, MS, RDN, LD
Clinical Research Dietitian,
The Ohio State University Wexner Medical Center
Columbus, OH

Carrie King, PhD, RDN, LD, CDE
Professor, Dietetics and Nutrition, University of
Alaska Anchorage
Anchorage, AK

Nicole M. Moore, MS, RDN, LD
Assistant Professor, Augusta University
Augusta, GA

Mary Rozga, PhD, RDN
Nutrition Researcher, Academy of Nutrition and Dietetics
Chicago, IL

Shey Schnell, MHA, RD
Director of Food and Nutrition Services
The University of Vermont Health Network-Champlain
Valley Physicians Hospital
Plattsburgh, NY

Kim S. Stote, PhD, MPH, RDN
Associate Dean, Health Professions State University of New York,
Empire State College
Albany, NY

Ashley Vargas, PhD, MPH, RDN, FAND
Health Scientist, Office of Disease Prevention, Office of the
Director, National Institutes of Health
North Bethesda, MD

Foreword

Research: Successful Approaches in Nutrition and Dietetics, now in its fourth edition, remains a touchstone for all nutrition and dietetics researchers. This text contains the collective knowledge of our field, with each chapter authored by a distinguished nutrition and dietetics researcher. This newest edition will continue to serve as a reference and educational foundation for our profession.

While the scientific method underpinning research has not changed in hundreds of years, the complexity of our research questions and research tools have increased appreciably. Professors Van Horn and Beto do an excellent job orienting readers to the full-spectrum of nutrition and dietetics research throughout this text, including clear indications of pros and cons for different tools and methodological approaches. Chapters 1 though 4 orient the reader, walk through the scientific method, describe how to obtain monetary support for research, and explain the ethical responsibility of researchers, respectively. The remaining chapters largely dive deeper into the array of different approaches, methods, and tools used in nutrition and dietetic research. This format easily allows the reader to simply choose topics of interest or to read through all topics for a more global understanding.

In 2017, the Academy of Nutrition and Dietetics celebrated its centennial, and, on behalf of the Research Dietetic Practice Group, I am beyond pleased to see the prominence of research within the Academy of Nutrition and Dietetics strategic plan. This is especially vital right now because research is more complex than ever and is being communicated to the public in smaller and smaller sound bites. Indeed, the Academy of Nutrition and Dietetics designated research as the first of four strategies to fulfill their mission to "Accelerate improvements in global health and well-being through food and nutrition." For over 25 years the Academy of Nutrition and Dietetics has committed to publishing this text, which demonstrates the long-standing dedication of the Academy of Nutrition and Dietetics, and its membership, to quality research.

Ashley J. Vargas, PhD, MPH, RDN, FAND
Health Scientist, Office of Disease Prevention, Office of the Director, National Institutes of Health;
Chair, Academy of Nutrition and Dietetics Research Dietetic Practice Group, 2018–2019

Acknowledgments

We are grateful to each of our talented authors. Their expertise is evident in these chapters, which provide the most current and credible information available in their respective areas of concentration. We highly respect these individuals for their hard work and creativity in presenting complex concepts in new and novel ways. We want to further give our appreciation to past authors whose contributions in earlier editions modelled certain topic areas.

We sincerely thank the Academy of Nutrition and Dietetics for supporting the development of this new edition. Specifically, the Publications, Resources, and Products team is recognized for its commitment to excellence, ongoing involvement, and dedication. Without them, this book could not have been produced.

We also wish to remember our former colleague and past editor of the *Journal of the Academy of Nutrition and Dietetics*, Elaine Monsen, PhD, RD, whose initiative launched the first edition of this book. Her commitment to teaching and training nutrition researchers has inspired countless investigators to take the tools and tips provided to design, implement, and publish remarkable findings and new discoveries.

Finally, we thank you, the readers, for your interest, scientific curiosity, and ambition. We encourage each of you to discover "successful approaches" to developing high impact nutrition research of your own!

Linda Van Horn, PhD, RDN
Judith Beto, PhD, RDN

About the Fourth Edition

The fourth edition of *Research: Successful Approaches in Nutrition and Dietetics* is a timely and comprehensive update on designing, conducting, and evaluating nutrition research. This text strategically targets nutrition students, their professors, and practitioners who seek a deeper understanding of the evidence base that forms nutrition policy and practical applications. There is an emphasis on the modern integration of nutrition science, epidemiology, clinical translational relevance and food-based practices. Advances in biostatistical analyses, biological mechanisms, and newly emerging biomarkers are encompassed throughout.

The book's ten sections capture the excitement of research discovery, the importance of establishing a supportive research environment, and details specific to conducting observational, integrative, and translational research in the modern era.

Section 1 follows in the footsteps of the previous edition, laying a general foundation for the importance of discovery through research. Examples have been updated to give readers a glimpse of current research models to illustrate the main points.

Section 2 brings to the reader the most up-to-date information on advancing science through ethical research. Detailed information on writing proposals has been revised to feature the most current resources in grant writing and proposal funding resources.

Section 3 explores, in depth, the unique attributes of descriptive research with a new focus on efficiency in data collection.

Section 4 has been expanded to introduce the topic of consistency in study findings and includes new figures and illustrations to elaborate on clinical nutrition studies. Chapter 9 has been augmented to offer the latest in nutrition monitoring.

Section 5 includes a brand new chapter on bridging disciplinary boundaries and working on teams with members from varied backgrounds.

Section 6 incorporates key components relevant to evaluation and assessment methods in research, ranging from surveys to assessment methodology, as well as the importance of the food composition databases and dietary reference intakes that are essential to all aspects of nutrition research. A detailed and up-to-date review of existing biomarkers and how to apply them is included, as well as a specific focus on research involving appetite assessment.

Section 7 includes six chapters that are fundamental to the food, nutrition, and dietetics arena. New to this section is the subject of diet and human genetics, which is rapidly evolving. This topic is an essential component of understanding nutrition research in the modern era.

Section 8 concentrates on statistical applications that are vital to nutrition research and an invaluable component of understanding as well as writing nutrition research papers that merit publication in high impact journals.

Section 9 further describes best approaches to illustrate, evaluate, and integrate nutrition research data within the development of subsequent studies and their interpretation.

Finally, **Section 10** brings it all together in the process of applying research in practice. The importance of community–based research in implementing public health benefits is the new culminating chapter to further emphasize applied-side nutrition and dietetics.

Authors who have contributed their time and talents to the fourth edition are uniquely qualified to address each topic, and their individual areas of expertise are well recognized and respected in the published literature. This text aims to enhance, expand, and energize readers to embrace the excitement of nutrition research, ignite new ideas and approaches, and achieve a better understanding of the importance of diet and nutrition in health throughout the life course.

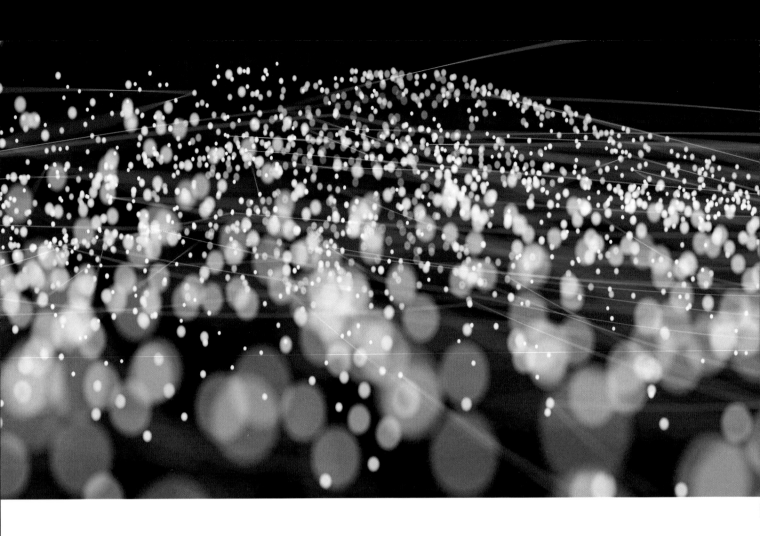

An Introduction to Discovery Through Research in Nutrition and Dietetics

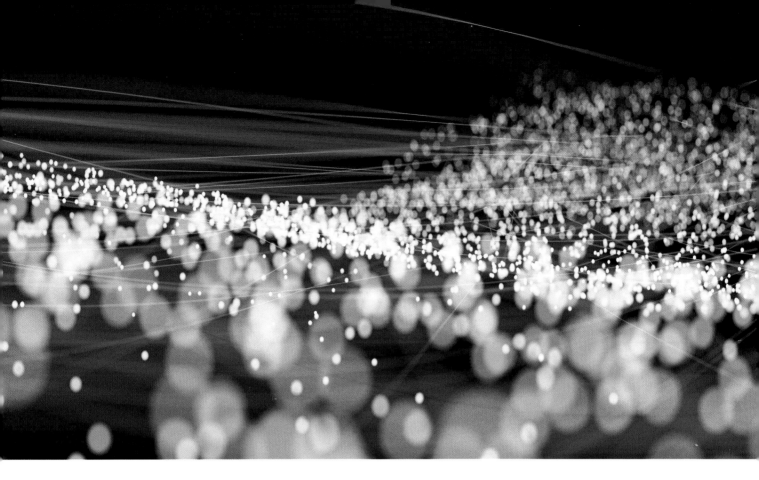

Chapter 1

Advancing the Research Continuum

Linda Van Horn, PhD, RDN

LEARNING OBJECTIVES

1. Introduce the overall premise of this book.

2. Highlight key topics and research elements addressed.

3. Encourage readers, whether novice or experienced, to apply these principles and strategies to their own research as they move forward with their careers.

Nutrition research is fundamental to the evidence-based practice of nutrition and dietetics. Well-designed, carefully executed, quality-controlled studies offer insights and breakthroughs that drive the field forward. Research fosters objective measurement of complex environments and demands rigorous evaluation of procedures, treatments and outcomes. Through research, associations can be identified, hypotheses tested, programs compared, and protocols validated. Research documents practice, monitors approaches, ensures credibility, and assesses cost-effectiveness. The strength of a discipline, whether in health sciences or management, is characterized by the quality and quantity of evidence in its research base. Strong and consistent research is essential to a vibrant profession, pending active involvement of professionals in keeping abreast of the dynamic findings.

FORCES FOR RESEARCH

Monsen[1] identified driving forces that continue to influence nutrition research today. These include recognizing unexpected findings, extending existing data, posing point-counterpoint comparisons, and responding to socioeconomic, political, and behavioral influences of a culturally diverse environment. Included in modern applications of research are the numerous influences conferred by social media and the rapid-fire communication of results that can undermine careful consideration of unintended consequences.

Recognizing the Unexpected

An exciting by-product of a research study is sometimes the hidden finding that launches new topic areas of study. This is more commonly known as the "Aha!" moment. Discovery of the first vitamin is a clear example. In the 1700s, a British naval surgeon, James Lind, gave a great deal of thought to the vast occurrence of scurvy among English sailors. The disease was particularly rampant on long voyages. In 1747, Lind completed the first controlled dietary study where he proved that citrus fruits cured scurvy. Six years later Lind[2] published his treatise, and in 1796, 43 years after his publication, the British navy officially introduced lemon juice as a prophylactic against scurvy.

More than a century later, in 1906, the concept of developing accessory food factors was introduced. In 1932, 185 years after Lind's first controlled study, crystalline vitamin C was prepared from lemon juice. While no one can plan for a breakthrough (such as the dietary importance of citrus fruit), investigators should always be alert for the unexpected. For example, the findings from the Women's Health Initiative reported completely unexpected results regarding the use of progestin-containing hormone therapy, which was long considered protective; the report found that progestin was adversely associated with increased risk of postmenopausal breast cancer.[3-5] These results changed the course of clinical postmenopausal management almost overnight. From 1988 through 1994, 44% of American women reported using hormone therapy, but this was reduced to 4.7% by 2010, with ongoing recommendations against its use in 2017 by the US Preventive Services Task Force.[6]

Extending Existing Data

Going beyond what is known to discover what is not known remains a compelling force of research. Another classic example is discovery of the second vitamin. When the idea of accessory food factors was introduced to the scientific community, researchers eagerly devoted attention to ascertaining whether other important food factors existed and their sources and functions. From 1913 to 1916, research teams led by McCullum et al[7,8] observed and isolated components from foods that they termed Fat Soluble A and Water Soluble B. Shortly thereafter, Fat Soluble A was partitioned into vitamins A, D, E, and K, and Water Soluble B developed into the long series of B vitamins.[9] This search for accessory food factors was a highly productive extension of the earlier discovery of vitamin C.

A more current example is the study of glycemic index and glycemic load. While the relevance and practical application of these two factors in regards to development of insulin resistance or type 2 diabetes remains somewhat mixed,[10,11] awareness of the potential role of these factors in impacting postprandial glucose/insulin response opened a new and compelling area for nutrition research.[12-14] The epidemiologic relevance of a topic like this and its importance in setting the stage for next generation research are addressed more extensively in Chapters 5 and 7.

One of the trending topics of today centers on the growing awareness of biomarkers, which can help provide objective measures of nutrient intake and help to identify biological pathways and processes related to digestion, absorption, and metabolism. Chapters 16 and 21 are particularly relevant to this topic and offer insights into how best to cross-check diet intake with metabolic outcomes.

Also, with the increasing interest in precision medicine and now precision nutrition, nutrigenomics and the myriad of diet-gene interactions are likely to become even more important to the understanding of prevention and diet therapy to meet the needs of the individual, including questions regarding weight control.[15] Chapter 19 is devoted to this topic and raises many hypothesis-generating research questions.

Point-Counterpoint Comparisons

The point-counterpoint concept involves actions and reactions. A current example is the explosion of "functional foods," including prebiotics and probiotics that have been developed by the food industry, presumably to conveniently meet nutrient needs of busy people without imposing the hassle of buying and preparing raw ingredients. Whether these foods and products prove helpful or harmful (perhaps due to extra calories, sugar, salt, or other factors) remains controversial,[16,17] but the presence of these products continues to have a growing influence on the modern diet.[18] The knowledge gap associated with their risk-benefit ratios—especially the gap based on age, sex, health status, and pharmacological influences—requires future study.

Responding to the Socioeconomic, Political, and Culturally Diverse Environment

The Special Supplemental Food Program for Women, Infants and Children (WIC) represents an outstanding response to the socioeconomic and political environment.[19] Evaluation and documentation of the WIC program and innovative new approaches are among the prime reasons that the program has been so successful.[20] Increasing cultural diversity and the accompanying increase in rates of homelessness raise challenges related to economic opportunity and adequate nutrition for underserved pregnant women. Qualitative research on these and associated topics is addressed in Chapter 6. Applied research on these topics offers promise for ameliorating these difficult problems.[21]

Research Now

Nutrition research has never been more exciting or more challenging. The forces of research are ever influencing new studies and their findings. Registered Dietitian Nutritionists (RDNs) are encouraged to take an active role in designing studies, both basic science and clinical, to document the benefits of nutrition in prevention and treatment of disease. Applied translational research is especially valued; it takes results from bench to bedside and even curbside, offering timely community health benefits derived from well executed experimental and clinical designs. Chapters 11, 18, 29, and 30 are especially relevant in this area. This book offers a wealth of tools and techniques for designing nutrition research studies of your own. Here are a few of the basics to get you started.

Prepare the Research Protocol

A research protocol is essential to direct the study in a manner that ensures meaningful results. The research protocol includes (1) specific aims and hypotheses that pose focused and concisely stated research questions, (2) a comprehensive literature review, (3) the merit and potential value or innovations of the research, and (4) the appropriate research design to adequately test the questions. Research design includes the study methods, data collection, and decisive statistical analyses to be used to test the hypotheses. See Chapters 8 through 10.

Research proposals must conform to a funding agency's requirements, as stated in its guidelines. Chapter 4 provides detailed guidance on securing funding. Many private and public agencies model their guidelines after those of the National Institutes of Health (NIH). Proposals are typically submitted electronically, requiring the authors to pay careful attention to all details, including the due date and time.

Conduct the Pilot Study to Produce Preliminary Data

A pilot study to generate preliminary results is essential in most NIH studies to demonstrate the feasibility and merit of the proposed study design and methodology. Testing instruments and validated methods permits researchers to make adjustments before launching the study, thereby assuring that data collection is efficient and accurate. All data collection needs justification. Providing preliminary data and demonstrating experience gained from the pilot study are crucial to successful review and funding for the proposed project. See Chapters 2, 8, 9, 12, and 13.

Ensure Ethical Research

Institutional Review Board (IRB) approval is required prior to initiating all research studies. Researchers must follow ethical procedures in all aspects of the design and conduct of their research. Everything, ranging from the choice of topic, to the samples collected, to the interventions designed, to the data collected, to—perhaps most important of all—gaining informed consent, must be considered ethical as judged by IRB approval. Data analyses and reporting of data are likewise subject to scrutiny. Chapter 3 provides a more detailed discussion.

These investigations must meet ethical guidelines to protect the rights, privacy, and welfare of the individuals. The Declaration of Helsinki, drafted in 1964 by the World Medical Association, serves as the basis for the ethical guidelines that are now detailed regulations issued by governmental agencies, such as the NIH. The local IRB is required to review all investigations using human subjects to ensure ethical conduct and evaluate potential risks and benefits.

As part of informed consent, the investigator must explain to potential participants the nature of the study, including the possible risks and discomforts they may experience. Confidentiality of all data is mandated by all review boards. Specific elements to be included in the informed consent procedure, including written and verbal descriptions, are designated by the local IRB. See Chapters 3 and 9.

Validity, Accuracy, Reliability, and Precision

Qualities critical to all research are validity, accuracy, and precision. Use of validated instruments is essential to ensuring accuracy, reliability, and precision of the data and the results.[22] The National Cancer Institute has developed a highly comprehensive Dietary Assessment Primer (https://dietassessmentprimer.cancer.gov) that provides detailed definitions and examples of these and other aspects of nutrition research as follows:

- **Validity:** The degree to which a tool measures what it claims to measure.
- **Accuracy:** The degree of closeness of measurements of a quantity to that quantity's true value.
- **Precision:** The degree to which repeated measurements under unchanged conditions show the same results.

Sensitivity and Specificity

The choice of a single cut point to categorize individuals may not always be clear when the test yields a continuous scale of values. A cut point selected to maximize sensitivity will unavoidably cause the test to be less specific. The selection of an appropriate cut point is aided by use of graph plotting true-positive against false-positive ratios, known as the receiver operating characteristic (ROC) curve. The ROC curve graphically displays the reciprocal relationship between sensitivity and specificity for values of a test measured on a continuous scale, and it allows investigators to choose a cut-point that maximizes the performance of the test for the needed levels of sensitivity, specificity, or both. See Chapters 17, 25, 28, for more detailed explanations.

National Health and Nutrition Examination Survey (NHANES) I, II, and III provide countless examples of valid survey testing. The mean intakes of certain vitamins by age and gender are useful for determining areas of weakness in the population's diet and indicating possible policies to apply. Limitations in survey results often include low response rate and cross-sectional design.[23] Randomized clinical trials and longitudinal cohort studies are considered more robust, but these also have limitations that require further considerations. Chapters 8, 9, 12, 13, and 14 offer further discussion and insights regarding these issues.

Researchers must also use discretion in applying inferential statistical tests to data from survey research. Because survey studies are designed to be descriptive rather than analytic, formal tests of hypotheses are undertaken after the data are viewed, and the test result is likely to be biased toward a spurious statistically significant result. Such inferential tests should be regarded as exploratory and useful in generating questions for future analytic studies. Chapters 21 and 25 offer further explanation of this topic.

ADVANCING YOUR OWN RESEARCH

The topics listed in this chapter represent only a few of the key aspects of nutrition research that are addressed in this book. The possibilities are endless, but the competitive nature of grant reviews and funding constraints often steer research proposals towards filling high priority knowledge gaps identified by the funding agencies.[24] A newly convened Dietary Guidelines for Americans Advisory Committee, with the assistance of the Nutrition Evidence Library, conducts systematic reviews of newly published nutrition research every 5 years as part of the process for developing the next edition of the Dietary Guidelines for Americans. Savvy researchers can begin with the end in mind by reviewing these priority areas and carefully developing testable hypotheses that will address them. Consider the population, intervention, comparator, and outcome (PICO) that form the criteria used in systematic reviews. Formulation of study questions, specific aims, and validated outcome measures that are consistent with these criteria can often make or break an investigator's chances of achieving a fundable score.

CONCLUSION

In this era, massive use of social media, blogs, tweets, and crowdsourcing to derive answers to countless questions has influenced public perception of what to believe and how to behave. The importance of evidence-based science to provide sound answers and guide public policy, including what to eat, is paramount. Take these tools and **go for it**!

REFERENCES

1. Monsen E. Forces for research. *J Am Diet Assoc.* 1993; 93:981-985.

2. Lind J. *A treatise of the Scurvy. In three parts. Containing an inquiry into the nature, causes, and cure, of that disease. Together with a critical and chronological view of what has been published on the subject.* Edinburgh, Scotland: Sands, Murray, and Cochran for A Kincaid & A Donaldson; 1753.

3. Modugno F, Kip KE, Cochrane B, et al. Obesity, hormone therapy, estrogen metabolism and risk of postmenopausal breast cancer. *Int J Cancer.* 2006;118(5):1292-1301.

4. Collaborative Group on Hormonal Factors in Breast Cancer. Breast cancer and hormone replacement therapy: collaborative reanalysis of data from 51 epidemiological studies of 52,705 women with breast cancer and 108,411 women without breast cancer. *Lancet.* 1997;350(9084): 1047-1059.

5. Chlebowski RT, Hendrix SL, Langer RD, et al. Influence of estrogen plus progestin on breast cancer and mammography in healthy postmenopausal women: the Women's Health Initiative randomized trial. *JAMA.* 2003;289:3243-3253.

6. Osborne T, Mendell, L. *Feeding experiments with isolated food substances.* Washington DC: Carnegie Institute; 1911:156.

7. Osborne T, Mendell L. Amino acids in nutrition and growth. *J Biol Chem.* 1914;17:325-349.

8. Stipanuk M. The vitamins. In: *Biochemical, Physiological and Molecular Aspects of Human Nutrition.* 2nd ed. St. Louis, MO: Saunders; 2006:661-663.

9. Campfield LA, Smith FJ, Rosenbaum M, Hirsch J. Human eating: evidence for a physiological basis using a modified paradigm. *Neurosci Biobehav Rev.* 1996;20:133-137.

10. Sacks FM, Carey VJ, Anderson CAM, et al. Effects of high vs low glycemic index of dietary carbohydrate on cardiovascular disease risk factors and insulin sensitivity: the OmniCarb randomized clinical trial. *JAMA.* 2014; 312(23):2531-2541. doi:10.1001/jama.2014.

11. Tay J, Luscombe-Marsh ND, Thompson CH, et al, Comparison of low- and high-carbohydrate diets for type 2 diabetes management: a randomized trial. *Am J Clin Nutr.* 2015;102(4):780-790. doi: 10.3945/ajcn.115.112581.

12. Shukla AP, Andono J, Touhamy SH, et al. Carbohydrate-last meal pattern lowers postprandial glucose and insulin excursions in type 2 diabetes. *BMJ Open Diabetes Res Care.* 2017;5(1):e000440. doi:10.1136/bmjdrc-2017-000440.

13. Le T, Flatt SW, Natarajan L, et al. Effects of diet composition and insulin resistance status on plasma lipid levels in a weight loss intervention in women. *J Am Heart Assoc.* 2016;5(1):e002771. doi:10.1161/JAHA.115.002771.

14. Shikany JM, Margolis KL, Pettinger M, et al. Effects of a low-fat dietary intervention on glucose, insulin, and insulin resistance in the Women's Health Initiative (WHI) dietary modification trial. *Am J Clin Nutr.* 2011;94(1):75-85. doi.org/10.3945/ajcn.110.010843.

15. Celis-Morales C, Marsaux CF, Livingstone KM, et al. Can genetic-based advice help you lose weight? Findings from the Food4Me European randomized controlled trial. *Am J Clin Nutr.* 2017;105(5):1204-1213.

16. Pandey KR, Naik SR, Vakil BV. Probiotics, prebiotics and synbiotics–a review. *J Food Sci Technol.* 2015;52(12):7577-7587. doi:10.1007/s13197-015-1921-1.

17. Hu FB. Do functional foods have a role in the prevention of cardiovascular disease? *Circulation.* 2011;124(5):538-540.

18. De Filippis F, Vitaglione P, Cuomo R, Canani RB, Ercolini D. Dietary interventions to modulate the gut microbiome—how far away are we from precision medicine. *Inflamm Bowel Dis.* 2018;24(10):2142-2154. doi:10.1093/ibd/izy080.

19. Phelan S, Hagobian T, Brannen A, et al. Effect of an internet-based program on weight loss for low-income postpartum women: a randomized clinical trial. *JAMA.* 2017;317(23):2381-2391. doi:10.1001/jama.2017.7119.

20. Walker L, Freeland-Graves JH, Milani T, et al. Weight and behavioral and psychosocial factors among ethnically diverse, low-income women after childbirth: II. Trends and correlates. *Women Health.* 2004;40(2):19-34.

21. May L, Borger C, McNutt S, et al. *WIC ITFPS-2 infant report: Intention to breastfeed.* Rockville, MD: Westat; 2015.

22. Walker JL, Ardouin S, Burrows T. The validity of dietary assessment methods to accurately measure energy intake in children and adolescents who are overweight or obese: a systematic review. *Eur J Clin Nutr.* 2018;72(2):185-197. doi:10.1038/s41430-017-0029-2.

23. Briefel RR, Johnson, CL. Secular trends in dietary intake in the United States. *Annu Rev Nutr.* 2004;24:401-31.

24. Dwyer JT, Rubin KH, Fritsche KL, et al. Creating the future of evidence-based nutrition recommendations: case studies from lipid research. *Adv Nutr.* 2016;7(4):747-755. doi:10.3945/an.115.010926.

Chapter 2

Building the Research Foundation: The Research Question and Study Design

Carol J. Boushey, PhD, MPH, RDN | *Jeffrey Harris,* DrPH, MPH, RDN, LDN, FAND

LEARNING OBJECTIVES

1. Identify the value of relevant research to elevate nutrition and dietetics practice.

2. Provide guidance to develop salient, focused, and measurable research questions.

3. Describe the relevance of different study designs to best answer research hypotheses.

Research, the backbone of nutrition and dietetics, supports practice, innovation, and progress. Research allows objective measurement of complex environments and rigorous evaluation of the outcomes of procedures and treatments. Through research, associations can be observed, hypotheses tested, programs compared, and protocols evaluated. Research procedures can be used to document practice, to monitor activities, to ensure quality, and to assess cost-effectiveness. The strength of any discipline is associated closely with its research base. Strong research supports a strong profession.

Research may be broadly classified according to its purpose as descriptive or analytic. Descriptive studies include qualitative research, case series (including case reports), and surveys. The designs of descriptive studies characterize the state of nature at a specific point in time. They are useful for generating hypotheses regarding the determinants of a condition or disease or the characteristic of interest. Descriptive studies provide baseline data and can monitor change over time, as is being done to monitor achievement of the Dietary Guidelines for Americans[1] and the Healthy People 2020 goals and objectives.[2] The intent of analytic research is to test a hypothesis concerning causal relationships—perhaps a hypothesis generated from an earlier descriptive study. Experimental design is often considered the gold standard of analytic research as it involves important factors being held constant save those factors manipulated by the investigator. Some observational designs, such as prospective cohort (follow-up) studies and case-control studies, are analytic but not experimental. Collectively, these research designs inform practice guidelines. No one study design can answer all research questions. An appreciation for the diversity of study designs available can aid in the decision-making process for applying dietary guidelines to practice.

DESIGNING A RESEARCH STUDY

Research begins when an investigator identifies a relevant important topic and develops a well-considered research question and hypothesis. After determining the research design, the investigator prepares the research protocol and, if necessary, undertakes a pilot study. Throughout each phase, researchers must consider the ethical implications of their actions. This chapter focuses on the development of the research question and study design. Other chapters cover research protocols and ethical considerations.

Select the Research Topic

Research is a problem-solving, decision-making process involving a series of interrelated decisions. When the researcher focuses on one decision at a time, the research process becomes manageable. Each option can be considered, and the most appropriate option can then be selected. Research projects should be meaningful; they should expand current knowledge and enhance the practice of the profession.

A registered dietitian nutritionist (RDN) can choose issues important to practice and thereby choose issues important to the dietetics profession. Research questions can evolve from many sources, such as ideas to improve patient health, suggestions to increase the effectiveness of services and products, untested concepts in published literature, the application of business research methods, and uncharted boundaries in basic research in all areas of advanced study.[3,4] An RDN can observe and thoughtfully consider the needs of his or her practice. Then, in addressing the overall topic, the RDN can divide the topic into smaller component parts and single out a component that is feasible to study in the given setting. The process should start with a simple question. Data generated in response to the initial question will lead to many other questions and aspects of the problem that subsequent studies can address.

Prepare for the Research Project

A good first step in pursuing a research plan is to review the published research literature related to the topic. A thorough review will emphasize current scientific literature, seminal articles, and early published papers on the topic. The US National Library of Medicine, located on the campus of the National Institutes of Health, is the premier bibliographic resource covering the fields of medicine, the health care system, nutrition and dietetics, and the preclinical sciences.[5] PubMed.gov is a publicly available database of more than 26 million citations; links to guidance and tutorials to aid efficient searching are available from the site's home page. A search for available systematic reviews or meta-analyses relevant to the topic is an additional important step as covered in Chapter 10.[5,6]

Finding multiple papers on the topic when examining the literature should not discourage forward progress. A critical review of previous work in the field can be the base upon which to build solid new research projects. New studies can improve upon shortcomings in study design or suggest new areas for development. The RDN may want to contact experts in the field and discuss the problem by telephone, social media, or email or may actively seek out useful information from colleagues in related fields.

Once the topic is solidified and the issue to address is identified, the investigator should assess available resources, such as patient populations, laboratory and library facilities, foodservice equipment, nutrient databases, data-processing capabilities, computer facilities, personnel, statistical and other consultants, and collaborative opportunities. Practicing RDNs can demonstrate leadership in research by directing team efforts. Team efforts are invaluable as they permit quality research that provides major benefits to the profession. The direct and indirect costs of performing the research need to be estimated. If a study is well designed and carefully developed, it may be implemented with existing personnel and facilities. If it is necessary to obtain funds, the investigator should consider a variety of funding sources, such as government agencies or foundations. Guidelines for obtaining funding are highlighted in Chapter 4.

Clearly State the Research Question

Preparing for a research project involves formulating the research question and evaluating its feasibility.[7] A concise, simple, straightforward statement of the research question focuses the research design process. The investigator should clearly define the question; strive to keep it uncomplicated; and use objective, measurable, and operational terms, such as *identify*, *compare*, *differentiate*, *assess*, and *describe*.

Components of the research question include the following:

● **Who (which)?** The patients, population group, or units being assessed should be defined in broad terms (eg, patients with diabetes, nutrition and dietetics students, mothers with newborn or infant, food items, tray lines, or foodservice costs).

● **What?** The factor of interest should be stated specifically (eg, body weight, nutrition knowledge, iron intake, tray error, or labor costs).

● **How assessed?** The outcome to be assessed should be stated specifically (eg, disease incidence, change in knowledge, alterations in food selection, tray errors per meal, or labor costs per patient day).

A well-developed and focused research question leads directly to a hypothesis. A hypothesis has six essential characteristics: it is measurable, specifies the population being studied, identifies a time frame, specifies the type of relationship being examined, notes the variables being studied, and defines the level of statistical significance.[7,8] Descriptive studies will often use a research objective rather than a hypothesis as these studies frequently define distributions of diseases and health-related characteristics in the sample population.

The difference between use of a research objective and a hypothesis can be clearly seen by comparing a descriptive study and an analytic study that each examined the same health problem of overweight and obesity. Ogden and colleagues[9] published the results from a descriptive study outlining the prevalence of obesity among adults and youth in the United States. Rather than a hypothesis, these investigators used a research objective. Their objective was posed as a question: What was the prevalence of obesity among adults and among youth aged 2 to 19 years from 2011 through 2014 using data from the National Health and Nutrition Examination Survey (NHANES)? Many of the essential components of a hypothesis are present in their research objective/question: it is measurable (estimates of prevalence), specifies the population (youth aged 2 through 19 years and adults aged 20 and older from NHANES), identifies a time frame (2011 through 2014), and notes variables (obese status). However, a relationship is not specified nor is a level of statistical significance defined. In other words, consistent with a descriptive study, no a priori statements about prevalence rates of obesity were suggested by the research objective.

In contrast, an analytic study will propose an expected difference between groups. Bacon and colleagues[10] hypothesized that among female chronic dieters who were obese and aged 30 to 45 years, those randomized to a "health at every size" treatment would show statistically significant ($P \leq .05$) improvements in blood pressure, blood lipid levels, energy expenditure, eating behaviors, and self-esteem compared with those randomized to a traditional weight loss treatment after a 6-month intervention and 2-year follow-up. Note that the six essential components of a hypothesis are present in each study. Nevertheless, though one was a descriptive study directed by a research objective and one was an analytic study driven by a hypothesis, both studies provided a valuable contribution to the knowledge base in the field.[9,10]

Design the Research Project

When the research question, with its accompanying research objective or hypothesis, has been stated clearly, the research project can be designed more easily. An investigator should consider several research designs to see which is best suited to the research question and the setting. Among items to consider are the dependent and independent variables, which are characteristics or attributes of the persons or objects that vary within the study population (eg, serum lipid levels and dietary fiber intake). The dependent variable is the outcome variable of interest (eg, serum lipid levels). The independent variable or the exposure (the presumed causal or predictive factor) is the variable that is thought to influence the dependent variable and that is manipulated in experimental designs (eg, dietary fiber intake).

Other study design characteristics relate to time and the direction of data collection. These characteristics differentiate (1) a cross-sectional study (a study based on data collected from a group of study participants at a single point in time); (2) a longitudinal study (a study based on data collected at more than one point in time); (3) a prospective study (a study that begins by examining a presumed cause or exposure, such as dietary fiber intake, and goes forward in time to an observed presumed effect or outcome, such as cardiovascular disease); and (4) a retrospective study (a study that begins with manifestations of an outcome, such as cardiovascular disease, and goes back in time to uncover relationships with a presumed cause, such as dietary fiber intake).

DESCRIPTIVE RESEARCH DESIGNS

Qualitative Research

A qualitative study often precedes other research designs.[11] Its primary purpose is to explore the phenomenon of interest as a prelude to theory development.[12,13] The design is necessarily flexible so the researcher can discover ideas, gain insight, and ultimately formulate a problem for further investigation. Qualitative studies are considered formulative or exploratory studies, characterized by an investigator with a receptive, seeking attitude and by an intense study of the individuals or groups of interest.[14] One approach is grounded theory research, where data "grounded" or based in real-life observations are collected and analyzed with the purpose of developing theoretical propositions.[15]

Study volunteers or participants are selected according to their experience with the phenomenon being explored. Thus, they have special characteristics and are not considered to be typical or representative of the population. Data are collected by such methods as observation, interviews, and questionnaires. The interview format may range from structured (restricting the range of responses) to less structured (permitting an unlimited range of responses). A less-structured or unstructured interview may focus on a particular topic or experience (a focused interview) or may have minimal direction (a nondirective interview).[15-17] A more in-depth discussion of qualitative research can be found in Chapter 6.

A focus group involves a group of respondents assembled to answer questions on a specific topic. Focus groups can be used to examine attitudes

EXAMPLE

The factors influencing the consumption of calcium-rich foods among adolescents were examined using focus groups. Using a structured interview, group facilitators conducted focus groups among 200 boys and girls in two age groups (aged 11 to 12 years and 16 to 17 years) representing three ethnic groups (Asian, Hispanic, or non-Hispanic white). The sessions were audiotaped and transcribed. Researchers coded the comments following the principles of grounded research theory. The results of the content analysis procedures highlighted the importance of family influence, stressing the benefits of calcium-rich foods to girls and focusing on the breakfast meal. Results were also used to develop a quantitative questionnaire for use in larger, more representative population samples.[20]

toward issues in consumer groups or other target populations.[18,19]

Case Series

A report of observations on one participant (a case report) or more than one participant (a case series) may be used in administrative, educational, and clinical settings.

Uses of Case Series

The purpose of a case series is to quantitatively describe the experience of a group of patients with a common disease or condition. Investigators using this research design attempt to identify the variables that are important to the etiology, care, or outcome of a particular condition.

A carefully prepared case series report helps generate hypotheses for future studies. The information gathered can provide evidence for an association between a disease or condition and a suspected etiologic or therapeutic factor. It also provides the data necessary to justify the need for future studies and can help determine the methods to be used in such studies. However, results from case series research

cannot be generalized unless the cases are representative of the target populations.

Case Series Features and Participant Selection

A case series comprises all cases of a specific disease or condition occurring or being presented to a particular clinic or locality during a specified time. For example, a series may consist of patients with gastric cancer who were referred to a nutrition support service for consultation over a 6-month period. It is important to recognize that this method of participant selection yields a convenience sample that cannot be considered representative (eg, all patients with gastric cancer); therefore, the results cannot be generalized to larger groups.

Data Collection in Case Series

Most commonly, existing records provide the data in a case series; however, data generated concurrently may be collected. The advantage of concurrent data collection is the opportunity to obtain complete information in a standardized way, although that goal may also be obtained with the use of existing data.

EXAMPLE

A case series design was used to describe clinical characteristics of individuals with inflammatory bowel disease (IBD) who were following the Specific Carbohydrate Diet (SCD). Men and women were recruited through clinics, message boards, and websites focusing on the SCD. Volunteers mailed their medical records; completed medical history, symptom, and quality-of-life questionnaires; and completed a 3-day dietary record. Diagnosis of IBD was confirmed by a board-certified gastroenterologist using reports provided by the enrollees. Data were obtained from 50 patients in remission (mean age=36 years). Among the highly educated sample, responses suggested that SCD can potentially be an effective tool to manage IBD. These observations supported the need for further evidence to confirm whether SCD and diet therapies in general can offer effective treatment for IBD.[21]

EXAMPLE

A concurrent case series determined the labor minutes per meal equivalent and the percentage of time spent in direct work, indirect work, delay time, and total time in a foodservice setting. A preliminary study identified 14 areas in which employees worked most frequently in the foodservice department, the average number of employees per work area, and an estimate of the required number of recorded observations needed for the projected study on labor time. Data were collected from activity sampling studies of foodservice workers in the same community hospital for 7 days (Monday through Sunday) during the second week of February for 12 consecutive years. The annual data collection provided an opportunity to assess trends in the distribution of labor time, examine patterns among work and delay activities, and identify factors in the foodservice environment that may affect labor productivity.[22]

Data concerning relevant factors are collected by chart or record review, questionnaires, interviews, or examination. A combination of collection methods may be used. The data usually cover a broad range of factors in depth, forming a detailed description of the cases. The variety and depth allow a number of factors to be considered but of necessity limit the number of individuals observed or involved or the number of objects under study.

Regardless of sample size, statistical tests for inference are usually not appropriate because hypotheses are not investigated in a case series. When the researchers interpret the results of a case series report, they must acknowledge that the sample is not representative of a larger population of cases. The investigators select the series of cases according to certain conditions, and the series may consist of cases unique in certain characteristics. Further study will determine whether the results can be generalized beyond the participants chosen for the case series.

Surveys

A survey is research designed to describe and quantify characteristics of a defined population. A survey

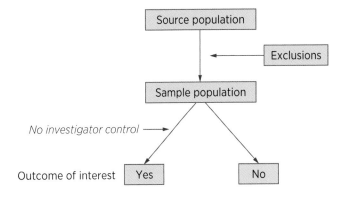

Figure 2.1 Basic cross-sectional study design (or survey) for determining prevalence rates of a health outcome (eg, hypertension) or a behavioral outcome (eg, fruit and vegetable consumption)

usually employs a research objective rather than a hypothesis. The purpose of a survey is to obtain a descriptive profile of a population.[9,23] For example, the study by Ogden and colleagues[9] described earlier in this chapter provided a statistical profile of obesity in the United States. A survey may be designed to assess the nutrient content of the food supply. A survey is an example of the cross-sectional study design, that is, individuals are measured at only one point in time (see Figure 2.1).

EXAMPLE

A survey was designed to describe clinical nutrition managers' perceptions of their access to sources of power (resources, support, information, and opportunity) and to explore how perceptions of power relate to such variables as time in the profession, years in management, education level, and work setting. Dietetics practitioners who were selected randomly from the American Dietetic Association (now the Academy of Nutrition and Dietetics) Clinical Nutrition Management dietetic practice group were sent a survey instrument designed to study empowerment in dietetics practitioners.[24]

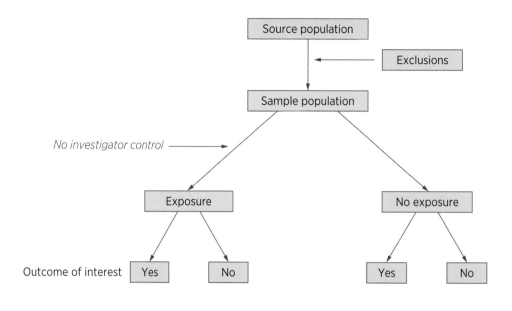

Figure 2.2 Basic cross-sectional study design (or survey) for examining a relationship between exposure and outcome

Uses of Surveys

A survey may be useful for establishing associations among variables or factors and often provides clues for further study (see Figure 2.2). Surveys can also provide baseline data about the prevalence of a condition or factor of interest in a population. A major use of the survey method is for planning health and dietary services. However, a survey does not allow investigators to draw conclusions about causal relationships

EXAMPLE

The clinical registered dietitian nutritionist (RDN) for a large prepaid health plan wants to know the proportion of the plan's enrollees interested in weight management. The RDN hopes to plan a weight management clinic and needs the estimated participation rates for budget purposes. A random sample of enrollees will be selected to receive a pilot-tested questionnaire regarding their interests. The results will be used to tailor the clinic to the participants' needs; thus, questions will cover the kinds of help enrollees want for weight management.

EXAMPLE

A patient survey can be designed for quality improvement in a hospital's dietary services. For example, in one hospital, randomly selected patients were asked about their satisfaction with tray presentation. Assessments of cold food, hot food, time of delivery, and tray appearance were included. The random survey was repeated periodically so that tray service could be monitored, trends could be observed, and actions could be taken to improve service.

Survey Participant Selection

It is usually not feasible to measure an entire population in a survey. Therefore, a sample is selected based on a probability design, which means that all individuals have an equal chance of being selected. Those who consent to participate are then questioned or examined for the disease or characteristic of interest and other relevant variables.

Results of a survey can be generalized to the entire population of interest with confidence only if the sample is representative of the target popula-

EXAMPLE

A survey was conducted to describe the food intake and food sources of macronutrients in the diets of older Hispanic adults in the northeastern United States as well as to explore relationships among acculturation, years in the United States, and macronutrient intake. The 779 participants in the Massachusetts Hispanic Elders Study sample were selected using a two-stage random cluster sampling technique that ensured a sample that was representative of the older Hispanic adult population in the state of Massachusetts.[25]

EXAMPLE

A survey was conducted to identify factors related to noncompliance with diet among patients treated for hypertension with medication plus diet. The study included a convenience sample of patients who returned for follow-up at a hypertension clinic. Unfortunately, this scheme selected those patients who were more likely to be compliant with the diet simply because they returned for follow-up. Investigators failed to meet the purpose of the research because the study generated no information on the patients who did not comply with follow-up visits.

tion. Thus, the target population must be defined and enumerated; then a sample is drawn at random from the target population. A simple random sample is devised by which all the individuals in the target population have a known chance of being included in the sample; that is, the chances of being selected are specified in the sampling scheme. A sampling method allows the investigators to calculate the sampling errors and increases the likelihood that the study is representative of the target population. A high rate of participation (response rate) increases the chances that the results are representative, as it is never certain that responders and nonresponders are similar.

Possible sampling schemes range from the simple random method to complex methods using varying selection probabilities among subgroups (strata) of the population. Elwood[26] discusses the rationale for probability sampling in nutrition research, and Moore and colleagues[27] provide details on methodology.

The appropriate sample size for a survey depends on many factors, including how precisely the sample should estimate the population parameters. Methods for calculating sample size requirements are covered in Chapter 24

A survey based on an accidental or convenience sampling scheme is of limited value because the results cannot be generalized. The reference population is undefined or is defined by the conscious or unconscious selection biases of the investigator. Further, the selection itself may be influenced by the condition or factor under study.

Survey Data Collection

Data in surveys are most frequently collected via questionnaires or interviews. Information may also be generated by physical examination (eg, anthropometric measurement; laboratory evaluation of specimens, such as blood analysis for hemoglobin levels; or direct observation, such as employee productivity).

One of the most difficult aspects of survey methodology is designing a questionnaire.[23,28] Depending on the research objectives, standard or tested instruments may be available. If questions must be developed, they must be unambiguous yet concise and tactful. The questionnaire length and format, as well as how it is to be administered, are also important considerations. The work of McColl and colleagues[23] and Dillman and colleagues,[28] along with the information in Chapter 12, present guidelines and suggestions for questionnaire development.

EXAMPLE

The study was designed to assess the nutritional status of 9- to 14-year-old girls living in Hawaii. Anthropometric measurements of height, weight, and skinfolds were collected during a clinic visit. After the visit, the girls completed dietary records over 3 days and physical activity records. Nutrient and food intakes were compared against recommended intakes, body mass index, and skinfold thicknesses.[29]

Surveys or cross-sectional studies are a valuable study design used extensively in nutrition research. Chapter 6 covers more information about descriptive research.

EXPERIMENTAL STUDY DESIGNS (RANDOMIZED TRIALS)

Experimental design is a powerful analytic research method, regardless of whether the participants are humans, animals, or inanimate objects. In each case, criteria for participation in the study need to be established, the appropriate sample size needs to be estimated, the treatment or treatments must be clearly defined, and end points must be identified. After a preliminary study has been conducted and the experiment has been designed, data need to be collected and analyzed suitably to permit appropriate interpretation and application.

Randomized Controlled Trials

Uses of Randomized Controlled Trials

The *randomized trial* is the most powerful experimental design for evaluating practices and medical treatments. This design is used to demonstrate the feasibility and safety of a treatment. After safety has been established, a randomized controlled trial (RCT) may be designed to determine the optimal treatment regimen to obtain the desired effect. Most commonly, an RCT is used to compare the efficacy of two or more treatments or practices. As noted previously, many RCTs are preceded by a pilot study to assess the efficacy as applied to a specific population sample or novel implementation.

Features of a Randomized Controlled Trial

An RCT has three general features. First, prospective study volunteers are informed about the study purposes and risks and are asked to participate. Second, individuals consenting to participate are assigned randomly to one or more treatment or intervention groups. Those randomized to receive the standard treatment or treatments constitute the control group. Participants randomized to receive the experimental treatment or intervention constitute the inter-

vention, experimental, or treatment group. The key feature is random assignment; that is, chance determines treatment assignment. Third, participants are observed for the occurrence of particular outcomes or end points following or concurrent with intervention or treatment (see Figure 2.3).

> **EXAMPLE**
>
> A Mediterranean-style diet (MedSD) has been associated with positive health outcomes. However, whether this dietary pattern could be effective with populations in the United States was an open question. A partial feeding and nutrition counseling pilot study was implemented with a one-group longitudinal design among women residing in the United States. The efficacy end point was changes in blood lipid levels. Over 12 weeks, the 16 participants increased adherence to a MedSD, and lipid profiles improved. The results confirmed the efficacy of applying this intervention as a randomized controlled trial among postmenopausal women living in the United States.[30]

> **EXAMPLE**
>
> Using a randomized controlled trial, the Women's Health Initiative examined how following a diet of 20% energy from fat, 5 or more servings of fruits and vegetables per day, and 6 or more servings of grains per day affected the incidence of breast cancer. Eligible women were randomized to either the intervention group (followed a low-fat dietary pattern) or the control group (followed their usual diet pattern). Randomization was done using a permuted block design. Effects were measured by monitoring incident cases of invasive breast cancer over a 12-year period.[31]

Selecting Participants

In an RCT, the degree to which a study group is representative of a reference population determines whether the results can be generalized. This issue

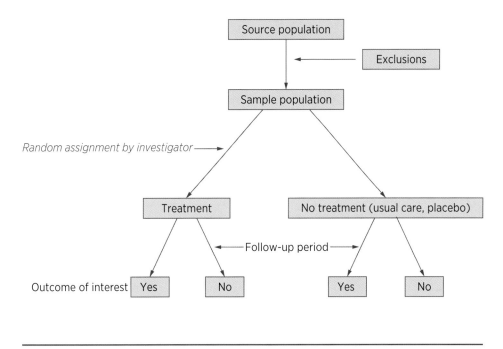

Figure 2.3 Basic randomized controlled trial study design

must be reconciled with the equally important requirement of a high degree of probability that the treatment effect be large enough that it can be measured. Therefore, if an intervention is directed to lowering dietary fat intakes and the recruited participants are already consuming a low-fat diet, additional lowering of dietary fat may not change the outcome enough to be detectable. On the other hand, if the recruited participants are consuming a high-fat diet, the probability of detecting a change in some biological outcome is higher. In general, the researcher should select participants who are relatively homogeneous in major characteristics (eg, diagnosis and nutrition status) so that extraneous sources of variation are eliminated. When selecting participants, other factors to consider are compliance, ease of follow-up, and cost of enrolling and monitoring participants.[32]

Compliance to the study protocol may be enhanced by offering appropriate incentives to all participants, such as special information or health care. Assessment of compliance prestudy may also be helpful; it can be done by including a prestudy requirement for all potential participants. Repeated 24-hour urine collections or several days of dietary intake records are useful requirements for judging compliance. Participants who are unable to complete the prestudy tasks are less likely to comply with study demands and should be excluded from the study before it begins. The resulting sample is necessarily biased, composed, as it is, of persons selected for their compliant behavior.

The ease of follow-up is related, in part, to the study setting. Follow-up is facilitated in highly restrictive settings or in settings in which the participant can be readily observed, such as in hospital settings. Unless the research question is relevant in such restricted settings, however, imposing severe restrictions on participants can impair the researchers' ability to create a study that corresponds to a natural setting and can decrease the study's usefulness.

The cost of enrolling and monitoring participants influences the number of participants in the study. In many cases, investigators can lower the cost per enrollee by using facilities and resources that are already available and using information that is collected routinely. Retaining participants for the duration of study is important to maintain the validity of the final results.

Choosing the Intervention or Treatment

As with participant selection, the intervention in an RCT is chosen to maximize the likelihood that an effect can be measured and detected statistically. The more the treatment of the intervention group differs from the treatment of the comparison or control group, within the range of safe or acceptable levels, the more likely measurable differences will be seen. As much as possible, the comparison or control treatment should have a reasonable expectation of benefit at least equal to that of the experimental treatment.[32] An untreated group as a control is valid only if there is no recognized treatment. Otherwise, the control group should receive the standard treatment or an accepted treatment for the disease or condition of interest.

If there is no recognized treatment and the investigators believe a psychological effect or observer bias is likely, a placebo is recommended. The result is a blind (masked) study in which the participants are unaware of the treatment assignment. The placebo, or sham treatment, must be inert and identical to the experimental treatment in appearance and mode of administration. The efficacy of blinding should be evaluated before and during the trial to ensure that blinding is maintained.[33] If both participants and investigators are unaware of the treatment assignment, the trial is a double-blind controlled trial—a powerful design because it eliminates expectation bias on the part of the participant and the investigative staff. The effect of expectation cannot be underestimated, as illustrated in the classic example in the Example box in the next column.

Assigning Treatment Groups

A random method of treatment assignment is essential in an RCT. Researchers are advised to avoid any treatment assignment method that is not random, such as allocation procedures based on characteristics associated with individuals (eg, birth dates or Social Security numbers) or odd-even or other systematic schemes.[34] The random method eliminates the selection bias that can occur if the participant or the investigator selects the treatment. It also mitigates unintentional bias or the chance formation of groups that are not comparable because of differ-

ences in factors that affect the response to treatment, such as age or sex. The random method does not guarantee comparable groups, however, and a chance imbalance between groups is possible, especially if the sample size is less than 200. Restricted randomization is a method of randomization that ensures that groups are equal or similar in numbers of study participants with certain characteristics, such as age and sex.

EXAMPLE

The National Institutes of Health conducted a double-blind randomized controlled trial (a trial in which neither participant nor investigator knows the study participants' assigned treatment groups) of the effectiveness of ascorbic acid on reducing the frequency and severity of the common cold. A lactose-capsule placebo that could be easily distinguished from a vitamin C tablet by taste was used, although the investigators gave little thought to the possibility that the study participants might actually bite into the capsules. Early in the study, the investigators learned that many of their curious volunteers had bitten into the capsules; as a result, a significant number of the participants knew which medication they were receiving. Although the study was no longer a double-blind study, the situation did illustrate an association between severity and duration of symptoms and knowledge of the medication taken. Among participants who tasted their capsules, those receiving vitamin C had shorter, milder colds, whereas the converse was true for the placebo group. Among the participants who remained blind to their treatment, no effect of vitamin C was observed.[35]

In a crossover design, participants serve as their own control rather than using a separate control group of matched participants. This design requires fewer participants because the within-participant variation is less than the between-participant variation, a concept that is important for sample-size calculations (see Chapter 24). When the study involves conditions that are chronic and the treatment effects, if present, are not long lasting, then the crossover design can be considered. In a crossover design, the

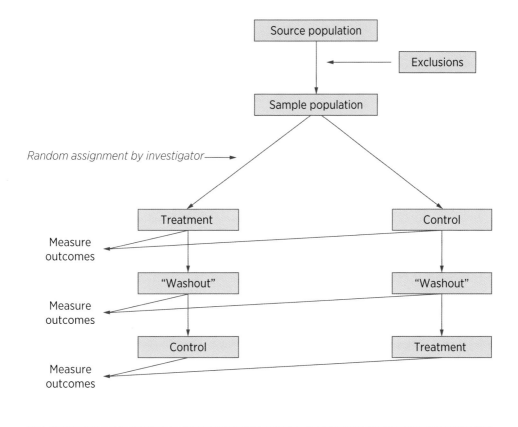

Figure 2.4 Basic study design for the crossover randomized controlled trial where participants are represented in both treatment and control (placebo) arms

eligible enrollees are randomly assigned to two groups differing in the sequence of treatments (see Figure 2.4). This assignment method ensures that an effect due to order of treatment is eliminated from the observed treatment effect as described in a classic article by Hills and Armitage.[36]

EXAMPLE

Diets low in fermentable oligosaccharides, disaccharides, monosaccharides, and polyols (FODMAPS) are recommended as a strategy to manage symptoms of irritable bowel syndrome. To investigate if there is a difference in gastrointestinal tolerance between juice from a high-FODMAP fruit (apple juice) and juice from a low-FODMAP fruit (white grape juice), fasting healthy volunteers were randomly assigned to consume one juice (treatment) before breath hydrogen testing and then a week later were switched to the other juice (treatment) and repeated breath hydrogen testing.[37]

Although seemingly simple and appealing, the crossover design is difficult to justify in many circumstances because the validity of the comparison rests upon the assumption that the participant enters each time period—treatment and control—in an identical state. There can be no carryover effects of the treatment and no appreciable change in the participant's condition. The crossover design is not appropriate when the treatment acts systemically or when the physical condition of the participant is unstable over the trial period. Hills and Armitage[36] discuss the relevant issues.

Instead of randomizing patients or previous study participants to a control group, it is often tempting to use a historical control group composed of individuals—usually patients—who were treated in some manner recognized as standard in the past. Unfortunately, it is difficult to establish the validity of historical controls. The biases present in such a series of patients are rarely completely identifiable and may irretrievably weight the outcome of the comparison in favor of the new treatment.[38] It is not possible to ensure comparability between current and previous patients and the treatments used. Despite these issues, ideas to incorporate historical control data remain of interest.[39]

Some clinical questions cannot be addressed by an RCT because a comparison group of internal controls cannot be formed for ethical or logistic reasons. Other comparison groups—external controls—are necessary. If those controls are well chosen, the studies can make valuable contributions. Bailar and colleagues[40] offer general advice on the proper use and interpretation of studies using external controls.

Sample Size

The ability of a clinical trial to detect a difference between treatment and control groups depends, in part, on the sample size. Procedures for determining sample size yield an estimate only and are based on several assumptions and judgments about circumstances of the study.[8]

If the resulting sample-size number is larger than is reasonable with available resources, the researcher should ask: given the available resources and the sample size feasible to accrue, what is the chance that a meaningful difference can be detected (ie, what is the power of the study)? The answer can be calculated by the same methods but by solving for power instead of sample size. A study may not be worth doing if there is a low probability of detecting a relevant difference. If the final analyses show that sufficient resources cannot be obtained, the project should be redesigned to require fewer assets. The Women's Health Initiative had a large sample size of 48,835, which turned out to be deceiving.[31] Despite the large number of study participants, the level of compliance with the diet was lower than expected, as was the number of incident cases of breast cancer. Thus, the lack of statistically significant results for the main outcomes may have been due to the unexpected reduction in study power.

End Points and Data Collection

The end point of a study is the variable by which the treatments are compared. The choice of a meaningful end point is often clear from the nature of the research question. However, the preferred end point for some research questions is not measurable; reasons may include the length of time required for the end point to occur or the sophisticated equipment necessary to measure the end point. In such cases, a surrogate for the end point is chosen, often an antecedent to the end point. The surrogate or antecedent condition must be highly predictive of the end point for it to serve as a valid answer to the study question.[32] Collecting more than a single surrogate may be advisable to help corroborate findings.

As Weiss[32] cautions, the treatment may affect only the antecedent or surrogate and not the end point of interest. In choosing the surrogate, researchers should consider all available information to help prevent that problem from occurring.

The choice of end point may be between "hard" (objective) and "soft" (subjective) evidence or data. For example, serum lipid concentration and body weight are hard data; degree of headache pain and severity of flu symptoms are soft data. Hard variables are preferred because they are more objective, more reliable, and easier to measure. Relevant soft variables should not be dismissed, however, because they are frequently the most interesting and important outcomes and can be useful in interpreting hard data. A useful approach is to combine a few carefully chosen hard and soft variables.

EXAMPLE

A randomized intervention trial was designed to evaluate the effectiveness of a behavioral intervention targeting sugar-sweetened beverage (SSB) consumption compared with an intervention targeting physical activity and to determine if health literacy influenced retention, engagement, or outcomes. SSB consumption was the primary outcome, and secondary outcomes included physical activity and anthropometry. Among the 301 participants enrolled and randomized, 296 completed measurements. Among the SSB intervention group, SSB consumption significantly decreased, and there was a small but significant reduction in body mass index compared with those in the physical activity group. An important discovery was that health literacy status did not influence retention rates, engagement, or outcomes.[41]

Statistical Analysis and Interpretation

Several excellent publications describe statistical procedures for testing hypotheses in experiments.[8,27,34,42] Among the major problems frequently encountered in analyzing and interpreting results of clinical trials are noncompliance and participants leaving the study.

Even with the best efforts to maintain strict adherence to the treatment protocol, noncompliance often occurs. Adherence to treatment should be monitored to learn about practical aspects of the treatment. All participants should be followed to the same extent, regardless of their compliance with treatment. At the time of analysis, participants should be retained in their originally assigned treatment group, whether or not they actually received the treatment.[34] This comparison, called the *intent-to-treat comparison*, reflects how the treatments perform in practice.[8] A selection bias is introduced if participants are excluded or analyzed in groups other than the group to which they were randomly assigned. A secondary analysis could evaluate the outcomes of the treatments actually received, but that analysis should not be given more weight or relevance than the primary intent-to-treat analysis.[27]

Withdrawal of participants presents another opportunity for selection bias to occur. Participants who withdraw from the study should be followed in the same manner as study participants, if possible.[8] As in the problem of noncompliance, these participants should be analyzed as part of the original treatment group. Reasons for withdrawal should be reported and compared among groups. One treatment may favor withdrawal because it is less acceptable or has unexpected adverse effects.

Reporting adverse effects will help investigators evaluate the practicality of the treatment and plan future studies. If follow-up is not possible and the outcome is not known, researchers can compare the known characteristics of the participants who withdraw with the characteristics of those who complete the study. This comparison may help determine the nature of the bias introduced into the results by the participants' withdrawal. As an additional step in estimating the effect of removing the participants, a secondary analysis could be done assuming an unfavorable outcome for those individuals. Investigators should compare this worst-outcome result with the result obtained with known end points.

Factorial Design

The study designs previously described in this chapter consider only one study question and investigate only one factor. Their simplicity makes them preferred designs in most settings. If the facilities allow, however, it may be useful and efficient to study more than one factor in a single study using a factorial design. A factorial design includes study groups for all combinations of levels of each factor under study. For example, a two-factor factorial design with two levels per factor would have four treatment groups (see Figure 2.5 on page 22).

The comparison of levels of factor A is achieved by comparing groups with factor A (cells 1 and 3) with groups without factor A (cells 2 and 4); the comparison of levels of factor B is achieved by comparing groups with factor B (cells 1 and 2) with groups without factor B (cells 3 and 4). These comparisons are made using two-way analysis of variance. This design also allows a synergistic effect (interaction) to be detected. Hulley and colleagues[8] provide details for the design and analysis of factorial experiments.

EXAMPLE

The impact of incentive programs on the effectiveness of employee training was assessed in a 2 × 2 factorial design in which awarding a monetary bonus was compared with awarding bonus points. All employees were enrolled in a course on customer service and given an audiocassette and a self-paced workbook. Employees were randomly divided into one of four groups according to their award: bonus points only, monetary bonus only, both bonus points and monetary bonus, or no bonus. Outcomes measured were knowledge and attitude scores before and after testing, reported customer satisfaction, and job performance evaluations before and 3 months after the course.

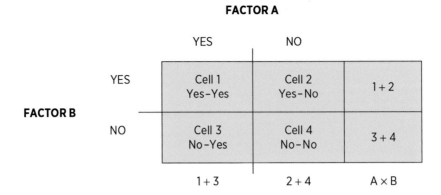

Figure 2.5 Example of a 2p factorial design in which two factors are at two levels each

The effects of factor A (cells 1 and 3 vs cells 2 and 4), factor B (cells 1 and 2 vs cells 3 and 4), and the interaction of A × B may be calculated using two-way analysis of variance

Partially Controlled or Quasi-Experimental Designs

All research involves a balance of the ideal with the feasible. In certain situations, it is impossible to randomize treatment assignment or assemble an appropriate control group. Other study design options are available, although each has limitations, and none is as convincing as the RCT. Experiments that compare groups that have not been randomized or that lack a control group are sometimes termed *quasi-experiments.*

Although these studies do involve the manipulation of a treatment or intervention, they are weak in terms of allowing researchers to make causal inferences. This is because quasi-experimental studies are far less satisfactory than RCTs in controlling for the influence of confounding or distorting variables. Of particular concern is the problem of unmeasured confounding variables, such as lifestyle.[8] Other research options to consider are observational analytic study designs (ie, cohort and case-control studies).

PROSPECTIVE (COHORT, FOLLOW-UP) STUDIES

Prospective (cohort, follow-up) studies are observational analytic studies that are designed to mimic an RCT. A prospective study does not involve investiga-

tor manipulation and thus is not categorized as experimental; however, it does test a hypothesis of a possible chronological or temporal sequence in the causal pathway, so it is analytic in approach.

A cohort is a group of persons followed over time who have a common characteristic or factor of interest. The cohort or group is assembled on the basis of factors thought to relate to the development of the end point under study and followed to observe its experience. This organization allows researchers to investigate a hypothesis concerning the etiology of the outcome of interest. The outcome studied most commonly is a disease; for convenience, the following discussion refers to the studied outcome as a disease. This design is by no means limited to the study of diseases, however. Many other conditions, such as overweight, can be studied in the same manner.[43] The possible causal factors under investigation, referred to as *exposures,* may cover a wide range of environmental and lifestyle characteristics (see Figure 2.6).

Uses of Prospective Studies

A cohort design is useful to determine the frequency of a newly diagnosed disease or a health-related event and to assess the exposure-disease relationship. In the cohort design, exposure to a suspected risk factor is identified when participants are free of detectable disease; that is, the cohort is identified on the basis

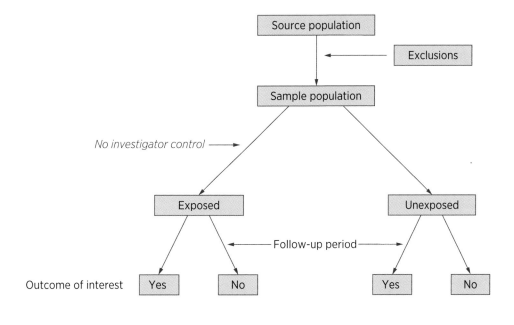

Figure 2.6 Basic prospective cohort study design

of exposure to certain factors thought to affect risk but without the presence of disease. Exposure to the factor of interest clearly precedes the detection of disease. Because it helps establish the temporal sequence of risk factor and end point, the cohort design is an appealing method for studying causes of disease. A drawback is that sufficient time must elapse between assessing the exposure and detecting the outcome; thus, a typical cohort study can be very long. Cohort studies are most useful when the time between exposure and detection of the end point is thought to be relatively short.

Unless the disease studied is extremely common in the study population, most individuals in a cohort will not develop it. Therefore, a large number of participants is required to compare incidence between exposure groups. This design is more feasible for conditions that are relatively common in the population studied.

EXAMPLE

Investigators used a prospective cohort design to assess the association between changes in nutritional status in hospitalized patients and the occurrence of infections, complications, length of stay in the hospital, and hospital charges. In patients admitted to the hospital inpatient service for a stay of longer than 7 days, nutritional status at the time of admission and discharge as well as change in nutritional status during hospitalization were assessed. Outcome measures included length of stay, complications, infections, and hospital charges.[44]

EXAMPLE

A prospective cohort study design was used to examine the ability of four diet-quality indexes (the Healthy Eating Index-2010 [HEI-2010], the Alternative HEI-2010 [AHEI-2010], the alternate Mediterranean diet score [aMED], and the Dietary Approaches to Stop Hypertension [DASH]) to predict the reduction in risk of mortality from all causes, cardiovascular disease, and cancer. The multiethnic cohort (n=215,782) was comprised of African American, Japanese American, Latino, Native Hawaiian, and white adults completing a validated food frequency questionnaire (FFQ). The baseline FFQ was used to compute scores for each dietary index and divided into quintiles. Results showed that high HEI-2010, AHEI-2010, aMED, and DASH scores were all statistically significantly inversely associated with risk of mortality from all causes, cardiovascular disease, and cancer in men and women.[45]

Features of Prospective Cohort Studies

The members of a cohort are apparently free of the disease under study and are selected on the basis of the presence or absence of a factor of interest, or exposure. Members are then followed forward in time to determine the occurrence of the disease or a specific end point serving as an indicator of the disease. The monitoring process can be concurrent or not concurrent. The direction of the study is always prospective because the exposure is identified before the disease is detected. However, the follow-up period may be concurrent (prospective) or nonconcurrent (retrospective). Follow-up may proceed at the same time as the study is conducted (concurrent follow-up), that is, current records generate data on disease occurrence. Alternatively, follow-up may have occurred earlier (nonconcurrent follow-up) where existing records yield data on disease occurrence. Clearly, the latter scheme alleviates the need to wait for the cohort to go through time.

EXAMPLE

A nonconcurrent (retrospective) cohort design was used to determine the association of patient characteristics and risk of hypoglycemia among patients receiving concomitant parenteral nutrition (PN) and insulin therapy. The cohort was assembled from a patient population older than 18 years and part of a PN quality improvement project in a tertiary care medical center over a specified time period. Investigators accessed the quality improvement database containing a nutrition-specific medical record for each patient receiving PN and obtained data about patient characteristics and treatment.[46]

Selecting Participants in Cohort Studies

Cohort participants must be at risk for developing the disease or outcome of interest but free of the disease at the start of the study. Participants may be members of a single cohort and classified according to their exposure to the factor of interest, or they may be members of different cohorts selected from special exposure groups so that the exposed cohort can be compared with the nonexposed cohort. The validity of the comparison between cohorts depends on the assumption that the cohorts are comparable in all relevant factors other than the exposure.

Assessing Exposure Status

Exposure to the factor of interest is observed or measured for each participant at the start of a cohort study. The technique of assessment should be standardized to improve reliability and validity. Information relating to exposure and other important characteristics can be collected from direct measurement, existing records, personal interviews, and questionnaires. Analytical epidemiology studies are discussed in Chapter 7

Assessing dietary intake poses special problems. Dietary intake methodology is the subject of continuing investigation, as no single method has been shown to be reliable and valid for all types of research. When selecting the method for collecting dietary data, the researcher should review these issues thoroughly, as discussed in Chapter 13.

A difficulty of cohort studies is that a change in exposure status may occur during the follow-up period. A change in exposure status may dilute the study's ability to detect a difference in risk between exposed and unexposed groups. To reduce this bias, investigators should measure the important exposure factors several times during the follow-up period.

Assessing Outcomes (Diseases)

The disease or health outcome in a cohort study should be defined in a way that is detailed, unambiguous, and reliable. The method and type of follow-up should be identical for all study participants, regardless of exposure status. To help ensure this goal, the evaluators should be unaware of the participants' exposure status (ie, blind assessment). Blinding ensures that follow-up efforts and the assessment methods used will be applied equally and will not be biased by the investigators' expectations.

Outcome events are counted as they occur during the follow-up period. However, outcomes occurring immediately after assessment of the exposure status cannot be counted when it is not clear that the exposure preceded the end point. This decision depends on what is known or believed to be true about the length of the induction or latent period for the disease or primary end point in question.

It is often useful to supplement the information about the outcome. Researchers should record the date the outcome is detected, as well as its occurrence, depending on the nature of the factor under study.

Complete follow-up on all members of the cohort is vitally important. Loss of participants can seriously distort the results, so researchers should make vigorous efforts to assess the outcome of each person at the end of the follow-up period.

The length of follow-up depends on the hypothesis and related knowledge of the latency period or the mechanisms of action of the risk factor. The longer the follow-up period, the more difficult the follow-up becomes due to changes of residence, death from other causes, changes in exposure status, and the added staffing expenses for monitoring study participants and collecting data. Those considerations must be balanced with the need to allow sufficient time for the proposed effect to become manifest.

Statistical Analysis and Interpretation

Baseline characteristics of the cohort are described using distributions and frequencies. The usual inferential comparative analysis of prospective studies involves determining the incidence of disease and estimating the incidence ratio for exposed vs unexposed participants. The incidence ratio, known as the *relative risk*, measures the strength of the association between the exposure factor and the disease or outcome of interest.[47] Thus, the results are stated as those with the exposure are more likely (or less likely) to develop the disease compared with those without the exposure.

The weakness in this observational study design is that a relationship is not clearly causal. All factors are not held constant, as they are in an experimental study design. These limitations need to be considered when interpreting the final results. The criteria for causation based on the collective results from observational and experimental studies are reviewed in Chapter 7

CASE-CONTROL STUDIES

Case-control studies involve observational analytic designs that investigate hypotheses of causal rela-

tionships. These designs are retrospective, historically oriented studies, also known as *case-referent studies* or *case-comparison studies*. Because case-control designs do not involve intervention by the investigators, they are not experimental but do adhere to as many principles of experimental design as possible.

Uses of Case-Control Studies

A case-control design is used to explore etiology by comparing the prevalence of exposure to factors of interest in persons who have a disease and persons who do not have the disease. The design is useful in studies of rare diseases or end points. In general, case-control studies are less expensive to conduct and require less time than cohort studies.

Features of Case-Control Studies

The case-control study design assesses exposure status after disease status is known and thus is retrospective. The comparison groups are formed on the basis of disease or outcome status, either with disease diagnosis (cases) or without disease diagnosis (controls). Study participants are then investigated for the current presence of, or previous exposure to, a factor or factors of interest. The prevalence of the factor or factors is compared between cases and controls (see Figure 2.7 on page 26).

EXAMPLE

The pathways involved in alcohol-related breast cancer are not clearly defined. A case-control study was designed to examine the association between low to moderate alcohol intake and breast cancer subtypes by tumor hormone receptor status. Over a 4-year study period, 585 women between 28 and 90 years old with new histologically confirmed breast cancer met the study criteria. Controls (n=1,170) were women without a history of cancer hospitalized in other departments (eg, ophthalmology). Both cases and controls completed a self-administered previously validated questionnaire so investigators could ascertain alcohol intake. The estrogen receptor and progesterone receptor levels were measured in breast tissue samples using immunohistochemistry.[48]

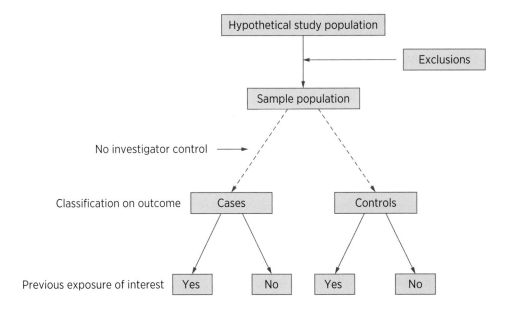

Figure 2.7 Basic case-control study design involves ascertaining cases after onset of disease and assessing exposure via recall of status before the onset of disease

Selection of Cases

In a case-control study, the goal in selecting cases is to obtain a sample that is representative of cases arising from a defined target population. This goal is difficult or impossible to attain in most circumstances. The ideal compromise is to select all incident (newly developed or detected) cases arising in a defined population over some specified period. Selecting incident cases rather than existing (prevalent) cases is preferred because factors related to survival, and thus to selection for the study, may differ from causal factors, but these cannot be distinguished from one another when prevalent cases are used. The definition of a case should be specific and objective to minimize the bias of personal judgment.

Selecting Controls

Selecting an appropriate comparison group in a case-control study depends largely upon the hypothesis. When selecting control participants, the goal is that controls should be representative of the population from which the cases arise. A random probability sample is ideal and is feasible if information is available on the sampling units (or community). A random

EXAMPLE

To investigate the hypothesis that a high intake of fruits, vegetables, and nutrients involved in antioxidant activities contributes to the risk of developing non-Hodgkin lymphoma (NHL), a case-control study was planned using the Surveillance, Epidemiology, and End Results cancer registry. Over a 3-year period, 1,321 of 2,248 potentially eligible incident case patients between 20 and 74 years old with NHL were enrolled as cases. Control participants ≤65 years old were identified by random dialing, and those ≥65 years old were randomly identified from Medicare files. Controls were frequency matched to cases by age (within 5 years), geographic location, race, and gender. All study participants were mailed a self-administered quantitative food frequency questionnaire to assess usual intake of foods and fruits and vegetables 1 year before NHL diagnosis for cases and the same time period for controls. The reported fruit and vegetable intakes (quantity and type) were compared between cases and controls.[49]

probability sample is also feasible if the population is closed, such as members of a prepaid health plan or patients in an institution. Convenience samples are often used, but the validity of the study rests upon the assumption that the selected participants are similar to the reference or target population with regard to the factors of interest; this assumption may or may not be reasonable.

Considerations in choosing a control group are cost, response rate, and interview setting. Investigators may have to compromise to reduce the cost of accessing a potential control participant while maximizing the response rate. Insofar as possible, the interview setting should be comparable to the setting for cases. Much of the information is elicited by recall and self-report, and factors bearing on those methods should be as identical as possible in the groups.

A selection bias in controls is undesirable but possible. Investigators can minimize bias by planning a structured selection system with established criteria for selecting the control participants. The criteria should be applied without the investigators' knowledge of the participants' exposure status. Other sources of bias, such as age, gender, or socioeconomic status, may be eliminated by matching in the selection process or by stratification in the analysis. The method for selecting appropriate controls is not always clear; Hulley and colleagues[8] and Breslow and Day[50] review problems and give suggestions.

EXAMPLE

Using a case-control design, researchers investigated a possible relationship between diet-related inflammation and risk of prediabetes among residents of Iran. The investigators examined the association between the dietary inflammatory index (DII) and risk of prediabetes in a clinic population-based study. Patients newly diagnosed with prediabetes (n=214) were selected as cases from specialized centers using a nonrandom sampling procedure. The controls (n=200) were randomly selected from the same clinics and frequency matched for age (±5 years) and sex. The DII scores were estimated from data collected using a validated and reproducible food frequency questionnaire. Logistic regression was used to estimate odds ratios.[51]

Assessing Exposure to the Factor of Interest

In case-control studies, historical information, including exposure to the factor of interest, is obtained from existing records, examinations, direct measurements, and personal interviews or questionnaires. The starting point for developing any data-gathering tool is a list of all pertinent variables, including the extent of detail needed. Methods for assessing past diet in case-control studies have been studied in a variety of settings.[52] Issues involved with selecting a dietary assessment method are covered in Chapter 13.

EXAMPLE

A population-based, case-control study was conducted to examine the association between selected nutrients, foods, and diet behaviors and bladder cancer. Patients diagnosed with bladder cancer within a 4-year period were identified from the Surveillance, Epidemiology, and End Results cancer registry for western Washington State. Controls were identified through random dialing for the same residential area. A food frequency questionnaire was used to estimate usual food intake. Study participants were asked to estimate food intake for the year that was the midpoint of the 10-year reference period (ie, 7 years before diagnosis for cases and a similar reference period for controls).[53]

Regardless of the instrument used, the procedure for gathering information should be the same for cases and controls. The comparability of the procedure is increased if the interviewer or evaluator does not know whether a participant is a case or a control. This goal may not be possible in a personal interview but may be feasible for a person gathering other objective data.

Statistical Analysis and Interpretation

In a case-control study, the frequencies of the exposure of interest are presented for cases and controls. The association between the exposure and the disease is expressed by estimating the odds ratio, a statistical comparison of the prevalence of exposure between cases and controls.[42,50] Thus, the results are expressed as a statement that those with the disease were more likely (or less likely) to have had the exposure compared with those without the disease.

The observational methodology and retrospective nature of case-control studies present limitations that researchers should keep in mind when interpreting the results. There are always alternatives to a causal explanation for an association. Chief among the alternatives are several issues. In a case-control study, it may be unclear whether the factor preceded or resulted from the disease. The self-report may be influenced by the presence of the disease, especially if the participant is aware of the hypothesis being tested. This recall bias may result in an observed association that overestimates the actual association. The comparability of cases and controls may be questionable, thus the choice of control group is crucial to a valid study.

CONCLUSION

Nutrition and dietetics offer many opportunities to pursue a compelling research question. To examine a proposed research question, an investigator must first summarize the literature on the topic and complement it with observations from the work environment. This step will help the investigator refine the hypothesis or research objective. Qualitative, descriptive, or analytic study approaches can be considered to address a variety of research questions. Selecting the best study design will allow investigators to infer valid conclusions from the data collected. The strengths and weaknesses of the different study designs need to be considered within the framework of available resources. Throughout the research process, the investigator uses brainstorming, attention to the detail of data collection, and teamwork.

REFERENCES

1. US Department of Health and Human Services, US Department of Agriculture. 2015–2020 Dietary Guidelines for Americans. 8th ed. Figure I-1. http:// health.gov /dietaryguidelines/2015/guidelines. Accessed November 17, 2016.

2. US Department of Health and Human Services. Healthy People 2020. Available at: www.healthypeople.gov. Accessed March 15, 2017.

3. Bryman A, Bell E. *Business Research Methods*. 3rd ed. New York, NY: Oxford University Press; 2011.

4. Blank SC. *Practical Business Research Methods*. Westport, CT: AVI Publishing Co; 1984.

5. National Library of Medicine. National Institutes of Health. PubMed website. www.ncbi.nlm.nih.gov/pubmed. Accessed February 2, 2017.

6. Cochrane Consumer Network. What is a systematic review? http://consumers.cochrane.org/what-systematic -review. Accessed March 26, 2017.

7. Boushey C, Harris J, Bruemmer B, Archer SL, Van Horn L. Publishing nutrition research: a review of study design, statistical analyses, and other key elements of manuscript preparation, Part 1. *J Am Diet Assoc*. 2006; 106(1):89-96.

8. Hulley SB, Cummings SR, Browner WS, Grady DG, Newman TB. *Designing Clinical Research*. 4th ed. Philadelphia, PA: Lippincott Williams & Wilkins; 2013.

9. Ogden CL, Carroll MD, Fryar CD, Flegal KM. Prevalence of obesity among adults and youth: United States, 2011-2014. *NCHS Data Brief*. 2015;219:1-8.

10. Bacon L, Stern JS, Van Loan MD, Keim NL. Size acceptance and intuitive eating improve health for obese, female chronic dieters. *J Am Diet Assoc*. 2005;105(6):929-936.

11. Aitaoto N, Campo S, Snetselaar LG, et al. Formative research to inform nutrition interventions in Chuuk and the US Pacific. *J Acad Nutr Diet*. 2015;115(6):947-953.

12. Cassel KD, Boushey CJ. Leveraging cultural knowledge to improve diet and health among affiliated Pacific Islander populations. *J Acad Nutr Diet*. 2015;115(6):885-888.

13. Kerlinger FN, Lee HB. *Foundations of Behavioral Research*. 4th ed. New York, NY: Harcourt College Publishers; 2000.

14. Hoyle RH, Harris MJ, Judd CM. *Research Methods in Social Relations*. 7th ed. New York, NY: Wadsworth Publishing Co; 2002.

15. Patton MQ. *Qualitative Evaluation and Research Methods: Integrating Theory and Practice*. 4th ed. Thousand Oaks, CA: SAGE Publications; 2015.

16. Sobal J. Sample extensiveness in qualitative nutrition education research. *J Nutr Educ*. 2001; 33(4):184-192.

17. Safman RM, Sobal J. Qualitative sample extensiveness in health education research. *Health Educ Behav*. 2004;31(1):9-21.

18. Dahlke R, Wolf KN, Wilson SL, Brodnik M. Focus groups as predictors of dietitians' roles on interdisciplinary teams. *J Am Diet Assoc*. 2000;100(4):455-457.

19. Frerichs L, Intolubbe-Chmil L, Brittin J, Teitelbaum K, Trowbridge M, Huang T-K. Children's discourse of like, healthy, and unhealthy foods. *J Acad Nutr Diet*. 2016; 116(8):1323-1331.

20. Auld G, Boushey CJ, Bock MA, et al. Perspectives on intake of calcium-rich foods among Asian, Hispanic, and white preadolescent and adolescent females. *J Nutr Educ Behav*. 2002;34(5):242-251.

21. Kakodkar S, Farooqui AJ, Mikolaitis SL, Mutlu EA. The specific carbohydrate diet for inflammatory bowel disease: a case series. *J Acad Nutr Diet*. 2015;115(8):1226-1232.

22. Matthews ME, Zardain MV, Mahaffey MJ. Labor time spent in foodservice activities in one hospital: a 12-year profile. *J Am Diet Assoc*. 1986;86(5):636-643.

23. McColl E, Jacoby A, Thomas L, et al. Design and use of questionnaires: a review of best practice applicable to surveys of health service staff and patients. *Health Technol Assess*. 2001;5(31):204-244.

24. Mislevy JM, Schiller MR, Wolf KN, Finn SC. Clinical nutrition managers have access to sources of empowerment. *J Am Diet Assoc*. 2000;100(9):1038-1043.

25. Bermúdez OI, Falcón LM, Tucker KL. Intake and food sources of macronutrients among older Hispanic adults: association with ethnicity, acculturation, and length of residence in the United States. *J Am Diet Assoc*. 2000; 100(6):665-673.

26. Elwood PC. Epidemiology for nutritionists: 2. Sampling. *Hum Nutr Appl Nutr*. 1983;37(4):265-269.

27. Moore DS, McCabe GP, Craig BA. Producing data. In: Moore DS, McCabe GP, Craig BA, eds. *Introduction to the Practice of Statistics*. New York, NY: WH Freeman and Co, 2016:163-214.

28. Dillman DA, Smyth JD, Christian LM. *Internet, Phone, Mail, and Mixed Mode Surveys: The Tailored Design Method*. 4th ed. New York, NY: John Wiley and Sons; 2014.

29. Daida Y, Novotny R, Grove JS, Acharya S, Vogt TM. Ethnicity and nutrition of adolescent girls in Hawaii. *J Am Diet Assoc*. 2006;106(2):221-226.

30. Bihuniak JD, Ramos A, Huedo-Median T, Hutchins-Wiese H, Kerstetter JE, Kenny AM. Adherence to a Mediterranean-style diet and its influence on cardiovascular risk factors in postmenopausal women. *J Acad Nutr Diet.* 2016;116(11):1767-1775.

31. Prentice RL, Caan B, Chlebowski RT, et al. Low-fat dietary pattern and risk of invasive breast cancer. *JAMA.* 2006; 295(6):629-642.

32. Weiss NS. *Clinical Epidemiology: The Study of the Outcome of Illness.* 3rd ed. New York, NY: Oxford University Press; 2006.

33. Farr BM, Gwaltney JM Jr. The problems of taste in placebo matching: an evaluation of zinc gluconate for the common cold. *J Chronic Dis.* 1987;40(9):875-879.

34. Meinert CL. *Clinical Trials: Design, Conduct, and Analysis.* 2nd ed. New York, NY: Oxford University Press; 2012.

35. Karlowski TR, Chalmers TC, Frenkel LD, Kapidian AZ, Lewis TL, Lynch JM. Ascorbic acid for the common cold. A prophylactic and therapeutic trial. *JAMA.* 1975;231(10): 1038-1042.

36. Hills M, Armitage P. The two-period cross-over clinical trial. *Br J Clin Pharmacol.* 2004; 58(7):S703-S716.

37. Erickson J, Wang Q, Slavin J. White grape juice elicits a lower breath hydrogen response compared with apple juice in healthy human subjects: a randomized controlled trial. *J Acad Nutr Diet.* 2017;117(6):908-913.

38. Sacks H, Chalmers TC, Smith H. Randomized versus historical controls for clinical trials. *Am J Med.* 1982;72(2): 233-240.

39. Hobbs BP, Carlin BP, Sargent DJ. Adaptive adjustment of the randomization ratio using historical control data. *Clin Trials.* 2013;10(3):1-19.

40. Bailar JC, Louis TA, Lavori PW, Polansky M. Studies without internal controls. *N Engl J Med.* 1984;311(3): 156-162.

41. Zoellner JM, Hedrick VE, You W, et al. Effects of a behavioral and health literacy intervention to reduce sugar-sweetened beverages: a randomized-controlled trial. *Int J Behav Nutr Phys Act.* 2016;13:38.

42. Rosner B. *Fundamentals of Biostatistics.* 7th ed. Boston, MA: Brooks/Cole, Cengage Learning; 2010.

43. Patterson KA, Gall SL, Venn AJ, et al. Accumulated exposure to rural areas of residence over the life course is associated with overweight and obesity in adulthood: a 25-year prospective cohort study. *Ann Epidemiol.* 2017;27(3):169-175.

44. Braunschweig C, Gomez S, Sheean PM. Impact of declines in nutritional status on outcomes in adult patients. *J Am Diet Assoc.* 2000;100(11):1316-1322.

45. Harmon BE, Boushey CJ, Shvetsov YB, et al. Associations of key diet-quality indexes with mortality in the Multiethnic Cohort: the Dietary Patterns Methods Project. *Am J Clin Nutr.* 2015;101(3):587-597.

46. Kinnare KR, Bacon CA, Chen Y, Sowa DC, Peterson SJ. Risk factors for predicting hypoglycemia in patients receiving concomitant parenteral nutrition and insulin therapy. *J Acad Nutr Diet.* 2013;113(2):263-268.

47. Rothman KJ. *Epidemiology: An Introduction.* 2nd ed. New York, NY: Oxford University Press; 2012.

48. Strumylaite L, Sharp SJ, Kregzdyte R, Poskiene L, Bogusevicius A, Pranys D. The association of low-to-moderate alcohol consumption with breast cancer subtypes defined by hormone receptor status. *PLoS ONE.* 2015;10(12):e0144680.

49. Kelemen LE, Cerhan JR, Lim U, et al. Vegetables, fruit, and antioxidant-related nutrients and risk of non-Hodgkin lymphoma: a National Cancer Institute-Surveillance, Epidemiology, and End Results population-based case-control study. *Am J Clin Nutr.* 2006;83(6):1401-1410.

50. Breslow NE, Day NE. Statistical methods in cancer research. Vol 1: the analysis of case-control studies. IARC Scientific Publications No. 32. International Agency for Research on Cancer. Lyon, France; 1980. www.iarc.fr/en/publications/pdfs-online/stat/sp32. Accessed February 5, 2018.

51. Vahid F, Shivappa N, Karamati M, Naeini AJ, Hebert JR, Davoodi SH. Association between dietary inflammatory index (DII) and risk of prediabetes: a case-control study. *Appl Physiol Nutr Metab.* 2017;42(4):399-404.

52. Thompson FE, Subar AF. Dietary assessment methodology. In: Coulston AM, Boushey CJ, Ferruzzi MG, Delahanty L, eds. *Nutrition in the Prevention and Treatment of Disease.* 4th edition, San Diego, CA: Academic Press; 2017:5-46.

53. Bruemmer B, White E, Vaughan TL, Cheney CL. Nutrient intake in relation to bladder cancer among middle-aged men and women. *Am J Epidemiol.* 1996;144(5):485-495.

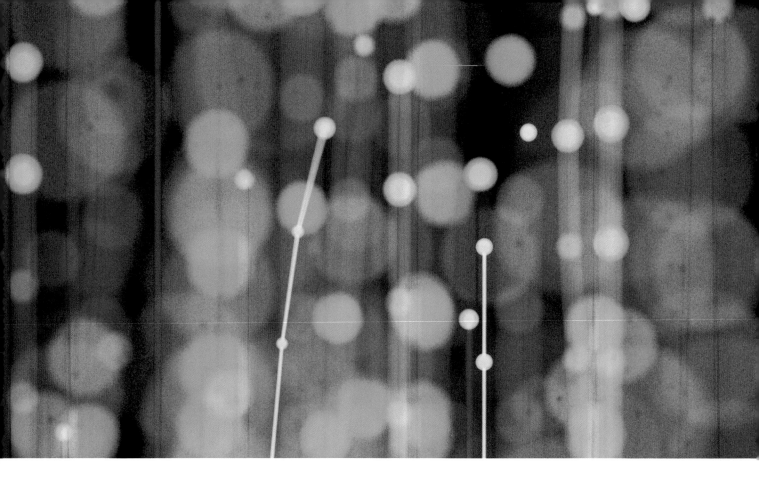

Establishing and Maintaining a Research Environment

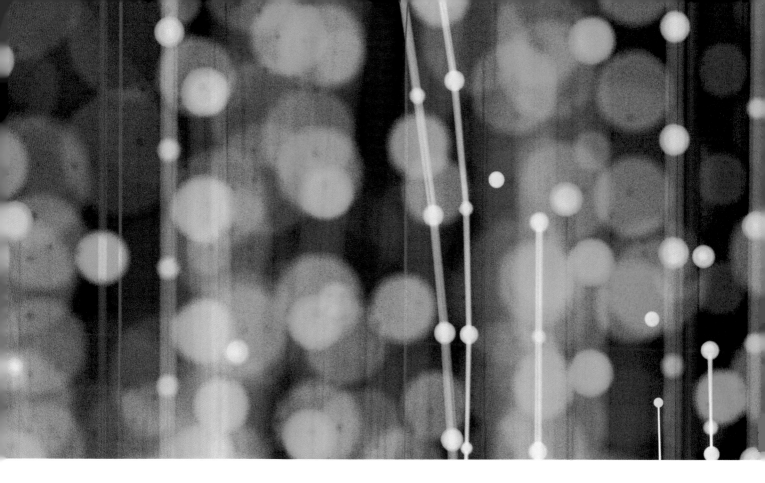

Conducting and Presenting Research Ethically

Rosa K. Hand, PhD, RDN, LD, FAND

LEARNING OBJECTIVES

1. Identify three types of errors and their relation to ethics in research.

2. Identify guiding documents in research ethics, both general and specific to nutrition.

3. Identify and describe how to avoid an ethical issue related to publication.

4. Explain ethical protections for human subjects, including institutional review board review and informed consent requirements.

EDITORS' NOTE
On January 21, 2019, after this chapter was written, the Common Rule was updated. Readers are referred to the resources in Table 3.1 and their own institutional policies for the most up-to-date information and guidance on Institutional Review Board policies.

Ethics encompasses the rules and principles that govern appropriate conduct as well as the values and guidelines that should govern decisions in science and medicine. Thus, ethical behavior and ethical decisions are of critical importance in conducting and presenting research. In the early 2000s, disclosures of scientific fraud in the field of stem cell research and cloning of human embryonic stem cells stunned the scientific community.[1] In 2006, Eric Poehlman, PhD, was sentenced to 1 year and 1 day in federal prison followed by 2 years of probation resulting from his history of falsifying and fabricating data related to the impacts of aging and menopause on body composition and energy expenditure.[2]

His most famous study, which claimed to follow 35 women longitudinally as they aged,[3] actually only followed two women; data for the other 33 subjects were made up.[2] Instances of modifying data to support hypotheses were also uncovered and resulted in 10 retractions or corrections of published information.[4] Besides serving prison time, Poehlman was fined and has a lifetime ban on receiving federal research funding.[2] Poehlman's actions negatively affected his colleagues and the overall body of science. While this example is particularly stark, it demonstrates that research misconduct is not unique to bench science.

Ethics also relates to the relationship between funders and researchers—although less blatant than data falsification or fabrication, there is concern in nutrition and dietetics about whether food and beverage industry funding influences scientific conclusions.[5] Such issues prompt a closer look at the ethics of conducting and presenting research. The concept of ethics encompasses the principles of conduct governing an individual or group; thus, it pervades all aspects of personal and professional life. The Academy of Nutrition and Dietetics and the Commission on Dietetic Registration have adopted a voluntary, enforceable code of ethics, as have other responsible professional groups. The current version of the Code of Ethics for the Dietetics Profession, which became effective in 2009, delineates 19 principles to guide dietetics practitioners in their commitments and obligations to "the public, clients, the profession, colleagues, and other practitioners." According to the Code of Ethics, practitioners act with objectivity and respect for the unique needs and values of individuals; avoid discrimination; maintain confidentiality; base practices on scientific principles and current information; conduct professional affairs with honesty, integrity, and fairness; and manage or reduce conflicts of interest.[6]

Ethical judgments frequently reflect divergent opinions, and clear reasoning is required to come to a decision. Each case may be evaluated on an individual basis using guiding professional principles and documents while acknowledging one's own opinions and beliefs.[7] Nonetheless, despite these differences, people of all cultures and eras agree on which actions are basically constructive—or destructive—to human interaction. Ethical conduct underscores behavior that supports positive relationships between persons and facilitates scientific progress.

At each step of research, ethical issues arise. Designing, conducting, reporting, and interpreting research, as well as planning future research, all involve decisions in which professional ethics are pivotal. Whenever human subjects are involved in research, the bioethics and regulations related to research must be recognized and carefully considered. To supplement the Code of Ethics, the Academy developed six scientific integrity principles that guide the organization's scientific activities.[8] These principles can be used to guide all dietetics practitioners in considering some of the issues discussed in this chapter, including authorship, publication, and conflicts of interest. These ethical issues and their statutory rules will be addressed along with key errors in research design and presentation. Case study examples of some of these issues are discussed in a 2017 *Journal of the Academy of Nutrition and Dietetics*.[9]

RESEARCH ERROR, HUMAN ERROR, AND FRAUD

Scientific errors can seriously impact scientific progress, whether the errors are consequences of flawed design, improper conduct of research, or unintentional or intentional human error. Repercussions of error are manifold. Time and funds can be lost in pursuing blind alleys, misapplication can be damaging to society, scientific careers can be severely thwarted, and education of future practitioners can be flawed.[10] Tainted literature, like an ocean blackened by an oil spill, requires time to be cleansed.[1,10] Poor and inadequate supervision is not acceptable in scientific enterprises. It is critical that researchers assume responsibility and enable investigation if misconduct is charged in any research projects in which they have participated.

Researchers need to, and generally can, circumvent research errors: those of design, execution, analysis, and presentation.[11] Research errors may be categorized into six types (discussed in more depth later in the chapter):

- sampling errors

- noncoverage errors
- nonresponse errors
- measurement errors
- errors of data distortion and overgeneralization
- errors of misrepresentation to human subjects, in authorship, and in conflicts of interest

Quality research demands that research errors be minimized; moreover, allowing such errors may cause major ethical dilemmas in the future. Depending on the intent of the researcher, these errors may or may not be a breach of ethical conduct.

Human errors are generally more hidden and less readily detectable than research errors.[12] Human errors are an unfortunate—and, it is hoped, infrequent—occurrence in research. Three sources of human error need to be differentiated:

- inadvertent behavior
- negligence
- intentional actions

Because scientists are fallible, inadvertent errors can occur.[12] An honest mistake is tolerable to the scientific community and the public if it is promptly and properly handled when uncovered. However, preventable mistakes attributable to carelessness or negligence are not tolerable to either science or society; sloppy science is a form of intentional error. It is critical, therefore, for researchers to be vigilant and maintain a strong leadership role throughout the research process.

Fraud (ie, intentional deception) destroys science by eroding trust and integrity. The scientific method is built upon hypotheses and honest observation; deception is anathema to science. Fraud comes in varying degrees, including concealing data that do not support a hypothesis and presenting only supportive data (referred to as "selective reporting" or "cooking data"),[12] revising observed data to conform to a hypothesis (known as "trimming data"), and blatantly fabricating data.[1,13] Examples of extensive intentional fraud have garnered significant media attention, such as those related to claims of successful cloning of human embryonic stem cells, originally published in 2004 and 2005 and retracted in 2006.[1] Each deception is intentional, though the extent of misconduct differs dramati-

cally. A meta-analysis of surveys showed that 2% of researchers admit to having participated in data falsification or fabrication, but 14% have observed colleagues falsify or fabricate.[1] Even these rates are unacceptable and can destroy laboratories, research groups, and institutions, as well as endanger patients and erode public trust in science. Plagiarism, where one puts forward the work or words of others as one's own, is a further category of intentional fraud.[1,14] The original authors and subjects feel the damaging effects of plagiarism keenly, and the perpetrators can face severe criticism from the scientific community and the public.

ETHICS IN RESEARCH INVOLVING HUMANS

Historical Basis and Guiding Documents for Protecting Human Subjects

Current guidelines and regulations regarding human experimentation have evolved since the middle of the 20th century in reaction to public and scientific outcry over cases of gross human injustice. One of the first areas to receive public scrutiny was the heinous behavior of physicians toward the inmates of Nazi concentration camps during World War II. Following the war, 20 doctors were tried in Nuremberg for war crimes and crimes against humanity before an international tribunal. The resulting Nuremberg Code of 1947 established 10 principles that must be followed in human experimentation to satisfy moral, ethical, and legal concepts.[15] These principles, for the first time, established that the informed voluntary consent of human subjects is essential.

The second major international code of ethics was the Declaration of Helsinki, adopted by the World Medical Association in 1964 with a proviso that the text be reviewed periodically.[16] The 12 basic principles delineated the concept of submitting experimental protocols to an independent committee for consideration, comment, and guidance. This concept was the genesis of the institutional review board (IRB), which has become a major force in ensuring the rights of human subjects (see further discussion later). The Declaration of Helsinki also counseled researchers to exercise caution in conducting research that could affect the environment and to respect the welfare of animals used for research. These first two documents govern research ethics internationally; outside the United States, the rights of human subjects are protected by ethics committees, which serve a similar purpose to IRBs. The rest of this chapter focuses on US research regulations and uses the term *IRB*.

A third important document supporting the rights of human subjects in the United States is the 1978 Belmont Report,[17] issued by the National Commission for the Protection of Human Subjects of Biomedical and Behavioral Research. Respect for persons, beneficence, and justice are the three basic principles evoked by the Belmont Report. This critically important report addresses the ethical conduct of research involving human subjects and argues for balancing society's interests in protecting the rights of subjects with its interests in furthering knowledge that can benefit society as a whole. The report argues that "respect for persons" incorporates at least two basic ethical convictions (or assurances): (1) that individuals be treated as autonomous agents and (2) that individuals in need of protection because of diminished autonomy are entitled to protection. Beneficence is understood to encompass acts of kindness and charity that go beyond strict obligation. Beneficent actions extend from doing no harm to maximizing possible benefits and minimizing possible harms. Justice, the third principle set forth in the Belmont Report, demands that each person be treated fairly. Justice requires that burdens and benefits be shared with equity and that those who may reap the benefits of the research are also those who should shoulder the risk. Collectively, these ethical convictions serve as the foundation of effective research that benefits human beings.

Reports issued by the National Commission for the Protection of Human Subjects of Biomedical and Behavioral Research established recommendations for protecting special categories of human subjects, including human fetuses, children, prisoners, and people with mental disabilities. To codify these protections for the rights of all human subjects, IRBs were empowered through 45 Code of Federal Regulations part 46, which has four subparts. Part A, also referred to as the Common Rule because it has been adopted by 15 federal departments and agencies, addresses IRBs and informed consent.[18,19] Other subparts that provide additional protections to specific vulnerable populations apply to some but not all participating agencies.[18] While technically these rules only apply to research funded by participating agencies, most institutions implement them across the board for consistency.

In all aspects of human experimentation, it is critical that researchers avoid misrepresentation to human subjects by following the aforementioned ethical principles of respect, beneficence, and justice. These principles affirm the importance of full and comprehensible disclosure to subjects; noncoercive consent; confidentiality[20]; protection of privacy; equity in subject selection; autonomous right of free choice, including the subject's right to terminate participation without penalty; and termination of the research project at any point if the data warrant such action.[21]

Most institutions require researchers to have formal training on these and other concepts before engaging in human subject research. While training requirements vary by institution, some examples are listed in Table 3.1 on page 38.

The Institutional Review Board's Role in Protecting Subjects

The role of the IRB is to protect human subjects.[22] To achieve this goal, IRBs review proposed research for social value, scientific validity, equity of subject selection, and risk-benefit ratio.[23] Federal rules govern the selection of IRB members and some IRB processes, but other processes vary from institution to institution. Some institutions have expanded the IRB's role to include minimizing legal risk to the institution, which can cause challenges and frustration to investigators.[22] As discussed later, 45 Code of Federal Regulations Part 46 changes to recognize new trends in research.[19] Although rules evolve, the goal of protecting human subjects remains the same. Researchers must stay up to date on national regulations and how their local institution enforces those rules.

Name	Website	Details
Collaborative Institutional Training Initiative (CITI) Program	https://about.citiprogram.org/en/homepage	Charges a fee unless the participant's institution has an agreement with CITI
National Institutes of Health (NIH) Office of Extramural Research Protecting Human Research Participants	https://phrp.nihtraining.com/users/login.php	Free NIH requires human subjects training, but not necessarily this particular training
Research Ethics for the Registered Dietitian Nutritionist	www.eatrightpro.org/research	Free to members of the Academy of Nutrition and Dietetics Not recognized by institutions but modeled on CITI and can be used to supplement CITI with nutrition examples[21]

Table 3.1 Resources for Training in Human Subjects Protection

The administration of the IRB with which researchers work is a good source of information; frequent interaction with the staff may smooth the approval process and ensure high-quality projects. In addition, the US Department of Health and Human Services Office for Human Research Protections maintains helpful frequently asked questions and decision guides on its website.[24]

Researchers must begin the IRB process early because research cannot begin until the IRB has reviewed and approved the project. The IRB may require multiple iterations of a proposal to address questions and concerns. Figure 3.1 outlines the IRB review process, and Box 3.1 on page 40 addresses the types of information the IRB requires.

Informed Consent Processes

Obtaining informed consent is the process of giving human participants all of the information they need to make a decision about whether or not they will participate in the research. Implicit to informed consent is that researchers clearly and accurately describe what the study entails, unless they have an IRB-approved justification for deceiving subjects or withholding information. Unless the IRB grants specific permission to modify the consent process, all information must be provided in writing, and participants must sign the consent document.[19,23] Informed consent documents must be written at a level that all potential participants can understand (typically about a fifth-grade reading level) and must contain information in lay terms rather than

scientific terms. For example, the amount of blood drawn should be stated in household measures, that is, tablespoons not milliliters. Reading level is based on number of syllables per word and words per sentence and can be calculated by copying and pasting text into a website or by using the spelling and grammar tools in word processing software. Using shorter words, bullet points, and short sentences helps achieve reading-level goals. A variety of resources are available to help rephrase medical terms into lay language for consent documents, including plain language materials and resources compiled by the Centers for Disease Control and Prevention.[25]

Informed consent is both a document (Box 3.2 on page 40) and a process—after being given the written material, researchers might verbally review the content with participants, who must always be given the opportunity to ask as many questions as needed. Once all questions have been answered, participants acknowledge their willingness to participate in the study by signing the informed consent document. The person from the research team who obtained the consent also signs the form (sometimes referred to as a witness); some institutions also require that the principal investigator sign the consent document, even if they did not participate in obtaining the consent. Individuals must be given a copy of the signed informed consent document so they can refer back to it throughout the study should they have questions. Part of the informed consent process is checking for the participant's understanding of the proposed research and allowing them to ask ques-

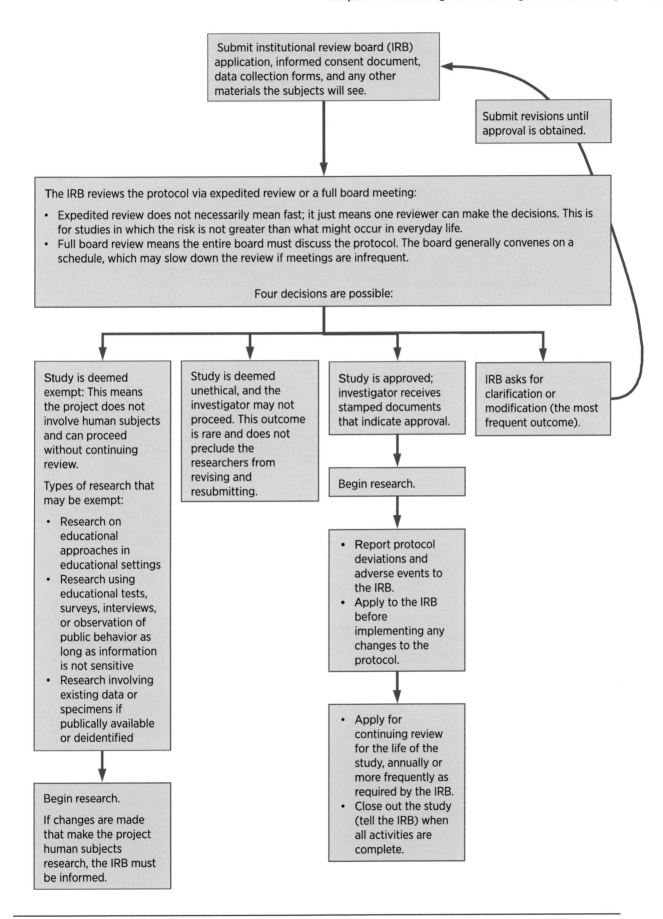

Figure 3.1 Institutional review board application and approval process

Though the wording will vary from institution to institution, the institutional review board will request the following information to consider a protocol:

- Purpose of research
- Background of research showing gap in knowledge
- Duration of study
  Subject characteristics (inclusion and exclusion criteria)
- Procedures for identifying and recruiting subjects
- All variables to be collected, including exact wording of questions and any forms that subjects will see
- Risks and benefits to subjects
- How and where the data will be stored (hard copy, electronically, or both) to maintain privacy and confidentiality
- What compensation will be provided and when
- Procedures for protecting vulnerable subjects, if included
- Any populations that will be purposely excluded (eg, minorities, non–English speakers) and justification
- Funding source for the project
- Names and roles of those working on the project

If the researcher cannot answer these questions, the project is not ready for institutional review board review.

Box 3.1 Information Requested in an Institutional Review Board Application

tions, confer with trusted advisers, and confirm their consent for each study visit or procedure. Participants should not be rushed into a consent decision—they must be allowed to take the information home to discuss with family or friends if they wish.

Possible modifications of the informed consent process, including waiving the requirement for a signature or obtaining consent verbally, are acceptable

Following are the basic elements of informed consent, which apply to all studies, as required by the Common Rule. There are other elements of informed consent that are required depending on the study details, which are not listed here. Note that most institutions have an informed consent form template that must be used.

- Statement that the study involves research
- Research purpose
- How long the subject's participation will take
- Procedures to be conducted:
  - identification of any procedures that are experimental
- Risks or discomforts to the subject
- Benefits to the subject/others as a result of the research (Compensation is *not* a benefit.)
- Any procedures or courses of treatment (including standard care) that are appropriate alternatives to the research (In a nonintervention study this may involve stating that the alternative to participation is to not participate, and that subjects will receive their standard care independent of research participation.)
- People or entities who will be able to access records identifying the subject (This may include research funding agencies or oversight boards in addition to investigators.)
- Contact information:
  - for questions about the research (investigator)
  - for questions about research subjects' rights (Institutional Review Board)
  - in the event of a research-related injury to the subject
- Statement that participation is voluntary
- Statement that the subject may stop participation
- Statement that if subjects don't participate or stop participating, they will still receive benefits to which they are otherwise entitled and will not be penalized
- Signature and date of participant signature
- Signature of witness (study personnel)

Box 3.2 Components of an Informed Consent Form[19]

in low-risk studies after IRB approval.[19,23] Modifications are granted when the usual informed consent process could endanger the participant, not simply for researcher convenience. For example, if the signature on a consent document is the only link between an otherwise anonymous participant and the study, then it is generally considered higher risk to obtain the signature. In this case the IRB could approve a modified consent process without signature. Waivers of informed consent are less frequent and are granted when studies are low risk and consent is not possible, such as retrospective chart review studies.[19] However, it is up to the IRB not the investigators to decide the type of consent required. If subjects cannot consent for themselves (eg, patients who are unconscious), the IRB must approve a plan for who can provide consent on behalf of the subject. Special consent processes are also required for minors: generally, children must be included in the decision-making process and must assent along with their parents providing signed consent.[26] Those who are not able to consent for themselves but later regain or gain that capacity must provide consent again (eg, when a subject awakes from a coma or when a child in a longitudinal study becomes old enough to assent). Again, these are complex issues, and the IRB with which a researcher works can provide valuable guidance.

The inherent rights for all human subjects who participate in a research study include the right to join or leave a research study whenever they wish to do so; people should never be pressured or coerced to join or leave a study. Subjects cannot lose access to their regular medical care, and they have the right to know about alternative options of care. The increasing complexity of the health care system has led to more rigorous regulations from IRBs and more detailed informed consent documents, although updates to the Common Rule are working to make these documents easier to navigate. For example, many clinical nutrition studies include genetic testing, which has created a new level of awareness about the disclosure of research findings and the linking of biological outcomes to personal identifiers of human participants.[19] Study participants must therefore know whether information gathered during a study will be provided to them for their own medical care. Implementing informed consent procedures appropriately bolsters subjects' confidence in the specific study and science in general.

Privacy and Confidentiality

Confidentiality of medical and personal information is a pillar of scientific ethics. Participants agree, through the informed consent process, to have specific clinical, psychological, or physiological data collected.[20] Researchers must manage the data in a manner that maintains subject confidentiality. Any records involving the identity of subjects must be maintained securely, with restricted access. This includes the code sheet or key that would allow researchers to reidentify information collected under a code. Institutions may require researchers to maintain locked barriers between the location of the code sheet and the coded data (eg, keeping them in separate locked file cabinets in separate locked rooms). Maintaining the security of electronically stored data is no less important, and best practices continue to evolve.

In the United States, data regarding an individual's past, present, or future health and health care are also protected by the Health Insurance Portability and Accountability Act (HIPAA).[27] Participants must grant permission to use protected health information (HIPAA authorization) as a special component of the informed consent process. Some institutions incorporate HIPAA authorization into the consent form, while others ask participants to sign a separate document. Information can be released without HIPAA authorization only if 18 identifiers are removed from the data set, known as the *Safe Harbor method* (see Box 3.3 on page 42), or if other methods, such as expert determination, are used to reduce the risk that participants may be identified.[20,27]

New modifications to the Common Rule clarify when it is allowable to use biospecimens without informed consent after IRB approval.[19] These samples of blood, tissue, and other material, known as *banked samples*, may be taken at the time of an ongoing experiment or for clinical care and carefully stored for subsequent analysis that may not be planned at the time of initial collection. Linking data sets introduces additional confidentiality concerns, and ways

The following identifiers of the individual or of relatives, employers, or household members of the individual, are removed:

(A) Names
(B) All geographic subdivisions smaller than a state, including street address, city, county, precinct, ZIP code, and their equivalent geocodes, except for the initial three digits of the ZIP code if, according to the current publicly available data from the Bureau of the Census:
 (1) The geographic unit formed by combining all ZIP codes with the same three initial digits contains more than 20,000 people; and
 (2) The initial three digits of a ZIP code for all such geographic units containing 20,000 or fewer people is changed to 000
(C) All elements of dates (except year) for dates that are directly related to an individual, including birth date, admission date, discharge date, death date, and all ages over 89 and all elements of dates (including year) indicative of such age, except that such ages and elements may be aggregated into a single category of age 90 or older
(D) Telephone numbers
(E) Vehicle identifiers and serial numbers, including license plate numbers
(F) Fax numbers
(G) Device identifiers and serial numbers
(H) Email addresses
(I) Web Universal Resource Locators (URLs)
(J) Social security numbers
(K) Internet Protocol (IP) addresses
(L) Medical record numbers
(M) Biometric identifiers, including finger and voice prints
(N) Health plan beneficiary numbers
(O) Full-face photographs and any comparable images
(P) Account numbers
(Q) Any other unique identifying number, characteristic, or code, except as permitted specifically for reidentification as outlined in the statue; and
(R) Certificate/license numbers

Box 3.3 The 18 Patient Identifiers That Must Be Removed to Meet the Health Insurance Portability and Accountability Act Safe Harbor Method

Reproduced from the US Department of Health and Human Services. Guidance Regarding Methods for De-identification of Protected Health Information in Accordance with the Health Insurance Portability and Accountability Act (HIPAA) Privacy Rule. 2012. https://www.hhs.gov/hipaa/for-professionals/privacy/special-topics/de-identification/index.html[27]

of managing this risk while maintaining statistical utility are evolving.[20]

Beyond the ethical necessity for these research regulations, proof that they have been followed is generally required to publish in reputable journals.[13]

ETHICS IN DESIGNING, CONDUCTING, AND ANALYZING RESEARCH

The scientific method is the basis for research design.[11] Initially, the existing body of scientific knowledge is carefully assessed. Questions important to science and society are formulated, and in response to the research questions, a vigorous and rigorous research design is crafted. Ethical scientific conduct includes accurately recording data in such a way that data are readily available and understandable to current and future colleagues. To ensure appropriate data accessibility, the data need to be correctly recorded at the time they are generated and in the detail necessary for ready comprehension. This means a codebook should be created and kept up to date so that variable names and calculated variables are interpretable in the future. Original records need to be carefully secured and retained as outlined in the IRB document. This is particularly important with the increasing interest in and requirements for public release of data upon publication.[10]

Throughout the research process, investigators must pay careful attention to details of subject selection, method choice, and execution.[28] If critical details are disregarded and sloppy science is allowed, ethical predicaments may develop.

Dillman,[29] recognized for his research on survey methodology, outlined four potential research errors that invalidate research: sampling error, noncoverage error, nonresponse error, and measurement error. The impact of such errors extends beyond survey design to other descriptive research techniques and to analytic research. By eliminating or minimizing these sources of error, research will be substantially more useful. In science, it is unethical to be aware of such errors and proceed as though they are of no consequence; thus, these errors are discussed along with the ethics of research. When researchers cannot overcome these errors, they must be clearly disclosed and discussed as limitations to the research.

Sampling Errors

Errors of sampling result from differences between the study sample and the actual population and lead to incorrect inferences from the data to the population, that is, poor generalizability.[28,29] To have a true probability sample, each individual in the study population must have an equal chance of being selected as a subject. Sampling errors may be random; that is, they may occur by chance as samples from the same populations are drawn. Ensuring that each individual within the study population has the same likelihood of participating will minimize random sampling errors.

Another key way to minimize sampling error is to ensure that the sample size is appropriate for the goals of the research (see Chapter 24). Random sampling errors generally decrease as the sample size increases. A useful guideline is that random sampling error will be reduced by half if the sample size is quadrupled.[29]

Noncoverage Errors

Noncoverage errors result from a sampling format that excludes some individuals within the study population when selecting subjects. Noncoverage errors, in general, are systematic and difficult to overcome and are caused by bias in specifying or selecting the study sample.[28,29] For example, subjects may be selected from outdated lists that exclude recent additions; from published telephone listings that exclude people with only cell phones; or from a group of people who are able to attend lectures in the evening, thereby excluding people who work at night. Recruiting from individuals who receive medical care is biased, as it excludes people who have a disease but do not receive care due to lack of access or their own choice. Bias generally occurs when convenience sampling is used—for example, members of a group, volunteers responding to advertisements, or people from different health care institutions in whom a specific disease is diagnosed. Such biases affect the degree to which the data generated may represent the population at large (generalizability) and should be addressed in reporting results. The ethical principle of justice requires that those who participate in research (ie, assume the risk) should be similar to the group that will benefit from the results (ie, accrue the benefits). Early research often only included white men as subjects, limiting the generalizability of important findings to minorities and women.[30] Conversely, researchers conducting studies with high levels of risk often preyed on minority groups.[31] Both of these historical injustices lead to lower participation in research. The National Institutes of Health has attempted to rectify this problem by requiring a statement about the inclusion of women, children, and minorities in all research grant applications, and funded projects must report on the enrollment of these groups.[32]

Nonresponse Errors

The third category of error is nonresponse. In surveys, the response rate is the percentage of people who actually answer the survey queries.[29] A low response rate has traditionally raised serious questions as to whether the observed data accurately represent the study population—that is, whether the nonresponders differ significantly from the responders. Newer research suggests that lower response rate is not always an indicator of nonresponse bias.[33] Still, it is important to attempt to improve response rate through proven strategies that motivate subjects to respond and to accurately calculate and report response rate so that readers can evaluate the results in context.[34]

One way to allay concern over a low response rate is to evaluate demographic and other available data of nonresponders and responders to ascertain whether important differences exist between the two groups. A further dilemma results when responders provide incomplete data sets, for example, omitting or providing partial responses to some questions in a survey. Researchers can decrease inadequate responses to survey questions by evaluating and pilot testing the survey carefully to ensure clarity of questions and ease of reply.

A corollary of nonresponse in clinical trials is an error resulting from loss of subjects to follow-up. To minimize such loss, researchers make valiant efforts to complete the data sets. For example, to secure 25 years of follow-up data, some researchers have commissioned private detectives to investigate the whereabouts and life or death status of individuals in cohorts. Other sources of nonresponse errors are missing data for laboratory values or anthropometric measurements, as well as incomplete food intake records. In each case, the complete and incomplete data sets must be evaluated to ascertain whether the missing data skew the apparent results.[35]

Unless the researcher is confident that inclusion of incomplete data does not misguide, the complete and incomplete data sets should be handled separately, rather than as a single, blended group of data. To do otherwise is to present the research in an unethical manner.

Measurement Errors

Whereas the first three types of research error result from nonobservation, measurement error is an error of observation.[29] As such, errors in conducting or executing research are akin to measurement error. For example, if a question is worded in such a way that it cannot be answered accurately or if a questionnaire is structured so that unequal emphasis is placed on certain questions, measurement error will result. The impact of the placement of questions is influenced by whether the respondent receives the questions verbally or visually. In all cases, it is critical to recognize that biased questions and biased organization produce biased answers. Subject characteristics may also produce measurement error. An all-too-common measurement error arises from instruments that lack reliability and validity. Instruments used in research need to be evaluated and validated before use.[36]

Other Sources of Bias Error

Other biases in executing research projects need to be avoided.[28] One frequent error results when the experimental group and control group are treated differently in ways beyond what is designated by the specified intervention, such as giving additional attention or care to the experimental group. When the control group does not receive care and attention equal to what the experimental group receives, differences in outcome may be inaccurately attributed to the intervention. A blinded study design in which both subjects and researchers are blinded to treatment and control group assignments can help avoid treatment biases. However, it is difficult to maintain the blinded design if certain end points (eg, body weight or blood pressure) are monitored during the study as a component of usual patient care and begin to change noticeably in one group.

Another type of research bias occurs when issues of efficacy become confounded with those of compliance, as may occur when the experimental design requires patients to adhere to specified therapies. For example, some subjects may have a low rate of attendance at the education sessions of a program being evaluated. As suggested in the section on nonresponse error, the researcher should compare the complete data sets with the incomplete data sets to determine whether the data can be merged. Similarly, subjects who withdraw or are withdrawn from an experiment may differ systematically from those subjects who remain, causing withdrawal bias if completer-only analysis is used. In cases of treatment noncompliance, the best ethical practice is to use intent-to-treat analysis, which groups participants based on the treatment to which they were assigned and, therefore, makes statistical significance harder to achieve.[35] Furthermore, confirmation bias is likely to occur unless the experimental design is blinded, allowing the investigation to proceed and data to be collected without influence or bias from subject or investigator. Even when interventionists cannot be blinded, efforts should be made for the person performing the clinical or statistical testing to be blinded as to the grouping of subjects.

Equipoise and Ethical Interventions

The ethics of randomization are based on the concept of clinical equipoise.[37] *Equipoise* is generally understood to mean that there is a lack of consensus among clinicians about which treatment is superior. Therefore, patients who enroll in a trial are not expected in advance to be advantaged or disadvantaged by their group assignment.[37] When there is no equipoise between interventions, it is unethical to perform (or continue) a randomized trial because researchers know which group will have superior outcomes. This is why clinical trials are sometimes stopped early—if one group's outcomes are clearly superior, there is no longer equipoise. This occurred in the nutrition field with the PREDIMED study of the Mediterranean diet as primary prevention of cardiovascular disease.[38] In nutrition, equipoise frequently cannot be achieved, especially between a placebo and an intervention. Therefore, many nutrition trials rely on head-to-head comparisons of interventions or unique study designs to ensure that the intervention with the expected benefit is provided to all participants. One study design that helps overcome the issue of equipoise is the stepped wedge design (see Chapter 8), which allows all participants to serve as their own controls and receive the intervention.[39] When obtaining informed consent, it is important that participants understand equipoise and not fall into the therapeutic misconception. This is particularly critical when the people who provide standard care to patients also recruit them to participate in research. Participants believe their care provider has their best interest at heart and, therefore, may fall into the therapeutic misconception, believing that they are certain to obtain better outcomes by participating in research and that the care is individualized to them, versus understanding that research is designed to answer a question.[40]

ETHICAL PRESENTATION AND INTERPRETATION OF RESEARCH

Honesty, truthfulness, and full disclosure are necessary in presenting research. The researcher's obligation is to publish valid data, to analyze the data objectively and dispassionately, and to present a fair and unbiased interpretation to readers.[35] Inference must be supportable by the data. Authors must recognize the power of inference and avoid misleading readers.

As a parallel, readers are obligated to use data ethically, without distortion, and to carefully consider the methods presented.[35] Equal care must be exercised by researchers and authors as to the message they send and by readers as to the message they receive and use.[41]

Presentation of the Whole Truth and Nothing but the Truth

Ethical investigators truthfully report and fully disclose research data and the methods whereby the data were generated. At all times, scientific proof must be rigorous and without bias. Limitations of the study design—for example, subject bias—should be clearly stated.[40] Ethical investigators objectively evaluate the data and provide a fair interpretation. To do more or less is ethically insupportable.

Several practices in handling data are considered unethical and may be considered errors of data distortion: data dredging, selective reporting of findings, fragmentation of reports, redundant publication, and inappropriate statistical tests. Data dredging or mining is the process of combing through a large pool of data to pick up purportedly significant findings from research that was not designed to produce those results.[1] Data dredging is particularly noxious when only positive results are reported and negative results are ignored, thus making the former appear to be important rather than merely significant by chance. Because the accepted level of statistical significance is a probability of 0.05 or less, the chance that a relationship would be considered significant is 1 in 20. Thus, if the number of comparisons were many, as could occur if researchers compared data collected from 10 laboratory values and the dietary intake of 10 nutrients, the potential comparisons would undoubtedly yield several seemingly significant relationships (perhaps 5 out of 100, in the example), most of which would be by chance and would lack relevance. Statistical approaches to account for this are discussed in more detail in Chapter 25.

The relationships that are appropriate to evaluate are those decreed by the original research design, driven by the research question and hypothesis. Chance observations may encourage further research and may be publishable if clearly identified as a chance or post hoc finding. Ideally, new research questions result in data that replicate the earlier positive post hoc results, justifying publication of the findings. Skipping or not reporting analyses that were specified in the analytic plan a priori is also inappropriate and can lead to selective reporting.[42] The ethical behavior to limit overanalysis and underanalysis is to register research studies in a public registry (such as clinicaltrials.gov) before they are initiated, so that the analysis plan is public record,[13] An adept reader of research will check to ensure that results of all of the analyses specified in the methods section or trial registry are reported in the publication.

Selective reporting of research findings is a form of intentional fraud, often motivated by efforts to support a hypothesis when the data do not clearly provide adequate support. Such actions as concealing data, presenting solely favorable data, or in any other way shaping or trimming data to accommodate the hypothesis disregards scientific and ethical principles.[12,42] Such conscious acts are ignoble, premeditated efforts to distort data and mislead colleagues and the public.

Reporting guidelines and checklists, such as CONSORT (Consolidated Standards of Reporting Trials)[43] for randomized controlled trials, PRISMA (Preferred Reporting Items for Systematic Reviews and Meta-analyses)[44] for meta-analyses, and MOOSE (Meta-analysis of Observational Studies in Epidemiology)[45] for observational and epidemiologic studies can help guide new and experienced investigators in what must be presented as the whole truth of a research project.[46] They can also be used in trial design to make sure that researchers consider all elements of a project that will need to be reported.

Research findings that are fragmented and published in multiple small units are a disservice to readers.[13] The whole picture is not visible, and interrelationships are lost. Scientific editors discourage submission of least publishable units, commonly called LPUs, and refer to such fragmentation as "salami science." A similar wasteful practice is duplicate or redundant publication—that is, presentation of essentially the same study in more than one place with little, if any, modification.[13,14] Copyright laws make such actions unlawful.

Statistics in Data Interpretation

Statistics is the art and science of interpreting quantitative data. Aspects of statistics include framing answerable questions, designing the study, exercising quality control of the data to reduce researcher-initiated variance and bias, drawing inferences from data, and generalizing results to other situations.[26,47]

Fienberg[48] suggests addressing the following eight points in a statistical review of a submitted manuscript. The following points are of equal usefulness in designing, conducting, and reporting research:

- What are the original data? How have they been transformed for use in the statistical analyses?
- Is information given on uncertainty and measurement error?
- How were the statistical analyses done, and are they accurately described in the paper?
- Are the statistical methods used appropriate for the data?
- Have the data or analyses been selected, and does such selection distort the facts?
- What population do the data represent? Does the design for data collection allow for the inferences and generalizations made?
- Would additional analyses be enlightening?
- Are the conclusions sensitive to the methodologic and substantive assumptions? If so, is this fact acknowledged? Do reported measures of uncertainty reflect this sensitivity?

Lang and Altman[49] published more detailed reporting guidelines that are specific to the planned analysis method and are valuable for readers and reporters.[9] The core of the scientific method, and hence of science, is inference: learn about unobserved phenomena by studying and interpreting relevant data on observed phenomena.[28,47] Inference must be protected, not abused by such distorting actions as selective reporting and data dredging. Data need to be honest and honestly presented.

Unethical or questionable analytic methods that may be used in biased presentation of results include reporting large effects in trials with only a few events, using faulty comparator groups (such as drugs of low efficacy or high toxicity), basing claims of equivalence on negative findings rather than true noninferiority studies, and emphasizing benefits rather than harms.[50]

ETHICS IN PUBLICATION

The researcher's responsibility is to submit manuscripts that are appropriate for publication consideration and peer review; in other words, the data need to be accurate, responsibly analyzed, and responsibly interpreted. The research design and the materials and methods used need to be clearly and fully presented. All relevant sources need full and accurate citation. As has been discussed, it is unethical and deceptive to present data selectively, to withhold contradictory data, or to revise data for more impact.

Questions often arise as to how much data should be presented in a manuscript. The goal should be to proffer the optimal publishable unit, not to disperse the data in a variety of LPUs. As tenure evaluations are turning toward quality per unit published and away from number of units published, LPUs will be a negative factor in a researcher's list of publications. When a researcher is allowed to offer five original publications for tenure consideration, the advantage will go toward a well-crafted and reasoned article rather than a single fragment of a research project.

Reporting guidelines for specific study designs (discussed previously) is another important way to ensure ethics in publication by setting uniform requirements for what should be reported in a manuscript.[13]

Peer review is the prime way science monitors itself.[13,14] Scientists accept the dual professional responsibility of submitting research for peer review and serving as objective, ethical peer reviewers for the work of others. Reviewers assume the responsibility of ensuring the scientific integrity of published literature, and confidentiality is necessary in ethical behavior toward an author. Should peer reviewers identify legitimate conflicts of interest between themselves and the paper under review, they should decline to review rather than jeopardize a sound review process. Obviously, it is unethical to take advantage of authors by invading the confidentiality of the peer review process or by using research before its official publication.[13]

When interpreting and applying data, it is tempting to over present them to the media and the public. The desire to make a point or to support a bias or preconception must not override accurate use of scientific data.[41] As discussed previously, research errors resulting from sample bias and noncoverage, nonresponse, and measurement errors determine, in large part, whether data may be generalized to other populations or even to the entire study population. For example, a research study showing lower serum cholesterol concentrations in men who consumed a diet low in saturated fat cannot be generalized to the population at large (all other men), let alone to infants, children, adolescents, women, or the elderly. The error of overgeneralization is an error of misrepresentation to colleagues and the public. To overgeneralize erodes the credibility of both the researcher and science. It is particularly disturbing when data are overgeneralized in an effort to perpetrate prejudices or patronage or because of a conflict of interest.[39] Honest differences of opinion exist; they should be stated clearly, while recognizing opposing views. However, inappropriately representing one's own data or the data of others is scientifically reprehensible, as it misleads others.[41] The Harvard School of Public Health and the International Food Information Council formed an advisory group to create guidelines about scientific communication to the media.[51] Their guidelines for scientists are shown in Box 3.4 (page 48); guidelines for journal editors, journalists, and industry, consumer and other interest groups are also available.[51]

Communication Guidelines for Scientists

1. Have you provided essential background information about the study in your written findings, or to journalists or others requesting it, in a language that can be understood?
   - Have you explained all details of the study including purpose, hypothesis, type and number of subjects, research design, methods of data collection and analysis, and the primary findings?
   - Are you reporting study findings consistent with the original purpose of the data collection?
   - Were appropriate scientific methods of inquiry used? Did you disclose any study shortcomings or limitations, including methods of data collection? Were objective health measurements used to help verify self-reports?
   - Was the study conducted in animals or humans? Are limitations of animal models noted in terms of their applicability to humans?
   - Have you waited to report the results until the study has been independently peer-reviewed? If

not, did you disclose to the media that the findings are preliminary and have not yet been peer-reviewed?

2. Have you clarified dietary risks and benefits?
   - Did you explain the dosage of a substance or amount of food or ingredient that was linked to the health outcome? Is this amount reasonably consumed by the average individual?
   - What was the original risk of developing the disease? Have you expressed the new level of risk in terms of both absolute and relative risk?

3. Have you met the needs of the media?
   - Are you available for media interviews the day before/after the release? Do you make every attempt to respond to media inquiries in a timely fashion?
   - Does the news release prepared for the study communicate the primary findings faithfully and without exaggeration? Have you reviewed and approved the final version of your institution's news release?

Box 3.4 Guidelines for Scientists in Communicating Emerging Science on Nutrition, Food Safety, and Health

Reproduced with permission from the *Journal of the National Cancer Institute*. Fineberg HV, Rowe S. Improving public understanding: guidelines for communicating emerging science on nutrition, food safety, and health. *J Natl Cancer Inst*. 1998;90(3):194-199.[51]

ETHICAL ISSUES RELATED TO AUTHORSHIP

Authorship implies a substantial contribution to a published article and conveys responsibility for the content.[13,14] The International Committee for Medical Journal Editors (ICMJE) delineates four criteria to determine whether someone has contributed sufficiently to be designated as an author. The criteria, all of which must be satisfied, are substantial contributions to (1) designing or analyzing and interpreting the data, (2) drafting or revising the article critically for important intellectual content, (3) giving final approval of the published version, and (4) agreeing to be accountable for all aspects of the work. Discussion continues on how extensive an individual's contribution must be to qualify as an author and

how accountable an author must be to peers and the public for the paper in its entirety. However, one guideline is that fulfilling the first two ICMJE criteria requires participation in two of four activities: study design, data analysis/interpretation, manuscript drafting, and revision. With increasing frequency, journals are requiring a statement of contribution to outline what each author did to merit his or her listing on the article or a signed statement agreeing to the publication with listed authors.[13]

Gratuitous or honorary authorship is neither appropriate nor ethically acceptable. Authorship is not a gift but a right founded on substantial contribution to the resulting manuscript. Authorship cannot be justified for a person whose participation is limited to acquiring funding, administering the department or unit, or collecting the data.[13] General, as opposed to specific, supervision of the research group is also considered inadequate to warrant authorship.

One of the obvious dilemmas is the extent of accountability an author assumes when collaborating with scientists and professionals in diverse fields. At minimum, individual authors are responsible for all aspects of work that are within and proximate to their fields of expertise.

Because conventions about authorship and the most important position vary from discipline to discipline, and even department to department, the ICMJE provides no guidance on order of authors, which can be a contentious topic. The primary author of the manuscript is customarily rewarded with the first author position. The person who has made the major intellectual input to the article also generally receives special placement, which may be as first or last author. Major intellectual input consists of outstanding, positive, and creative contributions; active participation in the work, data tabulation, and interpretation; and key scientific leadership throughout the research design, conduct, analysis, and presentation. The best policy is to discuss authorship early in a project in order to avoid disputes resulting from misplaced assumptions. Journals generally do not mediate authorship disputes; instead, these are referred to officials at the institution where the research was conducted.[13]

CONFLICTS OF INTEREST

Conflicts of interest occur in any situation in which financial or other personal considerations may compromise, or appear to compromise, an investigator's professional actions in designing, conducting, or reporting research.[14] Conflicts are generally understood to include an investigator's close family, such as spouse and children.[52] Conflicts of interest may also bias other aspects of an investigator's research activities, such as the choice of methods, length of time subjects are studied, purchase of materials, support staff hired, or choice of statistical analyses. Other scholarly activities are affected by conflicts of interest; for example, in preparing review articles, financial and personal interests may interfere with professional objectivity.

It is customary for investigators to disclose any and all possible conflicts. Professional journals expect acknowledgment of each author's funding sources and institutional and corporate affiliations on the title page of articles submitted for publication. In addition, consultancies, stock ownership, or other equity interests or patent licensing as well as potential nonfinancial conflicts, such as volunteer positions, should be disclosed to the journal editor in the cover letter or metadata at the time articles are submitted.[13,14] The error of misrepresenting conflicts of interests is averted when such interests are disclosed to readers. It is important for full disclosure to be made because the appearance of conflict may be as professionally damaging as known conflict.[14,52] Many reputable scientists have one or several actual or perceived conflicts of interest.[12] Disclosing them provides a platform for unbiased, open evaluation.

Fear of conflicts of interest should not deter an investigator from seeking ethical financial and corporate relations. Problems develop when financial interests and other conflicts of interest are not disclosed.[14,52] The Academy of Nutrition and Dietetics[43] and other organizations[53] offer guidelines to help manage conflicts related to industry-funded research. It is ethically irresponsible for a scientist, because of a personal conflict of interest and thus a potentially desirable or undesirable financial impact, to repress negative data, to expose only selected findings, or to distort the presentation of data in any way. Financial interest should neither impinge on professional objectivity nor drive professional activities.[52]

RESEARCH IN AN ETHICAL CLIMATE

Discovering the unknown, expanding horizons, updating perceptions and techniques, and devising and evaluating new applications all make research exciting. The investigator's profession and society are advanced concurrently. Ethical scientific conduct of research ensures the acceptance of new data and the positive assessment of the data's interpretation.

Throughout the many steps of research, highly ethical behavior is imperative. In selecting important questions and designing effective research protocols in which research errors are minimized, it is essential to keep in mind that research must be executed and presented in an ethical fashion. Throughout, researchers need to be accountable to the public.

Thoughtful and adequate supervision is essential in all research projects to ensure that the data are properly collected. Each person on a research team must assume responsibility for all aspects of the research in his or her domain and maintain awareness of the project in its entirety. The team involves graduate students, research assistants, intradisciplinary and interdisciplinary professionals, and faculty. Although the chief supervisor must assume ultimate accountability, responsibility for ethical conduct falls on everyone's shoulders.

CONCLUSION

The principles of respect for persons, beneficence, and justice are excellent guides not only when considering human subjects but also when interacting with close colleagues, professional peers, clients, the public, and the media. Conflicts of interest require full disclosure to avoid misleading others. In such an ethical climate, research accomplishments will grow and survive. Ethics in scientific research means investigators need to act responsibly in every aspect of research from design to presentation.

REFERENCES

1. Fanelli D. How many scientists fabricate and falsify research? A systematic review and meta-analysis of survey data. *PLoS One*. 2009;4(5):e5738.

2. Interlandi J. An unwelcome discovery. *New York Times Magazine*. October 22, 2006. www.nytimes.com/2006/10/22/magazine/22sciencefraud.html. Accessed January 14, 2018.

3. Poehlman ET, Tchernof A, Poehlman E. Effects of the menopause transition on body fatness and body fat distribution. *Obes Res*. 1998;6(3):246-254.

4. Stern V. 12 Years after researcher found guilty of misconduct, journal retracts paper. June 21, 2017. http://retractionwatch.com/2017/06/21/12-years-researcher-found-guilty-misconduct-journal-retracts-paper. Accessed August 1, 2017.

5. Kearns CE, Schmidt LA, Glantz SA. Sugar industry and coronary heart disease research: a historical analysis of internal industry documents. *JAMA Intern Med*. 2016; 176(11):1680-1685.

6. American Dietetic Association/Commission on Dietetic Registration code of ethics for the profession of dietetics and process for consideration of ethics issues. *J Am Diet Assoc*. 2009;109(8):1461-1467.

7. Fornari A. Approaches to ethical decision-making. *J Acad Nutr Diet*. 2015;115(1):119-121.

8. Tappenden KA, Elliott CH, Emenaker N, et al. A unifying vision for scientific decision making: the Academy of Nutrition and Dietetics Scientific Integrity Principles. *J Acad Nutr Diet*. 2015;115(9):1486-1490.

9. Byerley L, Lane H, Ludy MJ, et al. Ethical considerations for successfully navigating the research process. *J Acad Nutr Diet*. 2017;117(8):1302-1307.

10. Edwards MA, Roy S. Academic research in the 21st century: maintaining scientific integrity in a climate of perverse incentives and hypercompetition. *Environ Eng Sci*. 2017; 34(1):51-61.

11. Committee on the Conduct of Science National Academy of Sciences. *On Being a Scientist*. Washington, DC: National Academy Press; 1995.

12. Lomangino KM. Countering cognitive bias: tips for recognizing the impact of potential bias on research. *J Acad Nutr Diet*. 2016;116(2):204-205.

13. International Committee of Medical Journal Editors. Recommendations for the Conduct, Reporting, Editing, and Publication of Scholarly Work in Medical Journals. December 2017. www.icmje.org/recommendations. Accessed February 2, 2018.

14. Stein K. What the journal's publishing ethics mean for you. *J Am Diet Assoc.* 2009;109(5):793-795.

15. The Nuremberg Code. In *Trials of War Criminals before the Nuremberg Military Tribunals under Control Council Law No. 10, vol II.* Washington, DC: US Government Printing Office; 1949:181-182

16. World Medical Association. Declaration of Helsinki - Ethical Principles for Medical Research Involving Human Subjects. March 2017. www.wma.net/policies-post/wma-declaration-of-helsinki-ethical-principles-for-medical-research-involving-human-subjects. Accessed February 2, 2018.

17. The National Commission for the Protection of Human Subjects of Biomedical and Behavioral Research. The Belmont Report—Ethical Principles and Guidelines for the Protection of Human Subjects of Research. 1979. www.hhs.gov/ohrp/regulations-and-policy/belmont-report. Accessed January 30, 2017.

18. Office of Human Research Protections. Federal Policy for the Protection of Human Subjects ('Common Rule'). Updated March 18, 2016. www.hhs.gov/ohrp/regulations-and-policy/regulations/common-rule/index.html. Accessed August 1, 2017.

19. Code of Federal Regulations. Federal Policy for the Protection of Human Subjects: Final Rule. January 19, 2017. www.federalregister.gov/documents/2017/01/19/2017-01058/federal-policy-for-the-protection-of-human-subjects. Accessed January 15, 2018.

20. O'Keefe CM, Rubin DB. Individual privacy versus public good: protecting confidentiality in health research. *Stat Med.* 2015;34(23):3081-3103.

21. Hand RK, Lawless ME, Deming N, Steiber AL. Development and pilot testing of a human subjects protection training course unique to registered dietitian nutritionists. *J Acad Nutr Diet.* 2014;114(12):2009-2016.

22. Green LA, Lowery JC, Kowalski CP, Wyszewianski L. Impact of institutional review board practice variation on observational health services research. *Health Serv Res.* 2006;41(1):214-230.

23. Stang J. Ethics in action: conducting ethical research involving human subjects: a primer. *J Acad Nutr Diet.* 2015;115(12):2019-2022.

24. Office of Human Research Protections. Human Subject Regulations Decision Charts. February 16, 2016. www.hhs.gov/ohrp/regulations-and-policy/decision-charts/index.html. Accessed February 2, 2018.

25. Centers for Disease Control and Prevention. Plain Language Materials & Resources. December 19, 2016. www.cdc.gov/healthliteracy/developmaterials/plainlanguage.html. Accessed February 2, 2018.

26. National Institutes of Health. Research Involving Children: HHS Regulatory Requirements for Research Involving Children Described in Subpart D. https://humansubjects.nih.gov/children1. Accessed August 1, 2017.

27. US Department of Health and Human Services. Guidance Regarding Methods for De-identification of Protected Health Information in Accordance with the Health Insurance Portability and Accountability Act (HIPAA) Privacy Rule. 2012. www.hhs.gov/hipaa/for-professionals/privacy/special-topics/de-identification.

28. Riegelman RK. *Studying a Study and Testing a Test.* 4th ed. Philadelphia PA: Lippincott Williams & Wilkins; 2000.

29. Dillman D. *Mail and Internet Surveys: The Tailored Design Method.* 2nd ed. New York, NY: John Wiley and Sons. 1999.

30. Taylor HA. Inclusion of women, minorities, and children in clinical trials: opinions of research ethics board administrators. *J Empir Res Hum Res Ethics.* 2009;4(2):65-73.

31. Brandt AM. Racism and research: the case of the Tuskegee Syphilis Study. *Hastings Cent Rep.* 1978;8(6):21-29.

32. National Institutes of Health. Guidelines for the Review of Inclusion on the Basis of Sex/Gender, Race, Ethnicity, and Age in Clinical Research. Updated April 5, 2016. https://grants.nih.gov/grants/peer/guidelines_general/Review_Human_subjects_Inclusion.pdf. Accessed August 1, 2017.

33. Groves RM, Peytcheva E. The impact of nonresponse rates on nonresponse bias: a meta-analysis. *Public Opin Q.* 2008;72(2):167-189.

34. Groves R, Cooper MP, Presser S, et al. Experiments in producing nonresponse bias. *Public Opin Q.* 2006;70(5):720-736.

35. Johnston BC, Guyatt GH. Best (but oft-forgotten) practices: intention-to-treat, treatment adherence, and missing participant outcome data in the nutrition literature. *Am J Clin Nutr.* 2016;104(5):1197-1201.

36. Gleason PM, Harris J, Sheean PM, Boushey CJ, Bruemmer B. Publishing nutrition research: validity, reliability, and diagnostic test assessment in nutrition-related research. *J Am Diet Assoc.* 2010;110(3):409-419.

37. Rooshenas L, Elliott D, Wade J, et al. Conveying equipoise during recruitment for clinical trials: qualitative synthesis of clinicians' practices across six randomised controlled trials. *PLoS Med.* 2016;13(10):e1002147.

38. Estruch R, Ros E, Salas-Salvadó J, et al. Primary prevention of cardiovascular disease with a Mediterranean diet. *N Engl J Med.* 2013;368(14):1279-1290.

39. Brown CA, Lilford RJ. The stepped wedge trial design: a systematic review. *BMC Med Res Methodol.* 2006;6:54.

40. Morin K, Rakatansky H, Riddick FA Jr, et al. Managing conflicts of interest in the conduct of clinical trials. *JAMA*. 2002;287(1):78-84.

41. Berning JR, Karmally W. Ethics opinion: The RD and DTR are obligated to follow ethical standards when writing for the popular press. *J Acad Nutr Diet*. 2007; 107(12):2052-2054.

42. Nicklas TA, Karmally W, O'Neil CE. Nutrition professionals are obligated to follow ethical guidelines when conducting industry-funded research. *J Acad Nutr Diet*. 2011;111(12):1931-1932.

43. Schulz KF, Altman DG, Moher D, for the CONSORT Group. CONSORT 2010 Statement: updated guidelines for reporting parallel group randomised trials. *BMJ*. 2010; 340: c332.

44. Moher D, Liberati A, Tetzlaff J, Altman DG, The PRISMA Group. Preferred reporting items for systematic reviews and meta-analyses: The PRISMA Statement. *BMJ*. 2009; 339:b2535

45. Stroup DF, Berlin JA, Morton SC, et al. Meta-analysis of observational studies in epidemiology: a proposal for reporting. Meta-analysis of Observational Studies in Epidemiology (MOOSE) group. *JAMA*. 2000; 283(15): 2008-2012.

46. EQUATOR Network. Search for reporting guidelines. www.equator-network.org/reporting-guidelines. Accessed February 2, 2018.

47. Huth EJ. *Writing and Publishing in Medicine*. 3rd ed. Baltimore MD: Williams & Wilkins; 1999.

48. Fienberg S. Statistical reporting in scientific journals. In: *Ethics and Policy in Scientific Publications*. Bethesda, MD: Council of Biology Editors; 1990.

49. Lang TA, Altman DG. Basic statistical reporting for articles published in biomedical journals: the "Statistical Analyses and Methods in the Published Literature" or the SAMPL Guidelines. *Int J Nurs Stud*. 2015;52(1):5-9.

50. Guyatt GH, Rennie D, Meade MO, Cook DJ. *Users' Guides to the Medical Literature*. 2nd ed. Chicago, IL: American Medical Assocation; 2008.

51. Fineberg HV, Rowe S. Improving public understanding: guidelines for communicating emerging science on nutrition, food safety, and health. *J Natl Cancer Inst*. 1998;90(3):194-199.

52. Woteki CE. Ethics opinion: conflicts of interest in presentations and publications and dietetics research. *J Acad Nutr Diet*. 2006;106(1):27-31.

53. Alexander N, Rowe S, Brackett RE, et al. Achieving a transparent, actionable framework for public-private partnerships for food and nutrition research. *Am J Clin Nutr*. 2015;101(6):1359-1363.

How to Write Proposals and Obtain Funding

Dianne Neumark-Sztainer, PhD, MPH, RD | *Nicole Larson, PhD, MPH, RDN*

LEARNING OBJECTIVES

1. Explain the professional benefits of developing research ideas as a grant proposal.

2. Describe the steps involved in developing a research proposal.

3. Describe the components of a research proposal.

4. Identify what types of costs to include and justify within a proposal budget.

5. Discuss the review process and planning for a resubmission.

6. Select strategies likely to improve the chances that a proposal will be funded.

The primary reason for writing grant proposals is to obtain funding to implement a research idea. The grant proposal is the means to sell the ideas to potential funders.[1] Thus, ideas need to be conveyed in a manner that will spark enthusiasm among the reviewers and funding agency and will convince them that the proposal is innovative; the proposed research questions are worthy of exploration; the research team is qualified to implement the study; and the proposed methods are feasible, well planned, and appropriate for the research questions being addressed.

WRITE PROPOSALS TO ADVANCE SCIENCE

A grant proposal is a detailed blueprint of a research plan. Writing a proposal helps researchers clarify why the proposed study is important and guides the development of a polished, well-thought-out plan for addressing the research questions. To develop a strong plan, researchers must review the literature and conduct a needs assessment to justify the proposal. Choosing a theoretical framework can guide the selection of suitable objectives, intervention strategies, and evaluation targets, which helps link the different components of a grant proposal. Soliciting feedback on a proposal before its formal review allows the researcher to further refine and improve the plan. During the implementation phase of a study, researchers often refer back to the grant proposal to see how the protocol was originally designed. Thus, while the primary reason for writing a grant proposal is to obtain funding, a secondary benefit is that the process of writing the proposal helps the researcher develop a well-thought-out research plan and guides its implementation.

Writing grant proposals can also offer researchers benefits in terms of career development. Those who are able to write successful grant proposals will be more attractive to potential employers and may be more likely to progress up the career ladder. Furthermore, employees who can bring in money to fund their research ideas will generally have more independence on the job and be able to work on projects they view as important. For example, a registered dietitian nutritionist (RDN) working in a clinical setting may have reason to believe a particular type of dietary counseling is more effective than the current standard for care. If that RDN can write a research plan and obtain funding to examine differences in treatment outcomes, he or she may be given time to conduct a research study and write the findings on the job. As a result, the RDN's work is more interesting and has a broader impact.

Thus, learning how to write strong grant proposals is an important skill for researchers and practitioners who are interested in advancing science by carrying out their research ideas. Writing grant proposals can be a daunting and risky endeavor because it means expressing one's ideas for others to critique. Additionally, it consumes time and energy. Writing grant proposals is a skill that can be learned and that improves with practice. Both experienced and first-time grant writers can learn how to enhance their grant-writing skills to make the process of writing proposals easier, more enjoyable, and more successful.

DEVELOP AN IDEA AS A FUNDABLE RESEARCH PLAN

A successful grant proposal begins with a good idea that will be deemed worthy of funding. After determining a research idea, follow these steps to turn it into a workable and fundable plan:

1. **Clarify the plan.** Consider the idea and why it is important. Think about how to test the idea. Think broadly about how the idea contributes to science. Think about the specifics to ensure that the study will be feasible to implement and will truly address the research questions being explored. Thus, before developing and evaluating a program to reduce risk of overweight in elementary school children, consider how the approach is unique and whether it will move the field of obesity prevention forward; also, consider the number of schools needed for the study and how to recruit participants. After progressing to the next steps listed below, continue to come back to this first step to fully develop a clear research plan.

2. **Review the literature.** Determine if there is justification for the content area to be explored and the proposed methods. See what else has been done in related areas and determine what the next steps should be to advance science. Ideally, some related studies have already been done that demonstrate the importance of the topic, but the proposed research can address weaknesses in the knowledge pool. For

example, before studying a school-based obesity prevention idea, a researcher would need to determine if obesity is worth addressing and examine its prevalence, its health implications, and whether it may be changed. Previous school-based obesity prevention interventions and their evaluations should also be explored. In addition, the researcher should identify suitable target groups, novel intervention approaches, and appropriate evaluation strategies.

3. **Talk with others.** Talk with individuals who have been successful in writing grant proposals. Listen to what they say. Experienced grant writers may suggest refining the idea to increase its specificity and feasibility, and it is generally worthwhile to heed this advice. Also, talk with individuals who work directly with the target population to get their practical insights. For the school-based obesity prevention project mentioned above, this might entail speaking with other obesity researchers (about the study design and intervention content), a statistician (about the number of participants needed for statistical purposes), school staff (about perceived needs and logistics within schools), and children (about their interests).

4. **Explore funding possibilities.** Look for suitable funding agencies and grant opportunities related to the research plan. Read extensively about their mission, guidelines, and previously funded projects. Write a brief, clear description of the plan, and contact the funding agency to discuss the idea and assess its relevance to their funding priorities. The next section addresses how to explore funding opportunities.

5. **Go back and tweak the research ideas.** Use information learned from reviewing the literature, talking with others, and talking with the funding agency to strengthen the research ideas and the proposal.

IDENTIFY SOURCES OF RESEARCH FUNDING

Once a clear research idea has been established, the researcher will need to find a suitable funding agency. Online resources are listed at the end of this chapter. While there are many useful resources, exploring all of them can be overwhelming. Researchers may want to talk to others who have received funding for related ideas to learn about their experiences with different funding agencies. A number of funding possibilities are listed below.

● **Institutional or in-house funds** This form of funding is often available to new investigators who are just getting started in an academic setting. Many times these funds aim to help investigators implement small pilot studies that are likely to form the basis for larger grants down the road. This is an excellent place to begin the grant-writing process since institutes want to get their young investigators off to a good start. Institutes may offer grants from different internal funding sources that target new investigators or investigators who need seed money to change their direction of research. Students are particularly encouraged to apply for in-house student awards for small research studies. Some graduate school programs offer mechanisms for student research awards, and there may be less competition for these funds than those available from external sources.

● **Nonprofit and professional organizations** The Academy of Nutrition and Dietetics Foundation and the American Heart Association are examples of nonprofit and organizational sources of grant funds for practitioners at different levels of their careers, including students. Nonprofit and professional organizations offer funding opportunities to young investigators to promote research careers within their respective fields.

● **Foundations** The Robert Wood Johnson Foundation and Susan G. Komen are examples of foundations that solicit and fund research proposals. Funding from a foundation might

Type of Grant Program	Funding Period Limit	Direct Cost Limit
Research Grant Program (R01)	3–5 years	$500,000 per year
Small Grant Program (R03)	2 years	$50,000 per year
Exploratory/Developmental Research Grant Award (R21)	2 years	$275,000 for 2 years combined
Clinical Trial Planning Grant (R34)	1 year	$100,000
Research Project Cooperative Agreement (U01)	Not specified	Not specified

Table 4.1 Types of Grant Programs of the National Institutes of Health[2]

be available for projects of local interest or within specific content areas. Foundations may address a particular topic area (eg, infant health) or may serve a local community. In contrast to other funding agencies, foundations are often interested in funding projects that receive funds from multiple sources, thus demonstrating wider support for a project.

- **Industry** Industries often have foundations for research in areas that companies have identified as important. For example, the National Dairy Council and United Soybean Board are sources of competitive funds for research proposals. Usually, the funds are for a topic that will somehow be useful to the particular industry, although that is not always the case. Aside from their foundations, industries may have particular research interests of direct relevance to products they are developing. Food industries, for example, can be an excellent source for nutrition-related research funding; however, before accepting funds, it is important to clarify mutually acceptable conditions with regard to investigator independence in reporting study findings.

- **Government state and regional grants** This form of funding is available for all levels of researchers and comes in varied amounts from diverse sources. Topics of interest may be specified by the different funding agencies in the forms of program announcements, priority areas, or specific requests for applications. Alternatively, researchers may submit proposals based on their own interests. The largest funding agency for health-related research is the National Institutes of Health (NIH). The NIH offers numerous mechanisms

for funding that should be carefully investigated to ensure a good fit for the timeline and level of funding needed for a proposed project—a detailed summary of these mechanisms is maintained online as a resource for investigators, and commonly used mechanisms are briefly described in Table 4.1.[2] Other significant federal agencies for nutrition-related research include the National Science Foundation, the US Department of Agriculture, and the US Food and Drug Administration.

UNDERSTAND THE PROPOSAL REVIEW PROCESS

Before writing the grant, the researcher should consider who will review the proposal and how the review process works. While the process will differ across funding agencies and particular grant mechanisms, there are a number of commonalities involved in the review process.

Review panels are often formed to evaluate grant proposals. Reviewers on the panel read the proposals individually and discuss them in a face-to-face meeting or via a conference call. Review panels generally include researchers with some level of expertise in an area related to the content of each proposal. Grant proposals are distributed to reviewers who prepare an evaluative summary of the proposal and give it a score based on established criteria. Sometimes all the reviewers on a panel read the proposal and their scores are averaged to provide a summary score. More often, one to four primary reviewers will read the proposal and provide a description of the proposal and their evaluations to a larger panel of reviewers who have not read the proposal. The larger panel will contribute to the decision-

Significance: Does the proposal address an important problem or critical barrier to progress in the field? Is there a strong scientific premise for the proposal?

Innovation: Does the proposal challenge and seek to shift current research or clinical practice paradigms by using novel theoretical concepts, approaches or methodologies, instrumentation, or interventions?

Investigators: Are the investigators and collaborators well suited to carry out the proposal?

Approach: Are the overall strategy, methodology, and analyses well reasoned and appropriate to accomplish the aims of the proposal?

Environment: Will the project site and scientific environment contribute to the success of the proposal?

Box 4.1 Review Criteria for National Institutes of Health Proposals[3]

making process of how the proposal should be scored based on the primary reviewers' comments and the ensuing discussion.

For example, Box 4.1 lists the overarching criteria the NIH uses to evaluate proposals.[3] Researchers should take the time to become familiar with the scoring criteria reviewers will use and carefully consider the review process when writing a proposal, particularly the following points:

In general, grant proposal reviewers do this work in addition to their regular work. They may review proposals in the evening after a full day of work, on a weekend, or on an airplane. Even if they are able to review the grant proposals assigned to them during the regular workday, they may have to read an enormous amount of proposals in a short period. Furthermore, they are probably not being paid or are only receiving a small honorarium for their time. Fortunately, most reviewers view the grant review process as an important part of the service work that they do to advance science. They take this work seriously and want to do a good job of presenting their review to other members of a

review panel. Reviewers appreciate a clear, well-written research plan that addresses an important topic. While it is the reviewers' job to do a thorough evaluation of each proposal, it is the applicants' job to make the proposal stand out from others and be as easy to read as possible. Thus, in writing a proposal, researchers need to think about how best to get their ideas across to the reviewers. Tactics that can help a reviewer include a clear statement of the research questions and research plan at the beginning of the proposal; use of summaries and some repetition throughout the grant to emphasize major points; bolded subheadings to guide reading; diagrams to break up the text and clarify study designs and timelines; white space between sections and at margins; short, clear sentences; and correct spelling and grammar. Good ideas may be lost in a poorly written proposal.

The reviewer's level of expertise may be related to the topic of the grant proposal but not specific to the area being addressed. For example, a reviewer may have expertise in the field of nutrition but not in the design of school-based interventions for obesity prevention in adolescents. To increase the chance of receiving a strong review, researchers should not assume that the reviewer has a clear understanding of the topic at hand, why it is important, and how it should be studied. Clearly laying out a justification for the topic being studied and the proposed research design will help the reviewer understand the importance of the research questions and the appropriateness of the research methods. A well-written justification will also help the reviewer better explain the proposal to other members of the review panel if needed. The researcher should examine his or her proposal from the reviewer's perspective. The reviewer wants to appear in a positive light when presenting a proposal review to the other review panelists and does not want to appear to misunderstand the proposal or falsely judge its merit. A well-written proposal can help the reviewer make an accurate presentation of the proposal's aims and why it is important.

Pay special attention to how the abstract and study aims are framed. These first sections should clearly state what the study is about and why it is important as secondary reviewers on a panel may not read the full proposal. A strong abstract and study aims will make it easy for the primary reviewer to summarize the proposal in a succinct and convincing manner for other reviewers on the panel and the funding agency. Secondary reviewers can take a quick look at the abstract and be enthused about the study.

COMPOSE A STRONG RESEARCH PROPOSAL

The format and length of grant proposals depend on the funding agency and grant mechanisms. Guidelines regarding the components to include and the order of presentation differ, and length limitations may range from 1 to 25 pages. For example, NIH research applications are limited to one page for the specific aims; research strategy descriptions range from six pages for smaller grants (eg, R03 and R21 applications) to 12 pages for larger grants (eg, R01 and U01 applications) (see Table 4.1). All proposals, regardless of format or length, need to address the following questions[4]:

- What is the proposed study about?
- Why is the study worth doing?
- Who is on the research team and are the team members qualified to implement the study?
- How will the study be done, and is the study plan the best one for addressing the research questions?
- What are the anticipated research outcomes?

It is imperative that grant proposals sell both the investigative team and the research idea. The researcher needs to convince the reviewers and funding agency that the study needs to be done, the team is well suited to do the study, and the proposed methods are the best way to get it done.

Most NIH research applications include two main sections: specific aims and research strategy. The specific aims should describe what the proposed study is about without going into details of the design. The research strategy should address why the study is worth doing and who will do the study as well as provide important details regarding how the work will be done. The research strategy

should include information to answer each of the following questions:

- **Significance:** How is the research likely to advance the scientific field or have a positive impact on clinical practice or the health of the public?
- **Innovation:** Why is the research novel?
- **Approach:** Who will contribute to the study? How will it be implemented?

Although the primary purpose of each component of the proposal is to address the corresponding question, there will be some overlap. For example, the main purpose of the specific aims is to describe what the study is about, what the study aims are, and why the study is important. The specific aims and each component of the research strategy are described here, and examples of well-written research proposals may be accessed online through the National Cancer Institute and National Institute of Allergy and Infectious Diseases of the NIH.[5,6]

Specific Aims

The specific aims text within an NIH grant application allows the applicant to immediately address the question, "What is this study about?" This section helps the reviewer learn what the proposed study intends to accomplish right at the beginning of the review process.[4] Depending on the type of study, the applicant may choose to use goals and specific aims, study objectives, research questions, or hypotheses. Reviewers generally like to see hypotheses; however, if the study is descriptive in nature, hypotheses may not be appropriate. Regardless of whether the research questions are framed as statements or questions, they need to be clear.[1,7] A strong grant proposal will start with clear research questions and build on them throughout the proposal.[8]

Although the main point of the specific aims is to describe what the study hopes to achieve, it is also worthwhile to grab the reviewer's attention from the outset by stating why the proposed study is important. The researcher should show how the specific research questions will help advance the field in addressing a significant problem. Providing a succinct description of the study plan for addressing the research questions will give the reviewer a context for reading the proposal. Remember that this text may be the only section of the proposal some review panelists read, and it will be the first section read by all. This section should avoid too much detail; the details can come later, after the reviewer is convinced of the importance of this study and clearly understands what the proposed study aims to achieve.

Research Strategy

Significance

The research strategy section of the proposal should address the question, "Why is this study likely to have a positive impact?" The proposal should provide a clear justification for the proposed study that addresses the scientific basis and how successful completion of the aims will advance scientific knowledge and improve population health. For example, justification for a nutrition intervention study should provide support for the proposed strategies and address the needs of the target population. A strong statement about how the proposed study will move the field forward and contribute to the advancement of science should be included at the end.

This section is the researcher's opportunity to demonstrate familiarity with the literature and to clearly show that the study fills an unfilled niche; it is also advisable to search databases of funded grants for related activities.[9] Omitting a key study exploring a topic similar to that being addressed in the proposal will not be viewed favorably, and funding agencies generally will not fund two very similar proposals.[10,11] The researcher can show how his or her work will contribute to the topic being addressed in the proposal (and thus begin to address the question of "who?"). Remember that the purpose of this component is *not* to provide a thorough review of the literature but rather to provide a justification for the proposed study. This component should be written so that a sophisticated reviewer lacking expertise in the specific research area can easily identify the need for the proposed study without reading extraneous background information.[1] A focus on justifying the proposed study, instead of reviewing the literature, will make the applicant's work easier and lead to a more focused and successful proposal.

Innovation

The purpose of the innovation component of the grant proposal is to further build justification for the proposed study by addressing the question, "Why is it novel?" The NIH recommends that applicants provide information to help the reviewer determine whether a proposal challenges and seeks to shift current research or clinical practice paradigms by utilizing novel theoretical concepts, approaches or methodologies, instrumentation, or interventions. The novelty of the proposed study may be broad or specific in the application of concepts or approaches to the proposed field of research. It is also relevant to point out if the study proposes a refinement or improvement to previously applied theoretical concepts, approaches, instrumentation, or interventions.[3] For example, in proposing an observational study of nutrition and physical activity behaviors, the novelty of applying an assessment methodology originally developed for psychological assessments should be noted along with how the application may help to overcome biases associated with other more commonly applied assessment methodologies. The innovation component should conclude with a summary statement that clearly describes how the proposal could change practice or profoundly change the understanding of a disease process or health behavior.[1] To help ensure that reviewers can easily identify all the innovative aspects of the proposal, it may be helpful to use bold text for each key point or present key points in a bulleted list.

Approach

Text describing the approach is the core of most proposals and is typically the longest part. It is critical to describe relevant preliminary studies along with the research design and methods in a manner that will convince reviewers that the team of investigators is capable of successfully carrying out the proposed work. The researcher should build on the goals established within the specific aims section to answer the questions, "Who will contribute?" and "How will it be implemented?"

More specifically, in describing preliminary studies, the text should address the questions, "Who are the members of the research team?" and "Why are they qualified to do the proposed study?" First describe the research team and their qualifications, and then describe relevant work by the research team that has led to the study being proposed. Writing about preliminary studies can be particularly challenging for young investigators with limited experience in the field. New investigators should be encouraged to:

- begin with smaller grants to build up their record and demonstrate that they have the ability to successfully implement research studies;
- apply for grants that are specifically intended for young investigators; and
- include more experienced investigators on their research team as coinvestigators or consultants.

Coinvestigators are full-fledged team members who are involved in the study on an ongoing basis, whereas consultants are usually employed at a different institution or organization and are less involved. The role of consultant is typically included in a proposal to fill a gap in expertise among others on the team. If the researcher has difficulty writing this component and cannot demonstrate adequate experience in areas related to the proposal's content, it may be worthwhile to consider adding investigators to the study or implementing a pilot study before embarking on the proposed study.[10]

The applicant needs to convince the reviewers that the research team is highly qualified to implement the proposed study. This is not a time to be overly modest. It is best to use factual statements, as opposed to using adjectives, to describe team members' expertise. For example, discuss research team members' area of training, publication records, and previous studies. Research team members should discuss collaborative efforts in order to demonstrate that the team has successfully worked together in the past. Areas of complementary strengths should be emphasized; as a general rule, a diverse team representing multiple disciplines will strengthen a proposal.[10] Finally, resources available to the research team that will help in the study's implementation should also be mentioned.

A description of relevant research and pilot work done by the research team should be described in the approach component of the proposal. Details on what was done in and learned from pilot studies should be included. A description of how the proposed study will build on previous work done by the research team can also be useful. The text describing the team's preliminary work should provide a link to the description of the research design and methods by demonstrating the feasibility of the proposed study methodologies.

Text describing the research design and methods should include details regarding how the study will be implemented along with a discussion of study limitations and how they will be addressed. The details included within this component of the application will differ according to the specific study but will often include the following[10]:

- **Overview:** An overview should be provided to help orient the reviewer to the detailed plan to follow. A diagram that orients the reader to the overall plan can be useful.
- **Research design:** The design should be described and briefly justified as suitable for addressing the research questions.[11]
- **Study population and recruitment:** Details on exclusion and inclusion criteria and how participants will be recruited are absolutely essential.[10] Concerns about problems such as bias or lack of ability to generalize from the study population should be addressed. A brief description of procedures for obtaining consent for study participation and any incentives for participation should be included, although details on human participant procedures will need to be described in a separate section of the application.
- **Intervention:** If an intervention is part of the study, the theory underlying the intervention (see the Theoretical Frameworks section), components of the intervention, and differences between intervention and control conditions should be described. A diagram of factors being addressed in the intervention and intervention components can also be useful. Theoretical constructs addressed in the intervention should

Variable	Assessment Tool	Description	Psychometric Properties
Physical Outcomes; Body Composition			
Body fat percentage	DEXA[a]	Dual-energy x-ray absorptiometry	More information provided in the text of the proposal.
Body mass index (BMI)	Measurements	Height and weight will be measured and BMI calculated according to the formula: Weight (kg)/Height (m^2)	Pilot test-retest $r=0.99$
Behaviors			
Physical and sedentary activity	3 day physical activity recall	Participants will report the types of physical and sedentary activities that they did in half-hour blocks on a 3-day physical activity recall	Details are provided in the text of the proposal
Dietary intake	24-hour recall	Trained interviewers will ask participants about their dietary intake over the preceding 24 hours	Details are provided in the text of the proposal.
Healthy weight control behaviors	Project EAT survey	The EAT (Eating Among Teens) study assessed use of the following behaviors for weight control over the past month: exercise, more fruits/vegetables, fewer high-fat foods, fewer sweets	Pilot test-retest $r=0.69$
Unhealthy weight control behaviors	Project EAT survey	Use of the following behaviors for weight control over the past month: fasting, eating very little food, diet pills, vomiting, laxatives, diuretics, food substitutes, skipping meals, smoking more cigarettes	Pilot test-retest $r=0.83$
Binge eating	QEWP[b]	Questionnaire on eating and weight patterns (four items)	EAT test-retest $r=0.64-0.81$ for items

Table 4.2 Impact Evaluation Measures: New Moves[c]

[a] DEXA=Dual-energy x-ray absorptiometry
[b] QEWP=Questionnaire on Eating and Weight Patterns-5
[c] This is part of a table that was included in a grant proposal by Dianne Neumark-Sztainer for the New Moves study. The full table also included measures for personal and socio-environmental factors.

be clear, and there should be consistency across the theoretical framework, intervention, and evaluation plan.[10]

• **Data collection procedures and tools:** The text should include details on how data will be collected and what the tools will look like, including assurances, when appropriate, that the selected tools are valid, reliable, and adequately sensitive to detect change over time.[12] If a survey is being used, it may be useful to include a table that describes the global constructs to be assessed, specific variables, questions for each variable, psychometrics of questions and scales, and sources of questions. Although preparing such a table is a considerable amount of work, tables can be a good way to provide the level of detailed information needed to demonstrate within the established page limitations that the study has a strong measurement plan (see Table 4.2 for an example from a grant proposal for evaluating the New Moves obesity prevention program for adolescent girls).[13,14] Limitations of data collection tools (eg, collecting dietary data with one 24-hour recall or collecting self-reported data on height and weight) need to be addressed in a manner that justifies the selection of these tools.

• **Data analysis:** The analysis text should provide a clear plan that aligns with the type(s) of data to be collected and justification for the sample size. As applicable, the analysis text needs to describe how qualitative data will be coded and how quantitative data will be inspected and organized. If both quantitative and qualitative data will be collected, then it is important to describe any plans for using the data in combination to address specific aims. Often a statistician will help write about plans for analyzing quantitative data, but it is crucial for the principal investigator to review and edit the text to be sure it aligns with all other components of the proposal (see additional discussion in the Statistical Analysis section).

The researcher should provide a high level of detail throughout the approach component of the proposal. It may seem logical to first see if the proposal is going to get funded and then work out the details later. Unfortunately, it does not work that way. The level of detail will differ according to the type of study, length of the grant proposal, and amount of funding requested; however, the researcher needs to have a well-developed study plan before receiving funding. While this is a time-consuming process, it is far more efficient to invest the time in writing a strong grant proposal than to write numerous proposals because they are not funded.

Theoretical Framework

Most research proposals are guided by an underlying theory (eg, social cognitive theory, theory of planned behavior) or multiple theories in developing a tailored theoretical framework.[15,16] It is important to clearly and consistently describe guiding theoretical constructs throughout the proposal. In addition, it is effective to discuss the guiding theoretical constructs specifically in relation to the topic of the proposal. And it is often useful to represent this information in the form of a diagram. Diagrams should represent all of the main constructs to be investigated as part of the proposal or should help the reviewer understand how a complex theoretical framework will guide the investigation in regards to a relationship of particular interest. Diagrams, such as the example in Figure 4.1 from the Eating and Activity in Teens (EAT) study of changes in young people's eating and activity behaviors from 2010 through 2018,[17-19] should represent all of the main

constructs to be investigated as part of the proposal or should help the reviewer understand how a complex theoretical framework will guide the investigation in regards to a relationship of particular interest. The study design should be taken into account in developing the diagram(s) to ensure that reviewers are not confused by the illustration.

Timeline

A timeline should be included as part of the proposal to concisely describe when each aspect of the study will be carried out. This information can be effectively provided as narrative text for smaller proposals, such as those involving only data analysis, but it is often useful to include a diagram. Adequate time should be allotted for recruiting the sample; preparing intervention materials and evaluation tools; collecting, organizing, and analyzing data; and preparing the manuscript to disseminate the study's findings. See Figure 4.2 on page 64 for an example timeline for a grant proposal to continue another component of the Project EAT research program, specifically Project EAT-IV, involving a 15-year longitudinal, observational study of young adults' weight-related behaviors and parenting practices.[17]

Statistical Analysis

The statistical analysis text within the proposal should clearly describe how each of the specific aims or research questions will be addressed and should discuss potential mediators and moderators of the relationships to be investigated.[20-23] The text should follow the order of the specific aims section and use consistent terminology. If the specific aims are broad or the proposal will address many theoretical constructs, it may also be useful to include specific examples of models that will be used to investigate the study hypotheses. While some reviewers will have statistical expertise, it may be advantageous to write this section in language that is easily understood by most researchers with expertise in the content area. References should also be provided for all statistical approaches that are not commonly used and understood within the field of study. After discussion of the planned approach to modeling, power calculations should be included that address each study aim. Including power calculations is

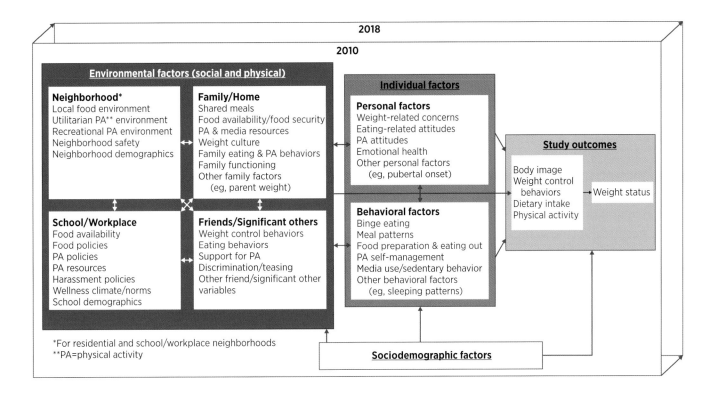

Figure 4.1 Theoretical framework example from the Eating and Activity in Teens (EAT) study of changes in young people's eating and activity behaviors from 2010 through 2018[17-19]

Adapted with permission from Dianne Neumark-Sztainer and Nicole Larson.

critical to demonstrate that attention has been given to determining a sample size that will allow for detection of an important effect (see Chapter 24).[24]

Summary and Future Directions

Concluding the proposal with a brief summary may be effective in reminding the reviewer about the strengths of the proposed study and why it is worthwhile. After reading details of the approach, reviewers should be provided with a concise description of why the proposed study is important, plans for disseminating the findings, and next steps for research building on the proposal. A couple of sentences about the study's significance will help to ensure that the proposal ends on an upbeat tone.

Other Project Information

In addition to the components of a proposal described previously, a few other components are fre-

quently required and should be carefully prepared. For example, the title of the grant is the first thing reviewers will see. Finding a title that is succinct, conveys the main message of the grant proposal, and generates interest on the reviewer's part may be challenging. Although the NIH allows principal investigators to request that a certain study section (eg, Community Influences on Health Behavior Study Section or Kidney, Nutrition, Obesity and Diabetes Study Section) review their proposal, the title may also guide the selection of an appropriate review panel and reviewer for the proposal. Note that some funding agencies limit the number of characters in a title.

The abstract or summary is also important for generating interest in a proposal and, as mentioned earlier, serves as the basis for assigning a proposal to a suitable review panel. The abstract provides reviewers with their first look into what a proposal is about, including long-term objectives,

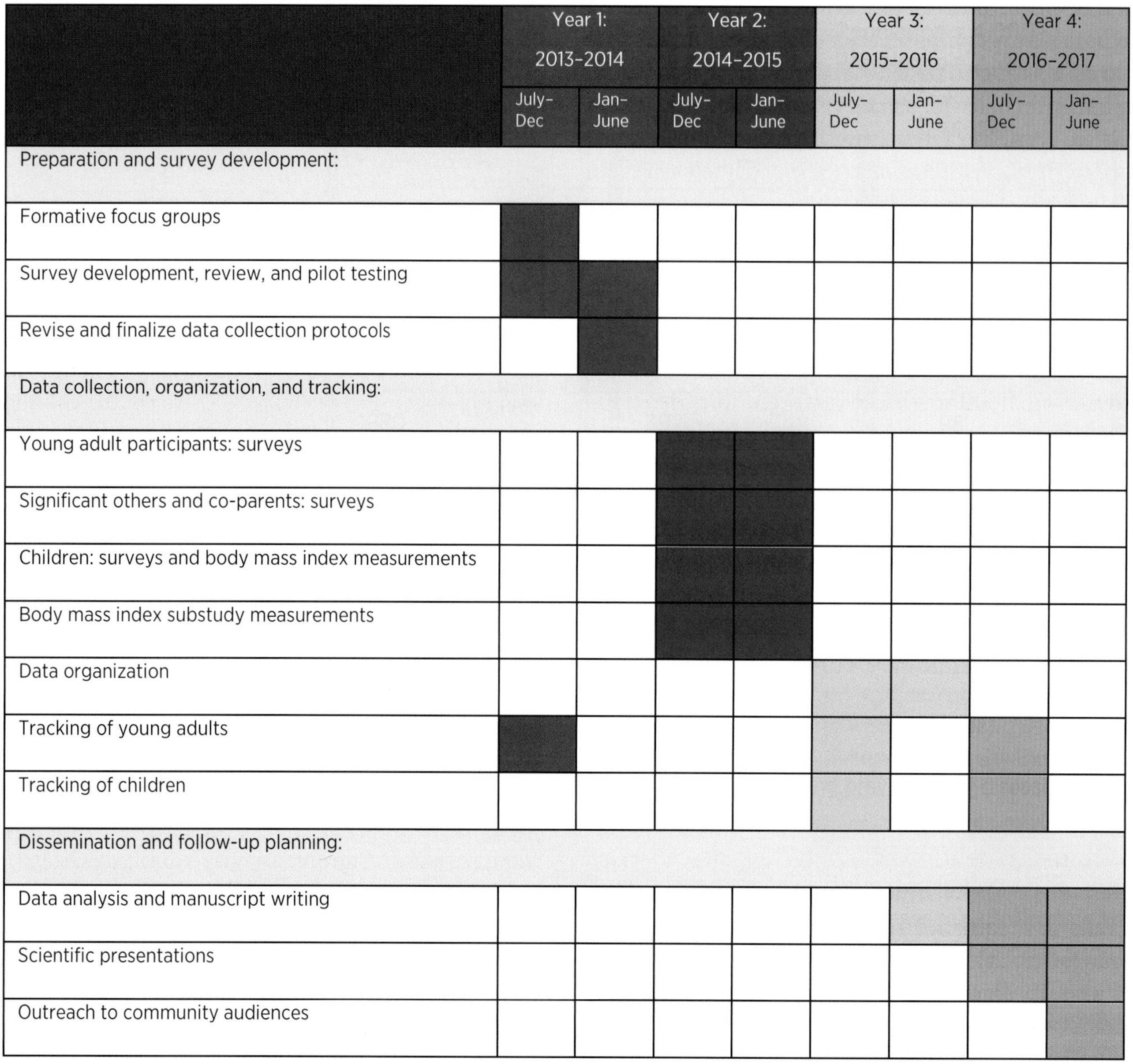

	Year 1: 2013-2014		Year 2: 2014-2015		Year 3: 2015-2016		Year 4: 2016-2017	
	July–Dec	Jan–June	July–Dec	Jan–June	July–Dec	Jan–June	July–Dec	Jan–June
Preparation and survey development:								
Formative focus groups	■							
Survey development, review, and pilot testing	■	■						
Revise and finalize data collection protocols		■						
Data collection, organization, and tracking:								
Young adult participants: surveys			■	■				
Significant others and co-parents: surveys			■	■				
Children: surveys and body mass index measurements			■	■				
Body mass index substudy measurements			■	■				
Data organization					▦	▦		
Tracking of young adults	■				▦		▦	
Tracking of children					▦		▦	
Dissemination and follow-up planning:								
Data analysis and manuscript writing						▦	▦	▦
Scientific presentations							▦	▦
Outreach to community audiences								▦

Figure 4.2 Timeline example

Adapted with permission from Dianne Neumark-Sztainer and Nicole Larson.

specific aims, research design, and methodology. For NIH applications, the abstract will be complemented by a project narrative that describes the relevance of the proposed work to public health in two or three sentences. The abstract and narrative may be the only parts of a proposal that some members of the review panel read, and these components often form the basis for the review that the primary reviewer shares with the larger panel. While the abstract and narrative are often written after most other components of a proposal, it is important to allow enough time to write a strong, convincing, and comprehensive summary that does not exceed any limits for word count or number of lines. For grant proposals that are being resubmitted, it is crucial to ensure that the abstract and narrative are revised with the rest of the proposal.

Other required components include those dealing with institutional supports for conducting the research and, particularly for early-stage investigators, protecting human participants, the use of animals, inclusion of women and minorities, and data and safety monitoring. The guidelines for completing these components vary across funding agencies and should be followed closely. It may be helpful to review what other investigators have written for these components in their grants. Some investigators are willing to share copies of their grant proposals, particularly if they have been funded.[5,6]

Appendix Materials

Appendix materials may play an important role in grant proposals, but decisions regarding what material to include should be made judiciously. Material should be supplementary and not required reading, as not everyone on the review panel will receive them. The funding agency or funding announcement may also provide specific guidance regarding what types of materials are allowed. For example, the NIH currently allows only the inclusion of blank informed consent and assent forms; blank surveys, questionnaires, and data collection instruments; and, when applicable, clinical trial protocols and information regarding an investigational new drug.[25] It is critical to follow these guidelines when submitting an NIH application; applications submitted with appendix material that is not allowed will be withdrawn and will not be reviewed. When specific guidance regarding appendix material is not provided, it may also be useful to include other materials, such as detailed information on planned survey questions and the investigators' relevant scientific articles that are not readily available but have been accepted for publication. Letters of support from those who will be involved in the work (eg, community partners, consultants, mentors) may be included within the appendix material or another designated section of the proposal.

Budget

The budget component includes a budget and budget justification. The budget usually includes three categories of costs:

● personnel costs,
● other study-related costs, and
● institutional overhead.

The specific costs to be included in a budget vary according to the study design. As an example, Box 4.2 on page 66 outlines the costs typically included in a grant proposal for a community-based nutrition intervention program. The budget presentation will also differ according to the funding agency and the home institution of the grant. Often a form will be provided to guide budget development and presentation. The researcher should carefully examine allowable expenses at the institution and funding agencies as there will be variations. It is not uncommon for funding agencies to prohibit costs related to the principal investigator's time, for example, and others do not allow for institutional overhead charges.

Unless a study requires expensive equipment, the major costs for a study are usually personnel expenses. Personnel costs are typically presented as percentages of time (eg, 50% of time in year 1 and 100% of time in years 2 through 4). For personnel working on a part-time basis (eg, interviewers) or as consultants on a grant, hourly rates may also be used. In developing a grant proposal. The researcher should take the time to carefully consider who will need to work on the project, how much time they will realistically need, the types of background(s) they should have, and how much they will cost. If the researcher has specific individuals with unique qualifications in mind, their names can be included in the budget justification.

The budget is generally followed by a budget justification that provides a more detailed explanation of how the funds will be used. For example, funds may be requested in the budget for a project director or study coordinator, and this person's role will be explained in the budget justification. The budget justification should be reviewed carefully before it is finalized to ensure that the text fully aligns with the

Personnel Costs

Principal investigator
Coinvestigators
Statistician/programmer
Study coordinator
Intervention staff
Graduate student assistants
Administrative assistant

Intervention Supplies

Materials development and printing
Supplies (eg, water bottles, pedometers)
Food for meetings/tasting/distribution

Evaluation and Dissemination Costs

Survey development and printing
Purchase of software (eg, for collecting and analyzing 24-hour recall data)
Data entry/coding
Participant incentives (recruitment, evaluation)

Audio recorders and transcription services
Publication and presentation costs
Scientific meeting travel

General Implementation Costs

Staff mileage
Office supplies
Rental of vehicles for participant transportation
Mailing costs
Phone and video conferencing
Photocopying
Translation of consent forms and other forms

Institutional Overhead

Amount based on prior agreements between institution and funding agency
May range from 0% to more than 50% of total study costs
Covers such costs as building upkeep, rental space, heating, and administrative expenses related to grants and overall institution

Box 4.2 Typical Budget Items for a Grant Proposal to Develop, Implement, and Evaluate a Community-Based Nutrition Intervention Program

approach component of the grant proposal. It is important to describe a unique role for each member of the research team and describe the use of materials, equipment, and incentives in the same manner as they are described in the research strategy.

A commonly asked question is "How much money should I ask for in my budget?" Ideally, the only question the researcher will need to address in order to determine how much money to request is the following: "How much money is needed to implement the study as I would like?" In an ideal world, the project will determine the budget and a funding agency (or a combination of funding agencies) will be willing to fund the study. In reality, however, the budget will also inform the study design. Before fully developing the study plan, the researcher should explore potential funding agencies and examine how much money

they typically give out. If there is an upper limit, the study will need to be planned in accordance. The final budget should reflect the true costs. A budget padded with unnecessary costs will not be viewed favorably. A budget that is too low may be viewed as unrealistic, and the investigative team may lose credibility. Reviewers and funding agencies generally have a good sense of how much it costs to implement studies. That said, it may sometimes be advantageous to take on a study that is inadequately funded, either for ideological reasons or because it is a necessary stepping-stone to a larger funding opportunity. In these cases, investigators may choose to donate their own time and find interested students or young investigators who are willing to contribute their time in return for a valuable learning experience.

ADHERE TO THE PLAN

A grant proposal should be viewed as a contract between the principal investigator and the funding agency. The funding agency agrees to give the requested funds to the principal investigator, who agrees to carry out the research plan outlined in the grant proposal. However, things may change as the plan goes into the field or the lab. Usually, small changes in methodologies do not pose a problem and may be implemented at the discretion of the principal investigator and the research team. Small changes may include changes in proposed questions on a survey, staff reassignments, and minor modifications to the proposed intervention. However, large changes to proposed methodologies, particularly changes that have implications for the key research questions, may not be permitted. If the original protocol needs to be modified and it is not clear whether the proposed change constitutes a major change, it is a good idea to contact the program officer or liaison at the funding agency. Put major changes into writing to ensure mutual understanding and agreement with the funding agency.

Sometimes a grant proposal will be approved for funding with a budget cut. In this case, determine if the study can be implemented as proposed at a lower cost or if protocol changes must be made to reduce study costs. If changes need to be made, they should be discussed with the liaison at the funding agency and put in writing. A number of options may be taken to modify the scope of work, and it is crucial to ensure that there is agreement on the best strategies.

REVISE AN UNFUNDED PROPOSAL

An important component of being a successful grant writer is paying attention to the details discussed in this chapter; it is equally important to learn how to cope with rejection. As only a limited number of proposals can be funded, applicants must become skilled at addressing the comments of reviewers in order to strengthen their proposals. The challenging nature of obtaining funding is particularly evident in reviewing the low and recently declining success rates of funding for NIH proposals.[26] To

eventually be successful, it is a reality that most investigators will need to follow this advice for dealing with rejection:

- **Don't blame the reviewer.** Often the first reaction to a rejection is to blame the reviewer. The applicant may think, "The reviewer didn't get it," or "Didn't the reviewer see where I explained that part?" However, it may be more effective to think in terms of how to improve the proposal so the reviewer will understand the project's importance and to ensure that the missing information will be more prominent in the a revised proposal.

- **Don't take the rejection personally.** This can be tough after a researcher has invested so much time and energy into a grant proposal. Try to avoid fatalistic thinking such as, "I don't have what it takes to be a good researcher" or "I'll never get funded." Instead, focus on the limitations of the proposal and what needs to be done to turn it into a fundable project.

- **Develop a plan for resubmission.** In collaboration with your research group, carefully consider whether a proposal should be submitted again; what changes should be made; and where the revised proposal should be submitted. Some funding agencies, such as the NIH, allow for one or more resubmissions. In fact, it is rare to be funded on a first submission to the NIH, and a responsive resubmission is often encouraged after a researcher has received a summary statement and conferred with the program officer for guidance.[10] If most or all of the weaknesses identified by reviewers are addressable and the research group decides to resubmit, read each of the reviewers' comments carefully, collectively identify the main issues to be addressed, develop a plan for addressing these issues, and establish a timeline for carrying out the plan. The timeline should allow several weeks or, even better, a few months of work in advance of the resubmission deadline. Recognize that a researcher's natural tendency may be to defend the original position. While that is an option, it will likely work in the researcher's favor to make the suggested modifications wherever possible. If a suggested change is not made, the researcher should justify the decision in a manner that demonstrates that the reviewer's suggestion has been carefully considered.

In a resubmitted proposal, pages may be allotted for a response to the reviewer. For NIH grants, one additional page of introduction should be included to indicate how the grant was revised and to direct reviewers to where changes were made within specific components.[27] The introduction should describe how the grant was modified in response to each suggestion made by the reviewers. Take the time to carefully plan responses and have others provide feedback on the content and tone.

If the proposal may not be resubmitted to the same funding agency, the researcher should look for other suitable funding agencies and tweak the proposal to ensure its suitability for a different audience. Although this can be a daunting task, it is generally worth doing.

It can be difficult to decide not to resubmit a proposal. If this is the decision, the researcher should take time to think about why the idea was not funded and what needs to be done to obtain funding next time around. One option is to do some pilot studies to learn more about the field and prove the worthiness and feasibility of the research ideas. The researcher should think about the content of research questions, research design issues, and writing styles. Some of the text in the significance and innovation components might even be used as a basis for a book chapter, review article, or lecture.

SET THE COURSE FOR SUCCESS

Since writing grant proposals is a time-consuming process, and since no one likes to have his or her ideas rejected, it is crucial to take advantage of various training opportunities offered by NIH or other reputable institutions and consider ways to increase chances for obtaining funding. The following suggestions are helpful when writing grant proposals. Try them out, find out what works best, and then add to the list.

● **Read and follow the directions carefully.** Grant proposals may not be funded because the font size was too small or the margins not wide enough. Read the directions carefully and know that there is no flexibility in abiding by them. Do not hesitate to contact the target funding agency if questions arise when developing the proposal.

● **Allow a lot of time.** Developing a research idea, pulling together a team of investigators, writing a grant proposal, and editing and reediting the proposal take a lot of time and energy. Start the process early and allow plenty of time to develop the document and get feedback on the initial draft of the aims before writing the full proposal. Leave time at the end for checking and rechecking. Try not to make any substantive changes immediately before submission; last-minute changes inevitably lead to careless mistakes and inconsistencies throughout the proposal. Write, get feedback, integrate feedback, rewrite, get more feedback, and rewrite. After the grant proposal is completed, take a little break to rejuvenate.

● **Work with a team.** Writing grant proposals can be a lonely experience. The proposal will gain from the shared expertise of others. The chief investigator should add other investigators to the research team whose skills complement theirs. Work with individuals who are hardworking, who will make valuable contributions to the study, and who are enjoyable to work with. New investigators should consider adding more experienced investigators to increase their likelihood of getting funded and to facilitate study implementation. Clarify roles and expectations with the team through an open discussion; raising issues early on can decrease conflicts down the road due to misunderstandings.

● **Get feedback at different stages.** Have others review the proposal at different stages of development for different types of feedback. At the beginning, have others review an outline or summary to get input on the big picture items, such as the research questions and proposed study plan. Have others review a near-final version at a stage when there is still enough time (and the writer has enough energy) to incorporate their suggestions. Keep in mind that the quality of the feedback will be in line with the quality of the proposal being reviewed. Thus, carefully check the proposal for sentence structure, grammar, spelling, and overall flow before asking others to review the proposal and provide meaningful feedback.

- **Start small and build on ideas.** Reviewers may be unlikely to grant a large sum of money to an inexperienced investigator or unexplored idea. Start small and build. For example, a grant might be built on smaller projects implemented incrementally over time.

- **Make things easy for the reviewer.** Make it easy for the reviewers to understand why the proposed study is worthwhile, grasp the main ideas, and read about the fine details. Although the researcher may want to include as much information as the page limit allows, it may be counterproductive to submit a proposal with crowded pages. Think like a reviewer and write from the reviewer's perspective.

- **Delve into the details.** While it may be tempting to leave the details until after funding has been received, a lack of attention to details will greatly decrease the chances that the study will ever being funded.

- **Aim for study enthusiasm.** Remember that the proposal is selling an idea. Though the writer should not sound like a cheerleader, the goal is to convince the reviewer and the funding agency that the proposed study is worth funding. The researcher must show that the idea is worth pursuing, that he or she is the best person to implement the study, and that the study design is optimal. Do this in a cautious and scientific manner. Do not get bogged down in the details and forget to convey enthusiasm for the topic.

- **Learn from the experience of others.** Talk with individuals who have written grant proposals to learn from their experiences. How did they come up with fundable research ideas? Budget their time? Read over other grant proposals. Participate in grant-writing classes. There is no one correct way to go about writing grant proposals. Observing how successful grant writers have navigated the process will help a researcher develop a unique style.

- **Learn through firsthand experience.** Look for opportunities to get involved with grants that are being written. Help out by offering to conduct literature searches or read different versions of the proposal. Ask to be part of meetings in which the grant proposal is being discussed in order to understand the big picture. Seek out opportunities to get involved in the grant review process. Although this can be time consuming, serving as a reviewer is a helpful way to understand the review process and what constitutes a strong grant proposal.

ONLINE RESOURCES

The following list of online resources for identifying research funding sources provides the website and a brief description for each resource:

- Grants.gov (www.grants.gov): This is the central site to find grants from government organizations. Researchers may complete applications through this portal.

- National Institutes of Health; Office of Extramural Research grants page (http://grants1.nih.gov/grants/oer.htm): This site has links to funding opportunities (requests for applications, program announcements, and notices), research training, programs, forms, application materials, submission dates, resources, award data, and policies. The site also links to the Electronic Research Administration (eRA), which has electronic submission, and enables applicants to check the status of grant proposals and view the results of the review process. An eRA Commons user name is needed to access this information.

- US Department of Agriculture National Agricultural Library Rural Information Center (www.nal.usda.gov/ric). This guide to funding sources provides information on different funding resources, links to funders and databases, and general guidelines.

- American Nurses Association Opportunities for Research Funding (http://nursingworld.org/research-toolkit/Research-Funding): This site has links to diverse funding sources in terms of funds available and research priorities.
- Nonprofit guides (www.npguides.org/links.htm): This site, which offers grant-writing tools for nonprofit organizations, provides general guidelines and links to funders and other resources for grant seekers.
- Catalog of Federal Domestic Assistance (www.cfda.gov): This site contains a database of federal programs available, links to information on writing grant proposals, and other information on assistance programs.
- US Department of Health and Human Services, Health Resources and Services Administration, Grants (www.hrsa.gov/grants/index.htm): This site provides information on Health Resources and Services Administration grant opportunities and information on getting funding.

CONCLUSION

Writing strong grant proposals is an important skill for RDNs interested in advancing the field of nutrition and their careers. A strong grant proposal begins with a good idea, which is transformed into a testable research question and a workable plan and then pitched to a funding agency as a project worthy of investment. A grant proposal should begin with and build on clear research questions. The proposal should address each of the questions outlined at the beginning of the chapter (see page 58):

The aim is to get the reviewer and the funding agency excited about the project and to provide enough details to show that there is a well-developed and feasible implementation plan.

When writing grant proposals, reseaarchers may find it helpful to look at them from the reviewer's perspective. A reviewer needs to be able to easily understand the project's aims and plan for implementation, be convinced of the project's importance and feasibility, and be able to explain it to others on the review panel. A clear summary/abstract is crucial. The overall appearance of the proposal is also important, and it should be reviewed many times before submission for clarity, grammar, and typos.

Writing grant proposals is both a daunting and a rewarding task. Rejections are to be expected and can be difficult, but if the reviewers' comments are taken as good advice and are not taken too personally, they can help improve future submissions. To be successful, it is usually best to start out with projects of a relatively small scope and gradually build on them.

REFERENCES

1. Liu JC, Pynnonen MA, St John M, Rosenthal EL, Couch ME, Schmalbach CE. Grant-writing pearls and pitfalls: maximizing funding opportunities. *Otolaryngol Head Neck Surg.* 2016;154(2):226-232.

2. National Institutes of Health Office of Extramural Research. Types of grant programs. https://grants.nih.gov/grants/funding/funding_program.htm. Accessed July 20, 2017.

3. National Institutes of Health Office of Extramural Research. Write your application. https://grants.nih.gov/grants/how-to-apply-application-guide/format-and-write/write-your-application.htm. Accessed February 21, 2017.

4. Arthurs O. Think it through first: questions to consider in writing a successful grant application. *Pediatr Radiol.* 2014;44(12):1507-1511.

5. National Institute of Allergy and Infectious Diseases, National Institutes of Health. Sample applications & more. www.niaid.nih.gov/grants-contracts/sample-applications. Accessed July 20, 2017.

6. Division of Cancer Control and Population Sciences, National Cancer Institute, National Institutes of Health. Sample cancer epidemiology grant applications. https://epi.grants.cancer.gov/funding/grantsmanship/sample-grants.html. Accessed July 20, 2017.

7. Ardehali H. How to write a successful grant application and research paper. *Circ Res.* 2014;114(8):1231-1234.

8. Seeman E. The ABC of writing a grant proposal. *Osteoporos Int.* 2015;26(6):1665-1666.

9. National Institutes of Health. Research Portfolio Online Reporting Tools (RePORT). Version 7.26.0. https://projectreporter.nih.gov. Accessed February 15, 2018.

10. Brownson R, Colditz G, Dobbins M, et al. Concocting that magic elixir: successful grant application writing in dissemination and implementation research. *Clin Transl Sci.* 2015;8(6):710-716.

11. Gholipour A, Lee E, Warfield S. The anatomy and art of writing a successful grant application: a practical step-by-step approach. *Pediatr Radiol.* 2014;44(12):1512-1517.

12. Gleason P, Harris J, Sheean P, Boushey C, Bruemmer B. Publishing nutrition research: validity, reliability, and diagnostic test assessment in nutrition-related research. *J Am Diet Assoc.* 2010;110(3):409-419.

13. Neumark-Sztainer D, Friend S, Flattum C, et al. New Moves—preventing weight-related problems in adolescent girls: a group-randomized study. *Am J Prev Med.* 2010;39(5):421-432.

14. Neumark-Sztainer D, Flattum C, Story M, Feldman S, Petrich C. Dietary approaches to healthy weight management for adolescents: the New Moves model. *Adolesc Med State Art Rev.* 2008;19(3):421-430.

15. Glanz K, Rimer B, Viswanath K, eds. *Health Behavior: Theory, Research, and Practice.* 5th ed. San Francisco, CA: Jossey-Bass Public Health; 2015.

16. National Cancer Institute. *Theory at a Glance: A Guide for Health Promotion Practice.* 2nd ed. Bethesda, MD: National Cancer Institute; 2005.

17. University of Minnesota. Epidemiology & Community Health Research. Project EAT. www.sphresearch.umn.edu/epi/project-eat. Accessed March 15, 2017.

18. Larson N, Wall M, Story M, Neumark-Sztainer D. Home/family, peer, school, and neighborhood correlates of obesity in adolescents. *Obesity.* 2013;21(9):1858-1869.

19. Graham DJ, Wall MM, Larson N, Neumark-Sztainer D. Multicontextual correlates of adolescent leisure-time physical activity. *Am J Prev Med.* 2014;46(6):605-616.

20. Breitborde N, Srihari V, Pollard J, Addington D, Woods S. Mediators and moderators in early intervention research. *Early Interv Psychiatry.* 2010;4(2):143-152.

21. Aschengrau A, Seage G. *Essentials of Epidemiology in Public Health.* 3rd ed. Burlington, MA: Jones & Bartlett Learning; 2013.

22. Lockwood C, DeFrancesco C, Elliot D, Beresford S, Toobert D. Mediation analyses: applications in nutrition research and reading the literature. *J Am Diet Assoc.* 2010;110(5):753-762.

23. VanderWeele T. Mediation analysis: a practitioner's guide. *Annu Rev Public Health.* 2016;37:17-32.

24. Boushey C, Harris J, Bruemmer B, Archer S. Publishing nutrition research: a review of sampling, sample size, statistical analysis, and other key elements of manuscript preparation, Part 2. *J Am Diet Assoc.* 2008;108(4):679-688.

25. National Institutes of Health. New policy eliminates most appendix material for NIH/AHRQ/NIOSH applications submitted for due dates on or after January 25, 2017. Notice Number: NOT-OD-16-129. https://grants.nih.gov/grants/guide/notice-files/NOT-OD-16-129.html. Accessed March 7, 2017.

26. National Institutes of Health. Success rates and funding rates. Research project grants: competing applications, awards, and success rates. https://report.nih.gov/NIHDatabook/Charts/Default.aspx?showm=Y&chartId=124&catId=13. Accessed July 20, 2017.

27. National Institutes of Health. Resubmission applications. https://grants.nih.gov/grants/policy/amendedapps.htm. Accessed March 2, 2017.

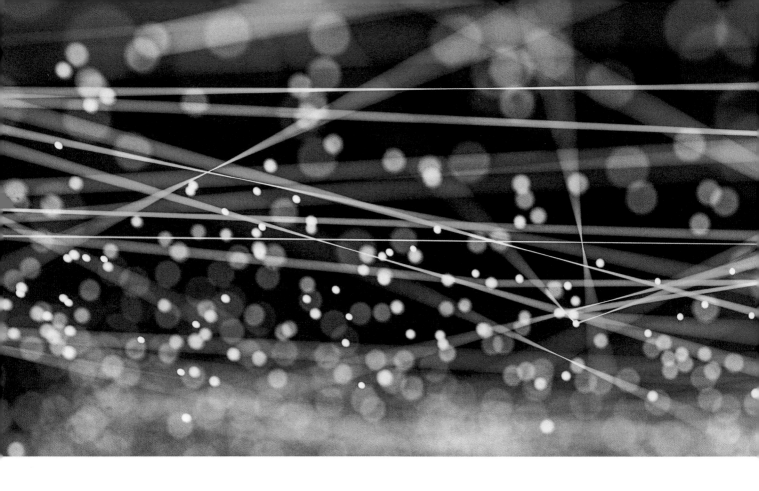

SECTION 3
Descriptive Research

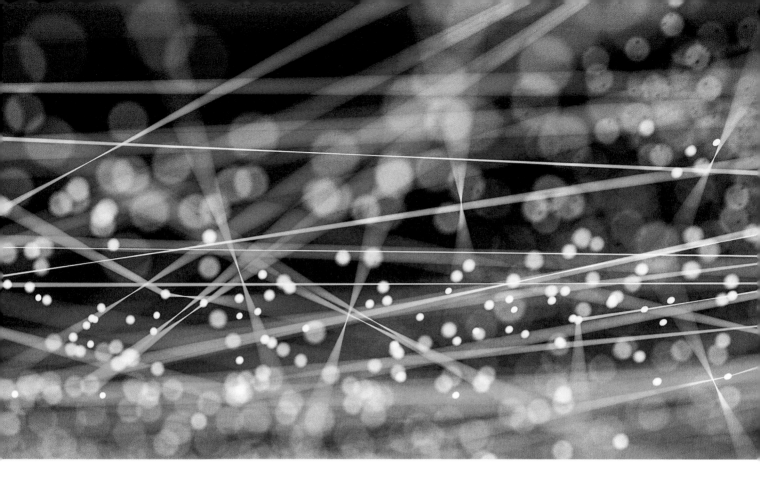

Chapter 5

Descriptive Epidemiologic Research

Maureen Brady Moran, MPH

LEARNING OBJECTIVES

1. Describe the concepts of validity and reliability of instruments used in epidemiologic research.

2. Construct a 2×2 table and demonstrate the relationships among prevalence, sensitivity, specificity, and positive and negative predictive value.

3. Select the appropriate descriptive research design to monitor specific health outcomes in a population over time.

Epidemiology is defined as "the study of the distribution and determinants of disease frequency."[1] The epidemiologic methods for study design, data collection, and analysis provide the conceptual framework for describing the distribution of disease and for testing etiologic hypotheses for a disease or health consequence. Descriptive studies provide information needed for public health programming and guide the development of hypotheses that may be tested using analytic methods. This chapter focuses on descriptive epidemiologic research measurements and study designs applicable to nutrition and dietetics. The advantages and limitations of measurements and designs are also presented.

TERMINOLOGY

Descriptive epidemiologic studies focus on the enumeration and description of person, place, and time. These studies can be used to quantify the extent and location of nutritional problems within a population and suggest associations between diet and disease that can be evaluated in analytic research.

Personal and behavioral characteristics can provide valuable insights into disease etiology. By examining who gets a disease, a researcher can determine whether a particular age, gender, racial, or cultural group is more likely to be at risk. Other person-associated attributes, such as socioeconomic status, family size, marital status, birth order, health behaviors, and personality traits, may be important to consider as well. For example, the personal and behavioral attributes of male sex, alcohol intake, red and processed meat intake, and cigarette smoking show a strong association with the incidence of colorectal adenoma.[2]

Place-associated characteristics may also provide valuable insights about potential risk factors for nutrition-associated problems. One study evaluated micronutrient status and neurodevelopment among internationally adopted children from post-Soviet states, Ethiopia, and China. The study reported that iron deficiency anemia and vitamin D insufficiency were greatest in children from post-Soviet states and less common in children from Ethiopia and China.[3] Such data will lead researchers to investigate reasons for these differences to help identify possible risk factors. The importance of place can also be illustrated in that urban or rural living may affect the availability and price of food items. Even with today's food distribution system, the availability and price of highly nutritious, perishable foods, such as fruits, vegetables, and fish, vary dramatically by geographic region and by urban and suburban or rural setting. This variability may have a significant impact on the poor.[4]

Time factors can also affect disease. Seasonal and interannual fluctuations in cumulative incidence, as well as secular trends, may indicate patterns that help elucidate causation. A longitudinal observational study of nutritional status and anemia among lactating mothers in two areas within rural Ethiopia reported that the prevalence of anemia increased dramatically to 40.9% during the preharvest season compared with 21.8% in the postharvest season.[5] Timing and length of exposure to a risk factor or the duration of the latency period may also be important considerations. An analysis of data from the Iowa Women's Health Study showed that women who had ingested water with higher levels of nitrate for more than 4 years were at higher risk of ovarian cancer compared with women without exposure at high levels.[6]

DISEASE FREQUENCY

Disease frequency measures the amount of disease or morbidity in a population and is expressed as incidence or prevalence. In practice, the amount of disease translates into risk of disease and becomes the foundation for all descriptive and comparative work. Knowledge of the amount of a given disease in different populations can be used to compare the relative importance of this disease in these populations, or it may be used as a basis for comparing populations with different exposures to possible etiologic factors.

Measurement of Incidence

Cumulative incidence, also known as *incidence rate*, is the term used to describe disease frequency in a population. Cumulative incidence is the number of new cases of a disease occurring in a population at risk within a specified time interval. Frequently, the observed period is 1 year. It is defined as follows:

$$\text{Cumulative incidence} = \frac{\text{Number of new cases in a time period}}{\text{Population at risk}}$$

Cumulative incidence is normally expressed as the number of cases per 100,000 per year; it can also be expressed as the risk of disease (see Box 5.1 on page 76). The population at the midpoint in the study period is used as the population at risk.

When cumulative incidence is calculated, the denominator is based on population defined by geographic area, and it can have an even more specific

$$\begin{aligned}
\text{Cumulative Incidence} &= \frac{\text{Number of persons in whom the disease develops}}{\text{Population at risk}} \times \text{Time period} \\
&= \frac{\text{Number of new cases of colon cancer in county A}}{\text{Midyear population of county A}} \times 1\,\text{year} \\
&= \frac{20 \text{ new colon cancer cases in county A in 2016}}{995{,}000 \text{ population } 07/01/2016} \times 1\,\text{year} \\
&= \frac{20}{995{,}000} \\
&= \frac{2.01}{100{,}000}
\end{aligned}$$

Or the risk of colon cancer in 2016 in county A is 0.002%

Box 5.1 Calculation of Cumulative Incidence: Colon Cancer Cumulative Incidence Expressed as Risk of Disease

focus, such as a particular sex, age, or ethnic group. Cumulative incidence is useful for documenting the relative importance of a disease in a population and for tracking changes in the occurrence of a disease over time. Cumulative incidence can also provide etiologic clues. A comparison of the cumulative incidence for populations that have different sex distributions, age groupings, ethnicities, or geographic locations can identify population groups with low or high rates of disease. This identification of groups with a high incidence of disease can be used to target intervention programs where they are most needed.

A specific application of cumulative incidence for registered dietitian nutritionists (RDNs) is quantifying the attack rate of an outbreak of food poisoning. *Attack rate* is the term substituted for cumulative incidence when the period of observation is short. In this situation, the population would be at risk for a short time, and the study period would encompass the entire epidemic. Such a study reported the foodborne outbreak of norovirus GII.17 at a military base in Poitiers, France. Civilians who made a 1-day visit to the base and military personnel were affected; all had consumed lunch on the base. To determine specific attack rates, the investigators divided the number of cases reported by the number who ate lunch on the base that day. Of 100 civilians and 200 military personnel, there were 37 and 66 cases, respectively, for an attack rate of 34.3%.[7]

Measurement of Prevalence

Prevalence is the proportion of the population that is affected by a certain disease or condition at a given time; it includes both new and existing cases. Prevalence can be expressed as point or period prevalence. Point prevalence depicts one point in time, as in a cross-sectional survey, and, unless otherwise specified, it is how the term *prevalence* is generally defined. Point prevalence is calculated as follows:

$$\frac{\text{Point}}{\text{prevalence}} = \frac{\text{Number of new, existing, and recurring cases}}{\text{Total population at risk}} \times \text{Time}$$

where time equals one point in time.

In contrast, period prevalence is calculated as follows:

$$\frac{\text{Period}}{\text{prevalence}} = \frac{\text{Number of new, existing, and recurring cases}}{\text{Total population at risk}} \times \text{Time}$$

where time equals a period of time.

Sometimes incidence data are not available for a disease, so prevalence data are calculated. This alternative is acceptable, as long as it is clear which is

Point prevalence

Number of all cases (new, existing, and recurring) in a population at a point in time

Period prevalence

The number of all cases (new, existing, and recurring) in a population over a specified period of time

Incidence

The number of new cases in a population in a time period

Box 5.2 Key Epidemiologic Calculation Terms

being used. See Box 5.2 for definitions. A lack of understanding of the difference between incidence and prevalence is a common mistake in scientific writing.[8]

Prevalence data are advantageous for assessing the frequency of diseases or conditions (eg, obesity) that do not have an acute onset. A series of cross-sectional studies that document point prevalence can be used to track changes in the burden of a disease to a population.

Prevalence is useful for identifying individuals at greatest risk and for planning health services because prevalence describes the burden of a disease or condition to a population. Findings from the continuing National Health and Nutrition Examination Surveys (NHANES) (1988–1994 and 2013–2014) indicate that the prevalence of obesity among American children and adolescents is increasing. Among children aged 6 to 11 years, obesity increased from 11.3% in the survey period from 1988 through 1994 to 19.6% in the 2007 through 2008 survey period. Obesity also increased among adolescents aged 12 to 19 years between 1988 and 1994 (10.5%) and 2013 and 2014 (20.6%).[9]

A researcher's lack of understanding of the difference between incidence and prevalence can introduce important sources of bias when he or she is evaluating the effect of a screening program where the identification of cases and the effectiveness of

an intervention both need to be examined. The first screening event detects new cases and undiagnosed cases of long duration. Subsequent screenings, if limited to those who have not previously been identified as having the condition of interest, identify only those cases that have developed since the previous screening. A decline in the number of cases identified in the population from the first screening to the second, in actuality, compares prevalence with incidence. A decline in the proportion of the population identified in the first screening compared with the proportion identified at the second may be attributable to the difference between prevalence and incidence rather than a successful intervention to reduce the burden of that disease in the population.

Reliability and Validity

Tests and tools used in descriptive epidemiologic research should be both reliable and valid. A *reliable* test gives the same results when the test is repeated on the same person several times. In other words, a reliable test gives reproducible results. A valid test measures what it is designed to measure.

Validity is used in epidemiologic studies to assess various methods of interest to RDNs, such as dietary assessment and anthropometric measures. Epidemiologic studies using a quantitative food frequency questionnaire typically test the validity of the dietary instrument by comparing the resulting data with data obtained by a gold standard or ideal measure. Validity addresses the question, "Does this measure what it claims to measure?" An example of reliability and validity is seen when dietary tools are tested in new populations. In a study testing a mindful eating questionnaire (MEQ) previously used in healthy adults in a sample of pregnant women, the test-retest reliability of the MEQ was assessed by repeated administration among study participants at two time points. The convergent validity was assessed by comparing responses to the MEQ with responses to similar, validated questionnaires designed to measure different dimensions of eating behavior and mindfulness. Discriminant validity was measured by comparing responses to the MEQ with responses to the neighborhood walkability scale, which

Disease or Condition

		Present	Absent
Test	**Positive**	a	b
	Negative	c	d

Sensitivity = Proportion of those with a disease who have a positive test

$$= \frac{a}{a + c}$$

Specificity = Proportion of those without a disease who have a negative test

$$= \frac{d}{b + d}$$

Figure 5.1 Schematic description of the screening test indexes sensitivity and specificity and their calculation

was not expected to correlate with mindfulness or eating behaviors.[10]

Increasingly, biochemical markers are being used in nutritional epidemiology as surrogates for dietary assessment measures or as correlates with dietary assessment because validation studies have shown that they are correlated with dietary intake and provide a valid measure of intake. One such study correlated biomarkers with breakfast and fast-food intake in adolescents. Eating breakfast more often was associated with lower insulin levels and lower percentage of body fat while more frequent fast-food consumption was associated with higher insulin levels and higher percentage body fat.[11]

Sensitivity and Specificity

Two parameters used to assess the validity of a test are sensitivity and specificity. *Sensitivity* is the proportion of persons with the disease or condition who have positive test results. *Specificity* is the proportion of individuals without the disease or condition who have negative test results. The higher the sensitivity,

the more likely a person with disease will have a positive test result. These screening tests are schematically described in Figure 5.1.

Sensitivity and specificity are used to establish cutoffs or reference interval limits for a test. The goal is to maximize sensitivity and specificity to minimize misclassification. Some individuals with positive test results do not truly have the disease. Conversely, some individuals with negative test results will have the disease. Siervo and colleagues[12] discuss how reference intervals are established to maximize sensitivity and specificity in their comparison of nutrition assessment techniques.

Predictive Value

The *predictive value* of a test is its ability to accurately distinguish individuals with or without the disease or condition. Thus, the positive predictive value is the probability of disease, given a positive test result, whereas the negative predictive value is the probability of no disease, given a negative test result (Figure 5.2).

Disease or Condition

		Present	Absent
Test	**Positive**	a	b
	Negative	c	d

Positive predictive value = Proportion of those with a positive test who have a disease

$$= \frac{a}{a + b}$$

Negative predictive value = Proportion of those with a negative test who do not have a disease

$$= \frac{d}{c + d}$$

Figure 5.2 Schematic description of the predictive values of a screening test

EXAMPLE

In a population where 100 individuals truly had malnutrition and 1,000 individuals truly did not have malnutrition, a test with 98% sensitivity and 95% specificity would correctly identify 98 individuals as having malnutrition, and 950 would be correctly identified as not having malnutrition. Two individuals who truly had malnutrition would not be correctly identified by the screening test, and 50 individuals who truly did not have malnutrition would be incorrectly identified as having malnutrition according to the screening test.

Predictive values are strongly affected by the prevalence of the condition or disease. Using a test with a given sensitivity and specificity, the differences in positive predictive values are notable as prevalence declines from 25% to 2.5% (Figure 5.3 on page 80). If the condition of interest is rare, even a highly sensitive and specific test will produce results with a very low positive predictive value. In such a case, many of those who test positive do not truly have disease. Further testing (using a gold standard) is necessary to distinguish true positives from false positives.

DESCRIPTIVE RESEARCH DESIGN

Descriptive studies are the simplest of all research designs. These studies simply report the characteristics of person, place, and time of a disease or a condition of interest, and they are used to identify patterns of a disease or condition. They may report on countrywide populations, small geographic areas, small groups of individuals, or individual participants. Following are the most common types of descriptive studies, which will be discussed in more detail in the next sections:

- ecological studies
- case reports and case series
- cross-sectional studies or surveys
- surveillance systems
- measurement of vital statistics and demographics

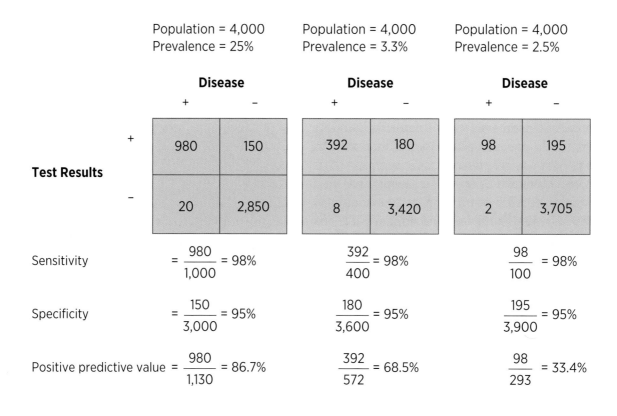

Figure 5.3 Comparison of positive predictive values in populations with differing prevalence of disease

Descriptive studies are also valuable for identifying potential associations between risk factors and a disease. Frequently, descriptive studies are less expensive and take less time than analytic studies because they use precollected data, such as the National Food Consumption Survey; NHANES I, II, and III; vital statistics; or clinical records. Results from descriptive studies can form the basis of hypotheses for analytic research. Analytic studies include prospective cohort studies and randomized controlled trials. Both of these designs require recruiting research participants, which always adds time and expense to a research endeavor.

Ecological Studies

Ecological studies are beneficial for examining patterns relating a possible risk or causative factor to a disease. Often, data from several countries are examined to identify these relationships. For example, investigators examined an association between individual dietary factors and chronic disease in more than 75 countries. Data on disease prevalence for the study were obtained from the World Health Organization Global Infobase. Data on food available for consumption came from Food Balance Sheets compiled from the Food and Agriculture Organization of the United Nations.[12] Physical inactivity, sugar consumption, and cereal consumption were significant predictors of obesity in a multivariate model.

Ecological studies show only associations between a factor and a disease or condition, however. They do not show causation or the effect of potential confounding factors, and they certainly do not document the biological processes involved in a disease or condition. In the earlier example, one cannot determine if cereal consumption *causes* obesity or use statistical analysis of the data to adjust for confounding factors that may contribute to obesity and be associated with higher cereal consumption.

Case Reports and Case Series

Unique experiences of one patient or a small group of patients with a similar diagnosis are reported in the literature as case reports or case series. These accounts can provide a basis for a more vigorous investigation and analytic approach to examining factors of interest. This brief documentation also alerts health care professionals to possible, but not proved, beneficial or life-threatening aspects of a disease or its treatment. To illustrate, a case series of 50 patients with inflammatory bowel disease who reported that they followed the Specific Carbohydrate Diet suggests that some highly educated patients with moderate to severe disease can discontinue immunosuppressive agents with the use of this diet.[13] Case reports or case series may also be used to document the beginning of an epidemic. Other uses for case reports include tracking toxicity reports of new foods.

A case series is of greater value than a single case report because it documents more evidence for the suggested hypothesis. Case reports or case series are never conclusive in establishing cause and effect, but they are useful for providing initial descriptions of a new disease or documenting the biological processes of a disease or condition.

Cross-Sectional Studies or Surveys

Surveys can provide a wide variety of descriptive information about a disease or condition, but their important contribution is in providing a view of the individuals studied at one point or period of time. Many national surveys have been done and are repeated periodically. Examples include the Continuing Survey of Food Intakes by Individuals and NHANES I, II, and III. Currently, the Continuing Survey of Food Intakes by Individuals and the NHANES have been combined and are being conducted annually.[14] These surveys have sophisticated sampling frames to provide representative information from all segments of the population or special high-risk population groups. (See more at the Centers for Disease Control and Prevention [CDC] website at www.cdc.gov/nchs/nhanes.htm.)

The primary advantage of surveys is that they can offer a representative overview of the health of the population (or cross-section). Their limitation is that the data cannot provide answers to questions about disease etiology. When a population is surveyed at one point in time, it may be difficult to determine whether exposure to a risk factor came before a disease unless questions about timing are included. For further discussion of surveys and using these large databases, see Chapter 12.

Surveillance Systems

Surveillance is a systematic, ongoing survey designed to monitor specific health outcomes in a population over an extended period of time.[15] Surveillance systems are used to identify and monitor public health problems. These data can be used for public health planning, program evaluation, policy development, or research purposes. Important components of a surveillance system include the cooperation and coordination of many individuals and groups, the collection of high-quality data, management of the data, and timely analysis and dissemination of the data for use. A pertinent example for RDNs is the Catalogue of Surveillance Systems collected by the National Collaborative on Childhood Obesity Research.[16]

Measurement of Vital Statistics and Demographics

Vital statistics are based on data from such records as birth certificates, death certificates, and censuses. Vital statistics are really a type of surveillance data, as they routinely monitor vital events. By law, birth and death certificates must be filed by the birth attendant or attending physician at the local town or city clerk's office; these data are also forwarded to county and state offices for compilation and reporting. At the beginning of each decade, the federal government collects population census data.

Birth and death certificate data are readily available from the vital records offices of counties or states. State vital statistics reports are published annually and can be obtained from the state office, and these reports are available in the public documents area of public, college, or university libraries. National vital statistics reports are also available on the internet from such agencies as the CDC, National Center for Health Statistics, and National Vital Statistics System. Examples of available data are age-adjusted death rates for selected causes, such as diabetes mellitus or cardiovascular disease, by race and gender; data for births in the United States, according to maternal and demographic characteristics; and infant health status (see the CDC website at www.cdc.gov/nchs/nvss.htm).

Vital statistics data are especially useful for documenting person, place, and time characteristics of a disease or condition, as well as for documenting the relative importance of a disease or health problem in a population. Cause-specific mortality rates can be used to identify the primary causes of deaths. This information can be used to target major problem areas, and in turn, as part of the follow-up, lead to the development of intervention strategies to reduce the risk of death from a particular cause.

Demographic data, such as the percentage of children living below the poverty level, can be useful for identifying the size of a target population for a public health program.

CONCLUSION

The two primary measures of disease frequency are incidence and prevalence. Cumulative incidence measures the rate of either the morbidity or mortality of a disease in a population over a specified period. Incidence density is similar to cumulative incidence, but it uses person-time as the denominator. In contrast, prevalence describes the burden of a disease in a population; it reflects the number of cases, both existing and new, at a specified point or period in time.

Screening tests are used to document the amount of disease that can be positively affected by early intervention. These tests must be reliable and valid. Specificity and sensitivity are used to evaluate validity. The predictive value of a test assesses its ability to accurately predict persons with and without a disease. Predictive values are strongly influenced by disease prevalence.

The major descriptive study designs include correlational studies, case reports and case series, surveys, and surveillance. The primary uses for descriptive studies are to provide information to develop priorities for health care planning and to generate hypotheses to be tested in analytic research.

REFERENCES

1. MacMahon B, Pugh TF. *Epidemiology: Principles and Methods*. Boston, MA: Little, Brown, and Co; 1970.

2. Kunzmann AT, Coleman HG, Huang WY, Kitahara CM, Cantwell MM, Berndt SI. Dietary fiber intake and risk of colorectal cancer and incident and recurrent adenoma in the Prostate, Lung, Colorectal, and Ovarian Cancer Screening Trial. *Am J Clin Nutr*. 2015;102(4):881-890.

3. Fuglestad AJ, Kroupina MG, Johnson DE, Georgieff MK. Micronutrient status and neurodevelopment in internationally adopted children. *Acta Paediatr*. 2016;105(2):e67-e76.

4. Bower KM, Thorpe RJ, Rohde C, Gaskin DJ. The intersection of neighborhood racial segregation, poverty, and urbanicity and its impact on food store availability in the United States. *Prev Med*. 2014;48:33-39.

5. Roba KT, O'Connor TP, Belachew T, O'Brien NM. Seasonal variation in nutritional status and anemia among lactating mothers in two agro-ecological zones of rural Ethiopia: a longitudinal study. *Nutrition*. 2015; 31(10):1213-1218.

6. Inoue-Choi M, Jones RR, Anderson KE, et al. Nitrate and nitrite ingestion and risk of ovarian cancer among postmenopausal women in Iowa. *Int J Cancer*. 2015; 137(1):173-182.

7. Sanchez MA, Corsostegui SP, DeBroucker CA, et al. Norovirus GIII.17 outbreak linked to an infected post-symptomatic food worker in a French military unit located in France. *Food Environ Virol*. 2017;9(2):234-237.

8. Flanders WD, O'Brien TR. Inappropriate comparisons of incidence and prevalence in epidemiologic research. *Am J Public Health*. 1989;79(9):1301-1303.

9. Ogden CL, Carroll MD, Lawman HG, et al. Trends in obesity prevalence among children and adolescents in the United States, 1988–1994 through 2013–2014. *JAMA*. 2016;315(21):2292-2299.

10. Apolzan JW, Myers CA, Cowley AD, et al. Examination of the reliability and validity of the Mindful Eating Questionnaire in pregnant women. *Appetite*. 2016;100:142–151.

11. Marlatt KL, Farbakhsh K, Dengel DR, Lytle LA. Breakfast and fast food consumption are associated with selected biomarkers in adolescents. *Prev Med Rep*. 2016;3:49-52.

12. Siervo M, Montagnese C, Mathers JC, Soroka KR, Stephan BCM, Wells JCK. Sugar consumption and global prevalence of obesity and hypertension: an ecological analysis. *Public Health Nutr*. 2014;17(3):587-596.

13. Kakodkar S, Farooqui AJ, Mikolaitis SL, Mutlu EA. The specific carbohydrate diet for inflammatory bowel disease: a case series. *J Acad Nutr Diet*. 2015;115(8):1226-1232.

14. Ahluwalia N, Dwyer J, Terry A, Moshfegh A, Johnson C. Update on NHANES dietary data: focus on collection, release, analytical considerations, and uses to inform public policy. *Adv Nutr*. 2016;7(1):121-134.

15. Teutsch SM, Churchill RE. *Principles and Practice of Public Health Surveillance*. New York, NY: Oxford University Press; 1994.

16. McKinnon RA, Reedy J, Berrigan D, Krebs-Smith SM, NCCOR Catalogue and Registry Working Groups. The national collaborative on childhood obesity research catalogue of surveillance systems and measures registry: new tools to spur innovation and increase productivity in childhood obesity. *Am J Prev Med*. 2012;42(4):433-435.

ADDITIONAL RESOURCES

Abramson JH, Abramson ZH. *Making Sense of Data*. 3rd ed. New York, NY: Oxford University Press; 2001.

Rothman KJ. *Epidemiology: An Introduction*. 2nd ed. New York, NY: Oxford University Press; 2012.

Weiss NS. *Clinical Epidemiology: The Study of the Outcome of Illness*. 3rd ed. New York, NY: Oxford University Press; 2006.

6 Qualitative Research

Judith Beto, PhD, RDN

LEARNING OBJECTIVES

1. Describe qualitative research.

2. Contrast qualitative with quantitative research methods.

3. Categorize methodology for sampling and data collection.

4. Distinguish among appropriate data collection and analysis choices.

5. Evaluate methods to interpret and report qualitative data.

Quantitative research is all about numbers! It focuses on the numeric measurement of standardized values, such as the number of grams of carbohydrate consumed derived from a 24-hour food record. Another quantitative measurement is the calculation of body mass index using actual measured height and weight with a validated mathematical formula. Quantitative research also tends to correlate measured variables with one another. An example of a quantitative correlation would be comparing changes in body weight with changes in estimated calorie intake.

Qualitative research, in contrast, is all about collecting information outside of the traditional measurement realm.[1] It has always been an integral part of cross-cultural comparisons and descriptions of food habits in the nutrition and anthropology literature.[2] Qualitative research often gathers data on health beliefs and practices from interviews and focus groups.[3,4] Some consider the qualitative research process to be subjective and descriptive fieldwork rather than objective and unbiased scientific discovery.[5] However, qualitative research is now recognized as a valid and reliable method to collect information and provide systematic analysis.[1]

The purpose of this chapter is to define qualitative research as a rigorous methodology, to describe when and why it should be conducted, and to review the necessary steps in qualitative inquiry. Examples will be provided of application to clinical nutrition, community nutrition, and foodservice management.

DEFINING QUALITATIVE RESEARCH

Qualitative research may be defined as any data-gathering technique that generates open-ended narrative data or words rather than numeric data or numbers.[1,3,4] For example, a researcher wants to understand the meaning of evolving terms such as "clean eating" in college students. A traditional quantitative approach might be to first create a set of possible researcher-created definitions. These definitions would be transformed into a multiple-choice question format and administered to college students, and then the responses would be numerically tallied. A qualitative approach to this research question might be to recruit college students to participate in semistructured interviews or focus groups. Sessions would be audio- or videotaped to collect, in the participants own words, descriptions of their understanding of the term "clean eating." The oral response data would then be coded and analyzed for common themes to determine the scope of the term rather than predefine it.

The primary caveat in qualitative research is that the words must reflect the point of view of the study participant, not the researcher.[6] In other words,

qualitative research assumes that findings about human interaction, thinking, and behavior are better understood and more scientifically valid when seen from the inside out than when viewed from the outside in.

CONTRAST AND COMPARISON OF QUALITATIVE AND QUANTITATIVE RESEARCH

Qualitative and quantitative research approaches have much in common. The most important similarity between qualitative and quantitative research approaches is a shared view that the world can be known through systematic, empiric observation. Both approaches can provide information that will add to either the conceptual or methodologic base of the field, contribute meaningful information to policy makers, or provide useful information to practitioners.[1,3]

Both qualitative and quantitative approaches may be descriptive, evaluative, theory building, and context sensitive. At the extreme ends of the continuum are the major differences between the research approaches, but in between there are numerous similarities. Although qualitative researchers start out with words, they may end up also using numbers to describe their results in a quantifiable way. Likewise, quantitative researchers may start out with numbers, but they often use words to describe their results. Thus, researchers from both traditions use both words and numbers, and both use interpretive analyses in one form or another, just in different amounts. One of the advantages of qualitative research, however, is that qualitative data can be analyzed as such. These data (words) can also be subsequently converted to quantitative data for future analysis—for example, by simply ranking or counting the number of statements within each category. Quantitative data rarely, if ever, exhibit the converse versatility.[1,7] Box 6.1 on page 86 illustrates the general similarities between qualitative and quantitative research.

Contrasting characteristics of qualitative and quantitative studies vary according to the issues of interest.[1,7] For example, qualitative approaches are

Descriptive
Evaluative
Sensitive to research context
Data at a single point or over a continuum
Use of rigorous and defined methodology
Methodology can be replicated

Box 6.1 General Similarities Between Qualitative and Quantitative Research

seldom appropriate in comparing the validity of two technical methods of calculating nutrient data, but they are often appropriate in the study of social behavior related to food choices made alone or in groups. Box 6.2 provides some contrasting characteristics of these two methods.

Primary differences between qualitative and quantitative research are sample size, data collection technique, and analysis approach. Sample size in quantitative research is determined prior to any data collection. A power analysis for sample size is required during the research planning phase to ensure statistical validity. In addition, large samples often require randomization strategies. The focus shifts in qualitative research to the depth of participant information. Participants are often selected specifically to answer a research question within grouping characteristics, such as mothers of children with diabetes or vegan college students. Data are collected until no new information is found and participants begin to repeat information shared by earlier participants.[1,3,7]

Data collection and analysis are unique with each research method. The qualitative emphasis is on relevance of participants/informants to the question, meaningfulness of their responses, and inductive approach to analysis. The quantitative focus is on random selection of participants, validity and reliability of the outcome measure (blood test, standardized test), and deductive analysis approach. Utilization of field notes, observations, and artifacts are common in qualitative research. Quantitative research uses objective measures that result in numeric parameters.[1,3,7-10]

The traditional research perspective is that an investigator must choose between a qualitative or quantitative approach because the fundamental differences between the philosophies make it impossible to combine methods. A mixed-methods approach, where both quantitative and qualitative data can be integrated to answer a specific research question, can also be used in specific situations. Therefore, mixed methodologies that incorporate both quantitative and qualitative approaches are not only permissible but are to be encouraged.[11,12] The scope of that integration is beyond the reach of this chapter but must be sufficiently rigorous to earn credibility for the results it produces.

Qualitative Research	Quantitative Research
Analysis: Content focused	Analysis: Statistical
Data: Analyzed thematically	Data: Analyzed numerically
Data: Audio, visual, textual	Data: Standardized measures
Exploration	Correlation
Inductive	Deductive
Participants: Smaller number, often chosen	Participants: Large number, often random
Settings: Naturalistic	Settings: Controlled
Study of less known or unknown phenomena	Study of well-known phenomena
Unique to population sampled; not generalizable	If prospective, can be applied to other populations; if retrospective, not generalizable

Box 6.2 Contrasting Characteristics of Qualitative and Quantitative Research[1,3,7-10]

REASONS TO DO QUALITATIVE RESEARCH

There are multiple reasons to perform qualitative research, but the most common is to provide meaning to an experience or lifestyle practice.[6] Many problems do not have established objective measures. For example, dietetics practitioners cannot measure the frustration of a person newly diagnosed with diabetes about the new diet parameters, but they can listen to that person. By listening to several individuals newly diagnosed with diabetes and analyzing their responses, qualitative researchers can often more fully understand the problem. This qualitative inquiry can then help them design a more effective education program. Box 6.3 illustrates some selected examples of the qualitative research approach.[13-20]

Answering New or Unique Questions

The most common reasons investigators perform qualitative research are to ask new questions, answer unique questions, and ask existing questions to new audiences. Qualitative research yields data that are richer in description and, presumably, deeper in insight and understanding than closed-ended quantitative measures can produce. Qualitative researchers are often interested in asking (1) What is happening? (2) How do we know it is happening? and (3) What does it mean? They seek to understand the context of the question rather than seeking a single answer. Qualitative methods can be used to discover pertinent questions, variables, concepts, and problems. Qualitative data can generate hypotheses or even theories that can then be tested by a practitioner-researcher.[1,3,6-8]

Qualitative Research Approach	Example
Conduct a complete formative evaluation	Assess an education program by interviewing program participants[13]
Describe an unfamiliar community or culture	Explore the body weight issues of adult lesbian women by a noncommunity researcher[14]
Describe the context of a phenomena	Survey opinions of individuals living in a food desert rural environment[15]
Determine causal explanations of phenomena in their natural settings	Collect situation-specific data from affected participants after an event such as the natural disaster Hurricane Katrina[16]
Generate tentative theories and hypotheses	Identify unmet needs of family caregivers of cancer patients with eating problems[17]
Study the process of natural history of a phenomenon	Gather information on how the concept of "good food" is evolving in the foodservice setting[18]
Understand the culture, traditions, symbols, perception, emotions, language, and meaning of a phenomenon to participants	Describe decision-making processes within Maasai families in Kenya[19]
Validate theory	Examine successful health coaching theories on behavioral impact in practice[20]

Box 6.3 Examples of Qualitative Research Approach

The most common situations in which investigators choose a qualitative research approach are highlighted in the following list:

- The use of traditional quantitative approaches is inadequate to improve practice or understanding of a problem issue. An example might be to understand why diverse undergraduate students are less likely to match in a computer program to a supervised-practice setting.
- The research problem is very new and not enough is known about the situation to formulate testable hypotheses or select a suitable theory to address it. An example is the public reaction to genetically modified corn or rice in staple core foods vs occasional or extra foods, such as dessert items.
- The researchers are interested in both outcome and process variables. When studying obesity in childhood, a researcher may decide to look at certain outcome variables, such as a child's weight, stature, and energy expenditure. However, certain process variables are important and may lead to the other outcome variables. These process variables may include a child's perceptions of weight and exercise, parents' perceptions of weight and exercise, and how parents convey these perceptions to their children.
- The evaluation needs to be extremely audience specific or very detailed in nature. An example is whether a needs assessment is to be done for a group of women with diabetes mellitus and bulimia.
- The researcher needs data on social context, structure, and interactions within which a behavior pattern can be understood. These data may be particularly important in understanding aberrant dietary behavior expressed by individuals or groups with anorexia, nonorganic failure to thrive, food addiction, or binge drinking.

Collecting Data in More Efficient Ways

Quantitative survey data may be difficult to collect from certain groups of individuals, such as young children, those who speak English as a second language, or individuals who are unfamiliar with the testing procedures. Individuals may refuse to answer survey questionnaires because they distrust questionnaires, the source of the questionnaire (for example, private industry or government), or researchers in general. Yet many of these groups may readily participate in the more intimate and interactive data collection procedures offered by qualitative methodologies, particularly if conducted within peer groups.

A small in-depth qualitative study may also provide more useful information than a large-scale quantitative study during formative evaluations, such as during the design and development testing of new products or programs. Early open-ended discussions may provide insight as to how a future intervention program or product might be developed or improved before further investments of time, personnel, and money are made. This kind of study can result in an economy of effort in the long term whether the product is a new gastric tube, hospital menu, pamphlet, or weight-loss program.

One of the main reasons interest in qualitative research has grown in community settings is that the more traditional quantitative methods are often impractical or too costly. Hospitals and clinics have neither the staff, the resources, nor the expertise to mount a study with a sample size large enough to yield statistical power yet are interested in effect. For example, individuals cannot be randomly assigned to different clinics in different communities to assess the impact of a new educational or counseling intervention but could be interviewed to provide insight into personal impact.

Sometimes it is not ethical to randomly assign individuals to different interventions. For example, quantitative research has established evidence-based correlations between low folic acid intake during pregnancy and neural tube birth defects. It would be unethical to assign pregnant women to a control group of no folic acid and compare them to an intervention group of adequate folic acid and then assess the birth defects in the newborns. With qualitative research, communities with higher than normal neural tube birth defects could be interviewed to potentially identify lifestyle or other factors that may be contributing to the higher incidence.

Qualitative methods often present a more pragmatic approach to conducting research in a natural

Dietary intake assessment using digital photo imaging

Educational materials development

Food and nutrition marketing

Food product development and sensory evaluation

Influences of social media on food choices

Program evaluation and assessment

Box 6.4 Selected Qualitative Research Topic Areas in Nutrition

setting. These methods also offer researchers greater opportunities to obtain information about clients' behavior, attitudes, beliefs, and social influences using open-ended rather than closed-ended questions. The results in qualitative research, however, are specific to the study group and cannot be generalized to any other population. Box 6.4 illustrates the diversity of selected qualitative research areas.

QUALITATIVE RESEARCH DESIGNS

Research designs using qualitative inquiry still require rigor and careful attention to detail. The selection of a design is linked directly to the question being posed. Examples of selected qualitative research designs are shown in Box 6.5 on page 90.[21-27]

A qualitative research proposal contains all the same components as traditional quantitative research.[9] The research question should be clearly defined. The methods of data collection will be driven by the nature of the question. The sampling strategy is grounded in locating the pool of participants that will provide the most experience and opinion linked to the research question. The standardization of how the data are collected and analyzed needs to maintain rigor and integrity. The research protocol should be submitted to an institutional review board for the protection of human participants to comply with federal law. Finally, the interpretation of the findings requires unbiased re-

porting of the participants' voices without investigator influence.

Qualitative and quantitative research designs have an important major difference. In qualitative research, the investigator retains the right to modify or alter the study design in the field according to issues that become apparent only in the field. Any changes, however, need to be grounded in logic and carefully detailed. The quantitative research protocol, in contrast, is seldom if ever altered regardless of circumstances.

QUALITATIVE DATA COLLECTION

Data collection for qualitative research evolves from the actual words and actions of the participants. The recording and documentation of this process is the basis of qualitative inquiry. The most common form of data documentation is audio- or video-recording of participants during data collection. Often another researcher will take field notes while the primary researcher conducts the data collection. A simple checklist, along with narrative field notes, may be more appropriate when there is no participant direct interaction. Rigorous training of the research team is required to maintain consistent methods and procedures that will result in valid and reliable data. This may include the preparation of participant research consent forms with permission to record sessions, standardized scripts to describe the purpose of the research, procedural checklists, interview guides to direct open-ended inquiry, and observational data forms. This section will discuss the importance of participant selection and the ways in which data can be collected.[1,3,7,8,28,29]

Participant Sampling

In qualitative research, sampling directly relates to the trustworthiness of data. The first principle is appropriateness, or the extent to which the sample includes all relevant perspectives (eg, individuals, settings, times) that can inform the study or question in hand. The second principle is adequacy, or the extent to which enough data are available to provide a rich description of the phenomenon and the context

Qualitative Research Design	Description with Example
Case study	Assembling individual narrative case studies or reports to describe a specific issue[21]
Ethnography	Study of a social system and culture through observations of daily life, such as the cultural role of Latino mothers[22]
Grounded theory	Interviews with participants reveal new information rather than an idea being tested, such as exploring the meaning of scratch cooking across age groups[23]
Narratives	Collection of stories results in description of a common life experience, such as interviews with registered nurses about their work with elderly patients with poor nutritional status[24]
Participatory action research	Qualitative version of a clinical trial based on identification of a need, implementation to address the need, and then reaction of intervention[25]
Phenomenology	Focuses on understanding emotions, attitudes, and beliefs after a group experiences a common event, such as the sensitivity to behavior advice given at prenatal visits[26]
Symbolic interaction	Investigation of how individuals create meaning (symbolism) from a social interaction. such as evaluation of a new food label format and the perceived impact of its use[27]

Box 6.5 Examples of Qualitative Research Designs

in which it occurs from each relevant perspective. Adequacy is achieved when results become repetitive or redundant and additional interviews fail to provide fresh insights. This is commonly known as data saturation, and it helps determine when the sample size is adequate to examine the research question.[8,29]

Decisions regarding sample size in qualitative research often rest on a compromise between the scope of topics and perspectives explored vs the depth to which each topic or perspective is studied. Studies that encompass a broad number of topics and perspectives are not likely to afford researchers the opportunity to explore each topic or perspective in depth with each participant or group. In contrast, studies that address issues in depth with each participant or group may need to be limited in the number of topics or perspectives covered and the number of participants involved because of the usual constraints of time and money.

Qualitative sampling is unique from quantitative sampling. Box 6.6 outlines some common qualitative sampling methods with examples.

Investigators carefully choose the qualitative sampling method that will match the research question with the participant group most likely to respond with relevant opinions. Researchers may stop periodically during the data collection phase or at the end of the first round of planned data collection to determine if more participants are needed to fully explore the research question. For example, if it is important to hear the voice of both fathers and mothers on parenting practices with adolescents who are overweight, then data collection should initially include a plan to interview similar numbers of parents from each gender. If interim data collec-

Sampling Method	Example
Extreme case	The sample is from an extreme scope of potential viewpoints to compare the full spectrum of an issue, such as a hot topic, ensuring inclusion of all variations of pro and con diverse opinions.
Homogeneous	The sample is from a cohort with common exposure to a phenomena or event, such as mothers of adolescents with epilepsy.
Maximum variation	The sample is from a wide variety of participants to get a balanced exposure, such as the impact of changes to a federal food policy program using participants from all 50 states.
Purposeful	The sample intentionally represents specific characteristics, such as African American women who have lactose intolerance.
Selective	Sampling is based on preconceived notions of when, where, and from whom the most fruitful data might come. An example is collecting data from women of child-bearing age about their dietary intake from an area with a high neural tube birth defect rate.
Snowball	An initial purposeful sample is selected for a topic, then participants identify others to sample. The process is repeated until data saturation occurs. An example is asking registered dietitian nutritionists interested in learning more about the electronic nutrition care process to identify others they know who share the same interest.
Theoretical	Sampling includes individuals who hold a theory, belief, or external locus control system in response to evolving action research. An example is exploring the theory of planned behavior by interviewing adults who purchase home-delivered meal preparation packages of ingredients with recipes.

Box 6.6 Common Qualitative Research Sampling Methods[1,3,7,10,29]

tion shows similar attitudes and practices being voiced by both fathers and mothers, the researcher might then justify ending the data collection since data saturation has occurred. In an alternative scenario, a researcher might stop interviewing mothers when similar comments are being repeated but continue to recruit more fathers because their voices continue to provide new theories and insights.[3,7,8]

In sampling for group interviews, additional considerations related to group dynamics may apply. Thus, it is often advisable to assemble relatively homogeneous groups (homogeneous with respect to age, educational background, ethnic group, language, status, or income, for example) so that group mem-

bers are comfortable expressing their views in front of other members of the group. For example, if studying breastfeeding perceptions, the researcher may separate men from women to alleviate discomfort and encourage participants to freely discuss the topic in their respective groups. If a variety of perspectives is required, additional groups may be formed, each representing a potential different perspective. By the same token, it may be best for group members to be strangers to one another so that the social liability of candid discussion is minimized.[3,7,8,30]

All sampling decisions must be adequately justified and made explicit in reporting qualitative research. Only then can reviewers judge whether the sample was appropriate and adequate to support valid conclusions.

Data Collection Methods

Individual interviews, group interviews, structured observations, and analysis of documentation (newspaper stories, reports, diaries, photographs, films, transcripts of speeches, stories, and other narratives) are basic qualitative data collection methods. An exhaustive list of methods and all their variations would fill this chapter and many more. It would also be dated because new methods are always being developed. Therefore, this section is intended only to introduce readers to fundamental methods.

Two primary methods of qualitative data collection are observations and interviews. In their classic form, these methods are applied in naturalistic settings, where study participants live, work, and play in everyday life. Naturalistic settings are important because qualitative research hinges on the fundamental notion that events and observations can be understood only within the context in which they occur. An example would be the naturalistic researcher sitting anonymously in a public fast-food restaurant to observe the patterns of mobile device use by caregivers and children during mealtimes.[31]

In their less classic form, observations and interviews are conducted in the researcher's setting. The loss of context that occurs when qualitative research is moved into the laboratory limits its potential, but data collected in nonnaturalistic settings can be useful nonetheless. The data can be especially useful if the context is addressed methodologically by recreating it in the laboratory. An example would be the controlled setting of a cooking workshop to directly observe the food preferences of a cohort of patients undergoing chemotherapy.[13]

Qualitative data collection using internet or social media methods is not discussed as part of this chapter. Currently, the use of this data collection method lacks the software methodology control to truly identify and sample the participants with the rigor necessary for publication. Online and mobile device surveys, however, may be valuable to identify opinions on a topic or an idea worth investigating using a qualitative research proposal. Guidelines are evolving.[32]

Observations

Systematic observation of individuals and events in their natural settings is used to discover and describe behaviors and interactions in context. Observation can help researchers explore and understand the apparent gap between what individuals know or say and what they are really doing. An important dimension of observation is the extent to which the researcher interacts with the participants. The continuum of interaction ranges from covert observation, where the individuals observed are not aware of the researcher's presence, to direct participant observation, where the researcher interacts freely with the individuals while collecting data.

Interviews

Interviews are planned interactions in which one person systematically obtains information from one or more other individuals via questioning and discussion. Interviews may be conducted one-to-one with individual study participants or in a group setting with multiple participants. One of the key points of the interview method is communication trust. This may include conducting the interview in the native language of the participants or using a setting that is neutral and unbiased. The researcher should select an interviewer of similar gender or common ethnicity as appropriate.

Individual interviews are one-to-one verbal exchanges with a trained researcher using a preplanned open-ended set of questions to guide and standardize the process. Individual interviews may vary in depth depending on the number of times each study participant is interviewed and the duration of each interview. In-depth interviews may require multiple, extended sessions to explore issues in detail. Most individual interviews consist of guided conversations, but they may also involve specially designed activities like cognitive response tasks. Cognitive response tasks involve the use of stimulus cues, often in the form of persuasive messages or illustrations, to elicit thoughts. These thoughts are labeled "cognitive responses" and are presumed to mediate the persuasive impact of the message via the content and structure of memory.

The group interview is the most widely used qualitative research method. Group interviews include the focus group interview, nominal group process, and Delphi process. Focus group interviews are designed to stimulate and facilitate topic- or product-relevant discussion among small groups of representatives of the target audience. Group dynamism is used to help draw out information about behaviors, attitudes, and opinions that may not be divulged as readily in one-to-one interviews. Participants can build on one another's comments and views, help clarify them, and contrast them with their own. The role of the focus group researcher is to facilitate, guide, and manage the group discussion. This management involves introducing issues, encouraging participants to discuss the issues among themselves, gently drawing out quiet participants and discouraging those who might dominate the conversation, introducing exhibits and activities, and making sure all issues are covered in the time allotted. The goal is not to conduct one-to-one interviews simultaneously in a group setting but to foster discussion among group members around the topics of research interest.[3,8,30]

Focus groups are often used as a part of audience assessment in planning nutrition education materials and programs. Researchers conduct focus groups to develop insight into participants' perceived needs and preferences, and they then use that information to develop strategies for intervention. Focus group research may be conducted with one interview per group or repeated interviews with groups that serve as panels.[30]

The nominal group process is a group method of soliciting and consolidating opinions in situations where decision-making is hampered by insufficient information or an overload of contradictory information. It is a consensus-generating technique designed to determine the extent to which experts or nonexperts agree about a given issue. The nominal group technique involves a highly structured meeting where each participant expresses opinions in writing, shares opinions with the facilitator one by one, reacts individually to all suggestions grouped by the facilitator according to some common characteristic, privately reevaluates personal opinions in light of what others have said, discusses differences within the group, and repeats the cycle until agreement is reached.[33] Another approach, photo elicitation, has been used by county extension workers to help understand barriers to farmers market use. Participants were asked to visit a local farmers market and take pictures. These pictures were then shared within a group discussion to help each participant visually explain what they saw while sharing their comments with the group. The group then jointly identified themes related to their observations and created a list of common barriers with potential solutions.[21]

The Delphi process, a similar technique, is often conducted by mail or email rather than in a group meeting. It sometimes uses anonymous participants, with the facilitator orchestrating the process and providing written summaries of input for consideration in subsequent rounds. This iterative process was used to help define the advanced practitioner credential of the Commission on Dietetic Registration.[34]

QUALITATIVE DATA ANALYSIS

Analysis of qualitative data requires the same attention to detail and rigor as quantitative research. Typically, data are coded by one or more researchers to identify common themes as a starting point for organizing the data. The planned method of data analysis should be cited in detail as part of the research proposal.[9,10]

Qualitative data analysis can proceed both inductively (moving from cases to generalizations) and deductively (moving from general to specific cases). In addition, (1) qualitative data analysis may be theory driven, theory generating, or both, and (2) qualitative data analysis lies on a continuum that ranges from purely qualitative (involving no numbers) to more quantitative (where a researcher counts the number of times a certain issue, opinion, or word arises in a document). It should also be understood that qualitative data include researcher-generated information (for example, field notes, annotations, study diaries, and other documents that make up the audit trail) as well as participant-generated information. These premises should serve as a foundation for understanding the following discussion of the basics of qualitative analysis.[3,10,29]

Content Analysis

Content analysis is the method by which the researcher systematically identifies and examines characteristics of the data collected. Historical qualitative research uses content analysis to interpret past events, drawing data from documents such as diaries, letters, poetry, music, and prose created at the time of the event.

Participant encounters are typically electronically recorded and transformed into written transcripts. Transcripts are usually verbatim accounts designed to preserve, as much as possible, everything that was said during the encounter. Transcripts, however, do not preserve nonlinguistic data, such as emphasis, mood, tone of voice, and other descriptive information that can be so crucial in elaborating meaning. Thus, it is important to listen to as well as read the data. It is also critical that the original interviewer edit each typed transcript carefully to check for accuracy, fill in the gaps using notes taken during and after the interview, and annotate the transcript appropriately. Annotations may be needed to clarify ambiguous situations.[10]

If the interview was recorded in a non-English format, it will need to be translated into English prior to analysis. Randomly selected passages should be back-translated by an independent professional to be sure the language-specific meaning has been captured. The technique of interpreter-facilitated cross-language interviews can also be used, which may provide interactive data collection and clarification.[35]

Transcribing tapes is very time consuming and therefore costly. A 60- to 90-minute audiotape takes approximately 6 to 8 hours to transcribe. One single interview can result in 20 to 40 pages of single-spaced text. Voice recognition software, an automated form of dictation and transcription, is a relatively new technological tool that qualitative researchers might consider in their work. It converts verbalizations into text via automated dictation. Randomly selected passages should be manually checked to ensure accuracy and meaning.

Box 6.7 lists an evolving cohort of selected software programs for qualitative data analysis. Each has unique strengths and limitations depending on the data-set format and the data variables that must be identified. Characteristics, content, and capabilities of software change frequently. The version used should be cited as part of the data reporting.

Coding

Coding facilitates the organization, management, and retrieval of qualitative data. It is used to link fragments of the data that share some commonality so that they can be viewed together to derive understanding. Coding helps the investigator extract meaning from qualitative data in a systematic way, uncovering patterns or themes that might otherwise be obscured by the sheer mass of information.

Unitizing is a step in the coding process whereby a recorded stream of verbalization (in the form of a transcript or document) is segmented into units of analysis that can be categorized. It is used primarily in cases where qualitative data are destined for quantitative analysis. Units may be defined in terms of time (for example, 20-second units for the analysis of television commercials), speaker (for example, all statements made by one speaker while holding the floor), or content (for example, each word, phrase, statement, or group of statements that express a single, coherent thought). Pilot testing should be performed to determine which type of unit is the most appropriate for a given project and how the units will be recorded. Recording of units should always include cross-references that trace each unit back to its original location in the transcript so that the surrounding context may be revisited as the need arises. Context is often needed to clarify the intent of ambiguous comments. Moreover, preserving and emphasizing context is a fundamental principle of qualitative research that makes it unique in its contribution to the body of knowledge.

Order and structure may be imposed on qualitative data in several ways, depending on the researcher's philosophy and objectives. Coding schemes may be developed inductively from the actual data or be driven by existing theory in a deductive manner.

The mechanical aspects of processing data involve a creative process that varies from researcher

Software Program	Manufacturer and Website
Atlas.ti	Atlas.ti (www.atlasti.com)
Dedoose	Dedoose (www.dedoose.com)
HyperRESEARCH	ResearchWare (www.researchware.com)
MAXQDA	VERBI (www.maxqda.com)
NVivo	QSR International (www.qsrinternational.com)
QDA Miner	Provalis Research (www.provalisresearch.com)
Quirkos	Quirkos(www.quirkos.com)
webQDA	webQDA (www.webqda.net)

Box 6.7 Selected Software for Qualitative Data Analysis[a]

[a] Information obtained from manufacturer websites, accessed on May 21, 2018.

to researcher and from project to project. There is no formula. Pilot work is needed to refine the proposed system and make sure that it works. An investigator may start with an elaborate coding scheme, only to find it too cumbersome to be practical. In contrast, an investigator may begin with a very simple scheme but find that it fails to cover or describe certain types of data adequately. In either case, adjusting or refining the coding system is necessary.

One way to maximize objectivity in qualitative data analysis is to use two or more independent analysts who can serve as cross-checks for one another. A subset of the data might be subjected to analysis by multiple, independent coders when researchers need some indication of interrater agreement but cannot afford to use multiple coders for the entire data set. The important point is that researchers must have a firm rationale for coding or organizing data in the way that they do. By specifying the rationale underlying the coding system, the investigator fosters consistency in the coding process and exposes the process to personal and peer scrutiny, thereby increasing the confirmability of the work.[3,8,10,35,36]

Once a coding system has been established, it may be judged according to two criteria: internal ho-mogeneity and external heterogeneity. Internal homogeneity refers to the extent to which all data within a category reflect the concept represented by that category: Does the data within each category follow the rules of inclusion for that category? External heterogeneity refers to the extent to which the categories are mutually exclusive: Are the differences between categories consistent?[36]

Unitizing and coding qualitative data can be a very subjective process requiring considerable judgment on the part of coders unless specific steps are taken to minimize this potential problem. Intercoder reliability is essential. For this reason, extensive pilot testing of the process is recommended to generate a well-defined set of instructions that can increase the reliability of the processes. The method of final data analysis needs to be clearly described as part of the research reporting process.

Displaying Data

Data display is a way to summarize data in a visual fashion to facilitate analysis and reporting. Some examples of data displays are matrixes, diagrams, flowcharts, and concept maps. Data displays can help researchers spot connections and relationships that might otherwise be obscured. They can also help researchers report data in ways that enhance understanding.

Data displays have been proposed as a major strategy for improving qualitative data analysis and reporting, but they are subject to drawbacks. The amount of information that may be included in a visual display is limited by available space. In developing displays, it is often necessary to summarize raw data or restrict the display to especially illustrative examples. These requirements call for subjective judgment on the part of the researcher, who must take care that displays represent the bulk of the data accurately and adequately. For example, it is tempting to select quotations that are particularly colorful, but selection on this basis alone can be misleading if the quotations reflect the views of only one participant. As with coding, investigators working on data displays are advised to record and report decision rules used to selectively display data so that the process remains open to review.

Interpreting and Verifying Data

This chapter separated data analysis from interpretation for the sake of discussion, yet the two often proceed simultaneously to some extent. For example, investigators involved in organizing and categorizing data will almost always find themselves discovering insights, coming up with hunches, and developing preliminary interpretations of the data. Indeed, preliminary interpretation may provide direction for further data collection and analysis. It is important, however, to remember that this interpretation is merely preliminary. The final interpretation must rest on a comprehensive evaluation of all the data.

One way to keep interpretation credible is by working with a research team whose members serve as devil's advocates for one another, helping to identify potential biases that can influence interpretation. All researchers have biases resulting from the personal and professional experiences that make up their lives. For example, in a study of food insecurity, a team member who has experienced food insecurity in the past may have biases that differ from team members who have not, but all members may be biased in some way.

Interpretation of results is valid to the extent that it accurately reflects the reality represented by data. Interpretations are verified by actively scrutinizing the data for evidence of disconfirmation (rather than confirmation). Interpretation is considerably easier if a variety of data collection strategies and analytic techniques have been used and yield similar conclusions. This concept, obtaining data from a variety of sources and using a variety of analytic techniques, is known as *triangulation* (assuming the use of at least three different techniques), and it is probably the best defense against criticism of investigator bias or subjectivity in qualitative research. As is the case with all processes described in this chapter, the methods used to interpret data and verify interpretation should be reported. Keeping a record of the route by which interpretations are arrived at and verified can help expose the process to fellow researchers and improve confidence in the conclusions. It also allows replication of qualitative research, which adds to its credibility and practice application.[3,8,10]

REPORTING QUALITATIVE RESEARCH

Qualitative research reporting follows the same guidelines as quantitative research. Following the research protocol format, sufficient details should be provided to allow replication. All methods should be reported with clarity. Attention should be given to the way data collection and analysis were performed to ensure data authenticity. Typically, selected quotes from participants are provided to support the content analysis themes. Since findings cannot be generalized, the participant characteristics are particularly important to understand the relationship between the observations and the interpretation by the research team.

EVALUATING PUBLISHED QUALITATIVE RESEARCH

The merit of qualitative research depends on the trustworthiness of its results and conclusions. Reviewing existing published qualitative research will provide a framework for reporting and understanding the qualitative research process. Four distinct aspects of trustworthiness defined in the literature are dependability, credibility, confirmability, and transferability.[10]

Dependability is the extent to which researchers accurately understand participants' meanings. It can be strengthened by the judicious use of follow-up questions and probes to clarify and confirm the meaning of what an interviewee says. Dependability can also be strengthened by member checks, in which participants are asked to review data summaries to see if they ring true from the insider perspective.

Credibility is the extent to which the phenomenon of interest has been adequately described. Data are credible when they provide a rich description of the phenomenon from a variety of perspectives rather than merely describing surface features from a limited number of critical vantage points.

Confirmability is the extent to which findings and conclusions are supported by evidence from the data. Confirmability can be enhanced by documenting the emergence and evolution of concepts and linking them with the data from which they are derived at each stage of the evolution. This process may be facilitated using study diaries.

Transferability is the extent to which findings from a qualitative study are useful in understanding how individuals experience the target phenomenon in other settings or under other conditions. Transferability of findings is determined after the fact by subsequent research with different audiences in different circumstances.[10]

Several checklists and guides are available for evaluating a qualitative research study.[37-39] These checklists can be used with a single study or when grouping several qualitative studies for a systematic or narrative review.[40,41] Investigators submitting a qualitative research study for publication may be required to complete a checklist specified by the publication.

Limitations and Concerns with Qualitative Research

Qualitative research has limitations. Perhaps the most obvious is that generalizations cannot be made from any one data set to larger populations, and it is often difficult to compare qualitative studies because they are context bound. In addition, qualitative data do not at present lend themselves to meta-analysis, although researchers are pursuing ways to solve this problem. Data collection is very dependent on personnel (as opposed to equipment and statistical software), and data quality subsequently depends entirely on the quality and training of personnel. Data analysis tends to be time-consuming and tedious. In fact, when qualitative and quantitative methods are used together, it is sometimes difficult to complete the qualitative analysis in time to be useful to the quantitative process.

CONCLUSION

Human events are far too complex to be viewed or analyzed from any single perspective. Researchers should explore the variety of methodologies offered by the qualitative approach to research, especially to develop and evaluate interventions or programs in clinical or community environments. Qualitative studies are becoming increasingly important, particularly in nutrition education and intervention. Qualitative research includes a wide variety of data collection and analysis approaches. Benefits of qualitative research are that it generates a deeper understanding to improve professional practice while yielding significant findings. In sum, qualitative research is a viable means of problem-solving in the nutrition and dietetics field.

REFERENCES

1. Ravitch SM, Mittenhelner-Carl N. *Qualitative Research: Bridging the Conceptual, Theoretical, and Methodological.* Los Angeles, CA: Sage Publishing; 2016.

2. Wilson B. *First Bite: How We Learn to Eat.* New York, NY: Basic Books; 2015.

3. Harris JE, Gleason PH, Sheean PM, Boushey C, Beto JA, Bruemmer B. An introduction to qualitative research for food and nutrition professionals. *J Am Diet Assoc.* 2009; 109(1):80-90.

4. Swift JA, Tischler V. Qualitative research in nutrition and dietetics: getting started. *J Hum Nutr Diet.* 2010;21(6):559-566.

5. Greenhalgh T, Annandale E, Ashcroft R, et al. An open letter to *The BMJ* editors on qualitative research. *BMJ.* 2016;352:i563.0.

6. Holloway I, Biley FC. Being a qualitative researcher. *Qual Health Res.* 2011;21(7):968-975.

7. Creswell JW, Poth CN. *Qualitative Inquiry and Research Design: Choosing Among Five Approaches.* 4th ed. Los Angeles, CA: Sage Publishing; 2017.

8. Guest G, Narney EE, Mitchell ML. *Collecting Qualitative Data: A Field Manual for Applied Research.* Los Angeles, CA: Sage Publishing; 2013.

9. Klopper H. The qualitative research proposal. *Curationis.* 2008;31(4):62-72.

10. Miles MB, Huberman AM, Saldana J. *Qualitative Data Analysis: A Methods Sourcebook.* 3rd ed. Los Angeles, CA: Sage Publishing; 2014.

11. Patton SR, Clements MA, George K, Goggin K. "I don't want them to feel different": a mixed methods study of parents' beliefs and dietary management strategies for their young children with type 1 diabetes mellitus. *J Acad Nutr Diet.* 2016:116(2):272-282.

12. Zoellner J, Harris JE. Mixed-methods research in nutrition and dietetics. *J Acad Nutr Diet.* 2017;117(5):683-697.

13. Ben-Arye E, Kechet Y, Shahbar IM, et al. The kitchen as therapy: qualitative assessment of an integrated cuisine workshop for patients undergoing chemotherapy. *Support Care Cancer.* 2016;24(4):1487-1495.

14. Garbers S, McDonnell C, Fogel SC, et al. Aging, weight, and health among adult lesbian and bisexual women: a metasynthesis of the multisite "healthy weight initiative" focus groups. *LGBT Health.* 2015;2(2):176-187.

15. Carnahan LR, Zimmermann K, Peacock NR. What rural women want the public health community to know about access to healthful food: a qualitative study, 2011. *Prev Chronic Dis.* 2016;13(E57):1-11.

16. Stanko KE, Cherry KE, Ryker KS, et al. Looking for the silver lining: Benefit findings after hurricanes Katrina and Rita in middle-aged, older, and oldest-old adults. *Curr Psychol.* 2015;34(3):564-575.

17. Hopkinson JB. The nourishing role: Exploratory qualitative research revealing unmet support needs in family carers of patients with advanced cancer and eating problems. *Cancer Nurs.* 2018;41(2):131-138.

18. Tsui EK, Morillo A. How cooks navigate nutrition, hunger, and care in public-sector foodservice settings. *Public Health Nutr.* 2016;19(5):946-954.

19. Pilla L, Dantas JA. Intra-household nutritional dynamics. *Qual Health Res.* 2016;26(6):793-806.

20. Thom DH, Wolf J, Gardner H, et al. A qualitative study of how health coaches support patients in making health-related decisions and behavioral changes. *Ann Fam Med.* 2016;14(6):509-516.

21. Misyak SA, Ledlie M, McFerren MM, Niewolny KL, Hosig KW, Serrano E. Exploring community and local food systems by means of photo elicitation. https://articles.extension.org/pages/70549/exploring-community-and-local-food-systems-by-means-of-photo-elicitation. Published May 2, 2014. Accessed May 21, 2018.

22. Martinez SM, Rhee K, Bianco E, Boutelle K. Maternal attitudes and behaviors regarding feeding practices in elementary school-aged Latino children: a pilot qualitative study on the impact of the cultural role of mothers in the US-Mexican border region of San Diego, California. *J Acad Nutr Diet.* 2014;114(2):230-237.

23. Lavalle F, McGowan L, Spence M, et al. Barriers and facilitators to cooking from "scratch" using basic or raw ingredients: a qualitative interview study. *Appetite.* 2016; 107:383-391.

24. Gholizadeh L, Yazdi K, Dehghan-Nayeri N, Mohammadi E. Nutritional care of elderly patients in acute care settings: a qualitative study. *Geriatr Gerontol Int.* 2016;16(3):374-379.

25. Schwingel A, Linares DE, Galvez G, et al. Developing a culturally sensitive lifestyle behavior change program in older Latinas. *Qual Health Res.* 2015;25(12):1733-1746.

26. Whitaker KN, Wilcox S, Liu J, Blair SN, Pate RR. Patient and provider perceptions of weight gain, physical activity and nutrition counseling during pregnancy: a qualitative study. *Womens Health Issues.* 2016;26(1):116-122.

27. Swartz JJ, Dowray S, Braxton D, Mihas P, Viera AJ. Simplifying healthful choices: a qualitative study of a physical activity based nutrition label format. *Nutr J.* 2013;12:72..

28. Draper A, Swift JA. Qualitative research in nutrition and dietetics: data collection issues. *J Hum Nutr Diet.* 2010; 24(1):3-12.

29. Merriam SB, Tisdell EJ. *Qualitative Research: A Guide to Design and Implementation.* 4th ed. San Francisco CA: Jossey-Bass; 2015.

30. Krueger RA, Casey MA. *Focus Groups: A Practical Guide for Applied Research.* 5th ed. San Francisco CA: Sage Publications; 2014.

31. Radesky JS, Kistin CJ, Zuckerman B, et al. Patterns of mobile device use by caregivers and children during meals in fast food restaurants. *Pediatrics.* 2014;133(4):e843-e849.

32. Agarwal S, LeFevre AE, Lee J, et al; for the WHO mHealth Technical Evidence Review Group. Guidelines for reporting of health interventions using mobile phones: mobile health (mHealth) evidence reporting and assessment (mERA) checklist. *BMJ.* 2016;352:i1174.

33. Mirosa M, Loh J, Spence H. The possibilities of reducing food choice to improve performance of college foodservices. *J Acad Nutr Diet.* 2016;116(7):1163-1171.

34. Brady RA, Byham-Gray L, Touger-Decker R, Passannante MR, O'Sullivan Maillet J. Identifying components of advanced-level clinical nutrition practice: a Delphi study. *J Acad Nutr Diet.* 2012:112(6):859-869.

35. Williamson DL, Choi J, Charchuk M, Rempel G, Pitre N. Interpreter-facilitated cross-language interviews: a research note. *Qual Res.* 2011;11(4):381-394.

36. Saldana J. *The Coding Manual for Qualitative Researchers.* 3rd ed. San Francisco CA: Sage Publications; 2015.

37. Clark J. How to peer review a qualitative manuscript. In: Godlee F, Jefferson T. eds. *Peer Review in Health Sciences.* 2nd ed. London, United Kingdom: BMJ Books; 2003: 219-235.

38. Hsieh H, Shannon SE. Three approaches to qualitative content analysis. *Qual Health Res.* 2005;15(9):1277-1288.

39. Tong A, Sainsbury P, Craig J. Consolidated criteria for reporting qualitative research (COREQ): a 32-item checklist for interviews and focus groups. *Int J Qual Health Care.* 2007;19(6):349 -357.

40. Raman S, Nicholls R, Ritchie J, Razee H, Shafiee S. Eating soup with nails of pig: thematic synthesis of the qualitative literature on cultural practices and beliefs influencing perinatal nutrition in low and middle income countries. *BMC Pregnancy Childbirth.* 2016;15:192.

41. Vanstone M, Kandasamy S, Gicomini M, DeJean D, McDonald SD. Pregnant women's perceptions of gestational weight gain; a systematic review and meta-synthesis of qualitative research. *Matern Child Nutr.* 2017;13(4). Epub November 21, 2016.

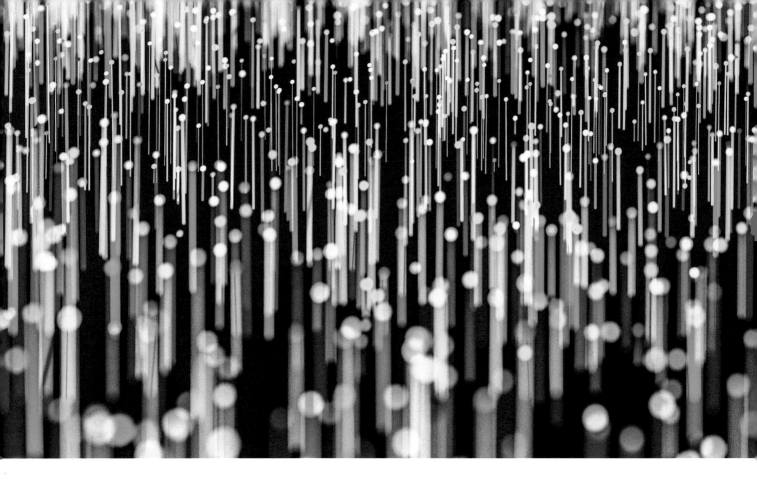

Observational and Experimental Research

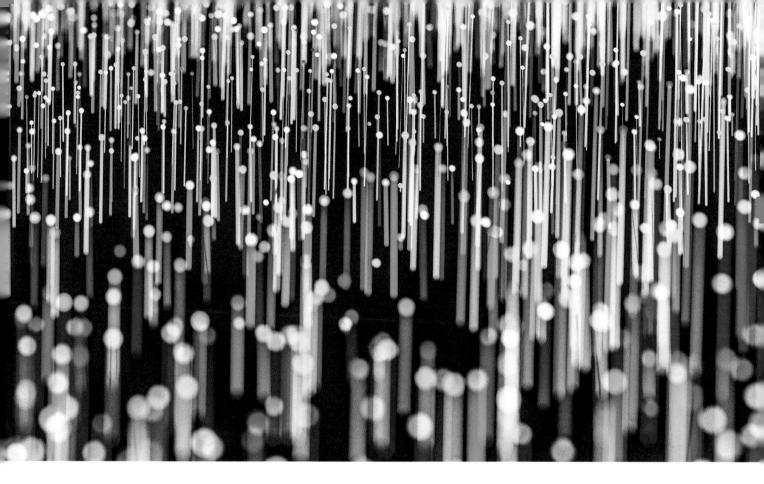

Chapter 7

Analytic Nutrition Epidemiology

Lyn M. Steffen, *PhD, MPH, RDN, FAHA*

LEARNING OBJECTIVES

1. Define analytic nutrition epidemiology.

2. Describe measures of association between a diet exposure and an outcome of interest.

3. Describe study designs for the association between a diet exposure and an outcome of interest.

4. Explain factors that may influence study results.

5. Explain potential inconsistencies between study results.

Nutrition epidemiology, a subdiscipline of epidemiology, addresses the fundamental question, "Does diet or nutrition influence health and disease?" The term *diet* as used here refers to dietary intake or items ingested, and the term *nutrition* refers to the resulting nutritional status of those ingested items. *Epidemiology*, the investigative basic science for health, studies "the distribution and determinants of health-related states or events and applies these to control health problems."[1] Operationally, epidemiologic studies can be categorized as descriptive or analytic. Descriptive epidemiology provides a bird's-eye view of disease focusing on a triad of key common features: time of occurrence, geography (place) of the occurrence, and individual traits of the persons affected. It depicts the frequency, distribution, and pattern of health-related states or events.[1] Analytic epidemiology examines whether a factor or exposure, such as dietary intake, is a source of risk or directly causes a health or disease effect.

Descriptive epidemiology findings, although important, are not definitive for disease associations or causal relationships.[2] Potential etiologic hypotheses can be generated from this descriptive information and its correlational findings. These etiologic hypotheses are the focus of analytic epidemiologic research. An analytic framework allows these descriptive findings to be rigorously examined and tested in observational or experimental study designs. Analytic nutrition epidemiology investigates whether diet exposures are significantly associated with, or have a causal linkage with, health or the risk, progression, or prognosis of disease.

This chapter provides an introduction to analytic nutrition epidemiology. First, an overview of analytic epidemiology is presented with a focus on analytic goals and measures. Next, key issues in designing and implementing analytic nutrition epidemiologic studies are discussed. Finally, analytic epidemiology study designs are covered, including uses, advantages, limitations, implementation issues, analytic considerations, findings, and diet and nutrition examples.

OVERVIEW OF ANALYTIC NUTRITION EPIDEMIOLOGY

Analytic nutrition epidemiology seeks to explain the described occurrence of disease or disease-related phenomena in relation to diet and nutrition.[2] It studies diet and nutrition as potential determinants of population health or disease patterns.[3] It asks if and what diet and nutrition factors independently contribute to, or are likely to cause, the pattern of health or disease identified in the population.

As noted, analytic epidemiologic studies can be classified as observational or experimental. Observational designs study potential health-related relationships as they occur in nature and examine evidence to explain why diseases are distributed the way they are.[4] Observational analytic designs include cross-sectional studies, surveillance studies, cohort studies, and case-control studies. Though descriptive epidemiologic studies also use cross-sectional and surveillance designs, the intent is to report characteristics of occurrences (ie, time, place, and individual traits). Additionally, analytic epidemiology uses experimental or intervention (etiologic) studies where the investigator intervenes and then examines the effect of the intervention on one or more specific health or disease outcomes. Experimental analytic epidemiology designs include randomized controlled trials (RCTs), group-randomized trials, and multicenter RCTs.

Nutrition epidemiology observational investigations examine whether health risks are significantly associated with diet and nutrition exposures.[3,5] Nutrition experimental investigations test whether diet or nutrition exposures are causally linked with health or disease outcomes. The researcher must select the study population and methods appropriate to answer the study question.[6,7]

GOALS OF ANALYTIC EPIDEMIOLOGY

Analytic epidemiology has two specific goals:

- Establish whether a significant association exists between a specific factor and a disease outcome.
- Examine or test evidence for a causal effect of a specific factor on a disease outcome.

Establishing Association

What Is an Association?

The first step in identifying the importance of a factor or exposure to health or disease is to examine whether an association exists between this specific factor/exposure and the disease in question.[1] The

$$\text{Relative risk} = \frac{\text{Cumulative incidence in the exposed}}{\text{Cumulative incidence in the unexposed}}$$

$$\text{Odds ratio} = \frac{\text{Exposed cases} \times \text{Unexposed controls}}{\text{Unexposed cases} \times \text{Exposed controls}}$$

$$\text{Etiologic fraction} = \frac{\text{Exposed cases} - \text{Unexposed cases}}{\text{Exposed cases}}$$

$$\text{Attributable risk} = \text{Cumulative incidence in the exposed} - \text{Cumulative incidence in the unexposed}$$

$$\text{Population attributable risk} = \text{Cumulative incidence in the population} - \text{Cumulative incidence in the unexposed}$$

Box 7.1 Measures of Association

analysis tests whether the risk associated with a particular disease is significantly different based on the presence or level of the factor. It examines the educated guess (hypothesis) that the specific risk factor is associated with a higher than normal or lower than normal risk of having a particular disease, disease prognosis, or disease progression.

What Are Measures of Association?

Epidemiology expresses disease association as risk of disease (see Box 7.1). This risk can be an overall risk or a risk specific to a particular exposure. Terms that express overall risk include risk difference, relative risk, odds ratio (or relative odds). *Risk difference* is the proportion with the disease in the unexposed group compared with the proportion in the exposed group.[6,7] *Relative risk* is the proportion of participants with the disease who have been exposed compared with the proportion not exposed. *Odds ratio*, sometimes called relative odds, is the ratio of the odds of exposure among cases compared with the exposure among controls. The choice of calculating a relative risk or odds ratio depends on the study design; odds ratios are calculated in case-control and cross-sectional studies, and relative risks are calculated in cohort (prospective) studies. Terms that focus on the impact of specific risk exposures (factors) include etiologic fraction, attributable risk, and population attributable risk.[7] The *etiologic fraction* is the proportion of participants exposed to a particular

factor who have the disease. *Attributable risk* is the amount of risk that can be assigned to a particular factor. *Population attributable risk* is the proportion of the disease incidence in a population (both exposed and unexposed) that can be associated with a specific exposure.[7]

What Study Designs Are Used to Study Associations?

Observational study designs can be used to study associations and collect observations of participants but do not include interventions. Epidemiologic observational study designs include cross-sectional studies, surveillance studies, cohort studies, and case-control studies. Cross-sectional studies are studies completed at one point in time (eg, the National Health and Nutrition Examination Surveys [NHANES]); those completed at designated intervals, typically for monitoring purposes (eg, the Pregnancy Nutrition Surveillance System [PNSS]); those that examine the same group of individuals repeatedly over time (eg, cohort studies such as the Coronary Artery Risk Development in Young Adults [CARDIA] study); and case-control studies (eg, the INTERHEART case-control study). Observational studies compare exposed and unexposed groups for case status (cohort studies), cases and noncases (case-control studies) for potential risk factors, or study populations for both case status and potential risk factors (cross-sectional studies and surveillance studies).[1,7] Measures of association are derived from these analyses. For example, data from the 1999 through 2002 NHANES, a cross-sectional study, were used to examine associations between chronic disease status and biomarker levels of nutrients.[8] In the CARDIA cohort, investigators observed lower risk of developing metabolic syndrome in study participants consuming a Mediterranean-style diet over 25 years of follow-up.[9]

Establishing Causation

What Is Causation?

Etiologic epidemiologic studies (ie, studies of disease causation) build on evidence to determine a significant association between a specific factor or exposure and a disease outcome where a possible causal relationship has been suggested. Although an association between exposure and outcome may be found to be statistically significant, this does not mean that the exposure causes the outcome but, rather, that cause is inferred. An experimental study is designed to test whether a causal relationship actually exists between the factor and the disease.

Criteria for Causation

For ethical and logistical reasons, epidemiologic studies are not pure experimental studies. Specific causal criteria have been suggested for epidemiologic studies. The eight classic criteria, commonly called the Bradford Hill criteria, are frequently cited for this purpose (Box 7.2).[10] Hill's first criterion is consistency of the association. Similar associations are found in a variety of studies (with different populations, study designs, and statistical methods). His second criterion is strength of the association. The magnitude of the association between the factor and the disease is significant. As illustrated in Figure 7.1, a relative risk of one indicates that the risk of a disease outcome is the same as expected. A relative risk with factor exposure substantially greater or less than one indicates that the disease outcome is likely to be associated with the factor. Hill's third criterion is specificity of association. A single cause results in a single outcome. With the fourth criterion, the temporal relationship, the exposure or factor precedes the disease outcome. The fifth criterion is evidence for a biological gradient. A dose relationship is seen with a specific threshold, or an increased effect is seen with an increased dose. The sixth criterion is biological plausibility, that is, biological evidence from relevant experiments (eg, in vitro cell systems, animal models, or human metabolic and clinical studies). Hill's seventh criterion is coherence. The causal relationship is congruent with existing knowledge about the disease or condition. The final criterion is evidence from experimentation where specific evidence is provided through controlled experiments, including laboratory studies, animal models, and randomized clinical trials.[7]

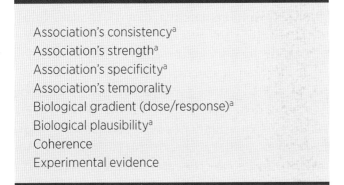

Association's consistency[a]
Association's strength[a]
Association's specificity[a]
Association's temporality
Biological gradient (dose/response)[a]
Biological plausibility[a]
Coherence
Experimental evidence

Box 7.2. Bradford Hill Criteria for Causation[10]

[a] Reduced criteria for diet and nutrition studies agreed upon by Potischman and Weed[11] and the Committee on Diet and Health, Food and Nutrition Board, National Research Council.[12]

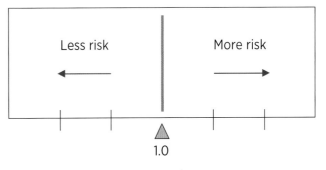

Figure 7.1 Relative risk

EXAMPLE

A highly significant association between salt intake and increase in blood pressure has been widely reported (strength of association). This finding is consistent regardless of the population studied (consistency of association). The association has been found regardless of other potential confounding influences, such as obesity or hypertensive vs clinically normal blood pressure (specificity of association). Higher salt intake has been shown to lead to higher blood pressure, and a reduction in salt intake has lowered blood pressures (temporal relationship). A dose-response relationship has been shown with salt intake: higher intake results in higher blood pressure, and lower intake results in lower blood pressure (biological gradient). Several well-known mechanisms for the salt and blood pressure relationship have been documented (biological plausibility). This association and its underlying mechanisms fit well with existing knowledge about blood pressure response (coherence). A large body of experimental evidence from animal studies and human clinical trials has documented this relationship (evidence from experimentation). An important caveat to this summary is that several key questions remain unresolved regarding the relationship between salt intake and blood pressure.[13] For example, the precise mechanism underlying the salt and blood pressure relationship is not definitively established.[14] Also, susceptible subgroups who elicit an even larger blood pressure response with salt need to be identified. Although evidence is consistent for the sodium and blood pressure association, findings have been inconsistent for the sodium and cardiovascular disease association in studies of various designs and methods.[13,15]

Diet and nutrition studies pose unique challenges in applying causal criteria.[11,12] Evaluation of associations for causal effects in diet and nutrition studies is complex because frequent exceptions to the Bradford Hill criteria are encountered.[2] Diet and nutrition factors have built-in measurement difficulties (eg, measurement error, possible lack of intake variation in population, and intake distributions unrelated to disease processes). Measurement problems can lead to serious underestimates of causal effects or can seem to produce evidence for causal effects that do not exist. Because everyone eats (ie, dietary exposures are common), somewhat small relative risks of 0.7 to 1.5 could be important.[3] In contrast, exposures from environmental contaminants or occupation would be uncommon because they would involve only a subset of the population. Note that there is considerable debate regarding the size of relative risk that should be considered important. Some epidemiologists argue that risks less than 3.0 (ie, three times expected levels) are likely to be spurious. Others argue that relative risks as low as 0.2 (ie, 20% greater than expected levels) may be important if the factor has widespread exposure and is likely to have significant measurement error. Diet exposures would fit that description. Weak associations, however, do not rule out a causal link.[16]

Absolute consistency of findings is not a realistic expectation,[3] and perfect specificity of associations is likely to be rare.[10] This imperfect consistency and specificity could be due to the complexity of the disease process, the imprecision of diet assessment and self-reported dietary intake, or the specific effects of diet components on organ systems or the disease processes.[12] Dose-response relationships are likely to be "nonlinear or almost any shape depending on the starting point on a hypothetical spectrum of exposure."[3] Thus, typical analytic approaches may not detect underlying relationships. Also, a clear dose-response relationship might easily be the result of bias or confounding.[3]

Arguments supporting biological plausibility that are developed "post hoc, should be viewed cautiously because they can usually be developed for most observations, including those that are later refuted."[3] Well-defined mechanisms are lacking for most cancers and many other chronic diseases.[3] This fact hampers the ability to meet criteria for biological plausibility and coherence for diet and nutrition studies. Finally, experimental studies, particularly in humans, might provide key evidence for causal relationships. However, practical considerations (eg, time and money constraints) and ethical considerations limit such investigations.

EXAMPLE

In the early 1990s, the US Food and Drug Administration reviewed evidence for the relationship between periconceptional folic acid intake and neural tube defects (NTDs) and subsequently implemented a policy for folic acid fortification of flours and cereals in the United States. Evidence from case-control studies and a prospective cohort study supported a consistent and strong association between occurrence of NTD and lower folic acid intakes, status, or both. A dose-response relationship was supported for prevention of NTD in women who have never had a child with NTD and women who previously delivered a child with NTD. The temporality criterion was met because folic acid supplementation appeared effective only when given during the critical neural tube fetal developmental period. Some experimental data were available from human studies (one British, one Chinese). Both provided credible evidence that folic acid supplementation in the periconceptional period significantly reduced the occurrence of NTDs in women who had previously delivered a baby with NTD (the British study) and those without such a history (the Chinese study). Although a 1996 critique[17] pointed to shortcomings in these experiments, newer, randomized double-blind supplement studies of folic acid alone are unlikely to be done because of ethical considerations.[1] Nonetheless, evidence supporting biological plausibility for folate and NTDs has continued to mount.[17,18] The positive outcomes in the wake of folate fortification have been substantial, including a reduction in the United States prevalence of folate deficiencies[19,20] and a substantial reduction in NTDs.[21]

In light of these many concerns, it has been strongly suggested that applying all Bradford Hill criteria to diet and nutrition studies is too stringent.[11,12] Instead, a minimum set of causal criteria has been recommended. This minimum set would include consistency of findings, strength of association, dose response, biological plausibility, and temporality. The Committee on Diet and Health (Food and Nutrition Board of the National Academy of Sciences) used this reduced set of criteria for its land-

mark publication *Diet and Health: Implications for Reducing Chronic Disease Risk* (see Box 7.2 page 105).[12]

Study Designs to Study Causation

Like other scientific disciplines, epidemiology uses experimental designs to study causation. In these studies, the investigator randomizes participants to a treatment or no treatment (control) group. General study designs (and relevant issues) for examining causation are discussed in detail in Chapters 2, 8 and 10 and elsewhere in this book. Epidemiologic investigations also include designs that involve multiple study centers and extended follow-up as well as designs that randomize groups rather than individuals to treatment or control status. In the case of multicenter studies with long-term follow-up, disease outcomes are compared for each randomization group controlled for center-specific effects. In the case of studies that randomly assign groups, disease outcomes are compared for each group rather than for each individual.

CONCEPTS IN ANALYTIC NUTRITION EPIDEMIOLOGIC STUDIES

Issues relevant to any analytic nutrition epidemiology study design include the analytic question, selection of the study population, choice of diet or nutrient exposures (or both together), problems resulting from poor exposure measurements, potential for other biases, and potential for confounding and multivariate relationships between diet and disease.

The Analytic Nutrition Epidemiology Question

From an epidemiologic perspective, diet and nutrition can be viewed as key factors that potentially influence health and disease or as a specific health/disease outcome. Nutrition studies often examine dietary intake/nutritional status as an outcome and analyze data for determinants of those outcomes. In epidemiologic studies, diet and nutrition are commonly studied as independent contributing factors/exposures (association) or independent etiologic factors/exposures (causation) of health/disease outcomes.

Diet or Nutrient as an Exposure

The term *exposure* refers to a factor's dose (ie, amount and concentration along with duration of exposure). To determine exposure, a method of measurement is needed that will sufficiently capture differences that truly exist.[1,3] The method or instrument used to assess dietary intake or nutritional status needs to capture measurements of potential active agents and their doses. Dietary exposure measurements are challenging and have been an active area of research for more than five decades.[3] Investigations of food-safety problems often use food information from one point in time. Investigations of chronic diseases, which are major causes of debilitation and death, require diet or nutrient exposures or both captured over an extended period of intake behavior. The term *usual intake* is often used to connote this type of diet exposure. Usual intake is difficult to capture in the heterogeneous US population, given the rapidly changing food marketplace and Americans' enthusiasm for changing food choices. Given existing measurement problems, investigators are encouraged to include more than one dietary assessment method or use other related measures of exposure, such as biological (eg, blood or urine) or molecular (eg, genetic) markers.[22,23] New approaches are being developed and studied. Various aspects of measurement methods for diet and nutrient exposures are discussed in Chapter 5.

The exposure measurement is meant to provide a reliable, accurate, and valid measurement of dietary intake or nutritional status exposure. Reliability is the characteristic in which repeated measurements done in a steady-state period yield similar results. *Accuracy* indicates that systematic error is minimized in the measurement.[3,6,7] *Validity* is the degree to which a test is capable of measuring what it is intended to measure.[3,6,7] None of these qualities can be corrected by increased sample size. To increase confidence in the reliability of the test, each participant can be tested at least twice.[3,6] Random error may be mitigated through careful measurement and large sample size. However, even then, random error cannot be completely eliminated and may be due to individual biological variation or residual sampling.[6,7]

Other considerations regarding diet or nutritional status exposure are important to the study design. Evidence for sufficient variation in diet or nutrient intake is needed. If everyone ate the same way, no differences in outcome with diet would be detected.[3,7] The latency period between diet exposure and disease outcome is needed. A negative result from a 5-year cohort study might be due to a latency period of 10 years or longer between diet exposure and disease outcome. Also, there may be a critical exposure period for a particular diet and disease relationship. For example, the critical period may be in childhood, with the disease manifesting in adulthood.[3] As previously described in the example, adequate folate intake before conception may reduce the risk of developing NTDs.[21] Finally, the effects of dietary intake or nutritional status exposure may be acute and transient rather than long term. For example, a double-blind placebo-controlled study found a significant lowering of blood pressure in the group supplemented with potassium compared with the placebo group after 6 weeks, but no blood pressure differences were found at 12 weeks.[24]

Choice of Nutrition Exposure Variable(s)

Nutrition can be represented as a single food or nutrient, components of these (eg, bioactive food element or active nutrient metabolite), groups of foods or nutrient classes, combinations of these groupings (either investigator determined or derived with statistical grouping methods), a score or scores based on specific criteria or as a marker that indicates that a particular critical diet/nutrient threshold has been met (ie, a biomarker). Deciding which exposure variable to investigate is pivotal and should be based on an a priori hypothesis since this choice can largely determine whether any true effect can be detected.[25] However, choice of diet assessment instrument is largely determined by the study question, study design, feasibility, ability of study participants, time available to administer the instrument, and budget.

If exposure variables are derived from the diet assessment instrument, diet assessment methods are important but problematic because they are complex, difficult, and imperfect. However, standardized collection methodology, research quality food-nutrient databases, and standardized coding and data processing mitigate some of these problems. Additionally, ongoing biometric advances have generated methods for performing adjustments to facilitate estimation of diet influences.[22,26-30]

Brief diet assessment methods, such as the food frequency questionnaire (FFQ), enjoy wide usage in epidemiologic studies because they minimize collection expense and participant burden, and many are formatted for automated scanners. Further, FFQs typically characterize usual food and beverage intake over a selected time period, usually the previous year. However, FFQs have intrinsic challenges.[31] Nevertheless, several FFQs have been constructed and are currently in use. Checklists are another brief diet assessment instrument that may be used to assess compliance in RCTs.[32] More comprehensive diet assessment instruments include the diet history, where usual dietary intake is obtained for a selected time period. Food records and the 24-hour recall interview obtain detailed information about dietary intake for the previous day, but multiple records are needed to characterize usual intake. It is essential that the diet assessment instrument selected for the study fits the population to be studied. For example, if that population includes important subgroups, such as Hispanics, Asians, and blacks, with each group having unique food choice behaviors, the question of whether and how much to tailor the FFQ or other diet assessment instrument is important.[33] Also important is whether the tailored FFQ should be validated. Pilot data would be important to answer these questions. Companion calibration studies are recommended for studies using FFQs.[22,23] These collect detailed dietary intake information from a subgroup to adjust FFQ intake estimates. Alternatively, or in addition, blood or urine markers of nutrient intakes and biomarkers related to nutrient intakes are recommended.[3,22,23] Furthermore, promising technologies, including metabolomics and gut microbiota analyses, continue to contribute to our understanding of the role that usual dietary intake and nutritional status play in health and disease.[34,35] Finally, improvements in collected dietary data have been achieved through training and cognitive insights developed from research in these areas.[36]

Regardless of the method used to generate diet/nutrition data, the underlying problem is the role that diet/nutrition plays in the development of disease outcomes, which is still under study, as are mechanisms for disease outcomes. Illustrative of this are supplement studies of single nutrients with strong evidence from observational studies and with well-defined mechanisms. Surprisingly, supplemented nutrients have not consistently predicted protective action with their associated disease processes. For example, in a large beta carotene supplement study of smokers, the supplemented group had a greater risk of developing lung cancer than the control group.[37] In another large study, increased dietary fiber intakes did not reduce the risk of recurring adenomatous colon polyps, a precursor lesion to colon cancer.[38] Some researchers have suggested that the nutrients or food components investigated in these studies were not the active players or had minor roles compared with others that were not studied. For example, recent analyses suggest that risk of colon cancer may be more strongly associated with folate intake than fiber intake.[39] Alternatively, the nutrient or food component that was analyzed could be part of a group that in concert represents the active unit. In the case of the dietary fiber study, recent analyses from the aforementioned study have identified dried beans as the potential active unit.[40] Another possibility is that the tested nutrient or food component is effective only in a subgroup. For example, in one report, the protective effect of dietary fiber on colon cancer risk was only seen in men.[41]

Interest in the technique of diet patterning has reemerged,[42] with positive findings from diet pattern trials like those testing the Mediterranean diet and the Dietary Approaches to Stop Hypertension (DASH) pattern. The patterns approach, therefore, may have an increased likelihood of capturing active diet/nutrition elements. The concept behind diet patterning is that empirically derived, objective, distinct food choices can be discerned with statistical techniques.[43] The method attempts to examine the effect of the diet as a whole rather than to examine the effect of a particular food/nutrient or food/nutrient component. Techniques such as factor analysis, principal components, and cluster analyses have been used for this purpose. The approach is appealing given the background of failed trials of single nutrients and diet components, the multiplicity of foods and nutrients associated with a single disease entity, and the variety of foods consumed by persons with low or high disease risk. The quality of the diet may be assessed using diet scores. For example, the Healthy Eating Index-2015 is a score characterizing adherence to the 2015 Dietary Guidelines for Americans.[44] Finally, proponents of these patterning methods suggest a future where healthy eating patterns may be derived through use of these techniques.[45] Publications about dietary patterns, however, have received mixed reviews. Some critics argue that these studies have not generated any new hypotheses[46] but rather identify patterns very similar to ones that might be constructed from general healthy eating advice. Other researchers suggest that the approach may be more productive than more traditional methods.[45] Because renewed diet patterning efforts are relatively recent, future advances in application of these techniques may provide those newer insights.

Problems Resulting from Poor Exposure Measurements

In analytic epidemiology studies, poor assessment of exposure (ie, dietary intake) in the study population will make it impossible to detect existing associations between exposure and outcome. Poor measurement of exposure or outcome can lead to findings of an association where none exists or an association in the opposite direction.[6,7] Diet and disease studies have inherent problems. Because of the limited range of dietary variation within most populations, in combination with the inevitable error in measuring intake (ie, self-reported dietary intake is susceptible to underreporting or overreporting of selected foods and beverages), very modest relative risks (0.5 to 2.0) are usually found for diet effects. Because dietary intakes are an obligatory human behavior (in other words, everyone eats), even small risks associated with diet should be important.[3] If risks were large,

less precise exposure measures would capture those differences. However, smaller risks would require more refined exposure measures. Willett[3] notes that typical dietary intake differences between cases and controls are only about 5%, and even a systematic error of 3% to 4% would seriously distort such a relationship. Furthermore, measurement errors would dilute or conceal any effect of diet on health/disease outcomes in experimental studies.

Potential for Other Biases

Systematic errors are also possible in epidemiologic studies through selection bias, other measurement bias, and analytic bias. Systematic errors are errors that occur regularly, occur in the same direction, and are reproducible. Methodologic sources of bias can obscure an existing relationship.[3,6,7] Selection bias occurs when there is a systematic difference between the characteristics of individuals chosen for the study and individuals who are not chosen for the study. For example, having a particular disease may reduce a person's chance of being selected for a study.[6,7] Several other participant selection biases are possible. The healthy-workers bias may be encountered in occupational epidemiology studies, where working individuals are likely to be healthier than individuals who are not working. There may be an increased likelihood that healthier or health-conscious and motivated individuals agree to participate in studies (volunteers' bias). An incidence-prevalence bias (Neyman bias) occurs where there is a loss of cases (by death or recovery) due to significant periods of time between exposure and development of the disorder.[3] Finally, spurious differences between exposure and the disease can be due to differential hospitalization of cases and those without the disease with the exposure (Berkson bias).[7]

Measurement bias occurs when individual measurements or classifications of disease or exposure are inaccurate. Measurement bias that occurs equally in the groups being compared (nondifferential bias) almost always results in an underestimate of the true strength of the relationship.[17] Recall bias can occur when the participant is aware of the study hypothesis. An information bias can occur where different quality or extent of information is obtained from exposed vs nonexposed participants.[1] A related problem is the Hawthorne effect,[4] where participants' performance changes because they are being studied. Measurement implementation problems can also occur (eg, quality control bias and nonstandardized measurement bias).[6] Blinding (where participants and research staff are unaware of whether participants are assigned to the treatment or the control group) is used in experimental studies to obviate participant measurement bias. Because knowledge about exposure status may bias assessment, outcome assessors may also be blinded to participant assignments or exposure status.[1]

Bias may also be encountered in the analysis phase. Unintentional bias may occur when analyzing data and interpreting study findings if the investigators have strong study preconceptions or financial conflicts of interest.[1,6] Finally, funding or sponsorship bias may influence the interpretation of study findings if the investigators are sympathetic to the sponsor's interests.

Potential for Confounding

As illustrated in Figure 7.2, confounding relationships are relationships where the exposure of interest is related to another factor that is also influencing the outcome of interest. With confounding, the association can be explained by another factor associated with both the exposure and the disease. Confounding is not strictly a type of bias because it does not result from systematic error in research design. Confounding occurs when there is a nonrandom distribution of risk factors in the source population that also occurs in the study population.[6,7] For example, smoking can confound a relationship between coffee drinking and a disease outcome because individuals who drink coffee may be more likely to smoke.[1] Confounders can obscure or exaggerate existing associations.[6,7] Another possibility is that an unmeasured third variable was related to the exposure and disease in an opposite direction, resulting in negative confounding.[3,7]

The inability to control for confounding is a major limitation of descriptive epidemiologic findings. Analytic studies are designed to consider potential confounding factors when testing associations or causal relationships between key factors and disease outcomes. Analytic studies accomplish this goal through design features (eg, randomization, restriction, and matching) and analysis strategies (eg, stratification and statistical modeling). In experimental studies, randomization can be used to randomly distribute confounders to treatment and control groups. Restriction limits the study to individuals who have particular characteristics. In case-control studies, controls are selected by matching them to cases on potential confounding factors to ensure that

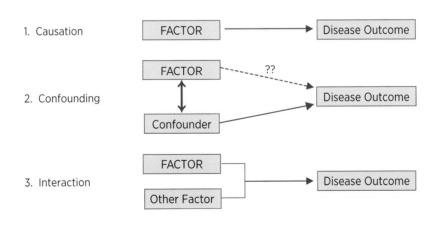

Figure 7.2 Comparison of predictive values

EXAMPLE

The following study illustrates a potential interaction between smoking and serum carotenoids in relation to incident diabetes. A subset (n = 4,493) of study participants enrolled in the Coronary Artery Risk Development in Young Adults (CARDIA) study[48] was examined. CARDIA was a large (n = 5,115), multicenter, prospective, epidemiologic study of black and white young adults that studied the development of cardiovascular disease risk. The subset of participants included in the analysis had baseline data for smoking status, serum carotenoids, plasma glucose, and known confounding factors; had completed follow-up surveys; and did not have diabetes at baseline. After 15 years of follow-up, 148 were diagnosed with diabetes. After adjusting for race, sex, study center, age, education, systolic blood pressure, ethanol intake, calorie intake, energy expenditure, vitamin supplement use, and serum lipids, researchers found that serum carotenoid levels were significantly inversely related to diabetes incidence, but only in nonsmokers. In other words, current smoking modified the relation between carotenoid levels and risk of developing diabetes.

confounders are evenly distributed in the two groups being compared.[6,7,23]

Potential for Effect Modification

An effect modifier (ie, an interaction) is a third variable that alters the association between an exposure and a disease outcome (see Figure 7.2 on page 111).[47] With effect modification, the exposure may not have the same effect in all settings or subgroups of the population.[28] For example, diet studies often separate sex and age groups because diet may have a different effect on a particular outcome for these subgroups. Sex and age, in these cases, are considered effect modifiers. Other effect modifiers may include genetic factors. A design strategy would be to randomize participants to ensure that groups are balanced or to match controls on effect modifier variables. In large studies, it is usually preferable to control for confounding in the analytic phase. Stratified analyses are performed where measures of the strength of association are examined in well-defined and homogeneous categories (strata) of the confounding variable.[6,7] Note, however, that diet and nutrition variables can also be effect modifiers. For example, the effect of a drug treatment on a disease might be enhanced or diminished as the result of diet or nutrition.

Multivariate Relationship of Diet and Disease

Willett[3] cautions that diet and disease relationships are likely to be "extremely complex for both biologic and behavioral reasons." Food and nutrients are biologically complex. Nutrients are largely provided by foods, and foods typically contain a variety of nutrients. Not surprisingly, specific nutrients tend to be intercorrelated. Nutrient-to-nutrient interactions occur where the effect of one nutrient depends on the level of another. What we eat and the quantity eaten are also related to other health-related but nondiet factors, such as age, sex, occupation, and behaviors (eg, smoking and exercise). All of these can distort, modify, or confound relationships of diet and disease.

Multivariate statistical methods are needed to tease out and clarify the effect of diet and nutrition on outcomes. Nonetheless, these effects can be complicated. Willett[3] points to the example of the effect of obesity on cardiovascular disease (CVD). When obesity is examined in a multivariate model that includes serum lipids, blood pressure, glucose tolerance, and body fat, the effect of obesity on CVD is diminished because obesity is likely to also be acting through the other factors. In other words, because of inherent data problems, multivariate methods are not foolproof in discerning diet/nutrient effects. Rather, new study designs and analytic modeling strategies are needed.

ANALYTIC EPIDEMIOLOGIC STUDY DESIGNS

The following sections describe the three types of analytic epidemiologic study designs: cross-sectional studies, cohort studies, and case-control studies. Table 7.1 shows the advantages and disadvantages of these observational study designs.

Characteristic	Cross-Sectional	Case-Control	Cohort
Relatively cost efficient	Yes	Yes	No
Relatively short duration	Yes	Yes	No
Able to determine time sequence of events	No	Unclear	Yes
Small sample size	Yes	Yes	No
Differential measurement bias	No	Yes	No
Yields prevalence	Yes	No	Yes
Yields incidence, relative risk	No	No	Yes
Useful to study rare outcomes	No	Yes	No
More bias/confounding because there are two samples	No	Yes	No
Only one outcome can be studied	No	Yes	No
Hypothesis generating	Yes	No	Yes
Useful to study many exposures/outcomes	Yes	No	Yes
Avoids dropouts from long-term follow-up	Yes	Yes	No

Table 7.1 Advantages and Disadvantages of Observational Study Designs[6]

Observational Study Designs for Examining Associations: Cross-Sectional Studies

Cross-sectional epidemiologic studies, also called prevalence studies or surveys, are those where participants are measured at approximately the same point in time.[49] Both the exposure to a particular risk factor and disease outcome (case status) are determined at the same time.[1,6] Although generally used for descriptive studies, they can also provide suggestive analytic information. Cross-sectional study data are commonly used to provide evidence for possible risk factors for disease outcomes.[1]

Advantages and Disadvantages of Cross-Sectional Studies

The key advantage of cross-sectional studies is that they are relatively simple and inexpensive because neither follow-up measures nor treatments are required.[6] However, several inherent problems make cross-sectional studies of limited utility in studying causal inference.[6,7,49] Because measurements are taken only at one point, the temporal relationship between exposure and disease outcomes cannot be tested.[1,6] The problem of reverse causality bias can occur where the disease outcome appears to precede the exposure in time.[6,7,49] Furthermore, cross-

sectional studies are likely to include survivors and new cases,[1] so early disease-related deaths are missed.

Cross-Sectional Study Implementation Issues

Key challenges in implementing cross-sectional studies include the ability to ensure and verify reasonable sample representativeness,[3,6] the ability to capture cases (those with the disease outcome of interest),[1,6] and the ability to capture adequate variation in key exposure variables.[4] Several analytic cautions are needed in examining cross-sectional data. Associations found may be related to survival rather than to disease development.[1] Furthermore, because early disease-related deaths would result in lost cases, there would be a reduced ability to find significant relationships between exposure and disease outcome.

Types of Findings in Cross-Sectional Studies

Associations between exposures or risk factors and disease outcomes can be suggested. In such studies, study participants with and without the disease can be examined in relation to exposures, other potential risk factors, or both. Cross-sectional studies identify factors that may affect the level of a risk factor.[6,7] The NHANES series provides examples of cross-sectional studies.[2]

Cross-sectional studies can also be multicentered. The International Study of Salt and Blood Pressure (INTERSALT), conducted in 52 population samples worldwide, tested whether salt intake (as assessed by urinary sodium levels) was associated with higher blood pressures.[50] INTERSALT found a linear positive relationship between sodium and blood pressure regardless of whether the participant was normotensive or hypertensive. Also, it found a rise in blood pressure with age only in those samples with higher salt intakes.

Suggestive evidence for the influence of other nutrients (eg, protein) on blood pressure led to the subsequent International Population Study on Macronutrients and Blood Pressure (INTERMAP),[51] a population-based epidemiologic investigation in 20 diverse samples from four countries (Japan, China, the United Kingdom, and the United States) from men and women aged 40 to 59 years. Two sets of consecutive 2-day, 24-hour recalls were collected for each participant, and dietary supplements were recorded in detail from patient interviews and supplement labels. Also collected were 24-hour urine specimens coinciding with day two of each recall pair. INTERMAP found that vegetable protein intakes were associated with lower blood pressures and animal protein intakes with higher blood pressures.[52] Further, analyses have shown that in INTERMAP, lower levels of education—frequently linked with higher blood pressure—were also associated with dietary intakes that typically lead to higher blood pressures.[53]

Observational Study Designs for Examining Associations: Cohort Studies

Cohort studies track health information of participants over a period of time.[51] They focus on disease development and survival or mortality[1,6,7] and allow the study of the natural history of disease.[49] An important feature of the cohort design is its time perspective on exposures. Concurrent cohort designs assess exposures as they occur during the study, but these studies are the most expensive.[1,6] Retrospective studies examine exposures backward in time, and prospective studies look forward in time for exposures. A combined approach determines past exposure and provides follow-up of future exposures.[1] Cohort studies are feasible for the study of common diseases where the exposure to risk factor(s) results in a measurable disease outcome within a reasonable time after the exposure. For practical reasons, cohort studies are not suitable for diseases with long latency periods (eg, 20 years) or for rare diseases requiring extraordinarily large sample sizes.[54]

Advantages and Disadvantages of Cohort Studies

Cohort studies offer several advantages. They can examine whether there is a temporal relationship between the exposure and the disease. Furthermore, they can provide direct information on the temporal sequence of events[6,7,51] and can establish timing and directionality of events.[6] Prospective cohort studies enable the measurement of dietary intake before disease onset.[3] Cohort studies are easier and less costly to conduct than experimental studies.[6] Finally, cohort studies can evaluate many diseases and exposures simultaneously.[54] Cohort study designs have several disadvantages. Although they are less complex and costly than experimental studies, cohort studies are nonetheless expensive, resource intensive, and difficult because they require the monitoring of large numbers of participants over an extended period.[54] Additionally, they are ill suited for studies with rare exposures, rare outcomes, or long latency periods.[47]

Cohort selection, recruitment, and retention are challenging, and selecting a random sample for the cohort is particularly tricky.[6] Individuals who refuse to volunteer may have particular characteristics, and their nonparticipation may bias the results.[7] If exposure is widespread, it may be difficult to find nonexposed individuals.[6,7] Groups may differ at the beginning of the study (the problem of confounding).[49] Over the course of the study, participants may change their behavior because they are being studied or their exposure to the factor of interest may change.[54] With long studies, participant nonresponse and loss to follow-up are likely problems.[1,6] If the loss to follow-up is correlated with disease, risks associated with exposure will be diminished. If this loss is correlated with exposure, risk estimates will be biased.[6,7]

Cohort Study Implementation Issues

Cohort studies are warranted when there is sufficient evidence that exposure leads to disease (eg, clinical observations, case-control studies) and a relatively short interval between exposure and development of disease.[1] However, there may be disagreement on what constitutes strong evidence, and diseases of interest may have low rates of occurrence.[1] To obviate problems with participant recall of exposures,[54,55] retrospective studies are possible if there are appropriate and adequate past records.[1] There are practical limits, however, because even common diseases such as heart disease require a cohort size in the thousands.[6,7]

It is increasingly common for large intervention studies to mount postintervention follow-up studies of participants after the main studies have been completed. Examples of these types of cohort studies include the Multiple Risk Factor Intervention Trial,[56] the Modification of Diet in Renal Disease study,[57] and the Trials of Hypertension Prevention study.[58] For example, 7 years after the Trials of Hypertension Prevention phase 1 study ended, Baltimore investigators[59] recontacted Baltimore participants and ascertained their hypertension status; measured their blood pressure, height, and weight; and collected 24-hour urine samples for sodium and creatinine measurement. About 40% had developed hypertension. However, the investigators found that participants who had previously lost weight and reduced sodium had 77% and 35% lower odds, respectively, of developing hypertension compared with controls. Approximately 19% of weight-loss participants and 22.4% of sodium-reduction participants had developed hypertension.

Among the analytic considerations in cohort studies, assessment of the disease outcome and selection of the nonexposed comparison group are key. Because there may be changes over time in relevant criteria and methods of assessment, ensuring comparability of repeated measures is crucial.[1] Key information on participants lost to follow-up (eg,

EXAMPLE

The Atherosclerosis Risk in Communities (ARIC) study, which examined the association between diet soda and incident end-stage renal disease (ESRD), is an example of a prospective population-based cohort study.[61] In this analysis, 15,369 black and white men and women aged 45 to 64 years and without ESRD at baseline from 1987 to 1989 were studied and followed through 2012. Dietary intake was assessed by a 66-item food frequency questionnaire at baseline and 6 years later. ESRD was defined as the initiation of kidney transplant or dialysis as identified by linkage with the US Renal Data System registry. In multivariate Cox proportional hazards regression, adjusting for demographic characteristics, physical activity, smoking, body mass index, energy intake, diabetes, systolic blood pressure, and estimated glomerular filtration rate, those consuming five to seven glasses of diet soda per week had an 80% higher risk of developing ESRD than those consuming less than one drink per week. In another study, diet soda was associated with incident metabolic syndrome.[63] The underlying mechanism that diet soda or artificial sweeteners may promote disease can be explained by the effect of artificial sweeteners on glucose intolerance via the microbiome as demonstrated in an animal model.[64] Further studies are warranted to elucidate whether these findings hold up over time.

disease occurrence or death) is important to capture. Specific analyses are required to account for such losses.

Types of Findings in Cohort Studies

In cohort studies, exposed and nonexposed groups measured at baseline and followed over time are compared for disease incidence or death. Data are collected at two or more distinct time points (at baseline and follow-up). Study participants presumably are comparable from one period to the next.[60] Data are compared between and among these periods, specifically for the incidence of disease (or new occurrence of the disease outcome) in participants exposed and not exposed to the risk factors of interest.

Measurements generated express the proportion of the exposed who get the disease (or die) compared with those not exposed. These measurements can be in terms of relative risks, odds ratios, and attributable risk ratios.[1,7] Cohort studies are usually prospective (ie, follow-up is forward in time) but can also be retrospective (ie, prior history is examined). The following example describes a prospective nutrition epidemiology study.[61] For an example of a retrospective nutrition epidemiology cohort study refer to the Vitamin and Lifestyle (VITAL) study.[62]

Observational Study Designs for Examining Associations: Case-Control Studies

Popular among epidemiologists examining diet and nutrition questions, the case-control design, examines cases (persons with the disease studied) and controls (those without the disease) for risk factor or prior exposure differences.[1,6,54] Controls are matched with cases on characteristics correlated with possible disease causes. These characteristics are not independent causes but are involved in the pathway through which the possible causes of interest lead to disease. Compared with a cohort study, which starts with exposure, a case-control study starts with identification of persons with a disease. Case-control studies compare individuals with and without a disease, whereas cohort studies examine exposed and nonexposed individuals. Case-control studies are well suited for studies of rare disorders and studies where the lag time between exposure and outcome is long.[7,49]

Advantages and Disadvantages of Case-Control Studies

Case-control studies offer several advantages. They are relatively quick and inexpensive, and they require smaller sample sizes than cross-sectional or cohort studies. Because investigators can set the criteria for selecting controls, they can untangle potential confounding factors and interactions more precisely.[1,54,55] Matching increases reliability and decreases the study costs.[6,55] Case-control studies also have a number of disadvantages. By design, case-control studies can investigate only one disease outcome. Information about relevant exposures may be problematic, and there may be significant differences in quality of information; that is, cases may be researched more thoroughly than controls.[54] Cases and controls are likely to have different recall of specific exposures and events relevant to the studied disease outcome.[6] For example, illness can affect recall of diet.[3] Reliance on records to determine exposure may be equally inadequate for determining exposure. Furthermore, because case-control studies do not involve a time sequence, it is not possible to demonstrate temporal causality between specific exposures and disease outcomes.[54]

Other disadvantages of case-control studies arise from their intrinsic complexity. The selection of cases and controls, although seemingly straightforward, is challenging. Case-control studies can suffer from bias error, given the problem of sampling controls.[54] Selection of controls is an ongoing area of methodologic concern.[49] Finding suitable control matches is especially difficult where multiple matching factors are required. Here the matching variable is related to the risk factor or disease under study but is not a true confounder or is so highly correlated with other matching variables as to be superfluous. Overmatching results in loss of efficiency and may also result in bias.[54]

Another disadvantage is that specific complex analyses are required for case-control data. Data analysis for matched analyses is more complex to compute and understand. Furthermore, any variable used as a matching variable cannot be estimated.[1,54] For example, if controls were matched on age and race, it would not be possible to examine the effect of age or race on the disease studied.

Case-Control Study Implementation Issues

Selecting cases and controls for case-control studies is a critical but complex issue. Given the problem of case misclassification, investigators need to specify how cases are identified or ascertained.[1,55] Case selection should be based on a formulated, precise disease definition[7,54] with inclusion and exclusion criteria specified to increase the likelihood of exposure to the risk factor of interest.[1,54] New (incident) cases are preferred because the risk factor being studied may be avoided by those who already have the condition (ie, existing cases). For example, diet changes may occur after diagnosis. Additionally, cases may be lost before or soon after diagnosis, and cases found may reflect survival rather than illness.[1,54]

A reliable source for cases needs to be identified, such as hospitals, primary care practices, clinics, and health maintenance organizations.[54] Disease-specific patient registries are an additional case source. However, case selection from a single source can be problematic. The patient population is likely to reflect referral patterns or other local factors and limit the ability to generalize study findings to other patients with that disease. For example, cases from a tertiary care facility may be severely ill,[1] whereas other cases may be less ill or have less complicated illnesses.

Controls are defined as persons who had an equal chance of exposure to a risk factor or had some potential for getting the disease but do not have the disease.[54] Ideally, controls are similar to cases in all respects other than having the disease in question. Conceptually, controls are representative of individuals without the disease from the same population as the cases. Controls are selected to match specific characteristics of cases, such as age, race, sex, or socioeconomic status.[1,6] The purpose of matching is to adjust for potential confounding. Cases and controls may have many differences besides exposure. Matched characteristics are those that potentially influence the disease outcome and are also related to the exposure being studied. For example, age and sex are commonly used matching factors because they often influence disease status. Controls are selected to match case characteristics that are of concern. Matching, by direct control of confounders, may reduce the required sample size or would support the use of a shorter exposure period for a risk factor.

Ideally, the controls selected would be a probability sample (ie, a random sample representative of the population). Recruitment can be resource intensive because only 60% to 70% of control eligibles are likely to complete study interviews.[3] In practice, controls are recruited from various sources. Hospital controls and controls drawn from patient care lists are convenient, are inexpensive, and presumably can provide comparable medical data. However, this source is not foolproof given the likelihood of differential rates of hospitalization (Berkson bias[3,7]) and potentially similar exposure to risk factors with different diseases[54]—for example, the use of antioxidant supplements for CVD and cancer.

Community controls are recruited from the same population as cases. Sources include school rosters, selective service lists, and insurance company lists, for example. Random-digit dialing is frequently used to draw a random community sample because the first three digits of telephone numbers generally match neighborhood boundaries. However, with high prevalence of cell phone use in the population, random-digit dialing may no longer be a feasible strategy for recruitment. However, the random-sampling frame is difficult, expensive, and time consuming to obtain.[54] Whatever recruitment frame is used, volunteers tend to be health conscious[4] and are not actually representative of the population. Other options include a "best friend" control, who is usually similar in age and other demographic and social characteristics. Alternatively, spouses or siblings (genetic controls) are sometimes used.

Some studies use multiple controls per case. These controls can all be of the same type or different types. In general, the greater number of controls per case, the greater precision in estimates and tests.[1] Power (one measure of precision) increases as the number of controls increases for a fixed number of cases.[6,7] Nonetheless, precision improvements are small beyond a case-to-control ratio greater than 1:4. Controls of a different type might be used for specific analyses.[1] For example, the investigator might be interested in using hospital controls to control for the effect of hospitalization but would also want neighborhood controls to control for social or environmental influences.

Alternative Case-Control Study Designs

Other approaches to the case-control design have been used, including nested case-control studies and the frequency matching approach. In the nested case-control study design, cases are identified from an ongoing cohort study, and controls are drawn from that same study. Cases and controls, therefore, are identified from the same cohort.[6,7,54] Baseline and follow-up data on exposures, risk factors, and disease status have already been collected from the cohort study. Cases are identified during the course of follow-up, and controls are selected from the cohort.[1] This design combines the efficiencies and strengths of the cohort and case-control designs. The Harvard studies (the Physicians' Health Study, Nurses' Health Study, and Health Professionals' Health Study), the Western Electric Study, and the Cardiovascular Health Study have used the nested case-control design with their cohorts.

Technically, frequency matching is not a case-control design. As such, it does not require the stringent analysis procedures of that type of design. This approach ensures that the control and case samples have a similar makeup.[54] Control matching is done so that the proportion with a certain characteristic is similar among cases and controls (group or frequency matching); for example, women comprise 50% of cases and controls.[1] With this type of matching, controls are selected after all of the cases are identified.[1]

Analytic Considerations in Case-Control Studies

The drawback to matching is that the matching factor's effect on the outcome cannot be estimated. For example, if marital status is a matching factor, distribution of marital status between cases and controls would be the same. Specific techniques for analyzing case-control data are detailed in several epidemiology methods texts. Refer to these for in-depth instructions in performing more advanced analyses beyond general odds ratios.

Types of Findings in Case-Control Studies

The case-control analysis generates an estimate of relative risk, known as the *odds ratio*, for having the disease with a specific exposure level or risk factor. Additionally, this type of analysis can provide an estimate of the attributable risk associated with the specific exposure level or risk factor.[49]

An example of a case-control study with hospital cases and population-based controls is presented next.[65] Refer to Kelemen and colleagues[66] for an example of a case-control study where both cases and controls are drawn from the population. Refer to

> ### EXAMPLE
>
> In a case-control study, investigators used a food frequency questionnaire to examine dietary intake, specifically *trans* fatty acid intake, in a series of hospital cases with age (within 5 years) and sex-matched controls randomly selected from residence rolls from the patient's town (population-based controls).[65] The cases were 239 patients with myocardial infarctions (MIs) who were admitted to six local hospitals. Controls were 282 individuals without a history of MI or angina. After controlling for age and energy intake, the highest quintile (compared with the lowest quintile) of *trans* fatty acid intakes was associated with a significantly higher risk of coronary heart disease (CHD) (odds ratio = 2.4; 95% confidence interval = 1.4 to 4.2). This means the odds of having an MI was 2.4 times greater in persons in the highest quintile of *trans* fatty acid intake compared with those in the first quintile (or referent group) and that the researchers are 95% confident the true value falls between 1.4 and 4.2. This relationship was still significant after controlling for other CHD risk factors and other dietary variables, including other fats, dietary cholesterol, vitamins C and E, carotene, and fiber. Because the intakes of cases were assessed after the patients had been hospitalized, the authors assessed the possibility that the hospitalization and MI diagnosis influenced recall of the usual diet. The investigators excluded individuals who reported that they had had high cholesterol before their MI, those who had changed their intake of butter to margarine in the previous 10 years, or those who were on a special diet.

Chasen-Taber and colleagues[67] for an example of a nested-case control study.

Etiologic Study Designs for Examining Causation: Randomized Controlled Trials

The RCT is the most efficient design for investigating a causal relationship between a treatment and its effect and is considered the gold standard for testing the effectiveness of clinical and public health therapeutic and preventive measures.[1,6] Its essential features are the planned allocation of participants to treatment (ie, randomization)[54] and the experimenter-controlled level of exposure.[6] Randomization is used to overcome selection bias and to ensure that confounders are equally distributed among groups. In other words, the goal of randomization is to ensure that the observed difference at the study's end can be directly attributable to the study factor,[49] that is, the experimental treatment. Other specific features of the RCT are discussed in Chapter 9 and elsewhere in this book.

Etiologic Study Designs for Examining Causation: Group-Randomized Trials

Group-randomized trials are clinical trials where identifiable groups, rather than individuals, are allocated to treatment or control conditions.[54,55] More trials of this type are likely to be fielded as effective prevention strategies and identified through usual RCT methodology. In the 1980s, three well-designed community trials for heart disease prevention were conducted in the United States: the Minnesota Heart Health Project, the Stanford Five-City Project, and the Pawtucket Heart Health Program. Each of these trials included a comprehensive intervention focusing on established risk factors and using state-of-the-art behavioral strategies.[68] The risk factors included cigarette smoking, hypertension, and elevated serum cholesterol levels. In the early 1990s, physician practice–based RCTs for heart disease prevention were conducted.[69,70] Neither the community trials[71] nor the physician practice–based trials[69,70] showed significant treatment effects. Building on that experience, substantial methodologic research on group-randomized trials has accelerated and continues to be pursued.[72] Issues needing more study include special sampling, outcome measures, and statistical techniques that may be required for this type of study.

Advantages and Disadvantages of Group-Randomized Trials

The group-randomized trial design allows the investigator to examine the effects of interventions that operate at the group level, where the physical or so-

cial environment is manipulated or cannot be delivered to individuals.[72] For example, the physician practice–based trials previously mentioned tested the efficacy of heart disease prevention interventions delivered by randomly selected physician practice groups compared with control practice groups. Group-randomized trials provide the opportunity to directly test the experimental treatment in its natural environment. Thus, group-randomized trials are more likely to provide key information on the generalizability of an intervention (ie, its external validity). External validity refers to whether a study's conclusions are applicable to other individuals at other locations and at other times. Such studies offer an experimental framework to test public health strategies.

Although group-randomized trials seem simple and straightforward, recent methodologic work has uncovered serious pitfalls in carrying them out. Important among these pitfalls are design and analysis issues. Given their inherent statistical properties, group-randomized trials require a larger sample size, careful attention to potential subgroups and outcomes, and a sophisticated analysis plan. Because of these previously underappreciated complexities, studies with null findings are common. Additionally, there is a need for stronger interventions that can produce detectable significant effects. Pooled analysis of the three community-based trials previously mentioned found that results were still below expectations even when adequate power was available.[71] Results below expectations were also found in subsequent group-randomized studies with strong design and analytic plans (eg, the Child and Adolescent Trial for Cardiovascular Health [CATCH]).[72,73]

Statistical Issues in Group-Randomized Trials

The specific statistical considerations for group-randomized trials are crucial. However, they are beyond the scope of this chapter. Instead, see Murray's seminal textbook[72] and the current literature in this area. Finally, although most research design and implementation would benefit from statistical advice, this type of input is a requirement for group-randomized trials because of the complexity and evolving nature of this method.

More research is needed to understand the best approaches to collecting outcome data that are likely to capture significant differences. Some investigators have suggested using end-point data at the community level (indicators) rather than measurements at the expensive individual level. Another approach is the use of more frequent, small surveys of randomly selected samples of the population or subgroups rather than infrequent, large surveys to capture end-point trends.[72]

Rooney and Murray[74] found that stronger intervention effects were detectable in studies with greater methodologic rigor. These studies were characterized by the use of appropriate group-randomized trial methods—that is, they were planned from the start to use the assignment unit for the analysis unit, used a sufficient number of randomized assignment units for each condition, adjusted for baseline differences in important confounding variables, and had extended follow-up and limited dropout and loss to follow-up. Also, smaller identifiable groups for assignment units (eg, worksites, physician practices, schools, and churches) may be better for detecting intervention effects. This makes sense, because it is likely to be more difficult to change the "health behavior and risk profile of an entire heterogeneous community rather than in smaller identifiable groups."[72]

Etiologic Study Designs for Examining Causation: Multicenter Randomized Control Trials

The essential and obvious difference between standard single-center RCTs and multicenter RCTs is the number of involved centers. Multicenter RCTs offer the ability to study questions that would be impractical for single-center RCTs due to sample size or resource limitations and for which there is an adequate pool of interested and qualified investigators.[6] The questions addressed by multicenter RCTs arise from observational basic science and evidence from small clinical trials, especially if these data are inconclusive or conflicting and indicate the need for a larger or more diverse participant pool.[6]

Advantages and Disadvantages of Multicenter Randomized Control Trials

Multicenter RCTs have several advantages. They can efficiently examine questions that require a larger number of participants or study groups (or both) or subgroups (eg, they can allow for minority inclusions, geographic spread, and rural/urban residence). They offer greater possibility for a more heterogeneous study population, thereby providing a broader basis for generalization of findings. Multiple centers are able to expedite the recruitment and follow-up of eligible participants to meet trial requirements. Also, economies of scale are offered. RCTs can afford central laboratory and reading centers, as well as dedicated resource centers for quality control, performance monitoring, and data analysis (eg, a data-coordinating center). Overall, these RCTs result in a lower cost per patient.

EXAMPLE

Child and Adolescent Trial for Cardiovascular Health (CATCH) was a multicenter group-randomized trial[73] conducted in four field sites (San Diego, Houston, New Orleans, and Minneapolis) over a 3-year period. Each site recruited 24 eligible schools with 56 of the 96 schools randomized to intervention. Half of these received school-based intervention alone and the other half received a family intervention. The study's primary end points were individual serum cholesterol levels and, at the school level, amounts of fat and sodium in school lunches and time spent in vigorous physical activity. A baseline survey was completed by 60.4% of eligible third graders (n ≈ 5,000 students) in the CATCH schools. Follow-up individual measures were done when these children completed the third, fourth, and fifth grades; about 80% completed final measurements. School measurements for school lunches and physical activity were completed at the same intervals. CATCH found a significant improvement in school measurements and a nonsignificant improvement in individual serum cholesterol measurements. The intervention group with additional family intervention showed greater dietary knowledge but were otherwise similar to the other intervention group. The investigators suggested that the limited time and resources for the intervention resulted in a weaker than desirable effect.[72,73]

Multicenter RCTs have several disadvantages. They require larger sample sizes than single-center RCTs, and the more heterogeneous sample that characterizes multicenter RCTs makes it is more difficult to detect treatment differences. Multicenter RCTs are administratively complex, involving multiple principal investigators, a steering committee, a data-coordinating center, an external safety monitoring board, and specific central laboratory and other measurement reading and coding centers. A complex organizational and communication structure is needed to link these components. (Web-based communications are now widely used to facilitate linkages.) These administrative complexities are cumbersome but essential.

Although less costly per participant, the overall cost of these studies is large, particularly in terms of participant recruitment. Data publication may be slowed or facilitated depending on the particular study teams and oversight committees.

Other Multicenter Randomized Control Trial Implementation Issues

RCTs are collaborative and require cooperative work, which is not easily accomplished when study personnel are located at various centers. It is necessary to maintain communications and decision-making structures because the study requires uniformity in study procedures. Performance of study methods and procedures requires supervision and documentation. Quality control requires standard application of measurements and intervention in multiple sites with many staff over several years.

Multicenter Randomized Control Trial Findings and Analysis Issues

In multicenter RCTs, issues of findings and analyses are similar to those of single-center RCTs. The one exception is the likely need to adjust for center-specific effects in the analyses.

INCONSISTENT STUDY FINDINGS AMONG NUTRITION STUDIES

Results from nutrition studies may be inconsistent for a variety of reasons, including systematic error (bias) or random error (variability) of exposure or

EXAMPLE

The Prevencion con Dieta Mediterranea (PREDIMED) study was a multicenter randomized, primary prevention trial that tested the effectiveness of the Mediterranean diet to lower risk of cardiovascular disease (CVD).[75] Study participants (n = 7,447) aged 55 to 80 years and at high CVD risk were recruited from 11 geographically dispersed clinics in Spain. Participants were randomized into one of three diet groups: low fat (control group), Mediterranean diet (MeDiet) plus extra virgin olive oil, and MeDiet plus tree nuts. All participants attended individual and group sessions for their assigned diet group every 3 months. A 14-item MeDiet checklist was used to assess compliance to dietary intake throughout the trial. Those randomized to either of the MeDiet groups significantly improved their CVD risk profile, including a lower rate of CVD events, compared with participants consuming a low-fat diet. After interim analysis showed beneficial effects of both MeDiets, the PREDIMED trial was stopped after 4.8 years. These study findings are in close agreement with the Bradford Hill criteria about causation[10]: the two MeDiet interventions protect against CVD.[76]

outcome measurement(s) as discussed earlier in the chapter. Another reason for inconsistent findings may be the differences between studies in their conduct, most importantly, study design, population, and methods of data collection.[77] In general, the selected population varies based on study design. For example, a case-control study about diet and hypertension would enroll individuals with hypertension (cases) and individuals without hypertension (controls). All participants in a cohort study would be free of hypertension at baseline, then followed over a period of time to see if they develop hypertension or not. In a cross-sectional design, participants who have or do not have hypertension are enrolled into the study keeping in mind that the information collected is obtained at one time point. Dietary intake collected in each of these study designs may or may not yield similar study findings. The cases in a case-control study may not correctly recall their dietary intake before developing hypertension, while in a cohort study dietary intake is obtained before hypertension develops, which leaves little chance of recall bias. For the cross-sectional study, it is not clear which came first—better diet after hypertension developed or poor diet with hypertension. Thus, study design may contribute to inconsistent results between nutrition studies.

Each diet assessment instrument (ie, 4-hour recall, food records, FFQ, and diet history) has its own measurement error issues.[3] Other explanations for diverse study findings include different population characteristics between studies, including differences in age, sex, race, education, socioeconomic status, and health status—all factors that influence a person's risk of developing hypertension (continuing with the example of hypertension as the outcome of interest). Studies of younger adults may yield a different diet-hypertension association compared with that of older adults. In addition, studying diet-hypertension associations between countries may yield inconsistent study results due to diverse food supply, culture, and food habits.[77]

Exposure and outcome definitions may differ between studies. For example, hypertension is typically defined as systolic blood pressure greater than or equal to 140 mm Hg or diastolic blood pressure less than or equal to 90mm Hg. However, some studies may use different cutoff points to define hypertension.

Methods may also differ between studies, including the diet assessment instrument used to capture dietary intake, protocols used to measure and represent blood pressure (ie, sitting at rest for 5 minutes and then measuring blood pressure three times vs no resting and measuring blood pressure only once), as well as the equipment used to measure blood pressure (digital device vs manual sphygmomanometer). Finally, quality control may differ between studies, including training and certification of data collectors, utilization of standardized procedures, calibration of equipment, and periodic monitoring of data collection quality (ie, recertification). When comparing results between studies of diet and an outcome of interest, it is important to compare study components across studies, including study design, population, exposure and outcome definitions, data collection methods and instruments, and quality control activities.

CONCLUSION

Analytic nutrition epidemiology provides a framework and tools to test whether diet or nutrition make a significant difference in health or disease outcomes. The tools provide tests for risk (association) and etiology (causation). Dietary intake or nutritional status exposure is a critical element in nutrition epidemiology studies, and considerable care is needed when choosing exposures for these studies. Analytic nutrition epidemiology studies consider health and disease outcomes from a multivariate perspective and examine potential risk factors, such as dietary intake and nutritional status, taking into account potential confounding and effect modifiers.

Analytic nutrition epidemiology uses two general types of study design: observational and experimental. Observational studies include cross-sectional studies, cohort studies, and case-control studies. In experimental studies, RCTs are considered the gold standard for etiologic investigations. Observational studies attempt to develop evidence for risk (association) of dietary intake and nutritional status as they relate to health or disease outcomes. Each type of design has advantages and disadvantages. The choice of design should be based on the study question, existing body of evidence relevant to the study question, and available study resources.

REFERENCES

1. Gordis L. *Epidemiology*. Philadelphia, PA: WB Saunders; 2004.

2. Centers for Disease Control and Prevention, National Center for Health Statistics. National Health and Nutrition Examination Survey. Updated September 15, 2017. www.cdc.gov/nchs/nhanes/about_nhanes.htm. Accessed November 1, 2017.

3. Willett W. Overview of nutritional epidemiology. In: *Nutritional Epidemiology*. 3rd ed. New York, NY: Oxford University Press; 2013:1-16.

4. Kelsey JL, Petitti DB, King AC. Key methodologic concepts and issues. In: Brownson RC, Petitti DB, eds. *Applied Epidemiology*. New York, NY: Oxford University Press; 1998:35-70.

5. Satija A, Yu E, Willett WC, HuFB. Understanding nutritional epidemiology and its role in policy. *Adv Nutr*. 2015;6(1):5-18.

6. Hulley SB, Cummings SR, Browner WS, Grady DG, Newman TB. *Designing Clinical Research*. 4th ed. Philadelphia, PA: Wolters Kluwer|Lippincott Willaims & Wilkins; 2014.

7. Szklo M, Nieto FJ. *Epidemiology: Beyond the Basics*. 3rd ed. Boston, MA: Jones and Bartlett Publishers; 2013.

8. Guallar E, Silbergeld EK, Navas-Acien A, et al. Confounding of the relation between homoscysteine and peripheral arterial disease by lead, cadmium and renal function. *Am J Epidemiol*. 2006;163(8):700-708.

9. Steffen LM, Van Horn L, Daviglus M, et al. A modified Mediterranean diet score is associated with a lower risk of incident metabolic syndrome over 25 years among young adults: the CARDIA (Coronary Artery Risk Development in Young Adults) study. *Br J Nutr*. 2014;12(10):1654-1661.

10. Hill, AB. The environment and disease: association or causation? *Proc Royal Soc Med*. 1965;58(5):295-300.

11. Potischman N, Weed DL. Causal criteria in nutritional epidemiology. *Am J Clin Nutr*. 1999;69(6):1309S-1314S.

12. Committee on Diet and Health. Methodologic considerations in evaluating the evidence. In: Food and Nutrition Board, Commission on Life Sciences, National Research Council, eds. *Diet and Health: Implications for Reducing Chronic Disease Risk*. Washington, DC: National Academy Press; 1989:23-40.

13. Whelton PK, Appel LJ, Sacco RL, et al. Sodium, blood pressure, and cardiovascular disease further evidence supporting the American Heart Association sodium reduction recommendations. *Circulation*. 2012;126(24): 2880-2889.

14. Blaustein MP, Zhang J, Chen L, Hamilton BP. How does salt retention raise blood pressure. *Am J Physiol Regul Integr Comp Physiol*. 2006;290(3):R514-R523.

15. Cook NR, Cutler JA, Obarzanek E, et al. Long term effects of dietary sodium reduction on cardiovascular disease outcomes: observational follow-up of the trials of hypertension prevention (TOHP). *BMJ*. 2007;334(7599):885-888.

16. Rothman KJ, Poole C. A strengthening programme for weak associations. *Int J Epidemiol*. 1988;17(4):955-959.

17. Rayburn WF, Stanley JR, Garrett E. Periconceptional folate intake and neural tube defects. J *Am Coll Nutr*. 1996;15(2): 121-125.

18. Tamura T, Picciano MF. Folate and human reproduction. *Am J Clin Nutr*. 2006;83(5):993-1016.

19. Dietrich M, Brown CJ, Block G. The effect of folate fortification of cereal-grain products on blood folate status, dietary folate intake and dietary folate sources among adult non-supplement users in the United States. *J Am Coll Nutr*. 2005;24(4):266-274.

20. Pfeiffer CM, Caudill SP, Gunter EW, Osterloh J, Sampson EJ. Biochemical indicators of B vitamin status in the US population after folic acid fortification: results from the National Health and Nutrition Examination Survey 1999–2000. *Am J Clin Nutr*. 2005;82(2):442-450.

21. Honein MA, Paulozzi LJ, Mathews TJ, Erickson JD, Wong LY. Impact of folic acid fortification of the US food supply on the occurance of neural tube defects. *JAMA*. 2001; 285(23):2981-2986.

22. Freedman LS, Commins JM, Moler JE. Pooled results from 5 validation studies of dietary self-report instruments using recovery biomarkers for energy and protein intake. *Am J Epidemiol*. 2014;180(2):172-188.

23. Day NE, McKeown N, Wong MY, Welch A, Bingham S. Epidemiological assessment of diet: a comparison of a 7-day diary with a food frequency questionnaire using urinary markers of nitrogen, potassium and sodium. *Int J Epidemiol*. 2001;30(2):309-317.

24. Whelton PK, Kumanyika SK, Cook NR, et al. Efficacy of nonpharmacologic interventions in adults with high-normal blood pressure: results from phase 1 of the Trials of Hypertension Prevention. *Am J Clin Nutr*. 1997;65 (2 suppl):652S-660S.

25. Fraser GE. A search for truth in dietary epidemiology. *Am J Clin Nutr*. 2003;78(3 suppl):521S-525S.

26. Kaaks R, Ferrari P, Ciampi A, Pummer M, Riboli E. Uses and limitation of statistical accounting for random error correlations, in the validation of dietary questionnaire assessments. *Public Health Nutr*. 2002;5(6A):969-976.

27. Freedman LS, Midthune D, Carroll RJ, et al. Adjustments to improve the estimation of usual dietary intake distribution in the population. *J Nutr*. 2004;134(7): 1836-1843.

28. Subar AF, Dodd KW, Guenther PM, et al. The food propensity questionnaire: concept, development and validation for use as a covariate in a model to estimate usual food intake. *J Am Diet Assoc.* 2006;106(10): 1556-1563.

29. Tooze JA, Midthune D, Dodd KW, et al. A new statistical method for estimating the usual intake of episodically consumed foods with application to their distribution. *J Am Diet Assoc.* 2006;106(10):1575-1587.

30. Kevin W, Dodd KW, Guenther PM, et al. Statistical methods for estimating usual intake of nutrients and foods: a review of the theory. *J Am Diet Assoc.* 2006;106(10): 1640-1650.

31. Subar AF, Thompson FE, Kipnis V, et al. Comparative validation of the Block, Willett and National Cancer Institute food frequency questionnaires: the Eating at America's Table Study. *Am J Epidemiol.* 2001;154(12): 1089-1099.

32. Martinez-Gonzalez MA, Garcia-Arellano A, Toledo E, et al, for the PREDIMED Study Investigators. A 14-item Mediterranean diet assessment tool and obesity indexes among high-risk subjects: the PREDIMED Trial. *PLOS.* 2012;7(8):e43134.

33. Nettleton JA, Steffen LM, Mayer-Davis EJ, et al. Dietary patterns are associated with biochemical markers of inflammation and endothelial activation in the Multi-Ethnic Study of Atherosclerosis (MESA). *Am J Clin Nutr.* 2006;83(6):1369-1379.

34. Milani C, Ferrario C, Turroni F, et al. The human gut microbiota and its interactive connections to diet. *J Hum Nutr Diet.* 2016;29(5):539-546.

35. Guertin KA, Moore SC, Sampson JN, et al. Metabolomics in nutritional epidemiology: identifying metabolites associated with diet and quantifying their potential to uncover diet-disease relations in populations. *Am J Clin Nutr.* 2014;100(1):208-217.

36. Zuniga K, McAuley E. Considerations in selection of diet assessment methods for examining the effect of nutrition on cognition. *J Nutr Health Aging.* 2015;19(3):333-340.

37. Omenn GS. Chemoprevention of lung cancer: the rise and demise of beta-carotene. *Annu Rev Pub Health.* 1998;19: 73-99.

38. Schatzkin A, Lanza E, Corle D, et al. Lack of effect of a low-fat, high-fiber diet on the recurrence of colorectal adenomas. Polyp Prevention Trial Study Group. *N Engl J Med.* 2000;342(16):1149-1150.

39. Bingham S. The fibre-folate debate in colo-rectal cancer. *Proc Nutr Soc.* 2006;65(1):19-23.

40. Lanza E, Hartman TJ, Albert PS, et al. High dry bean intake and reduced risk of advanced colorectal adenoma recurrence among participants in the poly prevention trial. *J Nutr.* 2006;136(7):1896-1903.

41. Jacobs ET, Lanza E, Alberts DS, et al. Fiber, sex, and colorectal adenoma: results of a pooled analysis. *Am J Clin Nutr.* 2006;83(2):343-349.

42. Hu F. Dietary pattern analysis: a new direction in nutritional epidemiology. *Curr Opin Lipidol.* 2002;13(1):3-9.

43. Ocke MC. Evaluation of methodologies for assessing the overall diet: dietary quality scores and dietary pattern analysis. *Proc Nutr Soc.* 2013;72(2):191-199.

44. Developing the Healthy Eating Index 2015. The Epidemiology and Genomics Research Program, National Cancer Institute, Division of Cancer Control and Population Sciences. Updated February 12, 2018. https://epi.grants.cancer.gov/hei/developing.html. Accessed November 6, 2015.

45. Jacques PF, Tucker KL. Are dietary patterns useful for understanding the role of diet in chronic disease? *Am J Clin Nutr.* 2001;73(1):1-2.

46. Kant AK. Dietary patterns and health outcomes. *J Am Diet Assoc.* 2004;104(4):615-635.

47. Freudenheim JL. Study design and hypothesis testing: issues in the evaluation of evidence from research in nutritional epidemiology. *Am J Clin Nutr.* 1999;69(6) :1315S-1321S.

48. Hozawa A, Jacobs DR Jr, Steffes MW, Gross MD, Steffen LM. Lee D-H. Associations of serum carotenoid concentrations with the development of diabetes and insulin concentration: interaction with smoking. The Coronary Artery Risk Development in Young Adults (CARDIA) Study. *Am J Epidemiol.* 2006;163(10):929-937.

49. Gerstman BB. Types of epidemiologic studies. In: *Epidemiology Kept Simple: An Introduction to Classic and Modern Epidemiology.* New York, NY: Wiley-Liss; 2003: 173-178.

50. Stamler J. The INTERSALT Study: background, methods, findings, and implications. *Am J Clin Nutr.* 1997; 65(2suppl):526S-642S.

51. Stamler J, Elliott P, Dennis B, et al, INTERMAP Research Group. INTERMAP: background, aims, design, methods, and descriptive statistics (nondietary). *J Hum Hypertens.* 2003;17(9):591-608.

52. Elliott P, Stamler J, Dyer AR, et al. Association between protein intake and blood pressure: the INTERMAP Study. *Arch Intern Med.* 2006;166(1):79-87.

53. Stamler J, Elliott P, Appel L, et al. Higher blood pressure in middle-aged American adults with less education—role of multiple dietary factors: the INTERMAP study. *J Hum Hypertens.* 2003;17(9):655-775.

54. Woodward M. Fundamental issues. In: *Epidemiology: Study Design and Data Analysis.* Boca Raton, FL: Chapman & Hall/CRC; 1999:1-30.

55. Friedman GD. *Primer of Epidemiology*. 4th ed. New York, NY: McGraw-Hill; 1994.

56. Stamler J, Neaton JD, Cohen JD, et al, The MRFIT Research Group. Multiple Risk Factor Intervention Trial revisited: a new perspective based on nonfatal and fatal composite endpoints, coronary and cardiovascular, during the trial. *J Am Heart Assoc*. 2012;1(5):e003640. doi:10.1161/JAHA.112.003640

57. Giles PD, Rylance PB, Crothers DC. New results from the Modification of Diet in Renal Disease study: the importance of clinical outcomes in test strategies for early chronic kidney disease. *QJM*. 2008;101(2):155-158.

58. Satterfield S, Cutler JA, Langford HG, et al, for the Trials of Hypertension Prevention Collaborative Research Group. Trials of hypertension prevention. Phase I design. *Ann Epidemiol*. 1991;1(5):455-471.

59. He J, Whelton PK, Appel LJ, Charleston J, Klag MJ. Long-term effects of weight loss and dietary sodium reduction on incidence of hypertension. *Hypertension*. 2000;35(2):544-549.

60. Sempos CT, Liu K, Ernst ND. Food and nutrient exposures: what to consider when evaluating epidemiologic evidence. *Am J Clin Nutr*. 1999;69(5):1330S-1339S.

61. Rebholz CM, Grams ME, Steffen LM, et al. Diet soda consumption and risk of incident end-stage renal disease. *Clin J Am Soc Nephrol*. 2017;12(1):79-86.

62. Gonzalez AJ, White E, Kristal A, Littman AJ. Calcium intake and 10-year weight change in middle-aged adults. *J Am Diet Assoc*. 2006;106 (7):1066-1073.

63. Lutsey PL, Steffen LM, Stevens J. Dietary intake and development of the metabolic syndrome: the Atherosclerosis Risk in Communities Study. *Circulation*. 2008;117(6):754-761.

64. Suez J, Korem T, Zeevi D, Zilberman-Schapira G, Thaiss CA. Artificial sweeteners induce glucose intolerance by altering the gut microbiota. *Nature*. 2014;514(7521):181-186.

65. Ascherio A, Hennekens CH, Buring JE, Master C, Stampfer MJ, Willett WC. Trans fatty acids intake and risk of myocardial infarction. *Circulation*. 1994;89(1):94-101.

66. Kelemen LE, Cerhan JR, Lim U, et al. Vegetables, fruit and antioxidant-related nutrients and risk of non-Hodgkin hymphoma: a National Cancer Institute-Surveillance, Epidemiology, and End Results population-based case-control study. *Am J Clin Nutr*. 2006:83(6),1401-1410.

67. Chasan-Taber L, Selhub J, Rosenberg IH, et al. A prospective study of folate and vitamin B*6* and risk of myocardial infarction in US physicians. *J Am Coll Nutr*. 1996; 15(2):136-143.

68. Shea S, Basch CE. A review of five major community-based cardiovascular disease prevention programs. Part I. Rationale, design, and theoretical framework. *Am J Health Promot*. 1990;4(3):203-213.

69. Caggiula AW, Watson JE, Kuller LH, et al. Cholesterol-lowering intervention program. Effect of the step I diet in community office practices. *Arch Intern Med*. 1996;156(11):1205-1213.

70. Keyserling TC, Ammerman AS, Davis CE, Mok MC, Garrett J, Simpson R Jr. A randomized controlled trial of a physician-directed treatment program for low-income patients with high blood cholesterol: the Southeast Cholesterol Project. *Arch Fam Med*. 1997; 6(2):135-145.

71. Winkleby MA, Feldman HA, Murray DM. Joint analysis of three U.S. community intervention trials for reduction of cardiovascular disease risk. *J Clin Epidemiol*. 1997;50(6):645-656.

72. Murray DM. *Design and Analysis of Group-Randomized Trials Design and Analysis of Group-Randomized Trials*. New York, NY: Oxford University Press; 1998.

73. Luepker RV, Perry CL, McKinlay SM, et al. Outcomes of a field trial to improve children's dietary patterns and physical activity: the Child and Adolescent Trial for Cardiovascular Health (CATCH). *JAMA*. 1996;275(10):768-776.

74. Rooney BL, Murray DM. A meta-analysis of smoking prevention programs after adjustment for errors in the unit of analysis. *Health Educ Q*. 1996;23(1):48-64.

75. Estruch R, Ros E, Salas-Salvadó J, et al; PREDIMED Study Investigators. Primary prevention of cardiovascular disease with a Mediterranean diet. *N Engl J Med*. 2013 ;368(14):1279-1290.

76. Mente A, Koning L, Shannon HS, Anand SS. A systematic review of the evidence supporting a causal link between dietary factors and coronary heart disease. *Arch Intern Med*. 2009;169(7):659-669.

77. Steffen LM, Hootman KC. A posteriori data-derived dietary patterns and incident coronary heart disease: making sense of inconsistent findings. *Curr Nutr Rep*. 2016;5(3):168-179.

ADDITIONAL RESOURCES

Bruemmer B, Harris J, Gleason P, et al. Publishing nutrition research: a review of epidemiologic methods. *J Am Diet Assoc*. 2009;109(10):1728-1737.

Heber D, Blackburn GL, Go VLW, Milner J. *Nutritional Oncology*. 2nd ed. Boston, MA:Elsevier-Academic Press; 2006.

Kelemen LE. Nutrition epidemiology. In: Talley NJ, Locke GR III, Saito YA, eds. *GI Epidemiology*. Malden, MA: Blackwell Publishing; 2007.

Weaver CM, Heaney RP, eds. *Calcium in Human Health*. Totowa, NJ: Humana Press; 2006.

Guidelines for Developing and Implementing Clinical Nutrition Studies

Alison L. Steiber, PhD, RDN | *Rosa K. Hand,* PhD, RDN, LD, FAND | *Constantina Papoutsakis,* PhD, RDN

LEARNING OBJECTIVES

1. Understand the key components and considerations in implementing a clinical nutrition study.

2. Compare and contrast common study designs.

3. Identify strategies for overcoming common barriers to ensure successful implementation of clinical nutrition–related trials.

Clinical nutrition studies have provided the defining research evidence that serves as the basis for the dietary guidance that is issued for health promotion and disease prevention as well as the treatment and management of a wide variety of clinical conditions. Findings from clinical nutrition studies have been central to defining nutrient requirements that are the basis for Dietary Reference Intakes issued by the Food and Nutrition Board of the Institute of Medicine in the

National Academy of Sciences.[1] Thus, the ongoing process of revising dietary recommendations is dependent upon high-quality clinical nutrition research studies. Exciting new frontiers in clinical nutrition research include elucidating the effects of bioactive compounds and foods on a multitude of established and emerging biomarkers of health and disease; expanding the focus from intermediate outcomes like biomarkers and nutrients to patient- and health-oriented outcomes; and collaborating with researchers in other disciplines to understand the behavioral, social, and economic underpinnings of food choices. The underlying impetus is to evolve dietary guidance that advances our ability to promote health and well-being and thus decrease morbidity and mortality and improve quality of life.

Clinical nutrition research is an overarching term that encompasses research conducted with human participants using many different experimental designs, participant populations, methods, and interventions. The central focus of controlled clinical nutrition studies is to evaluate the effects of a dietary or behavior modification on one or more end points. The study design, participant population, and methods are determined by the research question to be addressed. Studies range from very small scale clinical studies with just a few participants to large clinical trials involving thousands of participants and multiple research sites. Clinical nutrition studies also vary by length of study time and range from acute (hours to days) to intermediate (weeks to months) to long term (spanning years). The participant population may target specific groups, such as children or the elderly; specific disease states, such as hypertension or inflammatory bowel disease; or a participant population that is representative of the population at large. The diets and interventions used in clinical nutrition research studies are inherently variable because of the vast array of dietary factors that can be evaluated, including single nutrients or bioactive components; multiple nutrients or bioactive components; single and multiple foods, food groups, and beverages; enteral and parenteral products; dietary patterns, such as timing of diet; and behavior change techniques to help integrate these modifications

into daily life. Moreover, the approach used to deliver the interventions can vary appreciably. For example, nutrition interventions can be well controlled, where participants are fed all nutrients, bioactive compounds, foods, or meals in a highly controlled setting (such as a metabolic unit), or conducted with participants in a free-living environment with or without much oversight. In a less controlled setting, participants can be given some foods to consume on-site or off-site or given behavioral advice about the dietary pattern or foods to consume. It is evident that there are many different methodologies for conducting clinical nutrition research studies to determine the effects of a dietary or behavioral intervention on the end points of interest. Different methodologies that can be implemented are discussed in this chapter.

Regardless of whether the clinical nutrition study is conducted in an inpatient facility, academic setting, or other research setting, registered dietitian nutritionists (RDNs) play a key role in designing, implementing, analyzing, and interpreting the results of such studies. This chapter presents guidelines for developing and implementing clinical nutrition research and describes the important factors that must be considered to appropriately answer the experimental questions. Examples of various types of studies that have been conducted are discussed to illustrate how different experimental designs, intervention designs, and study populations have been used in clinical nutrition research studies. Readers are referred to other resources that provide comprehensive information about designing and conducting clinical nutrition research (see Box 8.1 on page 128). Consequently, this chapter provides a basic overview of clinical nutrition research and serves as a primer to learn more about how to do this research. The outline of this chapter follows the order of a protocol for a clinical nutrition trial.

IDENTIFYING IMPORTANT CLINICAL RESEARCH NEEDS

Thare are many resources available that provide information about important and timely clinical

Dennis BH, Ershow AG, Obarzanek E, Clevidence BA. *Well-Controlled Diet Studies in Humans*. Chicago, IL: American Dietetic Association; 1999.

- This book is out of print but is available online at https://sites.google.com/site/nabconnections /nutrition-research-book.

Kay CD, Kris-Etherton PM, Psota PM, Bagshaw DM, West SG. Clinical nutrition studies: maximizing opportunities and managing the challenges. In: Berdanier CD, Dwyer J, Feldman EB, eds. *Handbook of Nutrition and Food*. 2nd ed. Boca Raton, FL: CRC Press; 2007:693–714.

- There is a 3rd edition of this book. However, Chapter 41 from the 2nd edition has several practical suggestions and tools for implementing a nutrition study.

National Cancer Institute Measurement Error Webinar series

- This series is available at https://epi.grants.cancer .gov/events/measurement-error.
- This is a classic series of webinars that focus on how to understand and address measurement error in dietary intake data sets.

National Institutes of Health, Office of Disease Prevention, Pragmatic and Group-Randomized Trials in Public Health and Medicine

- This seven-part online course is available at https://prevention.nih.gov/resources-for -researchers/nih-methods-training/grt#part1.

Dietetics Practice Based Research Network (DPBRN), Academy of Nutrition and Dietetics

- The DPBRN conducts, supports, promotes, and advocates for practice-based research that answers questions important to nutrition and dietetics practice.
- See www.eatrightpro.org/research/projects-tools -and-initiatives/dpbrn.

Steps to Developing a Research Project: Resources to Help, Academy of Nutrition and Dietetics.

- ○ This Academy web repository of research resources focuses on how to conduct nutrition and dietetic research.
- ○ See www.eatrightpro.org/research/projects-tools -and-initiatives/dpbrn/steps-to-developing-a -research-project-resources-to-help.

Academy of Nutrition and Dietetics Informatics Infrastructure (ANDHII)

- ANDHII enables users to track nutrition care outcomes and advance evidence-based nutrition practice research.
- See www.eatrightpro.org/resources/research /projects-tools-and-initiatives/andhii.

Box 8.1 Resources for Conducting Clinical Nutrition Research Studies

nutrition research needs. A report from the Academy of Nutrition and Dietetics critically assessed gaps in research identified by the dietary guidelines committees.[2] There has not yet been an examination of other systematic reviews for conclusions with poor grades (ie, relevant studies have not been done; a limited number of studies is available; or available studies are of weak design or findings are inconclusive due to design flaws, bias, or execution problems), which can also help identify research gaps. The Evidence Analysis Library makes it easy to identify Grade V (insufficient evidence) questions on its website (http://andeal.org /grade-v).

Practitioners are also important sources of research questions. They identify clinical quandaries and notice patterns in their work each and every day. Practice-based research is built on the concept that practitioner-generated questions are important to answer.[3] Results from epidemiologic studies may be enhanced by validation from a clinical nutrition trial. Similarly, quality improvement projects at individual facilities can help researchers generate questions to address through more generalizable research methods, meaning the results would apply broadly to real-world settings. In an effort to reduce the selective reporting of results from clinical research trials, the International Committee of Medical Journal Editors has created a policy that any study submitted for publication must be registered as a clinical trial in a public registry (eg, ClinicalTrials.gov).[4] This resource informs researchers about clinical nutrition studies that are being conducted or have been completed and may not be published. Since it is sometimes difficult to publish papers that show no effect, this registry can be a useful resource to researchers in identifying research questions that merit study.

STUDY HYPOTHESES AND OBJECTIVES

A hypothesis is a proposition made as a basis for reasoning without any assumption of its truth. In research, investigators accrue existing but incomplete evidence to develop a hypothesis on a particular topic. Then that hypothesis is tested to determine whether it is accurate or needs further revision. Hypothesis-driven investigation is a core foundation for conducting clinical nutrition research and is always linked to specific aims that robustly test the study hypothesis or hypotheses. The aims of a clinical nutrition trial are generally presented quantitatively so that specific end points can be measured precisely. Aims are designed to evaluate the effect of an intervention on some number of end points. This can be done in one or more population groups. Thus, the hypothesis or hypotheses to be tested and corresponding aims determine the experimental design, methods to be implemented, and subsequent statistical analyses. Statistical tests are performed on the null hypothesis—that no association or difference exists. Examples of hypotheses and null statements are shown in Figure 8.1 on page 130.

Many clinical nutrition studies test a primary hypothesis and a number of secondary hypotheses. The primary hypothesis is the testable statement that is most important to the researchers and involves the outcome variables for which the study has been powered. Secondary hypotheses are often used to answer questions related to the primary hypothesis. These additional questions can be included to provide information about mechanisms of action or about the effects of an intervention on any number of other end points, all of which could generate valuable scientific information and, possibly, a novel discovery.

When defining the hypotheses and aims of a clinical nutrition study, it is important to estimate the expected response to the intervention in a very controlled setting vs a free-living setting. This information is important in shaping the study design. Researchers can use a controlled study design to evaluate the efficacy of the treatment and establish internal validity (ie, the maximum response achievable for the treatment under tight conditions). For the purpose of external validity, researchers can evaluate effectiveness using a free-living study design (ie, the response observed to an experimental design that mimics what can be implemented in a real-world setting). These two concepts are important to consider in the design of clinical nutrition studies. Defining whether the study will evaluate efficacy vs effectiveness will shape the study design.

If there is little evidence in the literature about the expected response to a specific level (ie, dose or duration) of the intervention, dose-response studies are a prerequisite to implementing a larger clinical nutrition study. Dose and duration are extremely important to understand when considering the length of the trial, impact of the intervention, and sample size to be tested. For example, a study using a strong dose of nutrition counseling (6 months of 3-hour weekly sessions) may be expected to be longer in duration, see a larger change in outcome, and perhaps need a smaller sample size compared with a study with a smaller dose of nutrition counseling. Not only is dose important but the timeline of end-point collection also has to be established.

Single nutrient

Hypothesis: Routine vitamin A supplementation prevents blindness in children compared with no supplementation.	**Null Statement:** Vitamin A supplementation does not decrease blindness more than no supplementation.

Bioactive compound

Hypothesis: Plant stanol/sterol esters decrease absorption of fat-soluble vitamins.	**Null Statement:** Plant stanol/sterol esters do not decrease absorption of fat-soluble vitamins.

Specific food and nutrient profile

Hypothesis: A diet high in alpha-linolenic acid from walnuts decreases inflammatory status as measured by C-reactive protein level.	**Null Statement:** A diet high in alpha-linolenic acid from walnuts does not decrease inflammatory status as measured by C-reactive protein level.

Multiple-nutrient manipulation

Hypothesis: Replacing dietary carbohydrate with dietary protein decreases plasma triglyceride levels.	**Null Statement:** Replacing dietary carbohydrate with dietary protein does not decrease plasma triglyceride levels.

Dietary pattern

Hypothesis: A diet that meets the food-based recommendations of the 2015–2020 Dietary Guidelines for Americans significantly decreases blood pressure and low-density lipoprotein cholesterol levels in individuals with stage 1 hypertension and hypercholesterolemia	**Null Statement:** A diet that meets the food-based recommendations of the 2015–2020 Dietary Guidelines for Americans does not decrease blood pressure and low-density lipoprotein cholesterol levels in individuals with stage 1 hypertension and hypercholesterolemia.

Route of feeding

Hypothesis: Early vs late enteral nutrition support decreases mortality in critically ill adults.	**Null Statement:** Early vs late enteral nutrition support does not decrease mortality in critically ill adults.

Counseling intervention

Hypothesis: Nutrition counseling to achieve a 500-kcal daily energy deficit decreases body weight of adults who are overweight.	**Null Statement:** Nutrition counseling to achieve a 500-kcal daily energy deficit does not decrease body weight of adults who are overweight.

Figure 8.1 Examples of hypothesis and null statements

STUDY DESIGN

When designing a clinical nutrition study, the scope of the study, time needed to detect a meaningful result, level of intensity or dietary control required, and demands placed on the study participants must be considered. The randomized controlled trial (RCT) study design is considered the gold standard for clinical nutrition research. RCTs use a comparative design that involves an intervention with one or more treatments. Each participant is assigned to a group based on a formal randomization procedure.[5] The RCT design has the following advantages:

● Randomization removes the potential of bias when allocating participants to the intervention or control group.
● Randomization tends to produce comparable groups.
● The validity of statistical tests of significance is guaranteed.

Within any RCT, the length of the treatment period should be sufficient to adequately test the treatment effects. For example, it is well established that serum lipids stabilize after 3 weeks of a particular nutrition intervention. Consequently, each intervention period should be at least 3 weeks, and preferably 4 weeks or more, to ensure that the end-point measurements are accurate. It may be necessary to conduct a pilot study to determine the length of the treatment period needed to ensure that the response has stabilized.

Another determinant of the clinical study duration is the number of interventions studied. Thus, the time required to see a treatment effect, the number of interventions studied, and the length of the washout periods or breaks between treatments are factors affecting the study duration. In considering the length of the trial, it is important to consider the lasting effect of the intervention. How long will participants adhere to the intervention without the structure of the study? Thus, it may be important to allow time for follow-up measurements even after the initial intervention has ended. For example, in the Selenium and Vitamin E Cancer Prevention (SELECT) trial, men took assigned supplements for 5.5 years. However, the researchers continued to follow the participants for an additional 18 months after the intervention ended to see whether the effect was lasting.[6]

In a parallel-design RCT, participants are randomized to a particular treatment group and remain on this treatment throughout the study (see Figure 8.2). In a crossover design study each participant serves as his or her own control (see Figure 8.3 on page 132).[5] In the simplest example, a two-period crossover design, each participant would receive either intervention or control (A or B) in the first period and the alternative treatment (A or B) in the second period. In a balanced design, half of the participants would receive A first, and the other half would receive B first. One of the major advantages of

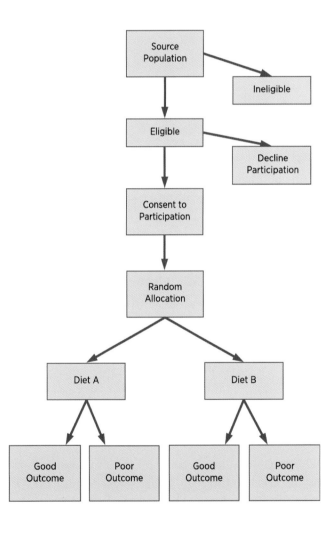

Figure 8.2 Parallel-design randomized controlled clinical trial

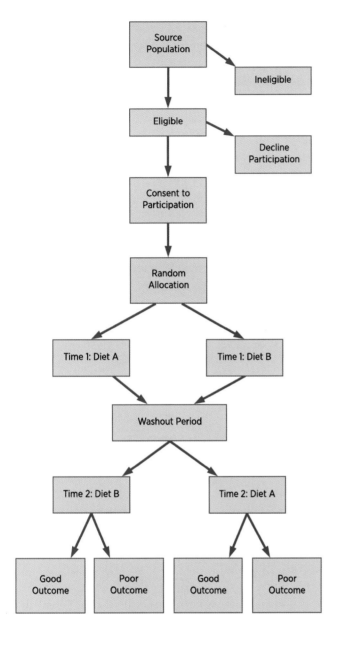

Figure 8.3 Crossover experimental trial design

the crossover design is that "variability is reduced because the measured effect of the intervention is the difference in an individual participant's response to intervention and control."[7] The decrease in variance allows researchers to use a smaller sample size than needed for a parallel-design RCT. Although a crossover design study is generally longer than a parallel-design study, there is an advantage in that each participant is exposed to all treatments tested in the study. This design is particularly powerful in

controlling for variation associated with overreporters and underreporters because they are on all interventions, which reduces interparticipant variation.

When using the crossover design, researchers must evaluate the assumption that there are no carryover effects from the first to subsequent periods.[5] This evaluation can rule out the use of a crossover design for many different circumstances. For example, if the intervention during the first period cures the disease, the participant would obviously receive no benefit from the treatment or control in the second period if the disease has been ameliorated. Frequently, a crossover design has a washout period or compliance break that separates the different periods within the study design. After completion of a crossover design study, statistical analyses can be conducted to test for any possible carryover effects.[8]

A major benefit of the parallel research design is that the total study duration is often shorter because participants receive only one treatment. While this may translate into a reduced cost to conduct the trial, oftentimes a larger sample size is required, and thus the cost may actually be the same as that of a crossover design, which generally requires a smaller sample size. Because participants receive only one treatment in the parallel design, the researcher relies on the randomization process to ensure that each group within the study is matched for pertinent baseline parameters. For example, if one group is significantly younger than the other at the initiation of the study, the results may be skewed based on age rather than treatments alone.

The use of a factorial study design allows the researcher to address multiple objectives within one study. In factorial designs, the *factor* is the major independent variable, and there are two or more *levels* as a subdivision of each factor (see Figure 8.4). For example, in a study designed to test whether increased carbohydrate intake increases triglyceride levels, researchers could also test whether or not the quality of the carbohydrate (ie, the amount of fiber) affects triglyceride levels. Using a factorial design, the following groups would be used to test the aforementioned objectives: (1) high carbohydrate/low fiber, (2) high carbohydrate/high fiber, (3) low carbohydrate/low fiber, and (4) low carbohydrate/high fiber. In this example, carbohydrate amount

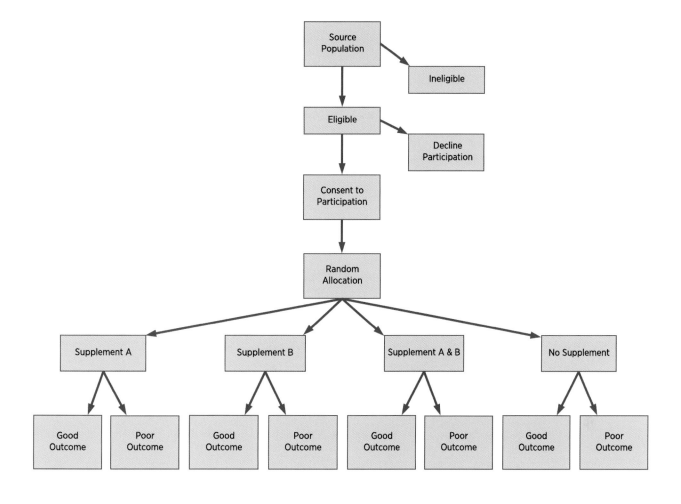

Figure 8.4 Factorial experimental trial design

has two levels, and fiber content has two levels; thus, it is classified as a 2×2 factorial design. This is the simplest form of the factorial design. In this notation, the *number of numbers* indicates how many factors there are, and the *number values* denote how many levels there are. A 3×4 factorial design would have two factors, one factor with three levels and the other with four levels. The number of different treatment groups in any factorial design can be easily determined by multiplying through the number notation. A classic example of the factorial design was the SELECT trial, which compared vitamin E and selenium, alone or in combination, for the prevention of prostate cancer. In this 2×2 factorial study, men received two placebo supplements, vitamin E + placebo, selenium + placebo, or vitamin E + selenium.[6]

In RCTs, blinding (ie, when the participant or researcher [or both] do not know which treatment the participant is receiving) and allocation concealment (ie, the researcher does not know or cannot guess in advance which group the next participant will be assigned to) are important for a high-quality study. However, these can be difficult to achieve in nutrition given that participants can readily ascertain what they are eating and whether they are receiving a behavioral intervention.[5] Whenever possible, the person collecting the outcome measures and conducting the statistical analysis should be blinded to the participant's study group.

Other study designs extend the previously explained principles to a group setting. For example, cluster randomization (see Figure 8.5 on page 134) extends the parallel RCT to a group setting. Inter-

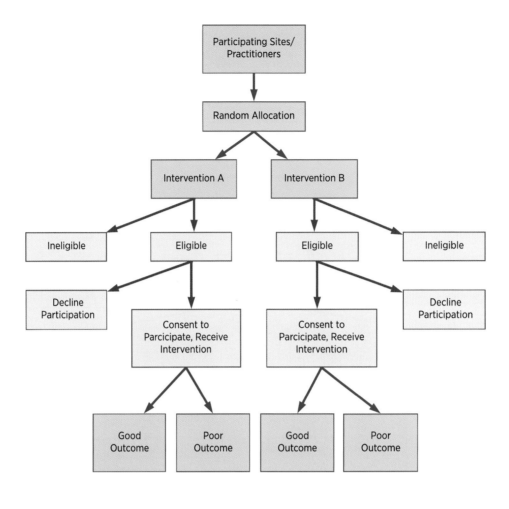

Figure 8.5 Cluster randomized experimental trial design

Note that the boxes in grey may or may not apply, depending on whether the intervention is provided to individuals (eg, a diet) or is based on a clinician-implemented or site-implemented change that would be applied to all patients (eg, use of the nutrition care process).

ventions might be assigned by group rather than by individual because of the risk of contamination (ie, one group receiving an unintended intervention because of social contact with a participant in another group) or because a single interventionist (ie, a practicing RDN) cannot provide both interventions without risk of contamination. For example, when providing a nutrition intervention in a dialysis unit, the investigator might decide that participants are social with one another, and therefore within a single dialysis facility, it is logical to provide only one intervention. Participants for the other intervention (or the control group) will come from another facility. School interventions are also frequently conducted using cluster RCT methods. For example the Academy of Nutrition and Dietet-

ics's Energy Balance 4 Kids with Play study was tested in two program schools and two control schools.[9] When using cluster randomization, statistical techniques are required to account for the known similarities of participants within sites (ie, the interclass correlation), which generally decrease the statistical power of a study.

The stepped-wedge design (Figure 8.6) extends the crossover design to groups or interventions in which the order of interventions cannot be reversed, or for which equipoise cannot be achieved.[10] For example, researchers cannot take away education after education has been provided. Even if a participant is told to ignore the education the interventionist provided previously, the participant is now aware of the education, and his or her future actions

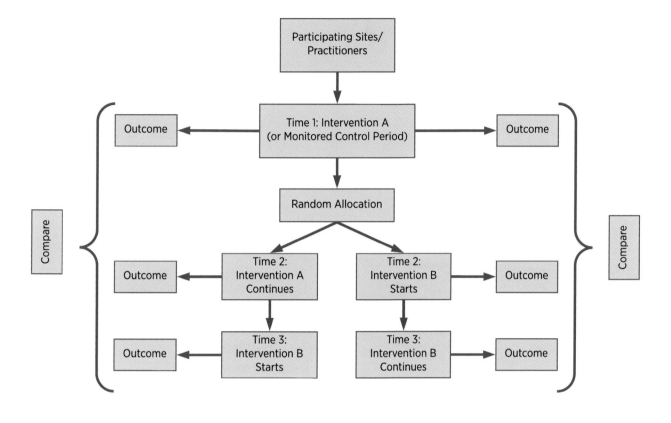

Figure 8.6 Stepped-wedge experimental trial design

In the stepped-wedge design, interventions are generally provided to all patients who are at the clinic, although this is not necessarily true. Outcomes are compared within the site over time and between interventions.

Note that while the outcome ascertainment in these figures is notated as dichotomous (good vs poor outcome), outcomes will generally be continuous, representing a range of outcomes.

may be informed by it. Therefore, it is illogical to conduct a control period after an intervention in a crossover design. Similarly, when working with a group of clinicians, after the researcher has introduced the nutrition care process, the researcher cannot ask participants to return to their old way of providing care. Instead, by introducing the intervention to different sites or individuals at different times, the researchers still have the benefit of the crossover in participants acting as their own controls. Introducing the intervention in steps (that is, at different time points) allows researchers to analyze change over time at multiple time points and can help the investigator logistically.[10]

Whatever trial design is chosen, it is wise to refer to the Consolidated Standards of Reporting Trials (CONSORT) statement, which helps increase the transparency of trial reporting (see Figure 8.7 on page 136).[11] Although the CONSORT statement was created with the publication process in mind, it is also a helpful checklist for those planning studies.[12] Researchers should ask themselves whether they know the answer to each question in the checklist or have a reason for not meeting a particular recommendation so they will be able to report on those factors when it is time to publish.

A free-living clinical nutrition study in which participants self-select their diet based on advice from the study personnel involves less control than an RCT. This type of free-living, self-selected diet study design has a higher level of external validity, that is, application to the real world. Free-living studies demonstrate effectiveness, whereas feeding studies demonstrate efficacy. Examples on this continuum are shown in Figure 8.8 on page 137. Free-living, self-selected clinical nutrition studies can be especially successful with counseling and motivation strategies. In fact, the purpose of the study may

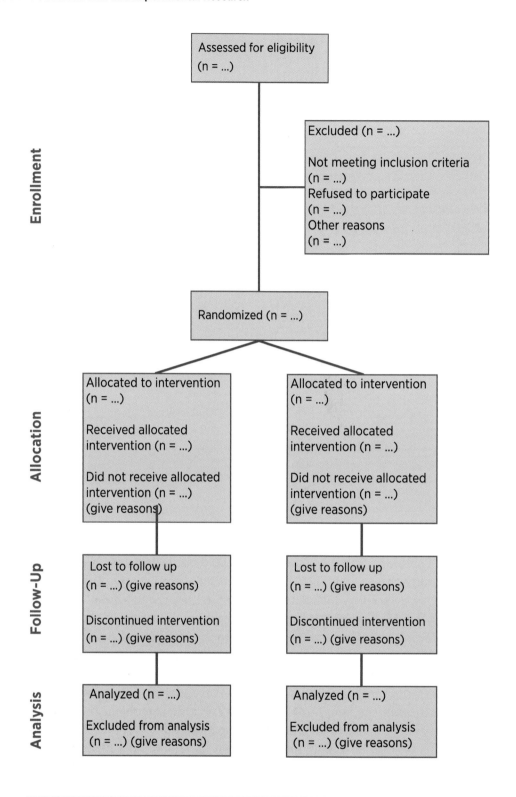

Figure 8.7 Sample template for the Consolidated Standards of Reporting Trials (CONSORT) showing the flow of participants through each stage of a randomized trial[1]

Examples

- PREDIMED (a Mediterranean diet intervention trial)
- PREMIER (lifestyle intervention for blood pressure control)
- WHI (Women's Health Initiative)
- DCCT (Diabetes Control and Complications Trial)
- SELECT (a vitamin E and selenium supplementation study to study prostate cancer risk reduction)
- DASH (Dietary Approaches to Stop Hypertension trial)

- Portfolio Diet Study
- DELTA (Dietary Effects on Lipoproteins and Thrombogenic Activity) trial
- OmniHeart (Optimal Macronutrient Intake Trial for Heart Health) randomized trial
- Overfeeding study in twins
- Energy requirements of burn patients
- Surgical patients on parenteral nutrition
- Liquid-formula diet
- Creatinine formula in patients receiving a heart transplant

Defining Characteristics

Degree of Nutrition Intervention Control

Low	High
Free living	Live in
Selection of own food	Food/nutrition provided
May focus on counseling or behavior change to encourage desired food choices	Eat in
Free living	Nutrient formula or defined whole food, special products (eg, pudding, cookies, cookie bars)
Food provided	
Eat in/take out	

Free Living

Adherence varies, often unknown

Diet/nutrient composition variable, often unknown

Easier to recruit

Long-term study is possible

Wider generalizability is possible

Metabolic Ward or Hospital Unit

Adherence is closely monitored

High degree of control

Difficult to recruit

Usually short term

Low generalizability

Figure 8.8 Nutrition intervention studies of varying control[1,6,13–24]

actually be to test the intensity of counseling or the particular behavior modification strategy that is required to achieve dietary change and resulting outcomes in the real world.

Postprandial studies enable researchers to evaluate the acute effects of a specific nutrient, food, or mixed meal on end points of interest. Although many biomarkers are typically studied in the fasting state, there is growing interest in identifying what occurs during the postprandial period because many individuals are in this period as much as 12 to 14 hours each day. Consequently, many research questions can be addressed during the postprandial period. In some cases, postprandial studies have been conducted to evaluate the acute effects of specific nutrients, foods, or nutrient profiles that have been tested chronically. For example, the postprandial effects of components of the Mediterranean diet on endothelial function have been studied.[25] Postprandial studies are important because they can build on the results of in vitro studies and longer-duration in vivo studies. For example, based on the results from a chronic feeding study, a study evaluated the effects of consuming particular tomato components and quantifying in vitro antiplatelet activity and ex vivo platelet function.[26] These studies can provide valuable information about the mechanisms associated with the diet-related pathophysiology of disease processes.

Dose-response studies are important because they provide information about the range of biological effects in response to different doses of nutrients or dietary constituent evaluated. Implicit to this type of study is that the maximally effective dose can be established. Consequently, all of this information is used to make dietary recommendations for preventing and treating diseases. For example, evidence from dose-response studies was used to support the recommendation that specific dietary intake levels of stanol or sterol esters can lower low-density lipoprotein cholesterol levels.[27] Some nutrition studies have inappropriately viewed diet as all or nothing. In free-living clinical nutrition studies, adherence to the diet may be a stand-in for dose.

Dose-response studies are required to determine nutrient levels or amounts of food required for health claims issued by the Food and Drug Administration and other government agencies. Numerous resources provide guidelines for conducting clinical nutrition research aimed at qualifying a food or nutrient for a health claim.[28-31]

RESOURCES

Sufficient resources are essential for conducting a clinical nutrition study. Self-selected diet studies require facilities for instruction, cooking demonstrations, and diet assessment; office space; and computer support. At the other end of the spectrum, facilities for food storage, preparation, serving, and cleanup are needed for well-controlled feeding studies. For studies that provide food but do not feed participants on-site, it is necessary to have a facility for storing meals, foods, or supplements that are picked up by or delivered to participants as well as for the food waste returned to the researchers for measurement. Location, accessibility, and ambiance of the feeding site or the facility where participants pick up the meals, foods, or supplements are important factors in recruiting and retaining study participants. Interventions involving supplements must have facilities for preparing and packaging foods, either in-house or through contractual arrangements with the manufacturer.

Most clinical nutrition studies collect clinical or biochemical end-point measurements or both ranging from simple measurements, such as body weight and skinfold thickness, to more complex procedures involving biochemical analyses of body fluids, tissue samples, or whole-body procedures, such as dual-energy x-ray absorptiometry. Resources must be available for carrying out these measurements or contractual arrangements must be made with other laboratories with established quality assurance procedures.

Essential resources for all studies are personnel, funding, and an adequate population from which to recruit. Nonessential resources can enhance the overall implementation of a study but are not necessary; some examples are participant incentives and exploratory end-point measurements. If possible within existing budget constraints, it is prudent to include additional study end points. Specifically, collecting additional biological samples that can be assayed at a later time, adding a questionnaire that could be administered easily and inexpensively, collecting information about physical activity level (eg, using a step counter), and gathering additional anthropometric data (eg, waist circumference in the supine position) are valuable additions to most nutrition studies when they are feasible without undue participant burden.

Many institutions recognized through the Clinical and Translational Science Awards (CTSA) Program from the National Institutes of Health have an RDN on staff who is an expert at these measurements and at producing food for controlled clinical trials.[32] They will also frequently have access to dietary/nutrient assessment software of the caliber required for research. CTSA sites have streamlined institutional review board (IRB) procedures, access to laboratories, and recruiting and data storage techniques that make them an excellent infrastructure for conducting clinical trials.[33]

BUDGET

An adequate budget that is sufficient to cover all study costs is essential. Although the actual cost depends on the study design, scope, and duration, there are some general guidelines. The major budget categories are personnel, supplies (including food costs), laboratory assays and procedures, equipment, and sometimes participant stipends. In most cases, an institution-specified percentage of the direct cost of the project must be added to cover overhead (ie, indirect costs). The research and grants office of the sponsoring institution provides this information.

Senior professional personnel are responsible for scientific decisions and control the budget. They also have an important role in compliance and building and sustaining staff and participant morale over the course of the study. Consistent day-to-day management by a study coordinator is necessary to supervise kitchen operations (where applicable), laboratory, and data collection. In studies involving diet instruction or counseling, RDNs are needed to provide the intervention. In feeding studies, personnel are needed to prepare food and food aliquots for assay. During the course of the study, work assignments may change; hence, some staff members should be prepared to assume various job responsibilities.

Well-controlled feeding studies require more extensive budgets, especially if food is prepared and served on-site. The budget may need to cover leasing kitchen and dining facilities and renting food storage and freezer space. High-precision scales for weighing food, high-powered blenders for preparing food aliquots for chemical analysis, and other specialized equipment may be required. In general, food is the most expensive item in controlled feeding studies. Dennis and colleagues[34] describe in detail resources required to conduct controlled feeding studies.

Most studies will also require a budget for the equipment and supplies associated with clinical, anthropometric, and laboratory measurements and for possible shipping costs for laboratory samples. Both statistical and computer capabilities, including specialized software, are required to manage and analyze the data and nutrient information. Clerical activities include preparing recruitment materials, creating and completing forms, handling communication, scheduling potential recruits, and preparing reports. Miscellaneous costs include forms, duplicating materials, monetary incentives for participants, transportation, parking for participants, social activities, closeout costs (celebration), and computer costs. If the plan is to collaborate with a CTSA site, there will still be associated costs; however, the staff at these centers are experts in accurate budgeting for trial needs.

STUDY PARTICIPANTS
Selecting the Participant Population

Inclusion and Exclusion Criteria

The study population should be defined in advance based on the hypothesis and should include specific inclusion and exclusion criteria. Inclusion and exclusion criteria are used to set parameters that more clearly define the study population and to focus the population or sample into one that is as homogeneous as possible. It is also important that selection of the participant population be determined by the hypotheses that are being tested. Following are typical inclusion criteria for consideration:

● age
● gender
● comorbidities
● pathophysiological condition (eg, presence of hypertension, AIDS or HIV, cancer, or burns)
● receiving certain treatment (eg, chemotherapy, dialysis)

Following are typical exclusion criteria:

● inability to perform a function or conduct a test
● taking a certain medication or receiving a particular treatment
● presence of comorbidities that might influence the primary outcomes

When considering which inclusion and exclusion criteria to use in a clinical trial, focusing on the parameters that may affect change in the primary outcome may be useful. For example, if a study is testing a nutrition intervention designed to improve hemoglobin A1c in patients who have type 2 diabetes mellitus, patients who are on insulin or oral hypoglycemic agents may need to be excluded, or participants may only be included based on their baseline hemoglobin A1c being within a certain range. Additionally, if a diet treatment is being tested to evaluate changes in a biological end point, some participants must be outside the range of normal or a diet response will not be observed. Participants with a clinically normal value may not be responsive to the diet intervention. However, if the abnormal end-point value is due to various comorbidities, it is essential to know this and to exclude these participants from the study as they could have a different intervention response. Thus, it is best to test the study hypothesis without the interference of underlying pathophysiological conditions that may overpower the effects of the intervention. One example that illustrates the importance of setting participant eligibility criteria appropriately is a researcher who wishes to study blood pressure responses to a diet intervention. The test diet studied may have little or no effect in normotensive participants but may significantly lower blood pressure in participants with hypertension. Likewise, a high-fiber diet may have no effect on C-reactive protein (CRP), a marker of inflammation, in participants who have low (ie, normal) values, whereas in participants with elevated CRP levels, a high-fiber diet would be expected to decrease CRP.

Number of Groups

Another consideration is whether more than one group of participants should be studied. Based on the results of previous studies, certain groups of individuals respond differently to an intervention compared with others. For example, individuals with elevated baseline triglyceride concentrations have decreased clearance of postprandial triglyceride-rich lipoproteins after a high-fat meal compared with individuals with clinically normal baseline triglyceride concentrations. A study that includes participants with elevated concentrations and participants with normal concentrations provides an opportunity to evaluate responses of different population groups to the diet intervention. Including multiple groups of individuals also allows researchers to generalize study results to a greater proportion of the general population. This is why it is important to include different age and sex groups that are representative of the population at large.

Sample Size

Sample size is both a functional consideration and an ethical consideration. Functionally, having a sample that is large enough to detect change but not so large as to make the study more costly is important. Ethically, studying too few patients makes the sacrifice of those patients who participate worth less; and similarly, studying too large a population can make the sacrifice of the participants above the needed sample worth less.[35]

Therefore, appropriate precautions must be taken to ensure that a study sample is large enough to detect differences between groups or treatments. Calculating sample sizes while providing for adequate levels of significance and power is an essential step in designing a study. When choosing the data to perform sample-size calculations, researchers need to be precise and choose not only a design but also outcome data that closely resemble the study in question. Data that are beneficial to power calculations are effect size, mean and standard deviation values between groups, and sample size of groups. These data can be used to calculate the needed sample size for one or more groups in order to detect a specific level of statistical significance. A common level desired is 80% power with an alpha of 0.05. However, for some studies high levels of power or lower alphas are needed. Although calculating sample size is an integral component of any study design, researchers must understand that these calculations provide only an estimate of the needed size of a study sample. Many software packages and some websites can help researchers calculate power (see Chapter 24 for more information on calculating sample size).

Once an estimate is obtained, investigators then need to account for other factors, such as participants lost over time (attrition) in clinical trials. A review of prior studies that are similar in design and length will provide information about the potential for attrition or withdrawal from a study. In determining the final sample size for the study, investigators should err on the side of being conservative within the resources of the design.

Participant Recruitment

When recruiting, the same ethical imperatives exist as for any study. See Chapter 3 for an in-depth discussion of ethical considerations.

Once the study population is defined, successful recruitment relies on a careful plan with multiple strategies.[7] Early in the planning stages of a study, the investigators must evaluate the likelihood of obtaining a sufficient number of study participants within an appropriate time frame and geographic area. If an important aspect of the study design or hypothesis is differential effects on diverse population groups, a second site may be required for the study to meet recruitment goals. For example, in designing a study to evaluate the effects of a dietary intervention on high blood pressure, researchers should attempt to recruit a population of black people, since this population is at higher risk for developing hypertension. A study such as this, conducted in a community with a small black population might necessitate including a second site in which a larger number of blacks could be recruited. However, no recruitment activity of any

kind can occur until the study has obtained IRB or ethics committee approval. All recruiting materials (eg, advertisements, flyers, emails, website postings) must be submitted and approved as part of the IRB application. The first step in the recruitment process is often an advertisement placed in a local newspaper or alternative media source (eg, listserv or website posting). When placing an advertisement for recruitment purposes, researchers should emphasize pertinent inclusion and exclusion criteria and a method for interested individuals to contact the study personnel (a toll-free phone number). Recruitment for clinical trials is often the most difficult part of the study, especially if the inclusion and exclusion criteria are narrow. Also, recruitment costs can be substantial and are often underestimated. For example, newspaper ads can run $250 to $500 per day, although ads can be disseminated at no cost via some methods, such as listservs. Technology also provides new opportunities for recruiting participants, for example, via internet interest groups related to a disease or condition or ResearchMatch (researchmatch .org), an initiative of the National Center for Advancing Translational Science that matches researchers and participants.

Participant Screening

After obtaining IRB or ethics committee approval for a study, it is important to have a process in place to screen potential participants for recruitment. Screening ensures that potential participants meet eligibility criteria. Individuals who are considering participation in a study need to be able to understand what will be required of them throughout the study and what they can expect from the researchers directing the study. Allowing potential participants time for questions and having answers to frequently asked questions lowers the chance of attrition later in the study. In general, a rigorous screening process is critical to study success. In addition to ensuring that potential participants meet eligibility criteria, screening provides an opportunity to evaluate subjective data, such as attitude, behavior, interest, commitment, maturity, and so forth, which are important attributes in retaining participants and maintaining adherence.

The complexity of the screening process depends on the specificity of participant exclusion criteria. Some studies require only a simple questionnaire, whereas others may require anthropometric, dietary, and laboratory data; information on lifestyle practices (such as smoking and physical activity behavior); and a medical examination to rule out underlying disease. It is particularly important that the screening process not prompt participants to make any behavior changes before the study. The interval between screening and study commencement should be minimized. Performing baseline assessments at the beginning of the study may be necessary to ensure that individuals have not made any behavior changes between the time they were screened and the time they begin the study. In addition, collecting baseline measurements assures the study staff that all participants are being assessed at a similar time point; in other words, if the screening process takes a number of months to complete before all participants are enrolled, baseline assessments should be taken for all participants within a short time period rather than over a period of months. Also, for some study questions seasonality may be a critical consideration; thus, time of year for screening and study initiation need to be considered.

The screening phase can be a multiple-step process such that participants who do not meet the eligibility criteria are eliminated early. As a result, the screening phase is more efficient and less costly. Depending on the nature of the study, the first stage in the screening process may include review of a patient's chart or questionnaires that can be mailed or completed by the recruitment team; these may be completed during telephone or personal interviews or on the participants' own time using online tools, for example.

It is important to document the number of patients screened, how many did and did not meet the inclusion criteria, and why they did not meet these criteria. This information should be reported in publications as it demonstrates that the sample selected was not biased or substantially different in some way from the overall population (see Figure 8.7). Additionally, this information may help determine barriers to recruitment. For example, during a multisite hospital-based pilot trial, the study team was having a very difficult time recruiting the desired number of participants. Close examination of the pilot screening data showed that the one criterion—patients to be enrolled within 24 hours of admission—was too difficult to achieve; thus, they extended enrollment to 48 hours.[36]

Some clinical studies have initial screening interviews. During the initial interview, it is important that participants learn what will be expected of them if they decide to participate. It is also important to ask questions about the individual's medical history that may exclude him or her from participating. If individuals still meet the eligibility requirements after this initial phase, researchers can proceed to a more in-depth screening appointment that often includes a clinic visit and collection of anthropometric and laboratory measurements that are of interest to the study staff. For example, if individuals with hypertension are being recruited for a blood pressure–lowering study, it would be important to establish that the potential participant has hypertension.

Participant Randomization

Participant randomization is used to remove systematic error and selection bias in clinical trials. In simple randomization, the most prevalent form of randomization, each participant is assigned to a treatment without any regard for previous assignments made to other participants. The main disadvantage of simple randomization is that it may lead to an imbalance in terms of participant characteristics that are known to be related to the variables under study (eg, more men in one group, lower or higher group mean values for a key baseline variable in one group) and, thereby, affect study results. When using stratified randomization, strata are constructed based on variables of interest, and a randomization scheme is performed separately within each stratum. For example, if a study is designed to evaluate the effects of a treatment in older vs younger individuals, participants would first be assigned to either a younger group or an older group and further randomized for treatment after this. In this way, stratified randomization ensures balance between the treatment groups with respect to various combinations of specific end-point measures. Constrained (or blocked) randomization, described by Hill,[37] is used to avoid imbalance in the number of participants assigned to each group. Within this randomization scheme, a sequence of blocks contains a prespecified number of treatments in a randomized order. This ensures that the randomization scheme is balanced at the completion of each block. For example, if groups of 10 participants are enrolled in a study every 3 weeks, a constrained randomization would ensure that the treatment allocations are evenly distributed across each enrollment group.

In a nonrandomized concurrent control study, the control group and the treatment group are not necessarily being treated at the same time. An example of this may be the comparison of survival rates of patients treated at two different institutions, with one institution using a new experimental procedure and the other practicing usual medical care. The major weakness of the nonrandomized design is the potential that the intervention and control groups may not be strictly comparable, making it difficult to elucidate effects of the treatment in question. Thus, integrating randomization is important.[38] Various randomization resources are available online. One free tool is the Research Randomizer, which generates one or more sets of random numbers from a specified range, with or without repeats, sorted or unsorted.[39]

Incentives

Incentives are important for participants in a clinical nutrition study. Although monetary incentives can be effective, other types of tangible incentives also encourage participation in the research process and may provide other benefits to participants. Examples of low-cost nutrition-related incentives include comprehensive nutrition assessment, dietary assessment analysis, a nutrition counseling session, a chronic disease risk profile, a pedometer, and recipes. The primary purpose of incentives is to facilitate participant recruitment and retention. Incentives can be as small as entry into a drawing for a prize item to as large as a substantial amount of money.

Incentives should be age- and gender-specific and appropriate for the time and effort required to participate in the screening process and research study. When designing a study that provides participants with nutrition information or education, researchers should present this as an incentive and convey the lasting influences that participation in the study could provide. Incentives should not be so grandiose that they encourage individuals with no intention of being study participants to participate in the screening process, and they should not imply or be perceived as coercion. However, participants should not perceive incentives to be worthless as this could have unintended consequences. Negative implications of incentives include selection bias (those who are interested in the incentive are different from the population that the sample represents) and a lack of participant commitment to the study.[40]

A distinction should be made between incentives for recruitment and incentives for retention. Incentives given throughout the study, such as recipes or laboratory results, often have a major impact because they demonstrate the effectiveness of the nutrition intervention to the participants. In contrast, incentives for recruitment are paid to the researchers executing the study at different sites and can lead to concerns about ethical recruitment if the incentives are large. Many IRBs mandate that participants be compensated for the time they spend participating in the study.

Participant Monitoring

Participants enrolled in a study must be adequately monitored. The extent of this is often a function of the overall intensity of the study design. For example, in an RCT feeding study, participants may be required to fill out daily and weekly monitoring forms where they have the opportunity to report any lack of compliance with the study protocol. On these monitoring forms participants can be prompted to report any study food they did not eat or any additional food consumed that was not included in the experimental diet plan. They can also be prompted to report any disruptions in normal activity, medication usage, or alcohol intake that may interfere with study outcomes. While the use of such forms provides a tool to monitor participants' level of adherence, the study staff should also take time to interact with participants and note any inconsistencies reported in conversations. In a free-living study, where study personnel may not interact with participants for a period of weeks or months, a more formal monitoring system may need to be implemented, such as weekly phone calls or emails to check in with the participants.

In studies with other types of interventions, strategies such as monitoring biochemical values, counting pills, and obtaining urine or stool samples provide evidence for participant adherence to the prescribed intervention or lack thereof. Actively involving participants in the research process means that participants are more likely to be committed to the project and adhere to the study protocol. It is important that participants in the control and intervention groups receive the same monitoring; if the intervention group receives more intensive monitoring, changes can result from the monitoring rather than the intervention.

Participant Retention and Adherence

Adequate resources are needed to ensure high participant retention and excellent adherence over the course of the study. Protocols must be developed that define retention policies and activities. Likewise, a protocol is needed for dealing with compliance issues, establishing policies for acceptable deviations from study protocol, and defining criteria for participant dismissal. The policy for participant dismissal must be shared with participants. Meticulous screening of potential participants will help identify those who will be cooperative and committed to all aspects of the study. The level of staff support provided to participants will vary depending on the design of the study. For example, the amount of personal interactions with participants will be greater during a controlled feeding study compared with a free-living study that has fewer staff-participant interactions.

Assessing adherence with the experimental protocol is important for meaningful interpretation of the treatment effects.[41] In some studies, adherence may be a significant outcome variable since the treatment effect may be biased by nonadherence. In either case, nonadherence must be accounted for in the final data analysis. For example, if a clinical

study is designed to evaluate the effects of iron supplementation on measures of iron status, and half of the treatment group takes only half of their prescribed supplement, this must be quantified and considered in interpreting the data analyses. A common approach to analyzing clinical trials is called "intent to treat." In this analysis, all data available for an individual are evaluated, even if the individual drops out early or is nonadherent. This analysis tests the effect of the mode of intervention but not the factors that could explain the effect.

Assessment of adherence must consider several variables that change as a function of the type and design of the investigation. In some studies, measuring adherence may entail a very simple, straightforward approach, whereas other studies may be dependent on measuring some biological variable that requires a more complex assay (eg, platelet phospholipid fatty acids to assess adherence with test diets high in certain fatty acids). Likewise, the sensitivity of the methods selected for assessing adherence may range from very sensitive (eg, measuring a urinary metabolite) to relatively insensitive (eg, participants' self-assessment of compliance). Another consideration is whether adherence is assessed objectively or subjectively. Examples of objective assessment are direct observation of participants' meal consumption on study premises or counting the remaining supplements in a bottle. Subjective assessment can be as simple as asking participants if they are adhering to the protocol. This approach is successful when the investigator and participants have established a friendly and trusting relationship. Often, investigators can ascertain adherence surprisingly well merely on the basis of participant attitude and behavior (eg, level of participation, punctuality). If there is any suspicion that participants are not adhering to the experimental protocol, this needs to be addressed promptly and in a nonconfrontational manner. If nonadherence is an issue potentially affecting the study outcome, the participant must be dismissed from the study.

Ideal adherence is the goal of all studies, but it is essential in metabolic studies. Not only must the participants consume all the allotted food (and not lose any through emesis) but they must also refrain from consuming any other food or substances that might bias the results of the study. However, it is not generally feasible to maintain study participants in an enclosed, supervised environment 24 hours a day over an extended period unless a CTSA site is involved in the study. Therefore, proxy measures are often used with varying degrees of sensitivity. For example, in the Women's Intervention Nutrition Study, adherence to a low-fat diet (up to 15% of energy from fat) was ascertained by unexpected collection of 24-hour recalls.[42]

Once energy equilibrium has been established, body weight changes may signal adherence problems. These changes, however, are a gross indicator of nonadherence. This method would not differentiate changes in energy expenditure, nor would it detect small deviations in food intake that could have a large effect if certain foods were systematically omitted or consumed outside the protocol.

A detailed description of various methods for assessing adherence is beyond the scope of this chapter. For more information, see Bingham.[43] Finally, it is important to note that human frailties and social needs being what they are, adherence is most likely not going to be perfect. It can be enhanced if overall morale is high and the investigators attempt to build some free choices into the protocol, for example, diet beverages that may be consumed at social gatherings.

NUTRITION INTERVENTION

Clinical nutrition studies can be designed to evaluate the effects of single nutrients, individual foods, dietary patterns, or behavioral interventions on end points of interest. The National Institute of Aging website offers the Clinical Research Study Investigator's Toolbox, a useful tool that offers a protocol template with a general format applicable to nutrition intervention studies, a template for a Manual of Procedures, and an Initial Proposal Concept Form (www.nia.nih.gov/research/dgcg/clinical-research -study-investigators-toolbox/startup).

Single nutrients can be provided by supplements (eg, n-3 fatty acids, eicosapentaenoic acid and docosahexaenoic acid)[44] or individual foods (eg, fatty fish).[45] Bioactive components can be provided via foods such as dark chocolate (eg, flavan-3-ols, procyanidins)[46] and processed tomato products (eg, lycopene).[47] When possible, researchers will

need to include a placebo group to maintain double-blinding. Studies can be conducted to evaluate the effects of specific foods on end points of interest (eg, extra-virgin olive oil).[48] In some instances, individual foods have been used to manipulate the nutrient profile of the diet (eg, walnuts).[49,50] Multiple nutrient manipulations can be evaluated. One such example of this approach is the OmniHeart Study, which evaluated how diets with different macronutrient profiles affected cardiovascular end points.[50] In other cases, manipulating the amount of a specific macronutrient in the diet (such as implementing a low-fat diet long term) is the focus of the dietary intervention.[42] Recently, there has been strong interest in evaluating the effects of dietary patterns on end points of interest. Examples of the latter include the Mediterranean diet,[1] Dietary Approaches to Stop Hypertension study,[13] the Portfolio Diet Study,[14] and a study evaluating the effects of the 2010 Dietary Guidelines for Americans diet on cardiovascular risk factors.[15] These various experimental approaches provide information about nutrients and bioactive components, foods, nutrient profiles, and dietary patterns and their effect on end points of interest. Thus, investigators can consider many different options when planning clinical nutrition studies; the choice of the nutrition intervention to be tested will depend on the hypothesis being evaluated. Figure 8.8 on page 137 shows how dietary control varies across a spectrum and provides examples of studies of varying dietary control.

In highly controlled studies, the menus for delivering the test diet should include popular, well-liked foods to facilitate achieving optimum adherence by study participants. Ideally, all foods in the test diets should first be tested for palatability. Also, it is helpful to include foods that are familiar to the study population (eg, kid-friendly foods for studies including children). Another useful practice is to present potential participants with a typical list of study foods during the screening phase to be sure they are able to consume these foods, as long as sharing this information does not interfere with the study protocol. Having a variety of foods on the menus helps avoid situations where specific food dislikes could be a reason for a potential participant to elect to not participate in the study. Some individuals may be willing to consume a food they do not like on occasion. Sometimes single foods on the menu can be substituted for others on the basis of nutrient content and study purpose. Researchers must also decide on the number of days for a menu rotation. Longer rotations of the study menu can be associated with greater nutrient variability. A shorter menu cycle (eg, 3-day cycle menu) may have less nutrient variability. However, if the cycle length is too short, participants may experience food fatigue, especially for a study of longer duration, thereby compromising adherence to the study protocol. To avoid serving the same meal on the same day each week, a 7-day menu cycle should be avoided. A 6-day menu cycle offers sufficient variety and has been shown to elicit good participant adherence over several months of a controlled feeding study.[17]

Nutrition Intervention Implementation Strategies

Investigators must consider a number of tradeoffs with the intervention design. As shown in Figure 8.8 (see page 137), the greater the dietary control, the more expensive the study, and the more difficult for potential participants. Liquid-formula diets or synthetic mixtures provide the greatest degree of consistency as each mouthful swallowed has the same composition. However, the relevance of the results to those that would be obtained with natural foods is limited. Nutrition intervention studies that require nutrition counseling need careful planning and substantial resources as they require well-trained interventionists (usually experienced in motivational interviewing), tailored intervention tools designed for the specific protocol, dietary assessment units that can collect dietary intake data over time, and elaborate collection of clinical data. Epidemiologic nutrition intervention studies in particular tend to be long term and require researchers to follow thousands of patients in several sites around the country for years.[17,42] Such studies come with a high financial cost to test the efficacy of nutrition counseling interventions. Again, the objectives of the study must be clearly delineated and, if necessary, revised to meet the limitations imposed by feasibility and reality. Once this is done,

the investigator can decide whether the attainable objectives justify doing the study. At the other end of the scale, studies that are more feasible in terms of cost and recruitment are more difficult to interpret because the results are confounded by variable adherence and variability in dietary composition.

Estimating Energy Requirements

In clinical nutrition studies, especially in controlled feeding studies, participants' energy requirements need to be assessed to ensure weight stability or weight change at a defined rate, depending on the goals of the study. This will affect the quantity of food needed and, hence, the budget in the case of feeding studies. Energy requirements can be estimated using a variety of methods depending on the age and health status of participants as well as resources available to conduct the study. The Academy of Nutrition and Dietetics Evidence Analysis Library project on energy expenditure is a comprehensive resource that provides different methods and conditions under which these estimating methods are appropriate to use (www.andeal.org/topic.cfm?menu=5299). Researchers should assess whether they need to measure resting metabolic rate vs estimating resting metabolic rate using predictive equations. When resources are limited, estimating energy requirements using predictive equations is common. The Harris-Benedict equation is frequently chosen, yet, more often than not, the caloric level defined for some participants needs to be adjusted.[24]Another equation that has been shown to predict energy needs better than the Harris-Benedict equation is the Mifflin-St Jeor equation.[52] This equation has provided the most accurate estimate of actual resting metabolic rate in the largest percentage of individuals, both nonobese and obese.[53] Predictive equations estimate participants' actual energy needs. Thus, it is highly advisable to have staff weigh participants daily or at every visit and to monitor feelings of hunger and fullness. Feelings of hunger and fullness are better short-term indicators of whether energy needs are being met with the test diet in a study where the goal is weight maintenance.

Determining Diet Composition

Several commercially available software packages estimate the nutrient intakes of individuals using data describing the nutrient composition of foods. Software packages most commonly include nutrient profile data available from the US Department of Agriculture's (USDA) Food Composition Databases (https://ndb.nal.usda.gov/ndb).[54] Researchers may look in the USDA Food Composition Databases for foods that may not be included in software package as the USDA continuously adds new data or provides data for less common food ingredients in commercially available software. However, nutrient databases are derived from average composition values that may not reflect what is being consumed, and actual nutrient content in foods can vary a great deal. For the highest precision, test diets need to be chemically analyzed, especially for the nutrients being studied. For studies in free-living participants, average values may be sufficient, but as the study moves toward greater control over the diet, the need for analytic values increases. A good plan is to analyze aliquots of the calculated diets and to make adjustments, if necessary, before the study begins. If differences are identified between calculated and assayed values, the food sources that account for the error must be identified and modified. If possible, aliquots should be collected and analyzed periodically throughout the study. Refer to Phillips and Stewart[55] for additional details on sampling and preparing composites. In addition, the American Oil Chemists' Society (AOCS)[56] and the Association of Official Analytical Chemists (AOAC) are valuable resources for selecting a food analysis laboratory.[57] The AOCS examination board provides a list of AOCS-certified laboratories. The AOAC provides methods and standards for analyzing foods, beverages, dietary supplements, and other products. Another important resource is USDA's Food Composition and Methods Development Laboratory, where content experts may be contacted and key publications can be accessed (www.ars.usda.gov/northeast-area/beltsville-md/beltsville-human-nutrition-research-center/food-composition-and-methods-development-laboratory/#).

POTENTIAL PROBLEMS
Random Error and Bias

While careful attention to detail will help eliminate the systematic error present in a clinical trial, random error cannot be controlled in the same manner. Random error is also known as random fluctuations or random variability. Despite the fact that the heterogeneity of the human population generally leads to a large random variation in clinical trials, the impact of this random error can often times be minimized by increasing the sample size. Examples of random errors that may be present in clinical trials are changes that occur based on seasonality or circadian rhythms. In addition to errors, clinical bias can yield point estimates that differ significantly from the true values. Sources of bias in clinical trials include the following:

- selection bias
- procedure selection bias
- postentry exclusion bias
- bias due to selective loss of data
- assessment bias (eg, when research staff are not or cannot be blinded to group assignment or when different groups are assessed at varying frequency)
- bias due to retroactive definitions (post hoc analysis wherein subgroups are defined after the data are analyzed)
- statistical bias

Any of these biases can diminish the external validity of the study and render the data and outcomes invalid.

QUALITY IMPROVEMENT AND DATA MANAGEMENT

A study can be a valuable addition to science only if the data supporting it were carefully collected. Every clinical nutrition study should incorporate a quality improvement program throughout all its stages (planning, implementation, data collection and management, and dissemination). A quality improvement program is a continuous process of monitoring and evaluating using predetermined criteria, feedback, and corrective actions. The quality control component is part of an overall management approach that utilizes written and oral reports, staff training, participant retention techniques, and budget monitoring.

Quality improvement relies on methods that provide the highest degree of accuracy and timeliness as is practically possible. Ideally, standards should be used, and routine monitoring should be included to ensure the continued accuracy of the methods used in a study. For example, a quality improvement system proactively plans for reanalysis of random subsamples (whether biomarkers, anthropometric measurements, or nutrient composition of foods) at different time points as a quality safeguard.

Quality improvement encompasses training staff; regularly maintaining and calibrating equipment; monitoring the performance of staff and equipment against performance standards; monitoring data quality; and documenting corrective feedback and changes throughout the collection, storage, and processing of data. Well-trained staff and repeated training are important for delivering standardized interventions and collecting complete data with minimal bias. Repeated training opportunities also minimize problems associated with staff turnover, especially in long-term trials.

Training is only one necessary component. Regular monitoring is also necessary. Over time, subtle changes in a procedure can cause considerable change in how or what data are collected, which can introduce bias in the results. The same is true for equipment. The tools and procedures for quality improvement should be developed and tested in the planning phase and should include a quality improvement protocol, written procedure and operations manuals, forms for data collection, and data management. Data management incorporates documentation of data quality, including protocol violations, missing and spurious values, and regular transmission of data to statistics staff. Visual inspection of completed forms, ranges for acceptable values, logic, and consistency checks are applied as data are collected so problems can be detected and corrected early (Box 8.2). Ideally, the quality assurance program prevents problems before they occur.

Throughout the study, efforts should be made to ensure that all data critical to answering the main questions of the study are high quality. Without quality data, conclusions are not evidence based or meaningful. The following types of problems are typically encountered during data collection: missing data; irrelevant, duplicate, or conflicting data; excess variability in the data; poor database format; poor documentation by staff; and insufficient time for proper data documentation. All of these problems can be minimized or even prevented by doing advance planning, training participating staff at different levels, and incorporating quality improvement measures throughout the study. For example, when performing anthropometric measurements on study participants, a training protocol must be in place, keeping in mind that more robust data are generated from multiple measurements performed (at least twice and optimally three times). Proper data collection and maintenance of quality control measures are integral in reducing the degree of systematic error in a trial or ensuring that the error is not a consequence of chance alone.

DATA ANALYSIS: PRIMARY AND SECONDARY

Data analysis is part of the statistical design of the study. The statistical design should be established during the study planning stages in order to control for and minimize biases, confounding factors, and random error as best as possible. Statistical testing of primary and secondary hypotheses should be specified up front in the study protocol. Issues such as deciding how to address missing or low-quality data, which participants to include or exclude in the analysis (due to nonadherence or drop-in/drop-out problems), which subgroup analyses to conduct, and how to conduct comparisons of multiple variables are critical for meaningful results and conclusions.[7] It is quite important that data analysis be conducted by scientists who are knowledgeable in statistical methodology and analysis for appropriate interpretation of the outcome variables.

A clinical study outcome is defined as a measured variable that allows investigators to determine if the null hypothesis of a study may or may not be accepted.[58] In a clinical study, according to the null hypothesis, there is no statistically significant difference between two treatment arms (con-

Aspects of the Study	Recommended Quality Control Procedures
Methods	Conduct advance statistical planning (power calculation and design randomization procedures, if applicable).
	Test instruments and intervention (materials and/or counseling approach) for validity, reliability, and usability.
Training and monitoring staff	Establish protocols.
	Establish written instructions for procedures and operations (a manual of procedures and a manual of operations can be extremely helpful for staff training and quality control).
	Provide initial training and repeat when necessary.
	Conduct regular site visits to audit clinic setup, protocol adherence, and quality of intervention, if applicable.
	Determine performance standards.
	Provide staff feedback.
Forms	Design data collection forms.
	Pilot test data collection forms for validity and reliability.
Study participants	Complete monitoring forms regularly.
	Receive feedback from staff who reviewed monitoring forms.
	Establish a retention protocol (especially important in intervention studies).
Data	Verify accuracy of data and data entry.
	Adjudicate questionable data.

Box 8.2 Recommended Quality Improvement Procedures in a Clinical Nutrition Study

trol vs intervention or intervention A vs intervention B) with respect to the stated outcome measure. Clinical study outcomes can be categorized as primary or secondary. Primary outcomes measure variables that will answer the primary (or most important) question being investigated, such as whether a nutrition intervention is superior to the usual diet in preventing a specific disease. In this case, the primary outcome would be based on the occurrence of disease during the study. The size of the study sample is determined by the power needed to detect a difference in this primary outcome. Secondary outcomes aim to answer other related questions in the same study; for example, whether there is also improvement in quality of life or whether the nutrition intervention reduces the overall length of hospital stay in patients. If secondary outcomes are also of high importance, the study must have enough power to detect a significant difference in both types of outcomes.

Today, clinical nutrition studies may include multiple primary and secondary outcomes for primary and secondary data analysis. If several hypotheses are tested, some are bound to end up statistically significant due to complete chance, even if all the hypotheses are actually false. Miller[59] has discussed in detail the problem of multiple comparisons and has provided various statistical approaches.

TRANSLATION

Researchers are obliged to communicate their study findings to the scientific community and the general public. Peer-reviewed papers published in the scientific literature are the gold standard for communicating study results to the scientific community. Other communications include abstracts, articles in the non–peer-reviewed professional literature and the popular press, as well as a final report. In addition, presentations at scientific meetings and conferences are important for rapidly communicating study findings.

The results of clinical nutrition studies have been used in setting dietary guidelines and establishing nutrient recommendations for the public. Accurate reporting and interpretation are crucial in translating the results of any study into dietary recommendations for the general public. Inherent to the evolution of dietary guidance is that a body of scientific evidence, not one study, is the basis for setting or modifying nutrition policy.[60] However, the ever-present reality is that one study can produce a novel discovery that greatly influences subsequent research efforts, which, in turn, grow the evidence base for making dietary recommendations for health promotion and the treatment of various diseases and conditions.

Nutrition is a critical component of translational research, that is, research that moves discoveries from laboratory and animal models into humans individually and as groups.[60] Clinical nutrition research may fall within many phases along the translational continuum, which is demonstrated by the importance of nutrition in many CTSA centers. When reporting results of clinical nutrition trials, researchers should indicate the next translational step.

CONCLUSION

The number and sophistication of clinical nutrition studies has rapidly evolved in recent years. However, key fundamental concepts remain the core for designing and conducting all clinical nutrition studies. The guidance presented herein, and elsewhere in the literature, provides a road map for all the necessary steps that need to be taken to carry out high-quality clinical nutrition research. A justified hypothesis guides the key aspects of the study. Crit-

ical considerations are the study and nutrition intervention designs, strategy for delivering the experimental nutrition interventions, statistical power, evaluations of the appropriate study population, appropriate statistical analyses, all logistics that pertain to carrying out all aspects of the study in a high-quality manner, and—importantly—the means of communicating study results. The success of a clinical nutrition study depends on a skilled and well-trained clinical staff, all of whom are adaptive and effective in interacting with study participants. Many opportunities are available for RDNs to be involved in all aspects of clinical nutrition research. Given their knowledge and expertise, RDNs understand the nutrition research needs that will advance clinical practice and health promotion efforts. RDNs are encouraged to be more proactive in seeking out leadership roles in conducting clinical nutrition research and, thereby, contribute substantively to the ongoing evolution of nutrition recommendations for health and treatment of disease.

REFERENCES

1. Otten J, Hellwig, JP, Meyers, LD. Dietary Reference Intakes: The Essential Guide to Nutrient Requirements. Washington, D.C.: The National Academies Press, 2006.

2. Myers EF, Khoo CS, Murphy W, Steiber A, Agarwal S. A critical assessment of research needs identified by the dietary guidelines committees from 1980 to 2010. *J Acad Nutr Diet.* 2013;113(7):971.e1.

3. Hand RK. Research in nutrition and dietetics—what can the academy do for you? *J Acad Nutr Diet.* 2014;114(1):131-135.

4. DeAngelis CD, Drazen JM, Frizelle FA, et al. Clinical trial registration: a statement from the International Committee of Medical Journal Editors. *JAMA.* 2004;292(9438):1363-1364.

5. Boushey C, Harris J, Bruemmer B, Archer SL, Van Horn L. Publishing nutrition research: a review of study design, statistical analyses, and other key elements of manuscript preparation, Part 1. *J Am Diet Assoc.* 2006;106(1):89-96.

6. Klein EA, Thompson IM Jr, Tangen CM, et al. Vitamin E and the risk of prostate cancer: the Selenium and Vitamin E Cancer Prevention Trial (SELECT). *JAMA.* 2011;306(14):1549-1556.

7. Friedman LM, Furberg CD, DeMets DL, Reboussin DM, Granger CB. *Fundamentals of Clinical Trials.* 5th ed. Switzerland: Springer International Publishing; 2015.

8. Grizzle JE. The two-period change-over design and its use in clinical trials. Biometrics. 1965;21:467-480.

9. Madsen K, Linchey J, Gerstein D, et al. Energy Balance 4 Kids with Play: results from a two-year cluster-randomized trial. Child Obes. 2015;11(4):375-383.

10. Brown CA, Lilford RJ. The stepped wedge trial design: a systematic review. *BMC Med Res Methodol.* 2006;6:54.

11. Moher D, Schulz KF, Altman DG. The CONSORT statement: revised recommendations for improving the quality of reports of parallel-group randomized trials. *BMC Med Res Methodol.* 2001;1:2.

12. Schulz KF, Altman DG, Moher D; CONSORT 2010 statement: updated guidelines for reporting parallel group randomized trials. *Ann Intern Med.* 2010;152(11):726-732.

13. Appel LJ, Moore TJ, Obarzanek E, et al. A clinical trial of the effects of dietary patterns on blood pressure. DASH Collaborative Research Group. *N Engl J Med.* 1997;336(16):1117-1124.

14. Jenkins DJ, Kendall CW, Faulkner D, et al. A dietary portfolio approach to cholesterol reduction: combined effects of plant sterols, vegetable proteins, and viscous fibers in hypercholesterolemia. *Metabolism.* 2002;51(12):1596-1604.

15. Schroeder N, Park YH, Kang MS, et al. A randomized trial on the effects of 2010 Dietary Guidelines for Americans and Korean diet patterns on cardiovascular risk factors in overweight and obese adults. *J Acad Nutr Diet.* 2015;115(7):1083-1092.

16. Appel LJ, Champagne CM, Harsha DW, et al; Writing Group of the PREMIER Collaborative Research Group. Effects of comprehensive lifestyle modification on blood pressure control: main results of the PREMIER clinical trial. *JAMA.* 2003;289(16):2083-2093.

17. Howard BV, Van Horn L, Hsia J, et al. Low-fat dietary pattern and risk of cardiovascular disease: the Women's Health Initiative Randomized Controlled Dietary Modification Trial. *JAMA.* 2006;295(6):655-666.

18. Implementation of treatment protocols in the Diabetes Control and Complications Trial. *Diabetes Care.* 1995;18(3):361-376.

19. Bouchard C, Tremblay A, Despres JP, et al. The response to long-term overfeeding in identical twins. *N Engl J Med.* 1990;322(21):1477-1482.

20. Coss-Bu JA, Jefferson LS, Levy ML, Walding D, David Y, Klish WJ. Nutrition requirements in patients with toxic epidermal necrolysis. *Nutr Clin Pract.* 1997;12(2):81-84.

21. Ahrens CL, Barletta JF, Kanji S, et al. Effect of low-calorie parenteral nutrition on the incidence and severity of hyperglycemia in surgical patients: a randomized, controlled trial. *Crit Care Med.* 2005;33(11):2507-2512.

22. Mustad VA, Jonnalagadda SS, Smutko SA, et al. Comparative lipid and lipoprotein responses to solid-food diets and defined liquid-formula diets. *Am J Clin Nutr.* 1999;70(5):839-846.

23. Delanaye P, Nellessen E, Grosch S, et al. Creatinine-based formulae for the estimation of glomerular filtration rate in heart transplant recipients. *Clin Transplant.* 2006;20:596-603.

24. Lin PH, Proschan MA, Bray GA, et al; DASH Collaborative Research Group. Estimation of energy requirements in a controlled feeding trial. *Am J Clin Nutr.* 2003;77(8):639-645.

25. Vogel RA, Corretti MC, Plotnick GD. The postprandial effect of components of the Mediterranean diet on endothelial function. *J Am Coll Cardiol.* 2000;36(5):1455-1460.

26. O'Kennedy N, Crosbie L, van Lieshout M, Broom JI, Webb DJ, Duttaroy AK. Effects of antiplatelet components of tomato extract on platelet function in vitro and ex vivo: a time-course cannulation study in healthy humans. *Am J Clin Nutr.* 2006;84(3):570-579.

27. Hendriks HF, Weststrate JA, van Vliet T, Meijer GW. Spreads enriched with three different levels of vegetable oil sterols and the degree of cholesterol lowering in normocholesterolaemic and mildly hypercholesterolaemic subjects. *Eur J Clin Nutr.* 1999;53(4):319-327.

28. Hasler CM. Functional foods: benefits, concerns and challenges—a position paper from the American Council on Science and Health. *J Nutr.* 2002;132(12):3772-3781.

29. Halsted CH. Dietary supplements and functional foods: 2 sides of a coin? *Am J Clin Nutr.* 2003;77(4 suppl):1001S-1007S.

30. Ferrari CK. Functional foods, herbs and nutraceuticals: towards biochemical mechanisms of healthy aging. *Biogerontology.* 2004;5(5):275-289.

31. Arvanitoyannis IS, Van Houwelingen-Koukaliaroglou M. Functional foods: a survey of health claims, pros and cons, and current legislation. *Crit Rev Food Sci Nutr.* 2005;45(5):385-404.

32. Kasim-Karakas S, Hyson D, Halsted C, van Loan M, Chedin E, Berglund L. Translational nutrition research at UC Davis—the key role of the Clinical and Translational Science Center. *Ann N Y Acad Sci.* 2010;1190:179-183.

33. National Center for Advancing Translational Sciences. Clinical and Translational Science Awards Program. https://ncats.nih.gov/files/CTSA-factsheet.pdf. Published November 2015. Accessed March 8, 2017.

34. Windhauser M, Ershow A, Obarzanek E, Dennis BH, Swain JF, Kris-Etherton P, Karmally W, Blackwell SE. The multicenter approach to human feeding studies. In: Dennis BH, Ershow A, Obarzanek E, Clevidence BA, eds. *Well-Controlled Diet Studies in Humans. A Practical Guide to Design and Management.* Chicago, IL: Academy of Nutrition and Dietetics; 1999:390-433.

35. Halpern SD, Karlawish JH, Berlin JA. The continuing unethical conduct of underpowered clinical trials. *JAMA.* 2002;288(3):358-362.

36. Hand RK, Murphy WJ, Field LB, et al. Validation of the Academy/A.S.P.E.N. Malnutrition Clinical Characteristics. *J Acad Nutr Diet.* 2016;116(5):856-864.

37. Hill AB. The clinical trial. *Br Med Bull.* 1951;7:278-282.

38. Kim J, Shin W. How to do random allocation (randomization). *Clin Orthop Surg.* 2014;6(1):103-109.

39. Urbaniak GC, Plous S. Research randomizer. Version 4.0. www.randomizer.org. Accessed August 13, 2017.

40. Goritz AS. The impact of material incentives on response quantity, response quality, sample composition, survey outcome, and cost in online access panels. *Int J Mark Res.* 2004;46:327-346.

41. Windhauser MM, Evans MA, McCullough ML, et al. Dietary adherence in the Dietary Approaches to Stop Hypertension trial. DASH Collaborative Research Group. *J Am Diet Assoc.* 1999;99(8 suppl):S76-S83.

42. Hoy MK, Winters BL, Chlebowski RT, et al. Implementing a low-fat eating plan in the Women's Intervention Nutrition Study. *J Am Diet Assoc.* 2009;109(4):688-696.

43. Bingham S. The dietary assessment of individuals; methods, accuracy, new techniques and recommendations. *Nutr Abstr Rev.* 1987;57A:705-742.

44. Dietary supplementation with n-3 polyunsaturated fatty acids and vitamin E after myocardial infarction: results of the GISSI-Prevenzione trial. Gruppo Italiano per lo Studio della Sopravvivenza nell'Infarto miocardico. *Lancet.* 1999;354(9177):447-455.

45. Burr ML, Fehily AM, Gilbert JF, et al. Effects of changes in fat, fish, and fibre intakes on death and myocardial reinfarction: diet and reinfarction trial (DART). *Lancet.* 1989;2(8666):757-761.

46. Keen CL, Holt RR, Oteiza PI, Fraga CG, Schmitz IIII. Cocoa antioxidants and cardiovascular health. *Am J Clin Nutr.* 2005;81(1 suppl):298S-303S.

47. Dutta-Roy AK, Crosbie L, Gordon MJ. Effects of tomato extract on human platelet aggregation in vitro. *Platelets.* 2001;12(4):218-227.

48. Garcia-Gavilan JF, Bullo M, Canudas S, et al. Extra virgin olive oil consumption reduces the risk of osteoporotic fractures in the PREDIMED trial. *Clin Nutr.* 2018;37(1):329-335.

49. Zhao G, Etherton TD, Martin KR, West SG, Gillies PJ, Kris-Etherton PM. Dietary alpha-linolenic acid reduces inflammatory and lipid cardiovascular risk factors in hypercholesterolemic men and women. *J Nutr.* 2004;134(11):2991-2997.

50. Appel LJ, Sacks FM, Carey VJ, et al; OmniHeart Collaborative Research Group. Effects of protein, monounsaturated fat, and carbohydrate intake on blood pressure and serum lipids: results of the OmniHeart randomized trial. *JAMA.* 2005;294(18):2455-2464.

51. Ginsberg HN, Kris-Etherton P, Dennis B, et al. Effects of reducing dietary saturated fatty acids on plasma lipids and lipoproteins in healthy subjects: the DELTA Study, protocol 1. *Arterioscler Thromb Vasc Biol.* 1998;18(3):441-449.

52. Mifflin MD, St Jeor ST, Hill LA, Scott BJ, Daugherty SA, Koh YO. A new predictive equation for resting energy expenditure in healthy individuals. *Am J Clin Nutr.* 1990;51(2):241-247.

53. Frankenfield DC, Rowe WA, Smith JS, Cooney RN. Validation of several established equations for resting metabolic rate in obese and nonobese people. *J Am Diet Assoc.* 2003;103(9):1152-1159.

54. US Department of Agriculture ARS, Nutrient Data Laboratory. Version Current: April 2018. USDA National Nutrient Database for Standard Reference, Legacy Release. https://ndb.nal.usda.gov/ndb.

55. Phillips K, Stewart KK. Validating diet composition by chemical analysis. In: Dennis BH, Ershow A, Obarzanek E, Clevidence BA, eds. *Well-Controlled Diet Studies in Humans. A Practical Guide to Design and Management.* Chicago, IL: Academy of Nutrition and Dietetics; 1999:337-366.

56. American Oil Chemists' Society. *Official Methods and Recommended Practices of the American Oil Chemists' Society.* 5th ed. Champaign, IL: American Oil Chemists' Society; 1998.

57. Association of Official Analytical Chemists. *Official Methods of Analysis of AOAC International.* 20th ed. Gaithersburg, MD: Association of Official Analytical Chemists; 2016.

58. Bakhai A, Wang D. Endpoints. In: Wang D, Bakhai A, eds. *Clinical Trials: A Practical Guide to Design, Analysis and Reporting.* London, United Kingdom: Remedica; 2006:37-45.

59. Miller RG. *Simultaneous Statistical Inference.* 2nd ed. New York: Springer-Verlag; 2011.

60. Zoellner J, Van Horn L, Gleason PM, Boushey CJ. What is translational research? Concepts and applications in nutrition and dietetics. *J Acad Nutr Diet.* 2015;115(7):1057-1071.

Chapter 9

Nutrition Monitoring in the United States: Sources of Data and Their Uses

Sharon I. Kirkpatrick, PhD, RD

LEARNING OBJECTIVES

1. Identify the key components of nutrition monitoring in the United States.

2. Appraise potential uses, strengths, and limitations of and gaps in available monitoring and surveillance data.

3. Recognize key considerations in conducting secondary analyses of monitoring data and interpreting the results.

4. Identify key resources relevant to nutrition monitoring data in the United States.

Integral to efforts to promote healthy eating among the population is the ongoing and comprehensive monitoring of nutritional status; patterns of consumption of foods, beverages, and supplements; and related factors, such as food security, food and nutrition assistance program participation, food-related knowledge and attitudes, characteristics of food environments, policies affecting foods available in different settings, and features of the broader food supply. For example, data from monitoring efforts provide the foundation for establishing nutrition standards and guidance, such as the Dietary Guidelines for Americans,[1] and for tracking eating patterns over time to examine how they align with such guidance.

Nutrition monitoring has been defined as "an ongoing description of nutrition conditions in the population, with particular attention to subgroups defined in socioeconomic terms, for purposes of planning, analyzing the effects of policies and programs on nutrition problems, and predicting future trends."[2] More broadly, within the context of public health, surveillance can be thought of as the continuous, systematic collection, analysis, and interpretation of health-related data to inform policy and practice.[3] A *nutrition surveillance system* "is used to collect, analyze, interpret and report information about the nutritional status of populations" and to "create appropriate response strategies."[4] Nutrition monitoring and surveillance in the United States consists of collecting, analyzing, and interpreting data from numerous surveys carried out at the national, state, and local levels that are used to assess the contributions diet and nutritional status make to the health of Americans and to learn about factors affecting dietary and nutritional status.[5,6]

The cornerstone of nutrition monitoring in the United States is the National Health and Nutrition Examination Survey (NHANES),[7] but a plethora of other data sources provide complementary information critical to understanding Americans' eating patterns and influences on those patterns. In recent years, researchers have seen increasing emphasis placed on surveillance of environments in terms of the extent to which they support and promote healthy eating.[1,8,9] This chapter provides an overview of the key sources of nutrition-related data available; highlights considerations related to analyses, utilization, and interpretation of the data; and identifies relevant resources available to nutrition and dietetics practitioners.

OVERVIEW AND BRIEF HISTORY OF NUTRITION MONITORING IN THE UNITED STATES

Information about the dietary and nutritional status of the US population and population subgroups, factors affecting dietary and nutritional status, and relationships between diet and health is provided by a variety of interconnected federal and state activities.[6] Data are collected in a number of measurement areas, detailed in this chapter, that are complemented by ongoing efforts to develop and maintain critical underlying databases, such as those relevant to food composition.[10]

The US National Nutrition Monitoring and Related Research Program (NNMRRP), previously called the National Nutrition Monitoring System (the updated name recognizes the importance of research to monitoring the nutritional status of the population),[11] is considered one of the best such systems in the world. Historical perspectives on the program are available elsewhere.[12-19] The Components of Nutrition Monitoring in the United States section and Table 9.1 (see pages 158 to 167) include information on historical nutrition monitoring activities (dating back to the 1930s). More recently, the National Nutrition Monitoring and Related Research Act of 1990[20] called for the development of a 10-year comprehensive plan, which was published for public comment in 1991[21] and finalized in 1993[22] with three primary goals:

● Provide for a comprehensive NNMRRP through continuous and coordinated data collection.
● Improve the comparability and quality of data across the NNMRRP.
● Improve the research base for nutrition monitoring.

These national goals were complemented by state and local objectives to strengthen data collection capacity; improve the quality of state and local data; and improve methodologies to enhance the comparability of data across national, state, and local levels. State and local government agencies have contributed by collecting data, for example, through the Behavioral Risk Factor Surveillance System (BRFSS), which is the largest continuously conducted health survey system in the world.[23]

In 1999, the National Academy of Sciences sponsored a symposium to discuss the future of nutrition monitoring and reauthorization. Despite this symposium, a report by the American Society for Nutritional Sciences Working Group,[16] and other efforts to gain support for reauthorization, the nutrition monitoring legislation was not renewed in 2002.[24] Monitoring activities continue, however, as described here, and in 2016, the Interagency Committee on Human Nutrition Research published a National Nutrition Research Roadmap that includes strategies for enhancing population-level food-related and nutrition-related health monitoring systems and their integration with other data systems.[8] The Roadmap calls for the development of a federal nutrition

---

Enhance our understanding of eating patterns and their correlates:

Enable dietary exposure estimates for nutrients, non-nutrient food components, and food groups and monitoring of intake in relation to recommendations for health, such as the Dietary Reference Intakes and Dietary Guidelines for Americans (DGA).[1,26-29]

Assess relationships among knowledge and attitudes, dietary and health behaviors, economic aspects of food consumption, and other nutrition-related behaviors.[30-34]

Examine how features of the food environment influence food consumption and the alignment between the food supply and dietary guidance;[35-39]

Expand the evidence on diet, health, and nutrient requirements:

Improve our understanding of the role of nutrition in the etiology, prevention, and treatment of chronic diseases and conditions.[40,41]

Advance our knowledge of nutrient requirements throughout the life cycle and inform the development and continued updating of the Dietary Reference Intakes.[28,29]

Inform guidance and standards:

Update the Dietary Guidelines for Americans[1] based on an understanding of the eating patterns of the population, factors influencing eating patterns, and evolving evidence on diet and health.

Develop reference standards related to nutritional status, such as growth charts.[42]

Inform and evaluate policies and programs:

Track food composition and consumption of nutrients of concern, such as sodium and added sugars,[43-45] as well as pesticides and other contaminants.[46,47]

Set targets and provide data to enable progress toward Healthy People 2020 objectives.[48]

Inform and evaluate fortification and labeling of the food supply.[49-52]

Monitor the prevalence and correlates of food insecurity and evaluate the impact of food assistance programs.[53]

Examine the environmental impact of current eating patterns.[54]

Box 9.1 Nutrition Monitoring Data Support Policy Making and Research in the United States in Different Ways

monitoring plan to address identified gaps, as noted later in this chapter. The National Institutes of Health (NIH) Nutrition Research Task Force is charged with developing a strategic plan to identify research gaps and promising opportunities, including the potential for interdisciplinary efforts to achieve common goals.[25] The task force met in June 2017 for the first time; future developments may highlight the relevance of nutrition monitoring and surveillance data to the task force's work.

USES AND VALUE OF NUTRITION MONITORING DATA

Nutrition monitoring is vital to policy making and research.[12,16,21,22] Box 9.1 on page 155, while not exhaustive, provides an overview of some of the myriad of ways in which monitoring data are used to develop standards; inform and evaluate policies, programs, and public health objectives; and enable research to understand Americans' eating patterns and other factors associated with nutritional status and food access. Box 9.2 uses Healthy People 2020 objectves as an example of how nutrition monitoring data may be used to assess progress toward public health goals.

While the purpose of monitoring data is mainly to enable inferences about populations or population subgroups (rather than about particular individuals), data may be collected at various levels, including from individuals (eg, dietary intake, height and weight); from households (eg, food security, food expenditures); from institutions, such as schools, universities, workplaces, and recreation centers (eg, policies related to vending machines); and at broader macro levels (eg, characteristics of the food supply). Indeed, information spanning the food stream from farm or factory to fork[55] is essential to building a comprehensive understanding of eating patterns and their influences or drivers, including those that operate at the level of the environment. In line with the social-ecological model, researchers and practitioners increasingly recognize that addressing these influences or structural factors is critical to shifting eating patterns toward recommendations.[1]

Healthy People provides evidence-based 10-year objectives for improving the health of Americans.[48] The Healthy People 2020 objectives related to nutrition and weight status fall under an overarching goal of promoting health and reducing risk of chronic disease through the consumption of healthy diets and the achievement and maintenance of healthy body weights.[56]

Researchers recognized that the factors influencing dietary behaviors and body weight are numerous and broad, including social and physical determinants. Thus, the objectives target not only individual behaviors related to food and nutrient consumption and weight status but also factors related to food insecurity and to the foods available in varied environments, including child care centers, schools, workplaces, and other settings in which healthy eating can be promoted.

Accordingly, data to evaluate progress toward objectives are gleaned from numerous sources, including data sets such as the National Health and Nutrition Examination Survey for indicators related to consumption of fruit, vegetables, whole grains, added sugars, solid fats, and sodium, as well as data sources relevant to child care, school policies, and physician practices related to assessment of body mass index.

The Healthy People website (www.healthy people.gov/2020/topics-objectives/topic /nutrition-and-weight-status) provides tangible examples of the use of complementary data sources to provide a more holistic picture of progress on nutrition-related objectives than could be obtained using any single source of information.

Box 9.2 Healthy People 2020 Objectives for Improving Health: An Example of the Use of Nutrition Monitoring Data for Assessing Progress on Public Health Goals

COMPONENTS OF NUTRITION MONITORING IN THE UNITED STATES

The first national dietary surveys in the United States were carried out in the 1930s. Since then, a multitude of surveys and surveillance systems have evolved in response to the information needs of federal, state, and local agencies and other users of nutrition-monitoring data. Table 9.1 (see pages 158 to 167) lists some of the key survey and surveillance activities at the federal level, organized by main measurement area or focus.

Areas of focus are derived from past listings of surveys and include (1) nutrition and related health measurements (such as indicators of nutritional status, food security, and participation in nutrition and food assistance program); (2) food and nutrient consumption; (3) knowledge, attitudes, and behavior assessment; (4) food composition and nutrient databases (expanded to include food patterns and supplements); and (5) food-supply determinations. To these, this chapter adds (6) information sources related to features of food environments and related policies reflecting current interest in this aspect of surveillance.[1,8,9,57,58] For each survey, the table includes details on sponsoring agencies, dates conducted, coverage of target populations, key nutrition-related variables, and URLs for websites for active or archived surveys. There is also an indication of whether the survey is part of the web-based Catalogue of Surveillance Systems (discussed later in this chapter) maintained by the National Collaborative for Childhood Obesity Research (NCCOR), a key compilation of data sources related to obesity that includes many resources considered part of the nutrition monitoring and surveillance system.[59,60] It should be noted that highlighted here are primarily surveys carried out or sponsored by the federal government. In a 2005 report, the Institute of Medicine Panel on Enhancing the Data Infrastructure in Support of Food and Nutrition Programs, Research, and Decision Making provided an overview of major federal and private-sector surveys related to food consumption, purchasing, and sales.[62] Elsewhere, Ng and Popkin[63] provided an overview of data sources for monitoring foods sold and consumed in the United States, considering both publicly available and commercial sources of data.

The sections that follow review some of the main surveys by area of focus. Later in the chapter, attention is given to such issues as the use of sampling weights to generate estimates that are representative of the population and other considerations related to appropriate analysis and interpretation of data.

Nutrition and Related Health Measurements

The cornerstone of nutrition monitoring and surveillance in the United States, the NHANES, provides population-level indicators of nutritional status, data on dietary and supplement intake, and various other health-related variables.[7,64] It enables researchers to perform analyses to estimate the prevalence of diseases and risk factors and, with consistent measurement and careful interpretation, allows examination of trends in nutrition and health status over time. For example, researchers have investigated trends in gluten avoidance over time.[65] Physical measurements, such as body measurements, blood pressure, findings of dental examinations, and results of biochemical and hematologic tests, allow for studying relationships among diet, nutrition, and health, such as associations between food insecurity and chronic disease[41] and levels of blood mercury concentrations and fish consumption among women of reproductive age.[66] The data also enable examination of patterns and disparities in nutrition and health related to sociodemographic characteristics. For example, a recent publication examined weight-loss strategies in relation to race and ethnicity.[67] The data are valuable to inform standards, such as the Centers for Disease Control and Prevention (CDC) Growth Standards[42] (see Box 9.3 on page 168).

Since 1999, the NHANES has used a continuous annual design and has included Americans of all ages.[72] Certain groups are sampled with higher probabilities than others to provide adequate sample sizes for reliable estimates; this is referred to as oversampling. From 2007 to 2010, oversampled groups included Mexican Americans, African Americans, low-income non-Hispanic whites, and persons

Survey[b]	Frequency (Date Initiated)	Department	Agency	Target Population/Sample
Nutrition and related health measurements				
National Vital Registration System	Continuously (1915)	Department of Health and Human Services (HHS)	Centers for Disease Control and Prevention (CDC)/National Center for Health Statistics (NCHS)	Total United States population
National Health Interview Survey (NHIS)	Annual (1957)	HHS	CDC/NCHS	Civilian, noninstitutionalized household population in the 50 states and Washington, DC
National Health Care Survey	Annually (1965)	HHS	CDC/NCHS	Record-based health care provider surveys capturing visits to hospitals and ambulatory surgical centers, office visits to nonfederal physicians, home health agencies, and nursing homes
National Health and Nutrition Examination Survey (NHANES)	Continuously in 2-year cycles since 1999; previous cycles were periodic (1971, with the addition of Nutrition to the NHANES)	HHS	CDC/NCHS	Civilian, noninstitutionalized individuals; all ages
National Survey of Family Growth (NSFG)	Continuously since 2006; previous cycles were periodic (1973)	HHS	CDC/NCHS	Noninstitutionalized individuals, 15–44 y; women only in 1973, 1976, 1982, 1988, and 1995
Pediatric Nutrition Surveillance System (PedNSS)	Continuously (1973–2011)	HHS	CDC/National Center for Chronic Disease Prevention and Health Promotion (NCCDPHP)	Children under the age of 5 y in federally funded maternal and child health programs 2010: 46 states, Washington, DC, and territories of the United States
Pregnancy Nutrition Surveillance System (PNSS)	Continuously (1973–2011)	HHS	CDC/ NCCDPHP	Low-income, high-risk pregnant women in programs operating in 2010; 29 states, Washington, DC, Puerto Rico, and three Indian Tribal Organizations contributed data
State and Local Area Integrated Telephone Survey (SLAITS)	Annually (1997)	HHS	CDC/NCHS	National and state estimates of target populations: subgroups such as persons with specific health conditions or from low-income households

Table 9.1 Federal Nutrition Monitoring Surveys and Surveillance Activities[a,6,61]

Sample Size and Characteristics	Response Rate[c]	Key Nutrition-Related Variables	Comments	Survey Website (Included in NCCOR[d] Catalogue)
All births and deaths in the United States	N/A[e]	Birth weight, mother's prepregnancy weight, and weight/height at child's birth	NCHS launched a project to modernize the National Vital Statistics System in 2016	www.cdc.gov/nchs/nvss.htm (Included in NCCOR Catalogue)
2006–2015: 35,000 households containing 87,500 persons (augmented by ~19% in 2015)	2015: 70% household 55% adult 63% child	Selected dietary variables (modules differ by cycle)	Survey redesign underway for 2018	www.cdc.gov/nchs/nhis /index.htm (Included in NCCOR Catalogue)
500 hospitals and 270,000 patient records; 1,500 nursing homes; 120,000 visits to 500 ambulatory facilities in a 3-year period; 1,800 home health and hospice agencies	Ranges from 70%–97% across surveys	Availability and utilization of dietary and nutrition services in health care settings, hospitalizations resulting from nutrition-related diseases	Comprised of separate surveys of hospitals, ambulatory medical care providers, nursing homes, hospice agencies, and ambulatory surgery providers since 1992	www.cdc.gov/nchs/dhcs /index.htm
~5,000/yr examined; 10,175 interviewed and 9,813 examined in 2013–2014	Interview response rate: 71% in 2013–2014 Examination response rate: 68.5% in 2013–2014	24-hour recall data, food security, measured height and weight, biochemical indicators	Data are released in 2-year cycles (eg, 2013–2014)	www.cdc.gov/nchs/nhanes /index.htm (Included in NCCOR Catalogue)
(~8,000–23,000) (10,205 in 2013–2015)	2015: 69%	Food assistance, breastfeeding practices, height, weight	Most recent data release: 2013–2015	www.cdc.gov/nchs/nsfg /index.htm (Included in NCCOR Catalogue)
2010: approximately 9 million children	N/A	Breastfeeding practices, participation in Supplemental Nutrition Assistance Program (SNAP) or Temporary Assistance for Need Families (TANF)	CDC discontinued compiling data in 2012; replaced with Special Supplemental Nutrition Program for Women, Infants, and Children (WIC) Participants and Program Characteristics	(Included in NCCOR Catalogue)
2010: approximately 1.2 million women	N/A	Breast feeding practices, use of maternal multivitamins	CDC discontinued compiling data in 2012	(Included in NCCOR Catalogue)
Varies	N/A	Includes National Survey of Children with Special Health Care Needs, the National Immunization Survey, and the National Survey of Early Childhood Health	Data collection mechanism to supplement national data collection initiatives	www.cdc.gov/nchs/slaits

(continued)

Survey[b]	Frequency (Date Initiated)	Department	Agency	Target Population/Sample
Food and nutrient consumption				
Consumer Expenditure Survey (expenditures on food purchases)	Continuously (1980)	Department of Labor	Bureau of Labor Statistics (BLS)	Civilian, noninstitutionalized, population and a portion of the institutionalized population
Survey of Income and Program Participation (SIPP)	Continuously (1983)	Department of Commerce (DOC)	Census Bureau (CB)	Civilian, noninstitutionalized population of the United States; aged 15 years and older
Continuing Survey of Food Intakes by Individuals (CSFII) and Supplement Children's Survey (Intake of Pyramid Servings and Servings database, 1994-96)	Periodically (1985-1998)	US Department of Agriculture (USDA)	Agricultural Research Service	Individuals of all ages residing in households nationwide in 1994-1996 and children aged 0-9 y in 1998; oversampling of individuals in low-income households; individuals 2+ y from CSFII 1994-1996
WIC Program Characteristics (PC)	Biennially (1992)	USDA	USDA/Food and Nutrition Service (FNS)	WIC participants using mail surveys of state and local WIC agencies, record abstractions at local WIC service sites
Current Population Survey (CPS), Supplement on Food Security	Annually (1995)	BLS, CB, USDA	USDA/FNS, Economic Research Service (ERS)	Civilian, noninstitutionalized United States population aged 16 y and older
FoodNet (surveillance of foodborne illnesses)	Continuous laboratory monitoring, periodic surveys (1996)	HHS, USDA	CDC; US Food and Drug Administration (FDA) Food Safety and Inspection Service (FSIS)	Laboratory, physician, and population surveys; special studies
What We Eat in America (WWEIA); dietary component of NHANES	Continuously (2002)	HHS, USDA	CDC/NCHS, Agricultural Research Service (ARS)	See listing for NHANES
Food composition, nutrient, food patterns, and supplement databases				
National Nutrient Database for Standard Reference	Continuously (1892-2018)	USDA	ARS	Basic and common foods available for consumption in the United States

Table 9.1 (cont.) Federal Nutrition Monitoring Surveys and Surveillance Activities[a,b,61]

Sample Size and Characteristics	Response Rate[c]	Key Nutrition-Related Variables	Comments	Survey Website (Included in NCCOR[d] Catalogue)
Targets: 7,500 households/quarter; 6,000 individuals/y	2015: Interview: 64% Diary: 58% (Response rates have been declining since 1990)	Expenditures on specific types of foods purchased for home consumption and consumed away from home	Quarterly interview survey of consumer units Diary survey of consumer units kept for 2 consecutive 1-week periods	www.bls.gov/cex/ (Included in NCCOR Catalogue)
29,835 households in 2014 SIPP Wave 1	70%	Food and nutrition assistance program participation, food security, frequency of family meals (breakfast and dinner)	Continuous series of panels with duration of 2.5–4 years; reengineered for 2014 panel	www.census.gov/sipp (Included in NCCOR Catalogue)
15,303 in 1994–1996 and 5,000 in 1998	76%	Dietary intake data	Integrated into What We Eat in America (WWEIA), the dietary component of NHANES, in 2002	N/A
9,303,253 records in 2014	N/A	Height, weight, nutritional risks present at certification	Near Census of WIC participants	www.fns.usda.gov/wic /wic-participant-and -program-characteristics -2014
2005 Supplement: 39,948 households	2015: 24% of households that completed CPS did not complete the Food Security Supplement	Food expenditure, access, and food quality and safety		www.census.gov/cps (Included in NCCOR Catalogue)
Varies	Varies	Incidence, attributes and burdens of foodborne illnesses Food eating patterns	N/A	www.cdc.gov/foodnet .index.html
See listing for NHANES	See listing for NHANES	See listing for NHANES	See listing for NHANES	www.ars.usda.gov/northeast -area/beltsville-md-bhnrc /beltsville-human-nutrition -research-center/food -surveys-research-group /docs/wweianhanes -overview/ (Included in NCCOR Catalogue)
SR-28 (2015): 8,789 food items and up to 150 food components. SR-Legacy (2018): up to 150 food components for over 7,793 foods.	N/A	Various micronutrients, vitamins, minerals, and food components	Updated approximately annually until 2015	www.ars.usda.gov/Services /docs.htm?docid=8964 (Included in NCCOR Catalogue)

(continued)

Survey[b]	Frequency (Date Initiated)	Department	Agency	Target Population/Sample
Total Diet Study (TDS)	Quarterly (1961)	HHS	FDA	Representative diets of specific age-sex groups
Food Label and Package Survey	Periodically (1977)	HHS	FDA	Food labels of processed/packaged foods
Food and Nutrient Database for Dietary Studies (FNDDS)	Continuously (1977)	USDA	ARS	Foods reported on the WWEIA, dietary component of NHANES
Food Patterns Equivalents Database (FPED)	Continuously (1994)	USDA	ARS	Foods reported on the WWEIA, dietary component of NHANES
Dietary Supplement Ingredient Database (DSID)	Continuously (2004)	HHS, USDA	ARS, National Institutes of Health (NIH)/Office of Dietary Supplements	Adult multivitamin/multimineral supplements available in the United States
Knowledge, attitudes, and behavioral assessments				
Health and Diet Survey	Periodically (1982)	HHS	FDA	Civilian, noninstitutionalized individuals in households with telephones, 18+ y, 50 states and Washington, DC
Behavioral Risk Factor Surveillance System (BRFSS)	Continuously (1984)	HHS	CDC/ NCCDPHP	Adults in all 50 states, Washington, DC, and 3 United States territories
Pregnancy Risk Assessment Monitoring System (PRAMS)	Continuously (1987)	HHS	CDC/NCCDPHP	Women with a recent live birth (sample of birth certificates)
Food Safety Survey	Periodically (1988)	HHS, USDA, FSIS	FDA	Adults in 50 states and Washington, DC
Youth Risk Behavior Survey (YRBS)	Biannually (1991)	HHS	CDC/NCCDPHP	Students in grades 9–12

Table 9.1 (cont.) Federal Nutrition Monitoring Surveys and Surveillance Activities[a,6,61]

Sample Size and Characteristics	Response Rate[c]	Key Nutrition-Related Variables	Comments	Survey Website (Included in NCCOR[d] Catalogue)
280 foods, including 50 infant foods, foods representative of dietary intake of specific age and sex groups	N/A	Nutrient elements, contaminants, and pesticides in foods	Does not estimate energy or macronutrient content	www.fda.gov/Food /FoodScienceResearch /TotalDietStudy/default.htm (Included in NCCOR Catalogue)
2006–2007: 1,227 food products regulated by the FDA	2006–2007: 94.5% of food brands purchased in the United States	Quantitative nutrient labels, ingredients, health/nutrient content claims of labels, allergen and food safety information	N/A	N/A
2013–2014: 8,536 food codes; 65 nutrients/ components	N/A		Updated for each 2-y cycle of NHANES/WWEIA Latest update was in 2013–2014	www.ars.usda.gov/Services /docs.htm?docid=12089 (Included in NCCOR Catalogue)
Food codes included in the FNDDS converted into 37 food patterns components	N/A	Dietary patterns and intake levels of food patterns components	Earlier version was MyPyramid Equivalents Database (1994–2004) Updated every 2 y corresponding with NHANES; most recent is 2011–2012	www.ars.usda.gov/Services /docs.htm?docid=23871 (Included in NCCOR Catalogue)
Commonly used multivitamin/multimineral and other supplements.	N/A	Levels of ingredients in dietary supplement products	Expansion planned to include single ingredient products and botanically based supplements	http://dietarysupplement database.usda.nih.gov (Included in NCCOR Catalogue)
2014: 2,480	2014: 30%	Knowledge/beliefs about diet and nutrition issues, use of food labels, dietary management practices	Most recent year conducted was 2014, first year to sample cell phone users	www.fda.gov/Food /FoodScienceResearch /ConsumerBehavior Research/default.htm (Included in NCCOR Catalogue)
2015: 441,496 interviews	2015: landline 17%, cell phone 18%	Food security status, dietary patterns (eg, sugarsweetened beverages, sodium, fruits and vegetables)	Most recently conducted in 2015; response rates vary by state; added cell phone sample in 2011	www.cdc.gov/BRFSS (Included in NCCOR Catalogue)
Annual sample sizes of 1,000 to 3,400 per state	83% of all United States births	Content/source of prenatal care, knowledge of nutritionrelated pregnancy information (eg, folic acid)	Joint project between state departments of health and CDC	www.cdc.gov/prams
2014: 4,196	21%	Food safety practices Attitudes, knowledge, and beliefs about food safety	Latest iteration was in 2016, first time cell phone interviews were conducted	www.fda.gov/Food /FoodScienceResearch /ConsumerBehavior Research/ucm529431.htm
2015: 15,624 to 16,000 students nationally	2015: School: 69%, students: 86%	Dieting practices, use of weight-loss aids, consumption patterns	Does not include United States territories; other components include middle school survey and methods studies	www.cdc.gov/HealthyYouth /yrbs/index.htm (Included in NCCOR Catalogue)

(continued)

Survey[b]	Frequency (Date Initiated)	Department	Agency	Target Population/Sample
School Nutrition Dietary Assessment Study (SNDA)	Periodically (1991–1992)	USDA	FNS	School food authorities and schools in the 48 states, students in grades 1–12 and their parents
Infant Feeding Practices Survey (IFPS) II	Periodically (1993–1994)	HHS	CDC FDA	Pregnant women and new mothers and healthy, full-term infants 0–1 y
Health Behaviors in School-Aged Children (HBSC)	Continuously (1997)	HHS	National Institute of Child Health and Human Development (NICHD)	Students ages 11, 13, and 15 y, attending school in the United States Administers an extended national instrument to youth in grades 6 to 10, with oversampling of minority youth
Food supply determinations				
Nutrient Content of the United States Food Supply Series	Periodically (1909)	USDA	ERS, ARS, Center for Nutrition Policy and Promotion (CNPP)	N/A
Fisheries of the United States	Annually (1909)	DOC	National Oceanic and Atmospheric Administration/National Marine Fisheries Service	N/A
Food Availability Data System	Annually (1971)	USDA	ERS	N/A
Nielson Scantrack and Homescan	Continuously (1980)	USDA	ERS, CNPP, The Nielson Company	Retail stores in the United States (Scantrack), households in the 48 states (Homescan)
Food environment and policy data				
National Survey on Recreation and the Environment	Periodically (1960)	USDA	National Forest Service	Civilian, noninstitutionalized individuals over the age of 16
School Health Policies and Practices Study (SHPPS)	Periodically (1994)	HHS	CDC	Education agencies and schools in all 50 states and Washington, DC

Table 9.1 (cont.) Federal Nutrition Monitoring Surveys and Surveillance Activities[a,6,61]

Sample Size and Characteristics	Response Rate[c]	Key Nutrition-Related Variables	Comments	Survey Website (Included in NCCOR[d] Catalogue)
2009–2010: 1,059 schools	2009–2010: 96%	District and school food policies, quality of meals offered in public schools, food sources, food consumption, family eating habits, participation in school meal programs	Most recent was SNDA-IV, conducted in 2009–2010; integrated into School Nutrition and Meal Cost Study in 2014–2015	www.fns.usda.gov/school-nutrition-dietary-assessment-study-iv (Included in NCCOR Catalogue)
2006: 4,000 pregnant women 2012 follow-up: 1,542 women	Follow-up: 52%	Breastfeeding, formula feeding, solid food intake, complementary foods	Year 6 follow-up conducted in 2012	www.cdc.gov/breastfeeding/data/ifps/index.htm
2009–2010: 12,649	N/A	Dieting practices, frequency of breakfast consumption, consumption of fruits and vegetables, sweets, sugar-sweetened beverages, alcohol	Contributes to a cross-national study, most recent data collection in the United States was 2009–2010	www.hbsc.org (Included in NCCOR Catalogue)
N/A	N/A	Nutrients per capita per day in food available for consumption, percentage contributions of nutrients by major food groups	N/A	www.cnpp.usda.gov/tools/IFS/default.htm www.cnpp.usda.gov/USfoodsupply
N/A	N/A	Annual estimates of fish and shellfish disappearance in the distribution system	N/A	www.st.nmfs.noaa.gov/commercial-fisheries/fus/fus15/index
N/A	N/A	Food availability data, loss-adjusted food availability data, nutrient availability data for over 200 commodities	Do not represent consumption but can complement intake data	www.ers.usda.gov/data-products/food-availability-per-capita-data-system (Included in NCCOR Catalogue)
100,000 households and 52 markets (Homescan)	N/A	Consumer packaged food purchase information, consumer eating patterns	The USDA ERS has acquired Homescan data for use in USDA-funded research, a partnership between the Nielsen Company and the University of Chicago Booth School of Business, which facilitates access for researchers	http://us.nielsen.com/ (Included in NCCOR Catalogue)
30,000 individuals between 2005–2010	N/A	Food sources: gardening practices, meals cooked at home, meals eaten outside of home	Most recently conducted in 2010	www.srs.fs.usda.gov/trends/Nsre/nsre2.html (Included in NCCOR Catalogue)
Varies	Varies	Availability and variety of foods/meals, food service evaluation (menu planning, promotion)	Collects data at the state, district, school, and classroom -levels	www.cdc.gov/HealthyYouth/shpps/ (Included in NCCOR Catalogue)

(continued)

Survey[b]	Frequency (Date Initiated)	Department	Agency	Target Population/Sample
SNAP Policy Database	Periodically (1996–2011)	USDA	ERS	SNAP rules or policies
Classification of Laws Associated with School Students (CLASS)	Annually or biennially (2003)	HHS	NIH/National Cancer Institute	State laws for the 50 states and Washington, DC
SNAP Retailer Locator	Bimonthly (2010)	USDA	FNS	SNAP-approved retail markets in the United States
MenuStat	Annually (2013)	HHS	CDC	Menu items from largest chain restaurants in United States

Table 9.1 (cont.) Federal Nutrition Monitoring Surveys and Surveillance Activities[a,6,61]

[a] Sources of information include the 2000 version of the Nutrition Monitoring in the United States directory (www.cdc.gov/nchs/data/misc/direc-99.pdf),[6] survey websites, and the National Collaborative for Childhood Obesity Research Catalogue of Surveillance Systems (https://tools.nccor.org/css/).[61] The National Collaborative for Childhood Obesity Research Catalogue provides access to information on over 100 publicly available data sets with relevance to childhood obesity research, many of which include data salient to monitoring of nutrition and related factors.
[b] Listings are in chronological order based on date of inception (in parentheses). Rows for surveys that are no longer active are shaded in grey. For studies no longer being conducted, the parenthetical date is the range from inception to the last year conducted.
[c] Percentage of sample population that responded.
[d] NCCOR=National Collaborative for Childhood Obesity Research
[e] N/A=not applicable

aged 60 years and older. In 2011, Asians were added to the oversampled groups,[73] recognizing the underrepresentation of this subgroup of the US population in surveillance and research more broadly.[74] This has enabled the generation of information on health indicators, including estimates of body mass index, hypertension, and abnormal cholesterol, among this fast-growing population.[75,76] Opportunities to leverage the nutrition-related data within NHANES are enhanced by linkages of particular cycles to geographic data, as well as Medicare and Medicaid data, the National Death Index, Social Security Administration data, and Department of Housing and Urban Development administrative data for rental assistance programs.[77]

Another survey that could be considered part of the cornerstone of nutrition surveillance in the United States is the National Health Interview Survey (NHIS).[78] This annual survey provides information about self-reported health conditions and, periodically, special nutrition and health topics, such as vitamin/mineral supplement use, food program participation, diet and nutrition knowledge, and food preparation. NHIS data collected in 2015 included the Adult Cancer Control Module encompassing the Dietary Screener Questionnaire developed by the National Cancer Institute (NCI), as well as supplementary questions on household food security. Large sample sizes enable estimates to be reported for the major racial/ethnic subgroups in the US population in addition to stratification by age group, sex, and income level. As with NHANES, oversampling is used to ensure that estimates can be generated for specific groups, including black, Hispanic, and Asian respondents. A redesign of the NHIS questionnaire is underway for 2019,[79] with proposed annual and rotating core topics along with supplements (eg, past supplements have focused on food security, cancer screening, and complementary and alternative medicine).

The Current Population Survey (CPS),[80] conducted by the US Census Bureau, represents an important component of nutrition monitoring in the

Sample Size and Characteristics	Response Rate[c]	Key Nutrition-Related Variables	Comments	Survey Website (Included in NCCOR[d] Catalogue)
50 states and Washington, DC	N/A	Rules or policies related to SNAP	Data gathered through legal/policy research and contacts with state administrators	www.ers.usda.gov/data-products/snap-policy-database.aspx (Included in NCCOR Catalogue)
N/A	N/A	State laws affecting competitive foods, pricing, advertising, promotion	Includes laws affecting nutrition and physical activity	https://class.cancer.gov/ (Included in NCCOR Catalogue)
Over 200,000 SNAP-approved markets	N/A	Food environment of SNAP beneficiaries	SNAP formerly known as Food Stamp Program	www.snapretailerlocator.com/ (Included in NCCOR Catalogue)
Information on nutritional content of over 35,000 food and beverage items sold at national chain restaurants	N/A	Macronutrient content of different menu items	Information retrieved from restaurant websites; information is not standardized; maintained by New York City Department of Health and Mental Hygiene, with funding in part from CDC	www1.nyc.gov/nyc-resources/service/3406/menustat-website (Included in NCCOR Catalogue)

United States due to an annual supplement focused on household food security. The 18-item measure was developed by the Federal Interagency Working Group for Food Security Measurement.[81] Using the CPS data, the US Department of Agriculture (USDA) Economic Research Service (ERS) publishes annual reports on household food security in the United States.[82] Inclusion of the measure in NHANES (beginning in 1999), the Survey of Program Dynamics (up to 2002), and the US Department of Education's Early Childhood Longitudinal Study (from 1998 to 1999) has allowed examination of indicators of household food security in relation to such variables as dietary intake[27] and academic performance in children,[83] as well as analyses of trends over time in exposure to food insecurity.[84]

Several monitoring efforts facilitate evaluation of characteristics of users of the USDA's nutrition and food assistance programs and the implications of program participation. A list of useful data assets for food and nutrition assistance research, with brief descriptions of each, can be found on the USDA's ERS website[85]; data sources relate to food consumption, availability, purchasing, and policy-related factors, among others. For example, the 2006 to 2008 American Time Use Survey included the Eating and Health Module, which ascertains information on food consumption occurring while engaging in other activities, such as watching television, and includes an indicator of participation in the Food Stamp program (now known as the Supplemental Nutrition Assistance Program, or SNAP) and measures of general health, height, and weight.[86] The Eating and Health module was also administered in the 2014 to 2016 American Time Use Survey.[87] The Consumer Expenditure Survey also includes information on SNAP participation,[88,89] while NHANES includes indicators of program participation and has been used to compare dietary intakes of program participants and nonparticipants.[90,91]

A number of studies have been conducted to evaluate the nutrition and health effects of participating in the Special Supplemental Nutrition Program for Women, Infants, and Children (WIC). Two relevant surveillance efforts conducted by CDC were the Pediatric Nutrition Surveillance System (PedNSS) and Pregnancy Nutrition Surveillance System (PNSS), which compiled information from the states and other contributors and were linked to one another through the infant data. Both systems were recently

Anthropometric data from the National Health and Nutrition Examination Survey were used to inform the 2000 Centers for Disease Control and Prevention (CDC) Growth Charts,[42] which include charts for infants through 20 years of age and body mass index for age charts.

Since the initial release of the charts in 2000, CDC has recommended the use of the 2006 World Health Organization (WHO) Child Growth Standards[68] for infants and children aged 0 to 2 years since they reflect growth patterns among children who were predominantly breastfed, provide a better description of physiological growth in infancy, and are based on a high-quality study with length and weight data measured at frequent intervals. This recommendation reflects a case in which the US data were not optimally suited to the purpose; integration of alternative resources appropriately reflect this.

To facilitate use of the charts and standards, CDC provides online training courses[69] and access to tailored software.[70] The interactive, self-directed training courses provide background on the growth charts and guidance on how to use them appropriately. The Epi Info software includes the Nutrition Project tool, which can be used to collect, analyze, and graph child age, weight, and height data using the WHO Standards or the CDC 2000 Growth Reference, as appropriate, to calculate percentiles.

The growth charts have been used in various studies, including surveillance of the proportion of American children affected by overweight and obesity.[71]

Box 9.3 Centers for Disease Control and Prevention Growth Charts: An Example of the Use of Nutrition Monitoring Data to Inform Reference Standards Related to Nutritional Status

discontinued,[92] but with appropriate analysis and interpretation, the data can be used to provide recent or historical insights. PedNSS was used to monitor key indicators of nutritional status (eg, anemia, birth weight, and weight status) among low-income, high-risk infants and children, with coverage reflecting the number of clinic visits in participating programs. Data can be analyzed at individual, clinic, county, state, and national levels. Information was also collected on breastfeeding status and television- and video-watching habits of children participating in WIC. The PedNSS had been used to monitor the proportion of toddlers from low-income families who are affected by obesity and has been replaced by the WIC Participants and Program Characteristics.[93-95] PNSS tracked nutrition-related problems and behavioral risk factors associated with low birth weight among high-risk prenatal populations. The PNSS data, collected for women participating in WIC, can be used to identify preventable nutrition-related problems and behavioral risk factors, such as weight gain during pregnancy, birth outcomes, and breastfeeding.[96] The coverage of PNSS reflected the number of pregnant women who participated in the programs contributing to the surveillance system.

Researchers should note that surveillance data related to women and children participating in publicly funded food assistance, nutrition, or health programs involve a self-selected population and are not representative of the community at large. Factors that differentiate members of this group from the general population include their meeting the income eligibility level, having a nutrition or health risk, and having the personal initiative or knowledge to participate in available programs. However, the data can be representative of program participants and thus may be useful for planning public health and nutrition programs and evaluating how these programs affect the nutrition and health status of the target populations. Another consideration is that eligibility criteria can vary from state to state and, over time, making comparisons across states and time difficult. Knowledge of program enrollment criteria and changes in criteria over time is important for appropriately interpreting the data. Information about programs administered by the USDA Food and Nutrition Service can be found on the website.[97] Data users may also need to consult state-specific resources.

Pertinent to school meal programs, the School Nutrition Dietary Assessment (SNDA) Study has been conducted periodically since 1991 and collects information on meals offered to and consumed by children participating in the National School Lunch Program and School Breakfast Program. The first cycle was followed by SNDA-II (1998 to 1999) and SNDA-III (2005), the latter of which collected information on the school food environment in addition to measures of students' heights, weights, and diets, with the findings published in a supplement to the *Journal of the Academy of Nutrition and Dietetics*.[98] The most recent cycle, SNDA-IV, was conducted from 2009 to 2010 and provides baseline data for measuring changes in school meals and associated measures in relation to standards issued by the USDA in 2012 as part of the Healthy, Hunger-Free Kids Act of 2010.[99,100] In 2014 and 2015, the goals of SNDA were integrated into the School Nutrition and Meal Cost Study.[92,100] The National Survey of Children's Health also includes indicators of school meal (and other food and nutrition assistance) program participation, as well as measures of the school and neighborhood context.[101]

Finally, the National Health Care Surveys, encompassing a number of record-based surveys of health care providers, provide data on the availability and utilization of dietary and nutrition services in health care settings, such as ambulatory surgical centers, hospital outpatient departments, emergency departments, hospices, and home health agencies.[102] For hospital outpatient department visits, nutrition-related data include physician-reported hypertension and obesity, as well as counseling services for diet, weight reduction, and cholesterol reduction. The survey also provides information on hospitalizations resulting from nutrition-related diseases.

Other surveys with relevance to monitoring of nutrition and health are highlighted in Table 9.1 (see pages 158 to 167).

Food and Nutrient Consumption

Food and nutrient consumption measurements include estimates of individuals' intakes of foods and beverages (nonalcoholic and alcoholic) and nutrition supplements, as well as levels of nonessential nutrients. In the context of monitoring, individual-level dietary data are typically used to make inferences about populations and population subgroups, not about particular individuals as would be the case in a clinical setting.

The main source of information on the food and nutrient consumption of Americans is What We Eat in America (WWEIA),[103] the dietary assessment component of NHANES. The WWEIA resulted from the integration in 2002 of NHANES and the USDA's Continuing Survey of Food Intakes by Individuals (CSFII), established to provide national estimates of food and nutrient intakes in the general US population and subgroups. The CSFII emphasized food and nutrient intake of the general population and the low-income population,[19] with collection of dietary intake data on two independent days as well as contextual information, such as where food was purchased and eaten. Beginning in 2002, the integrated survey, NHANES, included 2 days of intake per person to allow for the estimation of distributions of usual nutrient intake, which is critical for comparing with nutrient requirements and food group recommendations to assess adequacy of intake or the potential for excess intake.[104,105]

Prior to the integration to create WWEIA, the US Department of Health and Human Services and the USDA jointly implemented improvements in sample design, dietary methodologies, and related survey questionnaires. The National Center for Health Statistics (NCHS) evaluated telephone and in-person modes of administering 24-hour recall interviews within the NHANES survey environment. The Agricultural Research Service (ARS) developed a computerized dietary intake interview system (the Automated Multiple-Pass Method, or AMPM) and tested the accuracy and response rates of administering dietary recall interviews by telephone.[103,106-108] The ARS maintains and updates AMPM and the food composition database, processes the dietary recalls, and conducts and disseminates analyses.

The dietary intake data collected through WWEIA and, prior to that, NHANES and CFSII, can be linked to food, nutrient, supplement, and food patterns databases (described later), with the resulting data used in myriad ways to improve our under-

Data collected between 1988 and 1994 in the National Health and Nutrition Examination Survey (NHANES) III were used to assess folate status and the relationship between serum determinations, diet, and other nutrition and health variables prior to folate food fortification rule-making by the Food and Drug Administration.[49,117,118] The NHANES data were also used to compare serum and erythrocyte folate status and changes in food sources and dietary total folate intake among adults before and after fortification.[50]

Surveillance of rates of neural tube defects suggests that mandatory folic acid fortification of grain products has been an effective strategy to improve nutritional status and related health outcomes.[119]

Box 9.4 Nutrition Monitoring Data in Action: Mandatory Folic Acid Fortification and Neural Tube Defects

standing of current patterns of eating among Americans. For example, NHANES III data were used to inform mandatory fortification of grain products with folic acid (see Box 9.4). Recent uses of the data have included the examination of the extent to which American diets align with nutrient requirements[109] and federal dietary guidance,[26] including trends over time[110] and socioeconomic patterns in alignment.[111] The data have also been used to examine food sources of nutrients of interest, such as sodium and added sugars.[112-116] The NHANES data are also used to examine associations between diet and health, such as examining sodium intake in relation to blood pressure among children and adolescents.[40]

Others have used the NHANES dietary data in combination with complementary sources of data; for example, Ng and colleagues[34] illustrated the use of NHANES data along with Nielsen Homescan data (see the Food Supply Determinations section) on packaged goods purchases to examine whether purchasing patterns contribute to disparities in intake over time in relation to race/ethnicity and income. Similarly, Slining and colleagues[55] used data

from NHANES along with commercial food and beverage purchasing and nutrient databases to characterize the contributions of consumer packaged goods to intake, with implications for understanding how changes in the food environment affect dietary intake. Although combining NHANES data with other relevant information sources can be extremely useful and provide insights into novel areas of inquiry, it can also be challenging, and researchers must consider the implications of any assumptions made in the linking process. For example, food codes from food composition databases (described later) may need to be linked to commercially available products (sometimes manually), which may require expert judgments by registered dietitian nutritionists. For instance, Slining and colleagues[55] created a crosswalk approach to create nutrient profiles for items purchased by households that did not appear in food composition databases.

The NHANES data have also been used to examine exposure to pesticides.[46] The data are complemented by the Total Diet Study[47] conducted by the US Food and Drug Administration (FDA) (described in the Food Composition, Nutrient, Food Patterns, and Supplement Databases section), which provides the capacity to assess levels of additives and pesticides in diets consumed. Periodic assessments of food and nutrient consumption for specific subgroups of the population not adequately covered in national surveys have also been conducted, for example, among military populations, American Indians, children, and low-income populations.[6]

Food Composition, Nutrient, Food Pattern, and Supplement Databases

The USDA has maintained data on food composition since the late 1800s.[120] Significant efforts are dedicated to developing and maintaining such data, which are critical to the analysis of food consumption data. In 1997, the National Food and Nutrient Analysis Program was initiated by the USDA's Nutrient Data Laboratory (NDL) in collaboration with the NIH, CDC, and FDA.[120,121] The goal was to improve food composition databases in terms of the quality and quantity of data.[120] The underlying aims, which included developing databases for foods consumed by ethnic subpopulations, and the resulting standardized protocols and procedures are described in depth elsewhere and are reported to have enhanced the number of food items included in databases and the corresponding nutrient values.[120,121] In some cases, updates were driven by recommendations made by the Institute of Medicine in reports on the Dietary Reference Intakes (DRIs),[120] highlighting a reciprocal relationship between activities underpinning nutrition monitoring and usage of the data to set standards, which are then used to inform and evaluate policies and programs.

In collaboration with the National Food and Nutrient Analysis Program partners, the USDA's NDL[122] and Food Surveys Research Group (FSRG)[123] maintain four major databases (see Box 9.5): the National Nutrient Database for Standard Reference (SR), the Food and Nutrient Database for Dietary Studies (FNDDS), the Food Patterns Equivalents Database (FPED), and the Dietary Supplement Ingredient Database (DSID).[10] The USDA also periodically releases special interest databases (eg, flavonoids). Given the varied usages of these databases, illustrated in greater depth elsewhere,[10] the data are critical in terms of providing an infrastructure for nutrition monitoring and related research, policy, and practice in the United States, including interpretation of the data collected in the surveys described, such as NHANES, in terms of intakes of nutrients, food groups, and other dietary components.

The SR provides the foundation for most food composition databases in the United States.[43] The SR database is now referred to as SR-Legacy (containing 7,793 food items and up to 150 food components reported in SR28 [released in 2015], with select corrections and updates) and will be the last release of the database in its current form, with a modernized system under development.[43] Data were obtained from published and unpublished sources, including the food industry, other government agencies, USDA-initiated analytic contracts,[119] and the scientific literature. Recently, there have been special efforts to monitor foods (termed "sentinel foods") that are major contributors to dietary sodium.[43] The SR is used as the core of most nutrient databases developed in the United States for special purposes, such as those used in commercially available dietary analysis programs.[10] In addition, the

National Nutrient Database for Standard Reference (SR): Updated to 2015 and now incorporated into SR-Legacy, providing data on over 150 food components for over 7,793 foods.[43] Foundation for most commercial food composition databases in the United States. Recent efforts enhanced with industry data to develop the USDA Branded Foods Products Database.[124]

Food and Nutrient Database for Dietary Studies (FNDDS): Contains information for over 85 dietary components in over 8,500 food items.[125] Designed for the analysis of dietary intake data, particularly those collected in What We Eat in America (WWEIA), the dietary component of the National Health and Nutrition Examination Survey (NHANES).[10,126] Releases correspond to 2-year NHANES/WWEIA cycles.

Food Patterns Equivalents Database (FPED): Maps foods and beverages to 37 food groups,[127] allowing estimation of amounts of food groups derived from federal dietary guidance and examinations of diet quality in relation to dietary recommendations. Links to FNDDS and thus to WWEIA data. Releases correspond to 2-year NHANES/WWEIA cycles.

Dietary Supplement Ingredient Database (DSID): Contains information on ingredients found in supplements, including child, adult, and prenatal multivitamins/minerals.[128-131] Developed and maintained by USDA in collaboration with the National Institutes of Health Office of Dietary Supplements.

Box 9.5 Overview of Key Food Composition and Supplement Databases Developed and Maintained by the US Department of Agriculture and Its Partners

NDL has worked with a number of private and public partners to develop the USDA Branded Foods Products Database,[124] which complements SR with food composition data from the food industry. These data will allow researchers to track trends in food composition and can be used to support application software (apps) for consumers interested in the foods and beverages they consume.

Distinct from but based on the SR, the USDA's Food and Nutrient Database for Dietary Studies (FNDDS), maintained by FSRG, is designed for the analysis of dietary intake data and allows conversion of foods and beverages consumed into grams and determination of nutrient values.[10,126] The most recent release, corresponding with the 2013 to 2014 WWEIA, contains information for over 85 dietary components in over 8,500 food items.[125] The database is updated for each 2-year cycle of WWEIA. Though a major use is for coding of WWEIA dietary data, the FNDDS can be used with other survey data. FNDDS is also used to develop the Food Intakes Converted to Retail Commodities Database in collaboration with the USDA's ERS, which uses these data to estimate consumption of different retail commodities (eg, fluid milk) in relation to socioeconomic status.[10]

In addition to FNDDS, the FSRG maintains the FPED (formerly known as the My Pyramid Equivalents Databases), which allows estimation of amounts of food groups derived from federal dietary guidance (ie, USDA food patterns),[127] enabling examination of intake patterns in comparison to federal dietary guidance. As with FNDDS, the FPED is updated for each 2-year cycle of WWEIA. The most recent version for 2013 and 2014 maps foods and beverages to 37 food groups.[127] Using FPED, which can be linked to FNDDS and thus to WWEIA data, researchers can examine diet quality among the US population and population subgroups.[26,111] The FPED can also be used to support analyses examining the quality of the food supply and foods offered within specific environments, for example, using the Healthy Eating Index.[35,37,132,133] As well, the database informs nutrition guidance, such as the Thrifty Food Plan, and contributes to monitoring of Healthy People objectives.[10,110]

The fourth major database the USDA maintains is the DSID,[128-131] which is compiled by the NDL in collaboration with NIH's Office of Dietary Supplements and other federal agencies; it provides analytically validated information on the ingredients in dietary supplements. The DSID can be merged with NHANES, allowing estimation of total nutrient intakes from food and supplements.[10] The current version, DSID-3, contains information on multivitamins and minerals (including prenatal varieties) as well as n-3 fatty acid supplements.[128]

Complementing the USDA-maintained databases is the FDA's Total Diet Study, which provides annual food composition analyses based on the foods consumed most frequently according to NHANES.[47] Representative foods are collected from retail markets, prepared for consumption, and analyzed individually for nutrients and other food components at the Total Diet Laboratory to estimate consumption of selected nutrients, minerals, and organic and elemental contaminants. A recent analysis used data from the Total Diet Study to examine the contribution of food groups to intake of perchlorate (a contaminant that can interfere with iodide uptake) and iodine among the US population.[134]

Another relevant data source is the Food Label and Package Survey, sponsored by the FDA, which is conducted periodically to monitor labeling practices of US food manufacturers.[135] Facets of interest include the extent of labeling of nutrients, the prevalence of health claims, and allergen and food safety information. The Food Label and Package Survey was last conducted from 2006 to 2007, with the data used to track the prevalence of nutrition labeling and nutrient content claims related to trans fats[51] and to examine the extent and variety of structure function claims found on packaged foods.[52]

Knowledge, Attitudes, and Behavior Assessments

National surveys that measure knowledge, attitudes, and behavior about diet and nutrition and how they relate to health were added to the nutrition-monitoring program in the mid-1980s. As noted earlier, the BRFSS, initiated in 1984 by CDC in collaboration with states, is the largest continuously conducted health survey system in the world.[23] The focus is on preventive health practices and behaviors (such as diet, physical activity, and weight loss practices) and nutrition and health status.[23,92] State health departments have used data from BRFSS to plan, initiate, and guide health promotion and disease prevention programs and to monitor their progress over time. In 2002, BRFSS data became available for prevalence estimates of metropolitan (contains a core urban area of 50,000 or more population) and micropolitan (contains an urban core of at least 10,000 but less than 50,000 persons) statistical areas, allowing the CDC to make county estimates to assist local public health planners and program evaluators. In 2011, BRFSS began using cell phone surveys to produce a more representative data set. BRFSS includes modules on topics of special interest, such as the Sugar Sweetened Beverages and Menu Labeling module and the Sodium or Salt-Related Behavior module.[44,45] The Youth Risk Behavior Survey, also conducted by the CDC, is used to monitor priority health risk behaviors such as smoking, diet, physical activity, and weight loss practices among adolescents through national, state, and local surveys. Youth Risk Behavior Survey data have been analyzed to examine timely topics, such as trends in beverage consumption among adolescents.[136]

The NCI also monitors nutrition-related behaviors and attitudes, for example, through the Health Information National Trends Survey, initiated in 2003 to collect information about adults' use of cancer-related information, including data on attitudes, knowledge, and behaviors related to diet.[137,138] The Health Information National Trends Survey also captures information on the use of web-based resources, including social media. The NCI's Food Attitudes and Behaviors (FAB) Survey, conducted in 2007, was intended to assess factors associated with adults' fruit and vegetable consumption. Several analyses of the Food Attitudes and Behaviors data have been published.[30-32,139] Previously, NCI conducted the 5 A Day for Better Health Baseline Survey[140] in collaboration with the food industry to assess knowledge, behavior, and attitudes about fruits and vegetables.

The FDA also conducts surveys relevant to knowledge, attitudes, and behavior, including the Health and Diet Survey, which focuses on awareness of relationships between diet and risk for chronic disease, health-related knowledge and use of the Nutrition Facts label, and the Food Safety Survey, which measures trends in consumer food safety practices.[141]

Surveys addressing specific topics, such as infant feeding practices, weight-loss practices, and progress toward achieving related national health objectives, have been periodically conducted to meet specific data needs. Information on such surveys can be found in prior directories.[6]

Food Supply Determinations

Since 1909, the USDA has published annual food supply estimates indicating levels of foods and nutrients available for consumption.[142] These estimates, called the Nutrient Content of the US Food Supply Series, are used to assess the potential of the US food supply to meet the nutritional needs of the population and changes in the food supply over time. The data are also used to evaluate how technological alterations and marketing changes affect the food supply over time; to study relationships between food and nutrient availability and nutrient-disease associations; and to facilitate the management of federal marketing, food assistance, nutrition education, food enrichment, and fortification policy.

The Nutrient Content of the United States Food Supply Series makes use of data on food availability or disappearance (amount of food available for human consumption based on food supplies "moving from production through marketing channels"; referred to as disappearance data because they reflect the food supply after food "disappears" into the food marketing system[143]) as well as the databases on food composition described earlier. Since 1971, the USDA has maintained the Food Availability Data System, consisting of food availability data and loss-adjusted food availability data (both available through 2014), and nutrient availability data (available through 2010). The 2014 data include estimates for over 200 commodities, including individual fruits, vegetables, grains, added sugars and sweeteners, dairy products, nuts, meat, poultry, and seafood.[144] The data can be used to examine whether the amounts of various foods available for consumption are increasing or decreasing over time, as well as alignment of the food supply with federal dietary guidance.[35-37] While they do not represent actual consumption, they can be complementary to intake data in terms of understanding influences on eating patterns.[92] In addition, the Fisheries of the United States survey, conducted annually by the National Marine Fisheries Service since 1909, provides annual estimates of fish and shellfish disappearance in the distribution system.[145]

Complementing government-led surveys are the Nielsen Homescan (consumer panel data) and Scantrack (retail scanner data) Surveys, which are proprietary data sets that can be used to measure purchases of food products.[63,92] The supermarket scanner data (Scantrack) are limited to scannable packaged goods and do not reflect fruits and vegetables or prepared foods from supermarket, restaurants, or other food outlets. Households participating in the Homescan Consumer Panel transmit data on scanned purchases, including fresh foods, weekly. The USDA ERS has acquired Homescan data for use in USDA-funded research,[85] and a partnership between the Nielsen Company and the University of Chicago Booth School of Business facilitates access for researchers.[146]

Food Environment and Policy Data

Complementing the five measurement areas discussed earlier are a growing number of data sets that enable consideration of characteristics and influences of the food environment and policies that affect food availability and accessibility in different settings. As noted previously, the SNDA surveys have collected information about the school food environment.[98] The CDC conducts the School Health Policies and Practices Study, and the NCI has developed the Classification of Laws Associated with School Students data set to provide information on laws related to state nutrition and physical activity environments.[147] The SNAP Policy Database collected information about SNAP policies within the states and the District of Columbia.[148]

Also, given the inclusion of geographic indicators, data sets described in this chapter can be linked to sources of geographic data, such as the location of supermarkets and restaurants, to conduct analyses that consider the influence of environmental characteristics. For example, nutrition-related indicators from NHANES have been analyzed in relation to community characteristics.[149,150]

GAPS IN NUTRITION MONITORING AND SURVEILLANCE IN THE UNITED STATES

As noted, the US nutrition monitoring system is among the best in the world, and the United States is one of only a few countries with continuous programs for measuring food consumption.[151] Nonetheless, the National Nutrition Research Roadmap published by the Interagency Committee on Human Nutrition Research notes a number of gaps in the current monitoring system.[8] These include limited information on the influence of knowledge, attitudes, and social support on food choices as well as limited information on environments and policies in child care, worksite, and nutrition assistance program settings. Also noted is the paucity of data on the dynamics of dietary intake over time in relation to health outcomes, the lack of data on the composition of foods imported to the United States, and inadequate coverage of some population subgroups. Notably, the 2014 Agricultural Act mandated that the 2020–2025 Dietary Guidelines for Americans include guidelines for pregnant women and children younger than 2 years,[152] which may be challenging given that few data are available for these groups. The need for feasible measures of various aspects of nutrition and the need to collect high-quality data in addition to more frequent updating of dietary composition data were also noted. The committee noted the potential to use data collected for other purposes to advance nutrition monitoring and the utility of linkages between sources of data across the food system to improve our understanding of how different parts interact with one another as well as how changes to one part might affect others.

MONITORING RESOURCES AVAILABLE TO RESEARCHERS

Details on nutrition monitoring surveys, databases, and surveillance and research activities can be found on the respective agency websites (URLs are listed in Table 9.1 on pages 158 through 167 and in the references). For example, the CDC maintains a website with extensive details on NHANES, including documentation and downloadable data sets,[7] while the USDA's ARS provides details and documentation related to food composition and other databases online.

In addition to preparing, promoting, and distributing survey reports and data, increased efforts have been directed toward instructing users on how to access, process, and interpret data appropriately by providing training manuals, tutorials, and videos; documentation on survey methods and quality control procedures; and data user conferences at national and regional levels. For example, tutorials are available to guide analysis of NHANES (eg, accounting for the survey design), including modules specific to the dietary data.[72,153] Resources are also intended to build capacity in data collection to allow for results that are comparable to national data. For example, the CDC has a manual and a video regarding body measurements (anthropometry).[154] The NCI has also developed resources to help guide analyses of surveillance data, such as the Measurement Error Webinar Series.[105]

In addition to survey-specific websites, as mentioned earlier, NCCOR (an initiative of the CDC, the NIH, the Robert Wood Johnson Foundation, and the USDA to slow and reverse the epidemic of childhood obesity in the United States)[59] maintains a web-based Catalogue of Surveillance Systems that provides access to information on over 100 publicly available data sets salient to childhood obesity research, many of which include data relevant to nutrition monitoring and related factors.[60,92] The catalogue is searchable and allows filtering on the basis of key variables (eg, diet related), level (eg, individual, household), scope (eg, local, state, national), age and race/ethnicity of the target sample, and survey design (eg, cross-sectional, panel/longitudinal). Details provided include those relevant to sampling, key variables, data access and cost, and publications describing or using the data. Also highlighted are linkages between applicable surveys and other data sources (eg, other surveys, electronic health records), a potential means of enhancing monitoring identified within the Interagency Committee on Human Nutrition Research's National Nutrition Research Roadmap.[8] Given that the surveillance systems included are those that provide access to publicly available data released in recent years, the catalogue is a useful resource to identify sources of information relevant to different facets of nutrition, including health behaviors and determinants, policies, and environmental factors.

Previously, a directory of monitoring activities was developed and updated periodically by the Interagency Board for Nutrition Monitoring and Related

Research as part of an effort to improve the dissemination of information about nutrition-monitoring data and activities.[6] The directory was last updated in 2000 but provides historical information on a multitude of surveys, surveillance systems, and selected research activities at the federal level, as well as some state-level surveys. It provides a framework for organizing surveys by measurement area that was adapted here for consistency with past resources.

Online data tables can also be found on many websites. The NCHS releases short reports and Health-E Stats, and the CDC publishes the *Morbidity and Mortality Weekly Report* online. The ARS and NCI post numerous dietary intake data tables on their websites. See Box 9.6 on page 176.

Information on NIH activities related to nutrition can be found in Nutrition Research Reports[155,156] prepared by the Office of Nutrition Research, which was established in 2015 and replaced the Division of Nutrition Research Coordination.[157] The office is located within the National Institute of Diabetes and Digestive Kidney Diseases, which is NIH's largest funder of nutrition research.[157] The office oversees the NIH Nutrition Research Task Force, the Nutrition Research Coordinating Committee, and the Interagency Committee on Human Nutrition Research.[158] Other health resources at the NIH include Medline Plus (encompassing a medical encyclopedia; see https://medlineplus.gov), a registry of clinical trials,[159] science education resources, a health information page (www.nih.gov/health-information), and health information lines. The health information page is searchable and can help users find the NIH Institute(s) or center(s) that support research related to a given health topic. Research on dietary supplements, for example, can be found at the web page of the NIH's Office of Dietary Supplements, whereas information about the DASH (Dietary Approaches to Stop Hypertension) diet is available from the National Heart, Lung, and Blood Institute, and resources related to dietary assessment can be found on NCI's website.

The most relevant sources for nutrition research at the CDC include the NCHS, the National Center for Chronic Disease Prevention and Health Promotion, and the National Center for Environ-

Centers for Disease Control and Prevention (CDC): www.cdc.gov

National Center for Health Statistics (NCHS): www.cdc.gov/nchs

National Health and Nutrition Examination Survey (NHANES): www.cdc.gov/nchs/nhanes.htm

National Health Information Survey (NHIS): www.cdc.gov/nchs/nhis

Behavioral Risk Factor Surveillance System (BRFSS): www.cdc.gov/brfss

National Center for Environmental Health: www.cdc.gov/nceh

National Center for Chronic Disease Prevention and Health Promotion: www.cdc.gov/chronicdisease

Publications and products: www.cdc.gov/publications

Prevention Research Centers: www.cdc.gov/prc

US Food and Drug Administration's (FDA) Center for Food Safety and Applied Nutrition: www.fda.gov/AboutFDA/CentersOffices/OfficeofFoods/CFSAN

National Marine Fisheries Service surveys: www.st.nmfs.noaa.gov/recreational-fisheries/Surveys/survey-details

National Collaborative on Childhood Obesity Research (NCCOR): www.nccor.org

Catalogue of Surveillance Systems: www.nccor.org/nccor-tools/catalogue

National Institutes of Health (NIH): www.nih.gov

Office of Dietary Supplements: https://ods.od.nih.gov

Office of Nutrition Research: www.niddk.nih.gov/about-niddk/offices-divisions/office-nutrition-research/Pages/default.aspx

National Cancer Institute (NCI) National Data on Food Intakes: https://epi.grants.cancer.gov/diet/usualintakes/method.html

Health Information Index (includes health hotlines, clinical trials, and other information: www.nih.gov/health

MEDLINE—PubMed: www.ncbi.nlm.nih.gov/pubmed

PubMed Central: www.ncbi.nlm.nih.gov/pmc

US Census Bureau: www.census.gov

DataFerrett: https://dataferrett.census.gov

US Department of Agriculture (USDA): www.usda.gov

Agricultural Research Service (ARS): www.ars.usda.gov

Nutrient Data Laboratory (NDL): www.ars.usda.gov/northeast-area/beltsville-md/beltsville-human-nutrition-research-center/nutrient-data-laboratory

Food Surveys Research Group: (FSRG): www.ars.usda.gov/northeast-area/beltsville-md/beltsville-human-nutrition-research-center/food-surveys-research-group

Center for Nutrition Policy and Promotion: www.cnpp.usda.gov

Economic Research Service (ERS): www.ers.usda.gov

Food and Nutrition Service: www.fns.usda.gov/oane

AGRICOLA: www.ebsco.com/products/research-databases/agricola

Box 9.6 Selected Sources of Federal Information on Nutrition Research, Surveys, and Data Sets

mental Health. NCHS data systems include data on vital statistics, as well as information on health status, lifestyle, exposure to unhealthy influences, onset and diagnosis of illness and disability, and the use of health care. The National Center for Chronic Disease Prevention and Health Promotion carries out surveillance and behavioral research and demonstration projects on maternal and child health and chronic disease prevention. CDC's Network of Prevention Research Centers includes academic researchers, public health agencies, and community members that conduct applied research in disease prevention and control. Program and research activities at the National Center for Environmental Health, a part of the CDC, cover public health surveillance and applied research (epidemiologic studies, laboratory analyses, statistical analyses, and behavioral interventions).

The USDA Food and Nutrition Service provides information on published reports and ongoing research in the areas of food security, child nutrition programs, SNAP, and WIC. The USDA ERS also provides information on food and nutrition assistance programs and food security. The NDL and FSRG websites provide information on food composition databases, as well as WWEIA methods and results.

Thousands of scientific journals contain information on federal and nonfederal nutrition research. To find the most current listing of journals, researchers can use databases such as MEDLINE and AGRICOLA (AGRIcultural OnLine Access). AGRICOLA contains citations for journal articles, monographs, theses, audiovisual materials, and technical reports relating to all aspects of agriculture, whereas MEDLINE is a biomedical database consisting of citations from journal articles only; it contains more than 24 million citations dating back to 1946. To facilitate access to NIH-funded research, NIH has a public access policy that requires that articles describing such research be made freely available through PubMed Central, a free archive for full-text articles, within 12 months of publication.

The use of a database requires the development of a search strategy. A search strategy contains the key words, phrases, or terms of interest; synonyms for these terms; and how they should be combined. Research librarians working at universities and other institutions can be invaluable in terms of developing such strategies. The National Library of Medicine also provides a PubMed Tutorial[160] with tips on navigating and searching PubMed (which includes MEDLINE indexed journals).

CONDUCTING SECONDARY ANALYSES OF MONITORING AND SURVEILLANCE DATA

The collection of the vast amount of data within the monitoring and surveillance system presents an array of opportunities for those interested in nutrition and factors that influence eating patterns and nutritional status. Indeed, secondary analyses of existing data are extremely valuable for understanding dietary intakes and other nutrition-related phenomenon, particularly since in many cases, with appropriate weighting and attention to other survey-related aspects discussed later, findings may be representative of the US population or population subgroups of interest. Furthermore, although the researcher does not control the particular measures used within a survey, the analysis of secondary data can present a viable strategy to address important research questions in cases in which primary data collection is not feasible. For example, within the context of a dietetic internship, it may not be possible, from the perspectives of time, cost, and expertise, to collect detailed data using methodology such as 24-hour recalls (though this is increasingly viable with technological innovation). However, the use of existing data can enable dietetic interns or others to address a question of interest to dietetics practice and policy and to become familiar with issues related to complex data sets, cleaning and utilizing nutrition-related data, making appropriate inferences, and reporting findings in a robust and transparent manner. The appropriate analysis of secondary data also contributes a return on investment given the extensive resources allocated to maintaining monitoring and surveillance systems.

Data Sets and Related Resources

Surveys related to nutrition monitoring and surveillance in the United States generate a large amount of data. For selected surveys, agencies produce data sets for public use and publish survey findings in government and peer-reviewed reports. Data sets, along with documentation on sampling methods, survey design, sample sizes, and survey instruments and questionnaires, are often available online. DataFerrett, a computer search tool found on the US Census Bureau website, enables users to access and customize federal, state, and local data.[161] DataFerrett provides access to statistics from BRFSS; the Consumer Expenditure Survey; the CPS; the Survey of Income and Program Participation; and NCHS data systems, including NHANES, NHIS, and the Survey of Program Dynamics. Some agencies make data sets available through the National Technical Information Service. Still other reports and documents are available from the US Government Printing Office.

In addition, many agencies that conduct national nutrition surveys maintain lists of peer-reviewed research articles or bibliographies of survey findings. These references can be found by visiting survey websites. Many other agencies that use national survey data also list publications or links to publications on their websites.

Key Considerations for Analysis

When analyzing survey and surveillance data, one must consider whether the data are suitable for the questions being asked. The survey design, strengths and weaknesses of the methods used, and presence and degree of bias must all be considered. Bias in survey or surveillance data can arise from errors in the sampling process and coverage of the target population, lack of response to the survey by respondents or particular groups of respondents, and measurement error. Chapter 3 describes four types of research errors: sampling, noncoverage, nonresponse, and measurement; all can lead to biased results. For the purposes of this chapter, brief overviews related to sampling biases, nonsampling biases, and measurement error, particularly in regard to dietary intake data, are provided. It is critical for researchers to evaluate surveys and surveillance data to assess the types and extent of bias likely to be present and what can be done to minimize its effects on the analysis and interpretation of the data.

Population Coverage, Sampling Bias, and Response Rates

A number of considerations are important in evaluating the extent to which a sample represents the desired population. Following is a brief summary of some of these considerations, which are detailed in greater depth elsewhere, such as in resources accompanying NHANES and other data sets.

Examples of sampling bias include frame bias and consistent sampling bias. A frame is the sampling list used when listing the sampling units in the population is too difficult or tedious. Frame bias can be caused by the use of an incomplete list; for example, a list of telephone numbers for a particular city or geographic area would be biased in terms of excluding households without telephones and those with unlisted numbers. In the past, a sample based on such a list would likely have underrepresented low-income households, whereas with today's increased reliance on mobile phones vs land lines, there is also concern about other noncoverage biases, including underrepresentation of young adults.[162-164] Consistent sampling bias can be introduced by the mechanical procedures used to select units from the frame into the sample. In the telephone survey example, a consistent sampling bias could arise if the sample of telephone numbers were contacted from 9 AM to 5 PM on weekdays. Employed persons and students would be unlikely to be at home during those hours.

Sometimes researchers decide to narrow the areas covered in area probability samples to reduce the costs associated with collecting the data. These decisions can lead to noncoverage bias, that is, the failure to include elements in the sample that would properly belong in the sample.

Nonresponse bias results from the failure to obtain observations on some elements selected and designated for the sample. This bias occurs because people are not reached despite repeated attempts to contact them, they refuse to participate, or they are incapacitated and unable to participate. This bias also occurs because of lost data, such as lost interviews and laboratory accidents. Incomplete reporting is a potential for bias in survey and surveillance data. Decisions about excluding missing data elements from analyses must be made carefully, with consideration of the implications for biasing the sample.

Analysts frequently use the survey response rate as an overall indicator of the quality of a survey. When a substantial proportion of the sample selected for a survey does not participate, a potential for bias exists if the nonrespondents differ from the respondents in some systematic way. The greater the nonresponse, the greater the potential for bias. Even when a substantial proportion of the original sample does not participate in the survey, however, the sample may not be biased, and studies of nonresponse bias can be performed.

Bias (or systematic error) refers to consistent errors arising in the interview or laboratory method used to obtain the data. In 24-hour dietary recalls, bias can be introduced through imperfect recall of foods and beverages consumed the prior day, interview methods that may interact with social desirability biases (eg, when probing for sugary or alcoholic beverage consumption), coding assumptions (eg, rules for assigning default codes), and errors in the food composition database used to estimate nutrient levels, among other factors. Random error, primarily driven by day-to-day variation in intake, also affects data collected using short-term tools such as 24-hour recalls. While data from a single recall can be used to estimate mean intakes for a population, when the intent is to estimate distributions of usual intake, the repeat recalls and statistical modeling approaches must be used to account for day-to-day variation and arrive at appropriate results. Resources are available that explore sources of error in dietary intake data and strategies to mitigate them in detail.[105]

Other self-reported data are also subject to error. Inaccuracy may be related to poor recall, sensitivity to or not understanding the question, or lack of knowledge to answer the question. For example, research has shown that self-reported heights and weights can be biased; men report being taller than they are, and women report weighing less than they actually do.[165] In studies making use of proxies for children or others unable to respond for themselves, researchers must consider sources of bias that might influence the proxy's reporting. Interviewer training on how to ask sensitive questions and elicit responses can improve the quality of self-reported data.

Sample Weights and Design Effects

The statistical technique used to identify survey samples introduces complexities into the analysis of the data. In area probability sampling, some trade-offs are made in the randomness of the sample to minimize the costs of the survey. Area probability samples are not simple random samples, and the assumptions of simple random sampling do not apply when hypothesis testing is performed with survey data. The technique is multistage, and at each stage, sample elements with a known probability are selected. NHANES, for example, uses a clustered design that incorporates differential probabilities of selection.[71] Sample weights must be used to account for the sampling so as to avoid biased estimates and inflated significance levels. For weighted analyses, researchers can work with computer software packages that use an appropriate method for estimating variances for complex samples, such as SUDAAN (RTI International, Raleigh, NC), WesVar (Westat, Rockville, MD), STATA (StataCorp, College Station, TX), SAS (SAS Institute, Cary, NC), or R, a free software environment for statistical computing and graphics (The R Foundation, Vienna, Austria).

The design effect is the ratio of the true variance of a statistic (taking the complex sample design into account) to the variance of the statistic for a simple random sample with the same number of cases. Design effects differ for different subgroups and different statistics; no single design effect is universally applicable to any given survey or analysis. The design effect can be used to adjust estimates and statistics computed by using assumptions of simple random sampling for the complexities in the sample design.[166]

Determining whether a subsample is free of bias involves comparing the subsample with the overall sample for characteristics related to the subject of inquiry. Whenever analyses of this type are performed, it is essential that the analytic subsample be examined for bias and that the sample weights and design effects be used in the analysis.

Quality of Data

National surveys have extensive quality control and quality assurance programs, as well as well-documented data collection and laboratory protocols. However, assessment of data quality is a critical part of any research project. Researchers should review the survey methods and quality control procedures and data before they analyze and interpret the data. It is important that the variables and the questions used to construct them are a good representation for the constructs of interest. The degree of missing data should be considered and decisions regarding their treatment made carefully. Outliers should also be examined to assess their impact on study findings. When analyzing self-reported data, researchers must acknowledge that bias is likely to be inherent. This is the case for self-reported dietary data, which may be affected by under- or overreporting estimates of energy, nutrient, and food group intakes.[105] As noted previously, self-reported height and weight are also subject to reporting errors. It is crucial that considerations related to the quality of the data are noted in the interpretation of results from any secondary analysis of nutrition surveillance and monitoring data, along with an indication of how possible biases might have impacted results, so that users of the research (eg, policy makers) are able to make appropriate inferences and place the study findings in the context of similar research.

GETTING STARTED ON A RESEARCH STUDY

Define the Research Question and Identify the Appropriate Data and Analytic Approach

Before beginning any research initiative, researchers must clearly specify the question to be addressed, as this will dictate the data and methods to be used, along with other considerations. In some cases, data will not be available or appropriate for answering a particular question, so the question must be tweaked (for example, causality cannot be ascertained using cross-sectional data sourcs, such as NHANES). Possible research questions and topics that can be addressed using nutrition monitoring and surveillance data are many and may include examinations of means or distributions of usual intakes of a dietary component, such as added sugars, among various population subgroups; the contribution of different food sources or supplements to the intake of various dietary components; associations between variables such as income, race/ethnicity, or household food security status and dietary intakes; associations between implementation of an intervention and food-related knowledge or behaviors; and queries that can be pursued through linkages to other data sets, such as geographic information. Additionally, in some cases, analysis of nationally representative data sources may be undertaken to provide a comparison for estimates based on more localized data collection.

Answering different questions may involve unique considerations as far as data coding and analysis. The population(s) of interest may also vary, ranging from the general population to specific age groups (eg, children or older Americans), particular racial or ethnic groups, people with low incomes, or pregnant women. Another consideration is the sample size required to obtain estimates of interest; adequate power may be lacking for some population subgroups.

Match Available Resources and Expertise to the Research Question and Planned Analyses

Given the identification of a research question related to nutrition monitoring, it is useful to visit key sources, such as NCCOR's Catalogue of Surveillance Systems,[60,92] journals, and survey websites (see Table 9.1 on pages 158 through 167), to determine whether available data from a survey or surveillance system may include variables of interest and the consistency of measurement over time, if relevant to the planned analysis. NCCOR Catalogue entries, for example, include a section on key variables. Journal articles and federal agency websites provide information on recent analyses that may be pertinent to a given area of research and may help determine coding of variables, strategies to deal with missing data, and other considerations. Published analyses may also provide information on normal values or targets to which findings can be compared.

There are benefits and trade-offs to using public-access data sets as opposed to collecting primary data to address a particular research question. Surveys such as the NHANES, for example, provide a nationally representative sample, do not require investments of time and money collecting data, and are recognized as credible sources of data. However, in using these survey results, researchers are limited to variables that may not perfectly align with the research question, and data may be lacking about particular populations of interest. It is also possible that variables relevant to the research question across data sources are based on different measures, necessitating consideration of strategies for harmonizing the data; this may also pertain to attempts to examine trends over time in cases in which measures may vary.

Before embarking on a research project, researchers must consider financial and staffing resources and constraints. Conducting a research project requires significant financial, human, and labor resources. For example, researchers must determine if the research team possesses the expertise to analyze survey data that use a complex design. The length of time available to conduct a research project also has a bearing on study design. Whether researchers are collecting their own data or analyzing secondary dietary intake data, the NCI provides a review of dietary methods and considerations for selecting a dietary method to meet the needs of different research questions and study designs.[167,168] Other publications can help researchers apply the DRIs to dietary data for a population or subpopulation.[169]

Interpret and Report Results

Before beginning a research project, researchers must consider the potential implications for public health, clinical practice, or other applications. Some research can benefit consumers who are looking for information to inform decisions about their nutrition and health. Public and private policy makers might use research findings as a basis for creating dietary guidance materials and programs to enhance the nutrition quality of food supplies, provide food assistance, and evaluate policies. Health educators might use research findings to develop disease prevention guidelines. Physicians and other health professionals

might use research to keep abreast of current knowledge or to provide dietary recommendations to patients. Food, nutrition, and health associations may use knowledge gleaned from studies using nutrition monitoring data to set policy or to educate their constituencies. The media may use research studies as an educational tool or for background information. Finally, trade associations and those in industry may use research to develop guidelines for product development and improvement. Along with the potential application of the research findings, researchers must consider whether and how it can be translated for use by its intended audience. Therefore, knowledge of stakeholders and target audiences is important.

As noted previously, in interpreting and translating results for the intended audiences, it is critical to consider issues highlighted in this chapter and elsewhere in this book related to population coverage, consistency of measurement over time or across jurisdictions in studies making comparisons across these domains, and measurement error and other sources of bias that could affect the results and their generalizability. The source of the data, questions or procedures used to collect measures, coding and analysis techniques, and possible implications of sources of bias must be clearly articulated so that the research is interpretable and replicable and can be synthesized into the larger body of evidence on the diets and nutritional status of the US population.

CONCLUSION

The national nutrition surveys and state surveillance systems within the United States offer a broad array of information for policy making and research opportunities for nutrition and dietetics practitioners and researchers. For example, survey data can be used to study the relationship between dietary intake and nutritional status and obesity among high-risk groups, or the effect of changes in food fortification on the nutrient status of target groups. Surveillance data can be used to track dietary behaviors among population subgroups over time in relation to assessing or planning health promotion activities. Surveys and surveillance systems are also a source of well-tested survey instruments, methods, and data collection protocols that can be used or adapted for data collection in research studies.

Though gaps in the monitoring system have been identified, nutrition and dietetics practitioners and researchers working in the United States continue to enjoy access to a range of data that is unmatched in other countries in the world and provides the opportunity to link across data sets and to other sources of information to address novel questions of policy and program relevance. A number of resources are available on federal agency websites and elsewhere to help researchers locate and use monitoring data to advance our understanding of the nutritional status and health of the US population, influences on these, and how to intervene to promote nutritional health.

REFERENCES

1. US Department of Health and Human Services and US Department of Agriculture. Dietary Guidelines for Americans 2015–2020. 8th ed. https://health.gov/dietaryguidelines/2015/guidelines. Published 2015. Accessed April 1, 2017.

2. Mason JB, Habicht JP, Tabatabai H, Valverde V. *Nutrition Surveillance*. Geneva, Switzerland; World Health Organization; 1984.

3. World Health Organization. Public Health Surveillance. www.who.int/topics/public_health_surveillance/en. Accessed April 1, 2017.

4. World Health Organization. *Food and Nutrition Surveillance Systems: A Manual for Policy-Makers and Programme Managers*. http://applications.emro.who.int/dsaf/EMROPUB_2014_EN_1822.pdf. Published 2014. Accessed April 1, 2017.

5. Brown GE. National Nutrition Monitoring System: a congressional perspective. *J Am Diet Assoc*. 1984;84(10): 1185-1189.

6. Interagency Board for Nutrition Monitoring and Related Research. *Nutrition Monitoring in the United States: The Directory of Federal and State Nutrition Monitoring and Related Research Activities*. www.cdc.gov/nchs/data/misc/direc-99.pdf. Published 2000. Accessed April 1, 2017.

7. Centers for Disease Control and Prevention, National Health and Nutrition Examination Survey. www.cdc.gov/nchs/nhanes. Updated April 30, 2018. Accessed May 17, 2018.

8. Interagency Committee on Human Nutrition Research. *National Nutrition Research Roadmap 2016–2021: Advancing Nutrition Research to Improve and Sustain Health*. Washington, DC; 2016. www.nal.usda.gov/sites/default/files/fnic_uploads/2016-03-30-%20ICHNR%20 NNRR%20%282%29.pdf. Published 2016. Accessed April 1, 2017.

9. Story M, Kaphingst KM, Robinson-O'Brien R, Glanz K. Creating healthy food and eating environments: policy and environmental approaches. *Annu Rev Public Health*. 2008; 29(1):253-272.

10. Ahuja JKC, Moshfegh AJ, Holden JM, Harris E. USDA food and nutrient databases provide the infrastructure for food and nutrition, policy, and practice. *J Nutr*. 2013;143(2):241S-249S.

11. Briefel RR. Overview of nutrition monitoring in the U.S. Presented at the 17th Nutrient Databank Conference. June 7–10, 1992. Baltimore, Maryland. www.nutrient dataconf.org/PastConf/NDBC17/toc.htm. Accessed July 2, 2018.

12. Ostenso GL. National Nutrition Monitoring System: a historical perspective. *J Am Diet Assoc*. 1984;84(10):1181-1185.

13. Woteki CE, Briefel RR, Kuczmarski R. Federal monitoring of the nation's nutritional status. Contributions of the National Center for Health Statistics. *Am J Clin Nutr*. 1988;47(2):320-328.

14. Briefel RR. Assessment of the US diet in national nutrition surveys: national collaborative efforts and NHANES. *Am J Clin Nutr*. 1994;59(1 suppl):164S-167S.

15. Moshfegh AJ. The National Nutrition Monitoring and Related Research Program: progress and activities. *J Nutr*. 1994;124(9 suppl):1843S-1845S.

16. Woteki CE, Briefel RR, Klein CJ, et al. Nutrition monitoring: summary of a statement from an American Society for Nutritional Sciences Working Group. *J Nutr*. 2002;132(12):3782-3783.

17. Nestle M. National nutrition monitoring policy: the continuing need for legislative intervention. *J Nutr Educ*. 1990;22(3):141-144.

18. Kuczmarski MF, Moshfegh A, Briefel R. Update on nutrition monitoring activities in the United States. *J Am Diet Assoc*. 1994;94(7):753-760.

19. Tippett KS, Wilkinson Enns C, Moshfegh AJ. Food consumption surveys in the US Department of Agriculture. *Nutr Today*. 1999;34(1):33-46.

20. US Congress. H.R.1608 - National Nutrition Monitoring and Related Research Act of 1990. 101st Congress (1989–1990). www.congress.gov/bill/101st-congress/house-bill/1608. Accessed May 23, 2018

21. *Proposed Ten-Year Comprehensive Plan for the National Nutrition Monitoring and Related Research Program*. Washington, DC; US Department of Health and Human Services and US Department of Agriculture; 1991. Publication 91-25967:SS 716-55767.

22. *Ten-Year Comprehensive Plan for the National Nutrition Monitoring and Related Research Program*. Washington, DC; US Department of Health and Human Services and US Department of Agriculture;1993. Publication 58: 32752-32806.

23. Centers for Disease Control and Prevention. Behavioral Risk Factor Surveillance System. About BRFSS. www.cdc.gov/brfss/about/index.htm. Updated May 16, 2014. Accessed April 1, 2017.

24. Pennington J. Nutrition monitoring in the United States. In: Berdanier CD, Dwyer JT, Feldman EB, eds. *Handbook of Nutrition and Food*. 2nd ed. Boca Raton, FL: CRC Press; 2007:451-469.

25. National Institute of Diabetes and Digestive and Kidney Diseases, NIH Nutrition Research Task Force. www.niddk.nih.gov/about-niddk/advisory-coordinating-committees/nih-nutrition-research-task-force/Pages/default.aspx. Accessed August 14, 2017.

26. Krebs-Smith SM, Guenther PM, Subar AF, Kirkpatrick SI, Dodd KW. Americans do not meet federal dietary recommendations. *J Nutr*. 2010;140(10):1832-1838.

27. Kirkpatrick SI, Dodd KW, Parsons R, Ng C, Garriguet D, Tarasuk V. Household food insecurity is a stronger marker of adequacy of nutrient intakes among Canadian compared to American youth and adults. *J Nutr*. 2015;145(7):1596-1603.

28. Otten JJ, Hellwig JP, Meyers LD, eds. *Dietary Reference Intakes: The Essential Guide to Nutrient Requirements*. Washington, DC: National Academies Press; 2006.

29. Yates AA. Dietary reference intakes: a new approach to setting nutrition standards in the USA and Canada. *Bibl Nutr Dieta*. 2001;(55):4-13.

30. Erinosho TO, Moser RP, Oh AY, Nebeling LC, Yaroch AL. Awareness of the Fruits and Veggies—More Matters campaign, knowledge of the fruit and vegetable recommendation, and fruit and vegetable intake of adults in the 2007 Food Attitudes and Behaviors (FAB) Survey. *Appetite*. 2012;59(1):155-160.

31. Ferrer RA, Bergman HE, Klein WMP. Worry as a predictor of nutrition behaviors. *Health Educ Behav*. 2013;40(1):88-96.

32. Emanuel AS, McCully SN, Gallagher KM, Updegraff JA. Theory of Planned Behavior explains gender difference in fruit and vegetable consumption. *Appetite*. 2012;59(3):693-697.

33. Castner L, Mabli J. *Low-Income Household Spending Patterns and Measures of Poverty*. www.fns.usda.gov/sites/default/files/SpendingPatterns.pdf. Published April 2010. Accessed April 1, 2017.

34. Ng SW, Poti JM, Popkin BM. Trends in racial/ethnic and income disparities in foods and beverages consumed and purchased from stores among US households with children, 2000-2013. *Am J Clin Nutr*. 2016;104(3):750-759.

35. Miller PE, Reedy J, Kirkpatrick SI, Krebs-Smith SM. The United States food supply is not consistent with dietary guidance: evidence from an evaluation using the Healthy Eating Index-2010. *J Acad Nutr Diet*. 2015;115(1):95-100.

36. Wells HF, Buzby JC. Dietary assessment of major trends in U.S. food consumption, 1970–2005. www.ers.usda.gov/webdocs/publications/44217/12198_eib33_report summary_1_.pdf?v=41055. Economic Information Bulletin No. EIB-33. Published March 2008. Accessed April 1, 2017.

37. Krebs-Smith SM, Reedy J, Bosire C. Healthfulness of the U.S. food supply. *Am J Prev Med*. 2010;38(5):472-477.

38. Hennessy E, Oh A, Agurs-Collins T, et al. State-level school competitive food and beverage laws are associated with children's weight status. *J Sch Health*. 2014;84(9):609-616.

39. Fox MK, Gordon A, Nogales R, Wilson A. Availability and consumption of competitive foods in US public schools. *J Am Diet Assoc*. 2009;109(2):S57-S66.

40. Yang Q, Zhang Z, Kuklina EV, et al. Sodium intake and blood pressure among US children and adolescents. *Pediatrics*. 2012;130(4):611-619

41. Seligman HK, Laraia BA, Kushel MB. Food insecurity is associated with chronic disease among low-income NHANES participants. *J Nutr*. 2010;140(2):304-310.

42. Centers for Disease Control and Prevention, National Center for Health Statistics. Growth Charts. 2010. www.cdc .gov/growthcharts. Accessed April 1, 2017.

43. US Department of Agriculture, Agricultural Research Service. Composition of Foods Raw, Processed, Prepared: USDA National Nutrient Database for Standard Reference, Legacy (2018): Documentation and User Guide. www.ars .usda.gov/ARSUserFiles/80400525/Data/SR/sr28/sr28 _doc.pdf. April 2018. Accessed June 15, 2018.

44. Bowers KM, Suzuki S. Menu-labeling usage and its association with diet and exercise: 2011 BRFSS sugar sweetened beverage and menu labeling module. *Prev Chronic Dis*. 2014;11:130231.

45. Fang J, Cogswell ME, Park S, Jackson SL, Odom EC. Sodium intake among U.S. adults - 26 States, the District of Columbia, and Puerto Rico, 2013. *MMWR Morb Mortal Wkly Rep*. 2015;64(25):695-698.

46. Melnyk LJ, Wang Z, Li Z, Xue J. Prioritization of pesticides based on daily dietary exposure potential as determined from the SHEDS model. *Food Chem Toxicol*. 2016;96:167-173.

47. US Food and Drug Administration Center for Food Safety and Applied Nutrition. Total Diet Study. 2018. www.fda.gov /Food/FoodScienceResearch/TotalDietStudy/default.htm. Accessed June 15, 2018.

48. Office of Disease Prevention and Health Promotion. Healthy People 2020. www.healthypeople.gov/2020/topics -objectives/topic/nutrition-and-weight-status. Accessed June 15, 2018.

49. Lewis CJ, Crane NT, Wilson DB, Yetley EA. Estimated folate intakes: data updated to reflect food fortification, increased bioavailability, and dietary supplement use. *Am J Clin Nutr*. 1999;70(2):198-207.

50. Dietrich M, Brown CJP, Block G. The effect of folate fortification of cereal-grain products on blood folate status, dietary folate intake, and dietary folate sources among adult non-supplement users in the United States. *J Am Coll Nutr*. 2005;24(4):266-274.

51. Brandt M, Moss J, Ferguson M. The 2006–2007 Food Label and Package Survey (FLAPS): nutrition labeling, *trans* fat labeling. *J Food Comp Anal*. 2009 22(suppl):S74-S77.

52. Shimakawa T, Ferguson M. Prevalence of structure function claims: 2006–2007 Food Label and Package Survey. *Procedia Food Sci*. 2015;4:133-137.

53. US Department of Agriculture Economic Research Service. Food Security in the U.S.: Measurement. 2017. www.ers .usda.gov/topics/food-nutrition-assistance/food-security -in-the-us/measurement. Accessed June 15, 2018.

54. Hall KD, Guo J, Dore M, Chow CC, Leon A. The progressive increase of food waste in America and its environmental impact. *PLoS One*. 2009;4(11):e7940.

55. Slining MM, Yoon EF, Davis J, Hollingsworth B, Miles D, Ng SW. An approach to monitor food and nutrition from "factory to fork." *J Acad Nutr Diet*. 2015;115(1):40-49.

56. Office of Disease Prevention and Health Promotion. Healthy People 2020. Nutrition and Weight Status. www.healthypeople.gov/2020/topics-objectives/topic /nutrition-and-weight-status. Accessed April 1, 2017.

57. Vandevijvere S, Swinburn B. Towards global benchmarking of food environments and policies to reduce obesity and diet-related non-communicable diseases: design and methods for nation-wide surveys. *BMJ Open*. 2014;4(5): e005339.

58. McKinnon RA, Reedy J, Morrissette MA, Lytle LA, Yaroch AL. Measures of the food environment. *Am J Prev Med*. 2009;36(4):S124-S133.

59. National Collaborative for Childhood Obesity Research. www.nccor.org. Accessed April 1, 2017.

60. McKinnon RA, Reedy J, Berrigan D, Krebs-Smith SM; NCCOR Catalogue and Registry Working Groups. The National Collaborative on Childhood Obesity Research catalogue of surveillance systems and measures registry: new tools to spur innovation and increase productivity in childhood obesity research. *Am J Prev Med*. 2012;42(4): 433-435.

61. National Collaborative on Childhood Obesity Research. Catalogue of Surveillance Systems. Washington, DC: NCCOR; 2011. https://tools.nccor.org/css. Accessed August 17, 2018.

62. Panel on Enhancing the Data Infrastructure in Support of Food and Nutrition Programs, Research and Decision Making. *Improving Data to Analyze Food and Nutrition Policies*. Washington, DC: National Academies Press; 2005.

63. Ng SW, Popkin BM. Monitoring foods and nutrients sold and consumed in the United States: dynamics and challenges. *J Acad Nutr Diet*. 2012;112(1):41-45.e4.

64. Heimbach JT. Using the National Nutrition Monitoring System to profile dietary supplement use. *J Nutr*. 2001; 131(4 suppl):1335S-1338S.

65. Choung RS, Unalp-Arida A, Ruhl CE, Brantner TL, Everhart JE, Murray JA. Less hidden celiac disease but increased gluten avoidance without a diagnosis in the United States. *Mayo Clin Proc*. 2017;92(1):30-38.

66. Cusack LK, Smit E, Kile ML, Harding AK. Regional and temporal trends in blood mercury concentrations and fish consumption in women of child bearing age in the United States using NHANES data from 1999–2010. *Environ Health*. 2017;16(1):10.

67. Marquez B, Murillo R. Racial/ethnic differences in weight-loss strategies among US adults: National Health and Nutrition Examination Survey 2007–2012. *J Acad Nutr Diet*. 2017;117(6):923–928.

68. World Health Organization, Department of Nutrition for Health and Development. WHO Child Growth Standards: Methods and Development: Length/Height-for-Age, Weight-for-Age, Weight-for-Length, Weight-for-Height and Body Mass Index-for-Age: www.who.int/childgrowth/standards/technical_report/en. Published 2006. Accessed April 1, 2017.

69. Centers for Disease Control and Prevention, Division of Nutrition, Physical Activity, and Obesity. Growth Chart Training. www.cdc.gov/nccdphp/dnpao/growthcharts. Updated April 15, 2014. Accessed April 1, 2017.

70. Centers for Disease Control and Prevention, National Center for Health Statistics. Computer Programs. www.cdc.gov/growthcharts/computer_programs.htm. Updated May 16, 2014. Accessed April 1, 2017.

71. Ogden CL, Carroll MD, Lawman HG, et al. Trends in obesity prevalence among children and adolescents in the United States, 1988–1994 through 2013–2014. *JAMA*. 2016;315(21):2292-2299.

72. Centers for Disease Control and Prevention, National Center for Health Statistics. National Health and Nutrition Examination Survey. Main Continuous and Historical NHANES Tutorials. www.cdc.gov/nchs/tutorials. Updated March 29, 2012. Accessed April 1, 2017.

73. Broitman L. Ongoing Activities to Support the Asian Oversample in NHANES. American Public Health Association Annual Meeting and Expo, 2012. www.cdc.gov/nchs/ppt/nchs2012/ss-14_broitman.pdf. Accessed April 1, 2017.

74. Islam NS, Khan S, Kwon S, Jang D, Ro M, Trinh-Shevrin C. Methodological issues in the collection, analysis, and reporting of granular data in Asian American populations: historical challenges and potential solutions. *J Health Care Poor Underserved*. 2010;21(4):1354-1381.

75. NCHS Dataline. *Public Health Rep*. 2014;129(4):374-375.

76. Aoki Y, Yoon SS, Chong Y, Carroll MD. Hypertension, abnormal cholesterol, and high body mass index among non-Hispanic Asian adults: United States, 2011–2012. *NCHS Data Brief*. 2014;(140):1-8.

77. Centers for Disease Control and Prevention National Center for Health Statistics. NCHS Data Linkage Activities. 2017. www.cdc.gov/nchs/data-linkage/index.htm. Accessed June 15, 2018.

78. Centers for Disease Control and Prevention, National Center for Health Statistics. National Health Interview Survey 2018. www.cdc.gov/nchs/nhis. Accessed June 15, 2018.

79. Centers for Disease Control and Prevention, National Center for Health Statistics. National Health Interview Survey 2019 Questionnaire Redesign. 2018. www.cdc.gov/nchs/nhis/2019_quest_redesign.htm. Accessed June 15, 2018.

80. US Census Bureau. Current Population Survey (CPS). www.census.gov/programs-surveys/cps.html. Accessed April 1, 2017.

81. Bickel G, Nord M, Price C, Hamilton W, Cook J. *Guide to Measuring Household Food Security*. Washington, DC: US Department of Agriculture Food and Nutrition Service Office of Analysis, Nutrition, and Evaluation; 2000.

82. Coleman-Jensen A, Rabbitt MP, Gregory CA, Singh A. Household Food Security in the United States in 2015. Washington, DC: Economic Research Service, US Department of Agriculture; 2016. Economic Research Report No. 215.

83. Jyoti DF, Frongillo EA, Jones SJ. Food insecurity affects school children's academic performance, weight gain, and social skills. *J Nutr*. 2005;135(12):2831-2839.

84. Wilde PE, Nord M, Zager RE. In longitudinal data from the survey of program dynamics, 16.9% of the U.S. population was exposed to household food insecurity in a 5-year period. *J Hunger Environ Nutr*. 2010;5(3):380-398.

85. US Department of Agriculture, Economic Research Service. National Data Sets Useful in Food and Nutrition Assistance Research. 2018. www.ers.usda.gov/topics/food -nutrition-assistance/extramural-research/national -data-sets. Accessed June 15, 2018.

86. US Department of Agriculture, Economic Research Service. American Time Use Survey. www.bls.gov/tus/home .htm. Accessed June 15, 2018.

87. Hamrick K. 2014–16 Eating & Health Module User's Guide (2016 Edition). US Department of Agriculture, Economic Research Service, Administrative publication No. AP-070. www.ers.usda.gov/publications/pub-details/?pubid=42817. Published May 2016. Accessed April 1, 2017.

88. US Department of Labor, Bureau of Labor Statistics. Consumer Expenditure Survey. www.bls.gov/cex. Accessed April 1, 2017.

89. Mabil J, Maisberger R. Recent trends in spending patterns of Supplemental Nutrition Assistance Program participants and other low-income Americans. Bureau of Labor Statistics. Monthly Labor Review. September 2013. www.bls.gov/opub/mlr/2013/article/mabli-malsberger .htm. Accessed May 21, 2018.

90. Leung CW, Ding EL, Catalano PJ, Villamor E, Rimm EB, Willett WC. Dietary intake and dietary quality of low-income adults in the Supplemental Nutrition Assistance Program. *Am J Clin Nutr*. 2012;96(5):977-988.

91. Gu X, Tucker KL. Dietary quality of the US child and adolescent population: trends from 1999 to 2012 and associations with the use of federal nutrition assistance programs. *Am J Clin Nutr*. 2017;105(1):194-202.

92. National Collaborative for Childhood Obesity Research. Catalogue of Surveillance Systems. www.nccor.org/nccor -tools/catalogue. Accessed April 1, 2017.

93. Centers for Disease Control and Prevention. Overweight & Obesity Surveillance Systems. www.cdc.gov/obesity/data /surveillance.html. Updated November 17, 2016. Accessed April 1, 2017.

94. Pan L, Freedman DS, Sharma AJ, et al. Trends in obesity among participants aged 2–4 years in the Special Supplemental Nutrition Program for Women, Infants, and Children—United States, 2000–2014. *MMWR Morb Mortal Wkly Rep*. 2016;65(45):1256-1260.

95. Pan L, McGuire LC, Blanck HM, May-Murriel AL, Grummer-Strawn LM. Racial/ethnic differences in obesity trends among young low-income children. *Am J Prev Med*. 2015;48(5):570-574.

96. Joyce T, Racine A, Yunzal-Butler C. Reassessing the WIC effect: evidence from the Pregnancy Nutrition Surveillance System. *J Policy Anal Manage*. 2008;27(2):277-303.

97. US Department of Agriculture, Food and Nutrition Service. www.fns.usda.gov. Accessed August 14, 2017.

98. Story M. The Third School Nutrition Dietary Assessment Study: findings and policy implications for improving the health of US children. *J Am Diet Assoc*. 2009;109 (2 suppl):S7-S13.

99. US Department of Agriculture, Food and Nutrition Service. School Nutrition Dietary Assessment Study IV. www.fns.usda.gov/school-nutrition-dietary-assessment -study-iv. Published September 5, 2013. Accessed April 1, 2017.

100. Mathematica Policy Research. School Nutrition and Meal Cost Study (SNMCS). www.mathematica-mpr.com/our -publications-and-findings/projects/school-nutrition -and-meal-cost-study. Accessed April 1, 2017.

101. Health Resources and Services Administration Maternal and Child Health Bureau. National Survey of Children's Health. https://mchb.hrsa.gov/data/national-surveys. Accessed April 1, 2017.

102. Centers for Disease Control and Prevention, National Center for Health Statistics. National Health Care Surveys. 2017. www.cdc.gov/nchs/dhcs. Accessed April 3, 2017.

103. US Department of Agriculture, Agricultural Research Service. What We Eat in America. 2017. www.ars.usda.gov /northeast-area/beltsville-md-bhnrc/beltsville-human -nutrition-research-center/food-surveys-research-group /docs/wweianhanes-overview. Accessed June 15, 2018.

104. Dodd KW, Guenther PM, Freedman LS, et al. Statistical methods for estimating usual intake of nutrients and foods: a review of the theory. *J Am Diet Assoc*. 2006;106 (10):1640-1650.

105. National Cancer Institute. Measurement Error Webinar Series. https://epi.grants.cancer.gov/events/measurement -error. Accessed April 1, 2017.

106. Moshfegh AJ, Rhodes DG, Baer DJ, et al. The US Department of Agriculture Automated Multiple-Pass Method reduces bias in the collection of energy intakes. *Am J Clin Nutr*. 2008;88(2):324-332.

107. Blanton CA, Moshfegh AJ, Baer DJ, Kretsch MJ. The USDA Automated Multiple-Pass Method accurately estimates group total energy and nutrient intake. *J Nutr*. 2006;136(10):2594-2599.

108. Rhodes DG, Murayi T, Clemens JC, Baer DJ, Sebastian RS, Moshfegh AJ. The USDA Automated Multiple-Pass Method accurately assesses population sodium intakes. *Am J Clin Nutr*. 2013;97(5):958-964.

109. Ahluwalia N, Herrick KA, Rossen LM, et al. Usual nutrient intakes of US infants and toddlers generally meet or exceed Dietary Reference Intakes: findings from NHANES 2009–2012. *Am J Clin Nutr*. 2016;104(4): 1167-1174.

110. Wilson MM, Reedy J, Krebs-Smith SM, et al. American diet quality: where it is, where it is heading, and what it could be. *J Acad Nutr Diet*. 2016;116(2):302-10.e1.

111. Kirkpatrick SI, Dodd KW, Reedy J, Krebs-Smith SM. Income and race/ethnicity are associated with adherence to food-based dietary guidance among US adults and children. *J Acad Nutr Diet*. 2012;112(5):624-635.e6.

112. Reedy J, Krebs-Smith SM. Dietary sources of energy, solid fats, and added sugars among children and adolescents in the United States. *J Am Diet Assoc*. 2010;110(10): 1477-1484.

113. Shriver LH, Marriage BJ, Bloch TD, et al. Contribution of snacks to dietary intakes of young children in the United States. *Matern Child Nutr*. 2018;14(1):e12454.

114. Quader ZS, Gillespie C, Sliwa SA, et al. Sodium intake among US school-aged children: National Health and Nutrition Examination Survey, 2011–2012. *J Acad Nutr Diet*. 2017;117(1):39-47.e5.

115. Martínez Steele E, Baraldi LG, Louzada ML da C, Moubarac J-C, Mozaffarian D, Monteiro CA. Ultra-processed foods and added sugars in the US diet: evidence from a nationally representative cross-sectional study. *BMJ Open*. 2016;6(3):e009892.

116. Quader ZS, Zhao L, Gillespie C, et al. Sodium intake among persons aged ≥2 years—United States, 2013–2014. *MMWR Morb Mortal Wkly Rep*. 2017;66(12):324-238.

117. Wright J D, Bialostosky K, Gunter E , et al. Blood folate and vitamin B12: United States, 1988–94. *Vital Health Stat 11*. 1998;(243):1-78.

118. Centers for Disease Control and Prevention. Folate status in women of childbearing age—United States, 1999. *Morb Mortal Wkly Rep*. 2000;49(42):962-965.

119. Williams J, Mai C T, Mulinare J, et al. Updated estimates of neural tube defects prevented by mandatory folic acid fortification—United States, 1995–2011. *Morb Mortal Wkly Rep*. 2015;64(1):1-5.

120. Haytowitz DB, Pehrsson PR, Holden JM. The National Food and Nutrient Analysis Program: a decade of progress. *J Food Compost Anal*. 2008;21(S1):S94-S102.

121. US Department of Agriculture, Agricultural Research Service. National Food and Nutrient Analysis Program. www.ars.usda.gov/northeast-area/beltsville-md -bhnrc/beltsville-human-nutrition-research-center /nutrient-data-laboratory/docs/national-food-and -nutrient-analysis-program. Updated August 13, 2016. Accessed April 1, 2017.

122. US Department of Agriculture, Agricultural Research Service. Nutrient Data Laboratory. www.ars.usda.gov /northeast-area/beltsville-md/beltsville-human-nutrition-research-center/nutrient-data-laboratory. Accessed April 1, 2017.

123. US Department of Agriculture, Agricultural Research Service. Food Surveys Research Group: Beltsville, MD. www.ars.usda.gov/northeast-area/beltsville-md /beltsville-human-nutrition-research-center/food -surveys-research-group. Accessed April 1, 2017.

124. US Department of Agriculture, Agricultural Research Service. USDA Branded Food Products Database. www.ars.usda.gov/northeast-area/beltsville-md -bhnrc/beltsville-human-nutrition-research-center /nutrient-data-laboratory/docs/usda-branded-food -products-database. Updated 2017. Accessed June 15, 2018

125. US Department of Agriculture, Agricultural Research Service. 2013–2014 Food and Nutrient Database for Dietary Studies: Changes in Number of Codes and Nutrients. www.ars.usda.gov/ARSUserFiles/80400530/pdf/fndds /fndds_changes.pdf. Published October 5, 2016. Accessed April 1, 2017.

126. US Department of Agriculture, Agricultural Research Service. Food and Nutrient Database for Dietary Surveys. 2016. www.ars.usda.gov/northeast-area/beltsville-md -bhnrc/beltsville-human-nutrition-research-center /food-surveys-research-group/docs/fndds. Accessed June 15, 2018.

127. US Department of Agriculture, Agricultural Research Service. Food Patterns Equivalents Database. 2017. www.ars .usda.gov/northeast-area/beltsville-md-bhnrc/ beltsville-human-nutrition-research-center/food -surveys-research-group/docs/fped-overview. Accessed June 15, 2018.

128. National Institutes of Health, Office of Dietary Supplements, and US Department of Agriculture. Dietary Supplement Ingredient Database. Updated 2017. https://dietarysupplementdatabase.usda.nih.gov. Accessed April 1, 2017.

129. Roseland JM, Holden JM, Andrews KW, et al. Dietary supplement ingredient database (DSID): preliminary USDA studies on the composition of adult multivitamin /mineral supplements. *J Food Compost Anal.* 2008; 21(suppl):S69-S77.

130. Dwyer JT, Holden J, Andrews K, et al. Measuring vitamins and minerals in dietary supplements for nutrition studies in the USA. *Anal Bioanal Chem.* 2007;389(1):37-46.

131. Dwyer JT, Picciano MF, Betz JM, et al. Progress in developing analytical and label-based dietary supplement databases at the NIH Office of Dietary Supplements. *J Food Compos Anal.* 2008;21(suppl):S83-S93.

132. Guenther PM, Casavale KO, Reedy J, et al. Update of the Healthy Eating Index: HEI-2010. *J Acad Nutr Diet.* 2013;113(4):569-580.

133. Kirkpatrick SI, Reedy J, Kahle LL, Harris JL, Ohri-Vachaspati P, Krebs-Smith SM. Fast-food menu offerings vary in dietary quality, but are consistently poor. *Public Health Nutr.* 2014;17(4):924-931.

134. Murray CW, Egan SK, Kim H, Beru N, Bolger PM. US Food and Drug Administration's Total Diet Study: dietary intake of perchlorate and iodine. *J Expo Sci Environ Epidemiol.* 2008;18(6):571-580. doi:10.1038/sj.jes .7500648.

135. US Food and Drug Administration, Center for Food Safety and Applied Nutrition. Food Label and Package Survey 2006–2007. 2015. www.fda.gov/Food/FoodScience Research/ConsumerBehaviorResearch/ucm275404.htm. Accessed April 1, 2017.

136. Miller G, Merlo C, Demissie Z, Sliwa S, Park S. Trends in beverage consumption among high school students— United States, 2007–2015. *MMWR Morb Mortal Wkly Rep.* 2017;66(4):112-116.

137. National Cancer Institute, Division of Cancer Control and Population Sciences. Health Information National Trends Survey. https://hints.cancer.gov. Accessed April 1, 2017.

138. Nelson D, Kreps G, Hesse B, et al. The Health Information National Trends Survey (HINTS): development, design, and dissemination. *J Health Commun.* 2004;9(5):443-460.

139. Erinosho TO, Pinard CA, Nebeling LC, et al. Development and implementation of the National Cancer Institute's Food Attitudes and Behaviors Survey to assess correlates of fruit and vegetable intake in adults. *PLoS One.* 2015;10(2):e0115017.

140. Subar AF, Heimendinger J, Patterson BH, Krebs-Smith SM, Pivonka E, Kessler R. Fruit and vegetable intake in the United States: the baseline survey of the Five A Day for Better Health Program. *Am J Health Promot.* 1995;9 (5):352-360.

141. US Food and Drug Administration, Center for Food Safety and Applied Nutrition. Consumer Behavior Research. www.fda.gov/food/foodscienceresearch/consumer behaviorresearch/default.htm. Accessed June 15, 2018.

142. US Department of Agriculture, Center for Nutrition Policy and Promotion. Nutrient Content of the US Food Supply. www.cnpp.usda.gov/USfoodsupply. Accessed April 1, 2017.

143. US Department of Agriculture, Economic Research Ser-vice. Food Availability Documentation. 2018 www.ers .usda.gov/data-products/food-availability-per-capita -data-system/food-availability-documentation. Accessed June 15, 2018.

144. US Department of Agriculture, Economic Research Ser-vice. Food Availability (Per Capita) Data System. 2018 www.ers.usda.gov/data-products/food-availability-per -capita-data-system. Accessed June 15, 2018.

145. National Oceanic and Atmospheric Administration, Office of Science and Technology. Fisheries of the United States, 2015. www.st.nmfs.noaa.gov/commercial-fisheries/fus /fus15/index. Accessed April 1, 2017.

146. The University of Chicago, Booth School of Business. Neilsen Datasets at the Kilts Center for Marketing. https://research.chicagobooth.edu/nielsen. Accessed April 1, 2017.

147. National Cancer Institute, Division of Cancer Control and Population Sciences. Classification of Laws Associated with School Students (CLASS). https://class.cancer.gov. Accessed April 1, 2017.

148. US Department of Agriculture, Economic Research Service. SNAP Policy Database. 2018. www.ers.usda.gov/data -products/snap-policy-database. Accessed June 15, 2018.

149. Chai W, Fan JX, Wen M. Association of individual and community factors with C-reactive protein and 25-hydroxyvitamin D: evidence from the National Health and Nutrition Examination Survey (NHANES). *SSM Popul Health.* 2016;2:889-896.

150. Wen M, Kowaleski-Jones L. The built environment and risk of obesity in the United States: racial-ethnic disparities. *Health Place*. 2012;18(6):1314-1322.

151. De Keyzer W, Bracke T, McNaughton S, et al. Cross-continental comparison of national food consumption survey methods—a narrative review. *Nutrients*. 2015;7(5):3587-3620.

152. US Congress. H.R.2642 - Agricultural Act of 2014. 113th Congress (2013–2014). www.congress.gov/bill/113th-congress/house-bill/2642. Accessed August 14, 2017.

153. Centers for Disease Control and Prevention. NHANES Dietary Web Tutorial. www.cdc.gov/nchs/tutorials/dietary. Updated May 7, 2014.Accessed April 1, 2017.

154. Centers for Disease Control and Prevention, National Center for Health Statistics. National Health and Nutrition Examination Survey, NHANES III (1988–1994)–Reference Manuals and Reports. www.cdc.gov/nchs/nhanes/nh3rrm.htm. Updated November 10, 2015. Accessed April 1, 2017.

155. National Institutes of Health, Division of Nutrition Research Coordination. *NIH Nutrition Research Report 2015 & 2016*. Bethesda, MD; 2017. www.niddk.nih.gov/about-niddk/strategic-plans-reports/nih-nutrition-report. Accessed June 15, 2018.

156. *NIH Nutrition Research Report 2013 & 2014*. Bethesda, MD: National Institutes of Health, Division of Nutrition Research Coordination; 2015.

157. National Institute of Diabetes and Digestive and Kidney Diseases (NIDDK). NIDDK establishes Office of Nutrition Research. 2015. www.niddk.nih.gov/news/research-updates/Pages/niddk-establishes-office-nutrition-research.aspx. Published March 6, 2015. Accessed April 1, 2017.

158. National Institute of Diabetes and Digestive and Kidney Diseases (NIDDK). Office of Nutrition Research. www.niddk.nih.gov/about-niddk/offices-divisions/office-nutrition-research/Pages/default.aspx#category=strategic-plans-and-reports-on-nutrition. Accessed April 1, 2017.

159. National Institutes of Health. NIH Clinical Trials and You. www.nih.gov/health-information/nih-clinical-research-trials-you/finding-clinical-trial. Updated March 13, 2017. Accessed April 1, 2017.

160. US National Library of Medicine. PubMed Tutorial. www.nlm.nih.gov/bsd/disted/pubmedtutorial/cover.html. Updated August 25, 2016. Accessed April 1, 2017.

161. US Census Bureau. TheDataWeb. DataFerrett. https://dataferrett.census.gov. Accessed April 1, 2017.

162. Blumberg SJ, Luke J V. *Wireless Substitution: Early Release of Estimates from the National Health Interview Survey*. Atlanta, GA: Centers for Disease Control and Prevention; 2012.

163. Blumberg SJ, Luke J V. Reevaluating the need for concern regarding noncoverage bias in landline surveys. *Am J Public Health*. 2009;99(10):1806-1810.

164. Gundersen DA, ZuWallack RS, Dayton J, Echeverria SE, Delnevo CD. Assessing the feasibility and sample quality of a national random-digit dialing cellular phone survey of young adults. *Am J Epidemiol*. 2014;179(1):39-47.

165. Rowland ML. Self-reported weight and height. *Am J Clin Nutr*. 1990;52(6):1125-1133.

166. Rust K, Rao J. Variance estimation for complex surveys using replication techniques. *Stat Methods Med Res*. 1996;5(3):283-310.

167. Thompson FE, Kirkpatrick SI, Subar AF, et al. The National Cancer Institute's Dietary Assessment Primer: a resource for diet research. *J Acad Nutr Diet*. 2015;115(12):1986-1995.

168. National Cancer Institute, National Institutes of Health, National Cancer Institute. Dietary Assessment Primer. https://dietassessmentprimer.cancer.gov. Accessed April 1, 2017.

169. National Academy of Sciences. *Dietary Reference Intakes: Applications in Dietary Assessment*. Washington, DC: National Academies Press; 2000.

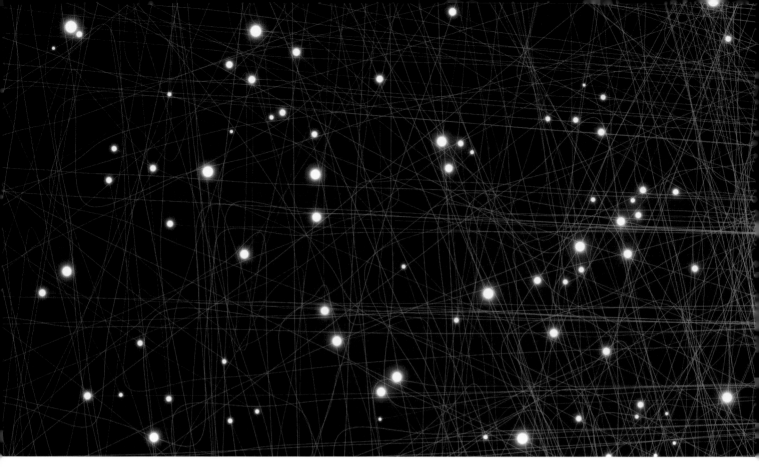

Integrative and Translational Research

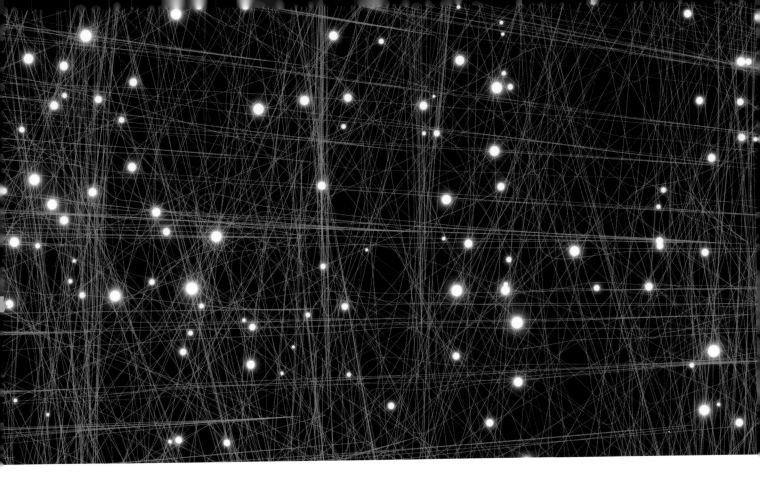

Systematic Reviews: Backbone of Evidence-Based Practice

Deepa Handu, PhD, RDN | *Lisa Moloney, MS, RDN* |
Feon Cheng, PhD, MPH, RDN, CHTS-CP | *Mary Rozga, PhD, RDN*

LEARNING OBJECTIVES

1. Differentiate between a systematic and narrative review.

2. Describe the basic steps in conducting a systematic review.

3. Describe the steps in developing an evidence-based practice guideline.

4. Identify strengths and limitations of systematic reviews and evidence-based practice guidelines.

5. Identify resources for systematic review and evidence-based practice guideline development.

The relationship between research and dietetics practice is a two-way interaction. Research findings are translated into dietetics practice, and dietetics practitioners identify questions that need to be researched. This dynamic relationship has become even more evident with the widespread adoption of evidence-based practice (EBP), which is defined as the conscientious, explicit, and judicious use of current best evidence in making decisions about the care of individual patients.[1] Evidence relative to a specific practice question is brought together through the process of a systematic review that includes searching for, selecting, critically evaluating, synthesizing, and disseminating the systematic review. The resulting document represents a summary and synthesis of the best available evidence, which is then used to develop evidence-based recommendations to aid practice decisions. Systematic review summary documents are intended to inform choices made by health care practitioners and policy makers. The procedures used in the systematic review and guideline development process must follow explicit, transparent, and rigorous scientific methodology.

This chapter provides an overview of evidence-based dietetics practice (EBDP), the systematic review process used to evaluate and present evidence, and guideline development. Examples and the resulting summary documents from the Evidence Analysis Library (EAL) of the Academy of Nutrition and Dietetics are included. The final section provides resources for conducting systematic reviews and developing guidelines.

WHY RESEARCHERS SHOULD USE EVIDENCE-BASED PRACTICE

Health care literature is being published at a rapid rate, and keeping up with it is challenging for practitioners. Practitioners recognize the need for using current, synthesized scientific evidence to improve patient-centered outcomes.

In the 1980s, EBP began appearing in the medical literature; it became common terminology in the 1990s and is an expectation of practice today.[1] The Academy of Nutrition and Dietetics has embraced the concept of EBP since 2004. Two major applications of EBP are especially relevant to dietetics practice: (1) review and synthesize the best available evidence to create recommendations for a defined area of practice (guidelines development and health policy making) and (2) search for scientific evidence to answer a specific question related to care for a specific patient or subgroup of patients (clinical decision-making). According to the Academy, EBDP: "involves the process of asking questions, systematically finding research evidence, and assessing its validity, applicability and importance to food and nutrition practice decisions; and includes applying relevant evidence in the context of the practice situation and the values of clients, customers and communities to achieve positive outcomes."[2]

Following are some of the key considerations of EBDP:

- EBDP is based on the best available evidence, including research, national guidelines, policies, consensus statements, expert opinion, and quality improvement data.
- The determination of "best available evidence" is based on the hierarchy of evidence.
- The systematic review of scientific evidence is an ongoing process.
- EBDP involves continuing evaluation of outcomes, which then becomes part of the evidence base.
- EBDP applies to individual clients, patients, and communities.
- Evidence-based Nutrition Practice Guidelines for dietetics practice are available on the Academy of Nutrition and Dietetics EAL (www.andeal.org).

To support practitioners in bridging the gap between research and nutrition care practice, the Academy has developed a rigorous process to conduct systematic reviews and develop clinical practice guidelines.[3,4]

CONDUCTING SYSTEMATIC REVIEWS

EBDP relies on systematic reviews of the best available evidence. A systematic review is a form of research that attempts to identify, appraise, and synthesize evidence that meets prespecified criteria to answer a specific clinical question using explicit methods.[5] In contrast, for narrative reviews authors (experts in the field) use informal, unsystematic methods to collect and interpret information. Search protocol, quality appraisal, and data synthesis are not usually described and, hence, narrative reviews are more prone to bias.[6] A basic requirement of the systematic review process used in EBDP is that a protocol—the methodology—must be articulated before beginning the evidence search, review, and synthesis.

Various groups have organized the process of systematic review of evidence into four to eight steps or components.[7-9] However, all processes incorporate the following essential steps, which will be discussed in this chapter:

1. Develop the question.
2. Gather and classify research.
3. Extract data from and critically appraise each article.
4. Summarize the evidence.
5. Grade the quality of evidence.

Step 1: Formulate the Evidence Analysis Question

Formulating an evidence analysis question is the crucial first step in the systematic review process. In EBDP, attention is focused on asking specific questions that can be answered using existing data and that are relevant to clinical decision-making. Questions about basic biological processes or background questions are not appropriate for EBDP and would be better answered by appropriate texts on the topic.[10] Question formulation is commonly driven by questions and uncertainties identified by practitioners with experience in the area of interest.

Formulating a high-quality research question for systematic review can be challenging. However, implementing standardized practices and utilizing available tools and resources can improve question quality. The following three frameworks are used to generate high-quality systematic review research questions[4]:

● **Nutrition Care Process (NCP):** to provide a systematic structure to scientifically manage patient-centered nutrition care[11]
● **Analytic framework:** to identify links between exposures and outcomes of interest in the NCP (see Figure 10.1)

■ **Population, intervention, comparative group, and outcome (PICO) question format:** to identify key question components

When formulating a systematic review question, it is important to consider how relevant factors in each stage of the NCP, including nutrition assessment, diagnosis, intervention, and nutrition monitoring and evaluation, will ultimately affect patient-centered outcomes of interest. One schematic tool that can be used to visually identify the relationships among these factors is an analytic framework template (see Figure 10.1).[12]

Analytic frameworks may also be constructed to visually show how subquestions relate to the overarching question.[12] In evidence reviews, four types of questions are used[13]:

● **Diagnosis and screening:** Is the nutrition-related problem or condition present?
● **Natural history and prognosis:** What is the progression of the nutrition-related problem before and after diagnosis?
● **Therapy, prevention and control, and performance improvement (treatment/intervention):** What action is effective in a given situation?
● **Etiology, causation, and harm:** What is the potential for positive and/or negative consequences of a specific aspect of nutrition care (or its absence)?

Though systematic review questions may focus on different areas, they include common key elements. Craig and colleagues[10] provided a PICO method for framing questions dealing with diagnosis, harm/etiology, prognosis, and intervention, all of which have a slightly different format for designing the question. Though the format may be altered depending on the question of interest, following are the key elements:

● Patient population of concern (P)
● Intervention being considered (I)
● Comparator to intervention (C)
● Outcomes, including anticipated measures, improvements, or effects (O)[13]

Here is an example of how the PICO format was used in question development for an Academy EAL proj-

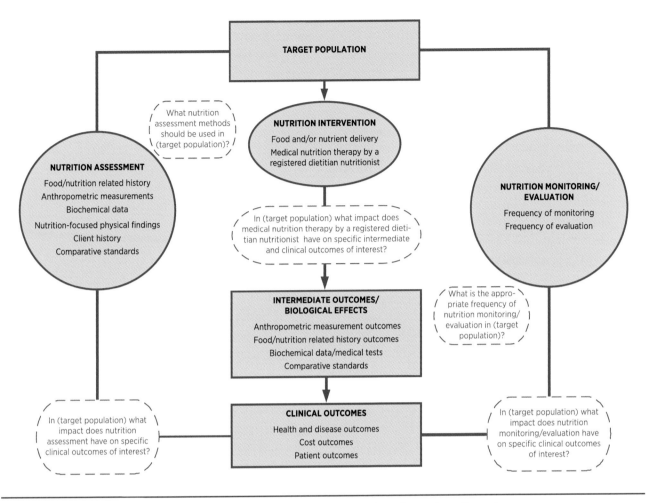

Figure 10.1 Example of an analytic framework to help develop questions for systematic review

Adapted with permission from Academy of Nutrition and Dietetics. *Evidence Analysis Manual.* www.andeal.org/evidence-analysis-manual. Published 2016. Accessed March 1, 2017.[12]

ect about medical nutrition therapy (MNT) in patients with diabetes.[14]

- Patient population of concern: Adults with type 1 and type 2 diabetes
- Intervention: MNT provided by a registered dietitian nutritionist (RDN)
- Comparator: Usual care
- Outcome: glycemia (hemoglobin A1c or glucose levels?)

The systematic research process often starts with a broad overarching question, which is then answered by several more specific subquestions that address various aspects of the overarching question.[8,12] Each question must be specific enough for research to be clinically applicable but broad enough to include all research relevant to the research question. Utilizing the PICO format ensures that research questions will address the project's goal.

Question formulation is an iterative process, and a research team may go through several versions of their research questions. To ensure that the systematic review project can be completed in a reasonable amount of time, the quantity and scope of the research questions must be manageable, which requires the research team to prioritize questions. Questions may be prioritized based on their importance to nutrition practice, impact on the patient/client and health care costs, ability to address confusing or controversial topics or variations in practice, likelihood to verify assumptions in practice, or availability of research studies to answer the question.

One technique used to examine availability of research is evidence mapping or scoping, which allows researchers to identify, organize, and summarize the literature on a broad topic in order to identify the current status of research on that broad topic and determine where there are gaps in the literature.[15] Evidence mapping and scoping follow the same initial steps as the systematic review process, including formulating questions and gathering, analyzing, and summarizing results.[16,17] However, in evidence mapping, data are not extracted from relevant articles, and the quality of the articles is not assessed. Instead, the goal of evidence mapping is to investigate the number and type of published studies on a topic, including the specific characteristics of the studies. The process is called mapping because results are mapped into tables or graphs to give the researchers an overall picture of the scope and direction of the current body of literature. This process allows researchers to prioritize research questions from the systematic review that can be answered by the literature to address EBP needs.

Step 2: Gather Research

Developing a Search Plan

After formulating the evidence analysis question that is the basis for the review, a search plan must be developed a priori to identify all relevant research studies to ensure an unbiased review. The search plan should identify the databases to be searched, initial key search terms, and the eligibility criteria (inclusion/exclusion criteria) for a research study to be included in the systematic review.

Eligibility Criteria

In addition to identifying a plan for finding the appropriate literature, researchers must establish explicit a priori eligibility criteria, called inclusion and exclusion criteria, which guide the selection of research studies to be included in the systematic review. Eligibility criteria can include a range of factors, such as publication year, study design, population age, study location, health status or condition, attri-

tion rate, and number of participants per treatment group. For example, inclusion criteria for a standard EAL systematic review are peer-reviewed human studies published in the English language; additional inclusion/exclusion criteria would vary depending on the evidence analysis question.[3] Most search strategies, similar to the EAL systematic review protocol, limit eligible evidence to published peer-reviewed research and studies with strong methodology Search protocol varies based on research topics. Some topics require more liberal inclusion criteria.

Search Terms

Search terms are key terms and outcomes of interest identified during the question formulation process. These terms are then used when conducting the literature search through identified databases. For EBP guidelines, selected outcomes should be measurable and patient focused.

Literature Search

After a search plan has been completed, the next step is to perform a literature search. Careful implementation of a sound search plan is critical to a high-quality systematic review. Introducing bias in the selection of the research to be reviewed or included will seriously flaw the final systematic review. As indicated in the Cochrane handbook, multiple databases should be used to ensure a comprehensive search.[8] The list of databases used may differ depending on the topic of the evidence analysis question. For instance, in the field of nutrition, some of the most common databases include Cochrane Library, MEDLINE (ie, PubMed), Excerpta Medica Database (EMBASE), Cumulative Index to Nursing and Allied Health Literature (CINAHL), and HEALTHSTAR.[3] It is important to note that search terms need to be specific to the databases being searched.[12] Reviewing references of included articles and other systematic reviews is an essential second step to ensure the comprehensiveness of a literature search.

Evaluate Search Results

Once the search is completed, the process of screening the search results is initiated. Cooper and Zlotkin[18] described the importance of the filtering process used to select the research articles to be reviewed. For a standard EAL systematic review, potential articles identified from the database searches will go through several rounds of screening to determine whether they meet the eligibility criteria (see Figure 10.2). Initial screening (first screening) usually involves screening titles and abstracts alone to exclude articles that are not relevant. The second screening involves reviewing full texts for inclusion/exclusion criteria and documenting reasons for excluding articles. Each round of screening includes at least two independent reviews of the article to determine whether it should be included in the systematic review per eligibility criteria. The Cochrane Collaboration recommends using one expert and one nonexpert in this process.[8] After evaluating search results, there should be a list of included and excluded articles from the second screening with exclusion reasons. All the included articles will then proceed to data extraction and critical appraisal (risk of bias).

Documentation

Each step of the search should be well documented to allow for transparency and reproducibility of the systematic review. All literature searches and results, such as search date, search terms, number of hits, number of duplicates, and included and excluded articles at each round of review, are recorded in the search plan. This is based on the Preferred Reporting Items for Systematic Reviews and Meta-Analyses (referred to as PRISMA), which provides a guide for reporting systematic reviews.[19]

Figure 10.3 on page 198 presents an example of a search plan for nutrition-related studies defined by the Academy of Nutrition and Dietetics Evidence Analysis Library.

Step 3: Extract Data and Critically Appraise Articles

Step 3 of the systematic review process involves two processes: data extraction and quality evaluation. Relevant data from each of the eligible research studies are extracted according to the protocol. Some methodologies suggest that the extraction process should vary depending on whether the question to be answered is related to prognosis, diagnosis, treatment, or economic impact.[7,20] The following types of data are usually extracted for each research report evaluated: author and date, methodology/type of study, number and characteristics of study participants, intervention, outcome measures, findings, author's conclusions, and study quality (design and execution). The Academy of Nutrition and Dietetics uses a web-based Data Extraction Tool (DET) for structured data extraction and storage (see Figure 10.4 on page 199). This tool provides standardized data entry fields (eg, study design, publication year) that are used in all EAL systematic reviews and allows users flexibility to customize other fields to meet the needs of different projects.

In addition to data extraction, the quality of each research study is evaluated using criteria relevant to the particular study design; see Box 10.1 on pages 200 through 203 for sample questions from the Academy of Nutrition and Dietetics risk of bias tool, the Quality Criteria Checklist.[12] The instrument includes 10 validity questions based on the Agency for Healthcare Research and Quality (AHRQ) domains for research studies. Listed under each validity question are subquestions that identify important aspects of sound study design and execution relevant to each domain.[21] Some of these subquestions are specific to research study design. Table 10.1 on pages 203 through 204 provides a brief description and hierarchy of study designs.

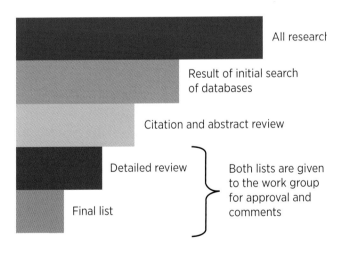

Figure 10.2 Steps to identify the best and most relevant research

Adapted with permission from Academy of Nutrition and Dietetics. *Evidence Analysis Manual.* www.andeal.org/evidence-analysis-manual. Published 2016. Accessed May 22, 2018.[12]

Search Plan and Results

Date of Literature Review

April 2013

Inclusion Criteria

Age: Adults over 18 years of age

Setting: Outpatient and ambulatory care

Health Status: Any

Nutrition-Related Problem or Condition: Overweight and obesity with or without comorbid conditions.

Study Design Preferences: Randomized controlled trials (Class A), cohort studies (Class B), nonrandomized clinical studies (Class C) and observational/noncontrolled Trials (class D) that have a study duration of at least 12 weeks or 3 months. The study designs were more inclusive for the Medical Nutrition Therapy studies because the Work Group was interested in the outcomes for that intervention only.

Size of Study Groups: The sample size must equal 10 individuals for each study group. For example, this would include 10 patients in the Intervention Group and 10 patients in the Control or Comparison Group.

Study Dropout Rate: Less than 20%

Year Range: July 2006 to April 2013

Authorship: If an author is included on more than one review article or primary research article that is similar in content, the most recent review or article will be accepted and earlier versions will be rejected. If an author is included on more than one review article or primary research article and the content is different, then both reviews may be accepted.

Language: Limited to articles in English

Exclusion Criteria

Age: Children and adolescents (under 18 years of age)

Setting: Inpatient or acute care

Health Status: Patients with a poor prognosis

Nutrition Related-Problem or Condition: Critical illness and other disease and conditions

Study Design Preferences: Narrative reviews and included study designs with durations of less than 12 weeks or 3 months

Size of Study Groups: Fewer than 10 individuals for each study group; for example, this would include 10 patients in the Intervention Group and 10 patients in the Control or Comparison Group

Study Dropout Rate: More than 20%

Year Range: Prior to July 2006

Authorship: Studies by same author similar in content

Language: Articles not in English

Search Terms: Search Vocabulary

Health Condition: diabet*

Intervention: RD, dietitian, dietician, nutritionist, Medical Nutrition Therapy, MNT

Type of Study Design: Randomized controlled trials (Class A), cohort studies (Class B) and nonrandomized clinical studies (Class C)

Electronic Databases

Database: PubMed

Search terms: (diabet*) and (RD or dietitian or dietician or nutritionist or "medical nutrition therapy" or MNT)

Hits: 622

Articles to review: 35

CENTRAL database not used

Other databases not used

Total articles identified to review from electronic databases: 35

Articles Identified from other sources:

Figure 10.3 Example search inclusion and exclusion criteria

Adapted with permission from Academy of Nutrition and Dietetics. Evidence Analysis Library. Diabetes Type 1 and Type 2. www.andeal.org/topic .cfm?menu=5305&pcat=5491&cat=5161. Accessed May 22, 2018.[14]

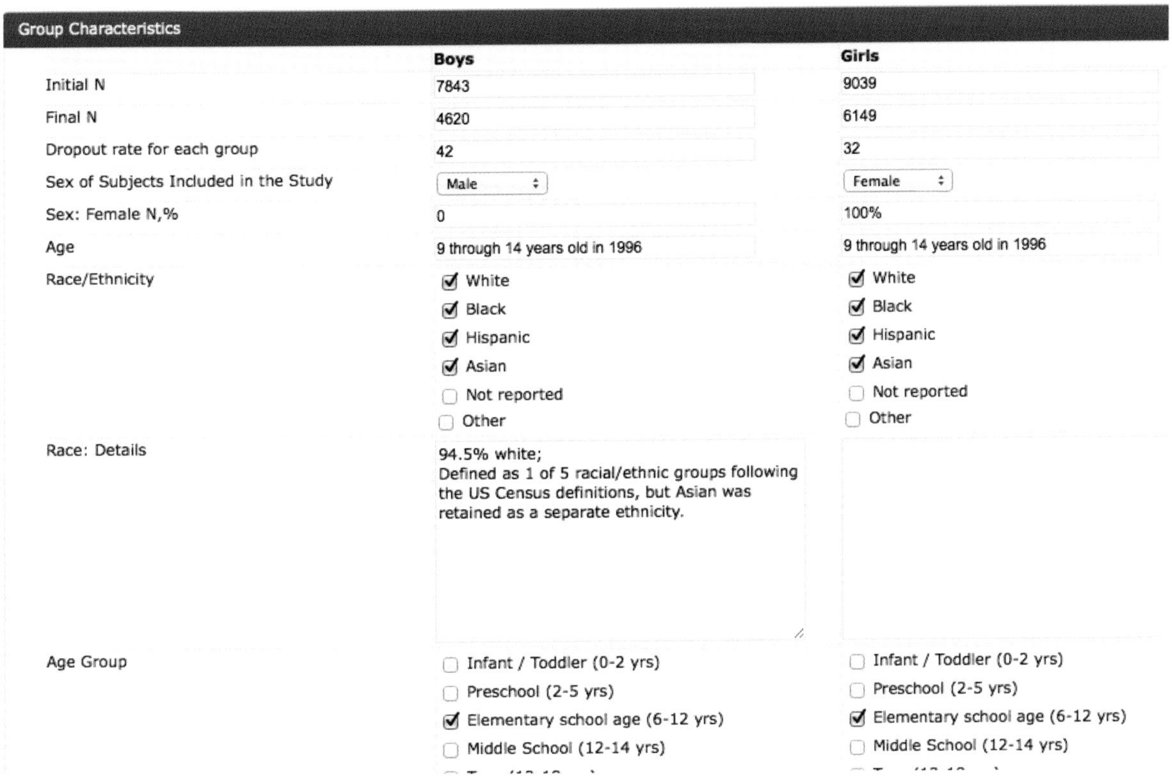

Group Characteristics		
	Boys	**Girls**
Initial N	7843	9039
Final N	4620	6149
Dropout rate for each group	42	32
Sex of Subjects Included in the Study	Male ⦂	Female ⦂
Sex: Female N,%	0	100%
Age	9 through 14 years old in 1996	9 through 14 years old in 1996
Race/Ethnicity	☑ White ☑ Black ☑ Hispanic ☑ Asian ☐ Not reported ☐ Other	☑ White ☑ Black ☑ Hispanic ☑ Asian ☐ Not reported ☐ Other
Race: Details	94.5% white; Defined as 1 of 5 racial/ethnic groups following the US Census definitions, but Asian was retained as a separate ethnicity.	
Age Group	☐ Infant / Toddler (0-2 yrs) ☐ Preschool (2-5 yrs) ☑ Elementary school age (6-12 yrs) ☐ Middle School (12-14 yrs)	☐ Infant / Toddler (0-2 yrs) ☐ Preschool (2-5 yrs) ☑ Elementary school age (6-12 yrs) ☐ Middle School (12-14 yrs)

Figure 10.4 Snapshot of the Academy of Nutrition and Dietetics Data Extraction Tool

In addition to the Academy of Nutrition and Dietetics Quality Criteria Checklist, there are other commonly used tools for assessing the quality of randomized controlled trials or observational studies. Some of the most recommended tools are Cochrane's Risk of Bias tool specifically for randomized controlled trials (Cochrane Handbook),[8] Jadad scale,[22] Newcastle-Ottawa Scale (NOS) for nonrandomized studies,[23] and the AHRQ checklist.[24] There are also tools for assessing the quality of systematic reviews, such as A Measurement Tool to Assess Systematic Reviews (AMSTAR).[25] Most of these tools focus on the core biases related to how the study is conducted. The Cochrane Handbook states these risks of bias domains as selection bias, performance bias, attrition bias, detection bias, reporting bias, and other bias.[8]

Step 4: Summarize the Evidence

After data extraction and critical appraisal of included research articles, researchers start the process of synthesizing the evidence. Different organizations have different tools or methods of synthesizing evidence. The objective of this step is to combine relevant and valid information into a brief, coherent, and easy-to-read summary. The most common method is presenting this information in tables supported with a narrative summary (plain language). These are typically called summary tables, summary of findings tables, study characteristics tables, or outcomes tables. Many variations of and combinations of these tables may be used.[3,26]

The Academy of Nutrition and Dietetics process includes presenting results in an evidence analysis summary table, evidence summary (narrative), and conclusion statement. The type of information included in a summary table depends on the type of project or research question being answered. However, the core data typically included are author/study information, study design, number of participants, intervention description, list of important outcomes, results for each outcome

Quality Criteria Checklist Domain	Primary Research Quality Criteria Checklist
Research questions	Was the research question clearly stated?
	Was the specific intervention(s) or procedure (independent variable[s]) identified?
	Was the outcome(s) (dependent variable[s]) clearly indicated?
	Were the target population and setting specified?
Participant selection	Was the selection of study participants/patients free from bias?
	Were inclusion/exclusion criteria specified (eg, risk, point in disease progression, and diagnostic or prognostic criteria), and with sufficient detail and without omitting criteria critical to the study?
	Were criteria applied equally to all study groups?
	Were health, demographic characteristics, and other characteristics of participants described?
	Were the participants/patients a representative sample of the relevant population?
Comparable groups	Were study groups comparable?
	Was the method of assigning participants/patients to groups described and unbiased? (Method of randomization should be identified if randomized controlled trial).
	Were distribution of disease status, prognostic factors, and other factors (eg, demographic characteristics) similar across study groups at baseline?
	Were concurrent controls used? (Concurrent preferred over historical controls.)
	If cohort study or cross-sectional study, were groups comparable on important confounding factors and/or were preexisting differences accounted for by using appropriate adjustments in statistical analysis?
	If case-control study, were potential confounding factors comparable for cases and controls? (If case series or trial with participants serving as own controls, this criterion is not applicable. Criterion may not be applicable in some cross-sectional studies.)
	If diagnostic test, was there an independent blind comparison with an appropriate reference standard (eg, gold standard)?

Box 10.1 Questions from the Quality Criteria Checklist: Primary (Original) Research *(continued)*

Withdrawals	Was method of handling withdrawals described?
	Were follow-up methods described and the same for all groups?
	Were the number, characteristics of withdrawals (ie, dropouts, lost to follow-up, attrition rate) and/or response rate (cross-sectional studies) described for each group? (Follow-up goal for a strong study is 80%.)
	Were all enrolled participants/patients (in the original sample) accounted for?
	Were reasons for withdrawals similar across groups?
	If diagnostic test, was decision to perform reference test not dependent on results of test under study?
Blinding	Was blinding used to prevent introduction of bias?
	In intervention study, were participants, clinicians/practitioners, and investigators blinded to treatment group, as appropriate?
	Were data collectors blinded for outcomes assessment? (If outcome is measured using an objective test, such as a lab value, this criterion is assumed to be met.)
	In cohort study or cross-sectional study, were measurements of outcomes and risk factors blinded?
	In case-control study, was case definition explicit and case ascertainment not influenced by exposure status?
	In diagnostic study, were test results blinded to patient history and other test results?
Intervention/exposure	Were intervention/therapeutic regimens/exposure factor or procedure and any comparison(s) described in detail? Were intervening factors described?
	In a randomized controlled trial or other intervention trial, were protocols described for all regimens studied?
	In observational study, were interventions, study settings, and clinicians/provider described?
	Was the intensity and duration of the intervention or exposure factor sufficient to produce a meaningful effect?
	Was the amount of exposure and, if relevant, participant/patient compliance measured?
	Were cointerventions (eg, ancillary treatments or other therapies) described?
	Were extra or unplanned treatments described?

Box 10.1 (cont.) Questions from the Quality Criteria Checklist: Primary (Original) Research *(continued)*

	Was the information for the previous three questions in this list assessed the same way for all groups?
	In diagnostic study, were details of test administration and replication sufficient?
Outcomes	Were outcomes clearly defined and the measurements valid and reliable?
	Were primary and secondary end points described and relevant to the question?
	Were nutrition measures appropriate to question and outcomes of concern?
	Was the period of follow-up long enough for important outcome(s) to occur?
	Were the observations and measurements based on standard, valid, and reliable data collection instruments/tests/procedures?
	Was the measurement of effect at an appropriate level of precision?
	Were other factors accounted for (measured) that could affect outcomes?
	Were the measurements conducted consistently across groups?
Analysis	Was the statistical analysis appropriate for the study design and type of outcome indicators?
	Were statistical analyses adequately described and the results reported appropriately?
	Were correct statistical tests used and assumptions of test not violated?
	Were statistics reported with levels of significance and/or confidence intervals?
	Was intent-to-treat analysis of outcomes done (and, as appropriate, was there an analysis of outcomes for those maximally exposed or a dose-response analysis)?
	Were adequate adjustments made for effects of confounding factors that might have affected the outcomes (eg, multivariate analyses)?
	Were clinical significance as well as statistical significance reported?
	If negative findings, was a power calculation reported to address type II error?
Conclusion support	Are conclusions supported by results with biases and limitations taken into consideration?
	Is there a discussion of findings?
	Are biases and study limitations identified and discussed?
Likelihood of bias	Is bias due to study's funding or sponsorship unlikely?
	Were sources of funding and investigators' affiliations described?
	Was there no apparent conflict of interest?

Box 10.1 (cont.) Questions from the Quality Criteria Checklist: Primary (Original) Research *(continued)*

MINUS/NEGATIVE (–)

If most (six or more) of the answers to the above validity questions are "No," the review should be designated with a minus (–) symbol on the Evidence Worksheet.

NEUTRAL (Ø)

If the answer to any of the first four validity questions (1 through 4) is "No," but other criteria indicate strengths, the review should be designated with a neutral (Ø) symbol on the Evidence Worksheet.

PLUS/POSITIVE (+)

If most of the answers to the above validity questions are "Yes" (must include criteria from the first four categories in the checklist), the report should be designed with a plus (+) symbol on the Evidence Worksheet.

Adapted from Academy of Nutrition and Dietetics. Evidence Analysis Manual. www.andeal.org/evidence-analysis-manual. Accessed March 1, 2017.[13]

Box 10.1 (cont.) Questions from the Quality Criteria Checklist: Primary (Original) Research

Study Design Type	Hierarchy of Study Design	Distinguishing Characteristics
Experimental and quasi-experimental trials		*Investigator-managed independent variable (the intervention)*
Randomized controlled trial	A	Randomization (at individual or site [a cluster of individuals] level) used to assign participants to two or more groups
Cluster randomized trial	A	
Randomized crossover trial	A	Participants receive two interventions in a random or nonrandom sequence, with a washout period between them
Non-randomized crossover trial	C	
Nonrandomized controlled trial	C	Participants assigned to two or more groups using a nonrandom method
Noncontrolled trial	D	Only one group studied, no comparison group
Descriptive studies		*No comparison, no intervention, describes "what is"*
Case study or case report	D	Detailed description of the unfolding course of events for one or a few participants, including treatments, intervening factors, and outcomes
Case series	D	
Other descriptive studies	D	In-depth quantitative and/or qualitative description
Observational studies		*Investigation of procedure, experience, or event with no researcher intervention*
Before-after study	D	Data collected at baseline and one or more times after a therapeutic or preventive procedure, experience, or event
Time series	C	Data from the same participants at a series of points over time, including prior to, during, and following the introduction of a therapeutic or preventive procedure, event, or natural exposure

Table 10.1 Study Design, Distinguishing Characteristics, and Important Quality Considerations *(continued)*

Study Design Type	Hierarchy of Study Design	Distinguishing Characteristics
Epidemiological analytic studies		*Comparisons constructed analytically, no researcher intervention, examines relationship among exposure factors and outcomes*
Prospective cohort	B	Enrollment based on defining characteristic or factor and screening to verify absence of outcome of interest
		Large number of participants tracked for long period of time
		Repeated data collection on "exposures" and status regarding outcomes of interest
Retrospective cohort	B	Existing database used to create a cohort and look back for a temporal relationship between exposure factors and development of the outcome
Case-control study	C	Cases with the outcome are identified then matched with noncases (controls) from the same population
		Looks back to determine if exposures differ between cases and controls
Cross-sectional study	D	One round of data collection where exposure factors and outcome status are measured at the same time
		Statistical tests used to examine association among variables
Trend study	D	Same data collected in different samples from the same population over time
		Like a series of cross-sectional studies
Diagnostic, validity, or reliability studies		*Comparison made with reference standard*
Diagnostic study	C	Used to determine the sensitivity or specificity of a diagnostic or assessment method
Validity study	C	
Reliability study	C	Used to determine the truthfulness or accuracy of a test, tool, or procedure used to measure or classify
		Comparisons made to determine consistency and reproducibility of results from a test, tool, or procedure

Table 10.1 (cont.) Study Design, Distinguishing Characteristics, and Important Quality Considerations

Adapted with permission from Academy of Nutrition and Dietetics Evidence Analysis Manual. Appendix 11: Important Considerations from Checklist by Study Design. www.andeal.org/evidence-analysis-manual. Accessed May 22, 2018.[5]

(eg, measure of risk, magnitude of effect), study quality, and overall conclusion. Table 10.2 shows an example of an evidence summary table. Concurrently, a narrative evidence summary is created that summarizes the trends in the data. Figure 10.5 on page 206 shows an example of the narrative evidence summary.

Statistical Analysis

Availability of the data determines whether quantitative statistics for a particular systematic review can be conducted. In situations where data are available, descriptive statistics and meta-analyses are conducted as appropriate. In a meta-analysis following a systematic review, data from individual studies may be pooled quantitatively and reanalyzed using established statistical methods.

Step 5: Grade the Evidence

The last step of the systematic review process is to answer the question in a statement called the conclusion statement (see Figure 10.6 on page 206).[3] The conclusion statement should be clear, to the point, and synthesize all evidence presented to answer the research question. The conclusion statement is graded to indicate the strength and quality of the supporting evidence. Figure 10.7 on page 207 shows the decision process that the Academy of Nutrition and Dietetics uses for determining grades for conclusion statements. The grade reflects the types of research in the hierarchy of evidence, the quality of the studies, and the consistency and magnitude of effect. The step of grading a conclusion statement is unique to the Academy of Nutrition and Dietetics process of systematic

Study, Year	Population	Intervention Duration	Intervention: number of RDN[a] encounters and length; MNT[b] intervention (type)	Major Findings: glycemia and cardiovascular risk factors	Major Findings: weight, medication changes, quality of life	Study Quality
Laitinen, 1993	n=86, type 2 diabetes, newly diagnosed	15 months	Intervention: 3 initial, 6 follow-up sessions; ↓ kcal, individualized, regular eating habits. Control: follow-up every 2–3 months for usual education (RCT[f])	HbA1c[c]: at 3-months baseline 8.4±2.2% ↓ SS[d] in both groups (P<.001) (as did FG[e]), at 15 months ↓ SS in intervention vs control (0.6% vs 0.3%); FG ↓ SS in intervention vs control (25 mg/dL vs 0 mg/dL); TC[g]: no change NS[h]; HDL-C[i] ↑ SS; in intervention vs control; TG[j] ↓ SS in intervention vs control	Weight at 15 months ↓ SS 5.1 kg vs 2.0 kg in intervention vs control (P<.05)	Positive
Franz, 1995	n=179, type 2 diabetes	6 months	NPG[k]: 3 visits, 2.5–3 hours; RDN determined nutrition prescriptions and care, ↓ kcal. Basic nutrition care of 1 RDN visit (RCT)	HbA1c: ↓ SS in both groups, 0.9% (NPG) and 0.7% (basic) (P<.001); FG: both ↓ SS (20 mg/dL and 11 mg/dL); HbA1c: in intervention in newly diagnosed ↓ 1.7% vs 0.4% in longer duration diabetes TC and TG: NPG SS ↓; LDL-C[l] and HDL-C NS changes	Weight at 6 months both SS ↓ (-1.7 kg)	Positive
Al-Shoorkir, 2012	n=200, type 2 diabetes	6 months	NPG: 3 sessions, 2.5–3 hours; ↓ kcal; individualized. Control: usual nutrition care (RCT)	HbA1c: NPG ↓ SS (1%, P<.01) vs NS change in control FG: NPG ↓ SS (22 mg/dL, P<.01) vs NS change in control TC & TG: NPG ↓ SS; LDL-C & HDL-C: NS	Weight NPG at 6 months ↓ SS (5.1 kg, P<.05) vs NS change in control	Positive
Battista, 2012	n=101, type 1 and type 2 diabetes	24 months	Intervention: RDN and endocrinologist; 3 sessions, first 6 months, 5 follow-up; ↓ kcal, healthy eating, and physical activity. Control: endocrinologist alone (RCT)	HbA1c: intervention ↓ SS 0.6% FG: intervention ↓ SS 13 mg/dL TC, LDL-C, HDL-C, TG: NS changes Blood pressure: intervention ↓ vs control↑	Weight, BMI[m], WC[n]: intervention vs control, ↓ SS weight (−0.7 kg vs +2.1 kg). BMI (−0.3 vs +0.7), WC (−1.3 cm vs +2.4 cm)	Neutral
Barakatun Nisak, 2013	n=104, type 2 diabetes	12 weeks	Individualized MNT, ↓ kcal; 3 sessions (cohort)	HbA1c: ↓ SS (0.4%, P<.001) FG: ↓ SS 5 mg/dL (P<.05) TC, LDL-C, TG: NS changes. HDL-C: ↑ SS (P<.05)	Weight, BMI: NS changes	Positive

Table 10.2 Example of an Evidence Summary Table (Summary of Findings Table)

a RDN=registered dietitian nutritionist
b MNT=medical nutrition therapy
c HbA1c=hemoglobin A1c
d SS=statistically significant
e FG=fasting glucose
f RCT=randomized clinical trial
g TC=total cholesterol
h NS=nonsignificant
i HDL-C=high-density lipoprotein cholesterol
j TG=triglycerides
k NPG=nutrition practice guideline
l LDL-C=low-density lipoprotein cholesterol
m BMI=body mass index
n WC=waist circumference
Adapted with permission from Academy of Nutrition and Dietetics. Evidence Analysis Library. Diabetes Type 1 and Type 2. www.andeal.org/topic.cfm?menu=5305. Accessed March 1 2017.[14]

EVIDENCE SUMMARY: In adults with type 1 and type 2 diabetes, how effective is medical nutrition therapy provided by a registered dietitian nutritionist on glycemia (Hemoglobin A1c or glucose)?

SYNOPSIS:

Hemoglobin A1c and Type 2 Diabetes

In adults with type 2 diabetes, 21 study arms, N=4,181 from 18 studies, N=5,434 [14 randomized clinical trials, N=3,835 (Al-Shookri et al, 2012; Andrews et al, 2011; Ash et al, 2003; Barnard et al, 2006; Barratt et al, 2008; Coppell et al, 2010; Davis et al, 2010; Franz et al, 1995; Goldhaber-Fiebert et al, 2003; Franz et al, 1995; Imai et al, 2011; Laitinen et al, 1993; Takahashi et al, 2004; UKPDS 1990; UKPDS 2000; Wolf et al, 2004), one nonrandomized clinical trial, N=44 (Battista et al, 2012), and three cohort studies, N=302 (Barakatun Nisak et al, 2013; Bastiaens et al, 2009; Lemon et al, 2004)] reported on the effectiveness of medical nutrition therapy (MNT) provided by registered dietitian nutritionists (RDNs) on hemoglobin HbA1c (HbA1c). HbA1c levels at baseline ranged from 6.6% to 10.3%. At three months, 13 study arms (Al-Shookri et al, 2012; Ash et al, 2003; Barakatun Nisak et al, 2013; Franz et al, 1995; Goldhaber-Fiebert et al, 2003; Imai et al, 2011; Laitinen et al, 1993; Lemon et al, 2004; Takahashi et al, 2004; UKPDS 1990; Wolf et al, 2004) reported decreases from baseline HbA1c levels ranging from 0.3% to 2.0%; at 6 months, nine study arms (Al-Shookri et al, 2012; Andrews et al, 2011; Barnard et al, 2006; Barratt et al, 2008; Bastiaens et al, 2009; Coppell et al, 2010; Davis et al, 2010; Franz et al, 1995; Imai et al, 2011; Laitinen et al, 1993; Lemon et al, 2004; Takahashi et al, 2004) reported decreases from baseline in HbA1c ranging from 0.3% to 1.8%; and with ongoing MNT support, at 12 months, six study arms (Andrews et al, 2011; Davis et al, 2010; Imai et al, 2011; Takahashi et al, 2004) reported decreases from baseline in HbA1c ranging from 0.3% to 1.6%; at greater than 12 months, four study arms (Battista et al, 2012; Davis et al, 2010; Imai et al, 2011) reported decreases from baseline in HbA1c ranging from 0.6% to 1.8%. %. In all 21 study arms, a minimum of three encounters with the RDN occurred during the first 6 months (range: 3 to 11); length of time for the total encounters ranged from 2 to 16 hours. Encounters with the RDN during the next 6 months ranged from two to six (Andrews et al, 2011; Battista et al, 2012; Davis et al, 2010; Imai et al, 2011; Laitinen et al, 1993; Takahashi et al, 2004; Wolf et al, 2004; UKPDS 1990); four to 12 additional encounters occurred in longer studies (Battista et al, 2012; Davis et al, 2010; Imai et al, 2011; UKPDS 2000). The largest decreases in HbA1c were in studies in which type 2 diabetes was newly diagnosed (Franz et al, 1995; Laitinen et al, 1993; UKPDS 1990), in which HbA1c levels decreased by 1.8% to 2.0%, and in studies in which HbA1c levels were over 8.0%, where decreases in HbA1c ranged from 0.5% to 2.0%. A variety of nutrition interventions such as individualized nutrition therapy, energy restriction, portion control, sample menus, carbohydrate counting, exchange lists, simple meal plan, and low-fat vegan diet were implemented and effective. All resulted in a reduced energy intake.

Hemoglobin A1c and Type 1 Diabetes

In persons with type 1 diabetes, three study arms (N=808) from three randomized controlled trials, (N=2,735; DAFNE 2002; DCCT 1993; Laurenzi et al, 2011) reported on the effectiveness of MNT provided by RDNs on HbA1c. In all studies, a series of MNT encounters with the RDN were provided (four to six during the first 6 months and monthly encounters with the RDN occurred throughout the DCCT study). At 6 months, two studies (DAFNE 2002; DCCT 1993) reported that individualized MNT using carbohydrate counting to determine premeal insulin doses and provided by RDNs assisted in decreasing baseline mean HbA1c levels of 9.4±1.2% and 8.8±1.2% to 8.4±1.2% and 6.9%, decreases of 1.0% and 1.9%, respectively. At 12 months, three studies (DAFNE 2002; DCCT 1993; Laurenzi et al, 2011) reported decreases in HbA1c ranging from 0.4% to 1.9%. In the large Diabetes Control and Complications Trial (DCCT 1993), ongoing monthly MNT support provided by RDNs assisted in maintaining the mean HbA1c level at 6.9% throughout the 6.5 years of the trial.

Glucose Levels and Type 1 and Type 2 Diabetes

In adults with type 2 diabetes, eight studies (Al-Shookri et al, 2012; Barnard et al, 2006; Coppell et al, 2010; Franz et al, 1995; Goldhaber-Fiebert et al, 2003; Laitinen et al, 1993; Lemon et al, 2004; UKPDS 1990) reported that MNT provided by RDNs decreased fasting blood glucose (baseline, 137 mg/dL to 223 mg/dL), ranging from 18 mg/dL to 61 mg/dL at 3 months, from 16 mg/dL to 56 mg/dL at 6 months, and with ongoing MNT support from 25 mg/dL to 60 mg/dL at 12 months. In persons with type 1 diabetes, the Diabetes Control and Complications Trial (DCCT 1993) reported the baseline mean fasting blood glucose levels of 230 mg/dL were decreased to a mean of 155 mg/dL (-75 mg/dL) and with ongoing MNT support were maintained throughout the 6.5 years of the study.

Figure 10.5 Sample evidence summary

Adapted with permission from Academy of Nutrition and Dietetics. Evidence Analysis Library. Diabetes Type 1 and Type 2. www.andeal.org/topic.cfm?menu =5305&pcat=5491&cat=5161. Accessed May 21, 2018.[14]

In adults with type 1 and type 2 diabetes, how effective is medical nutrition therapy provided by a registered dietitian nutritionist on glycemia (Hemoglobin A1c or glucose)?

In adults with type 2 diabetes, 21 study arms from 18 studies reported that medical nutrition therapy (MNT) provided by registered dietitian nutritionists (RDNs) significantly lowered hemoglobin A1c (HbA1c) levels. At 3 months, HbA1c levels decreased by 0.3% to 2.0% and with ongoing MNT support decreases in HbA1c levels were maintained or improved for more than 12 months. An initial series of RDN encounters (three to 11; a total of 2 to 16 hours) with continued RDN encounters throughout the studies were reported. Although nutrition therapy interventions were effective throughout disease duration, the decrease in HbA1c was largest in studies in which participants were newly diagnosed or had higher baseline HbA1c levels. RDNs implemented a variety of nutrition therapy interventions, all resulting in a reduced energy intake.

In adults with type 1 diabetes, three studies reported that MNT provided by RDNs contributed to significantly decreased HbA1c levels. At 6 months, HbA1c levels decreased by 1.0% to 1.9%. An initial series of RDN encounters (four to six) were reported. Ongoing MNT support resulted in maintenance of the reduced HbA1c levels at 1 year and in the Diabetes Control and Complications Trial (DCCT) throughout the 6.5 years of the trial.

In adults with type 1 and type 2 diabetes, nine studies reported that MNT provided by RDNs decreased fasting blood glucose levels at 3 months by 18 mg/dL to 61 mg/dL. With ongoing MNT support, decreased levels were maintained to 12 months and in the DCCT throughout the 6.5 years of the trial.

Grade I

Grade Levels: I, good/strong; II, fair; III, limited/weak; IV, expert opinion only; and V, grade not assignable.

Figure 10.6 Sample conclusion statement

MNT = medical nutrition therapy; RDN/RD = registered dietitian nutritionist/registered dietitian; HbA1c = hemoglobin A1c

Adapted with permission from Academy of Nutrition and Dietetics. Evidence Analysis Library. Diabetes Type 1 and Type 2. www.andeal.org/topic.cfm?menu =5305&pcat=5491&cat=5161Accessed May 21, 2018.[14]

Strength of evidence elements	Grade				
	I Good/strong	II Fair	III Limited/weak	IV Expert opinion only	V Grade not assignable
Quality Scientific rigor/validity Considers design and execution	Studies of strong design for question Free from design flaws, bias, and execution problems	Studies of strong design for question with minor methodologic concerns OR Only studies of weaker study design for question	Studies of weak design for answering the question OR Inconclusive findings due to design flaws, bias, or execution problems	No studies available Conclusion based on usual practice, expert consensus, clinical experience, opinion, or extrapolation from basic research	No evidence that pertains to question being addressed
Consistency Findings across studies	Findings generally consistent in direction and size of effect or degree of association, and statistical significance with minor exceptions at most	Inconsistency among results of studies with strong design OR Consistency with minor exceptions across studies of weaker design	Unexplained inconsistency among results from different studies OR Single study unconfirmed by other studies	Conclusion supported solely by statements of informed nutrition or medical commentators	Not available
Quantity Number of studies Number of subjects in studies	One to several good-quality studies Large number of subjects studied Studies with negative results have sufficiently large sample size for adequate statistical power	Several studies by independent investigators Doubts about adequacy of sample size to avoid type I and type II error	Limited number of studies Low number of subjects studied and/or inadequate sample size within studies	Unsubstantiated by published research studies	Relevant studies have not been done
Clinical impact Importance of studied outcomes Magnitude or effect	Studied outcome relates directly to the question Size of effect is clinically meaningful Significant (statistical) difference is large	Some doubt about the statistical or clinical significance of the effect	Studied outcome is an intermediate outcome or surrogate for the true outcome of interest OR Size of effect is small or lacks statistical and/or clinical significance	Objective data unavailable	Indicates area for future research
Generalizability to population or interest	Studied population, intervention, and outcomes are free from serious doubts about generalizability	Minor doubts about generalizability	Serious doubts about generalizability due to narrow or different study population, intervention, or outcomes studied	Generalizability limited to scope of experience	Not available

Figure 10.7 Criteria and definitions for grading the strength of the evidence for an Evidence Analysis Library conclusion statement[3]

reviews. Most other organizations conducting systematic reviews do not write or grade a conclusion. Organizations involved in developing guidelines do grade the quality and strength of evidence but use other systems to determine the level of evidence.

Evidence-Based Practice Guidelines

EBP guidelines are primary resources dietetics practitioners use to guide decision-making. According to the Institute of Medicine (IOM), "Clinical practice guidelines are statements that include recommendations intended to optimize patient care that are informed by a systematic review of evidence and an assessment of the benefits and harms of alternative care options."[27] Clinical practice guidelines take systematic reviews a few steps further by critically appraising the body of evidence, assessing potential benefits and harms, and providing clear statements relevant to patient care. EBP guidelines, have the potential to standardize practice, translate research into practice, and improve patient outcomes.[27]

Several organizations have developed standards for guideline development, including, but not limited to, the World Health Organization,[28] National Institute for Health and Clinical Excellence,[29] Scottish Intercollegiate Guidelines Network (SIGN),[30] National Health and Medical Research Council,[31] the IOM,[27] and Guideline International Network.[32] In general, most organizations recommend the same basic principles when developing a clinical practice guideline, including a diverse guideline development group with patient and public involvement, management of conflict of interest, transparency, use of systematic reviews, clear recommendations, external review, and a rating system to demonstrate strength and quality.[27,32]

The Academy of Nutrition and Dietetics EAL publishes stand-alone systematic reviews and systematic reviews that inform clinical practice guidelines. Whether or not a systematic review will be used to inform a guideline is predetermined in the scope of the project. EAL conclusion statements reflect what the evidence says, and recommendations guide what to do with the evidence. The EAL is unique in that conclusion statements and their grading are used to draft recommendations. Several organizations, such as the World Health Organization, use Grading of Recommendations, Assessment, Development and Evaluation (GRADE)[33] to draft recommendations. GRADE is described as a transparent and sensible approach to grading the quality of evidence and strength of recommendations.[34] In addition to evidence quality, potential harms and benefits, costs, and patient preferences are taken into consideration. EAL recommendations are written in two separate statements. The first states what the practitioner should do, and the second states why (see Figure 10.8 for a sample recommendation statement).[35] After researchers come

to a consensus on a recommendation, the Academy of Nutrition and Dietetics rates the recommendations using its Rating Scheme for the Strength of the Recommendation (Figure 10.9).[4] After rating, the Academy of Nutrition and Dietetics classifies recommendations as either *imperative* (applies to all of the guideline population) or *conditional* (applies only to certain circumstances). There are several guideline development organizations, many of which use different rating schemes, including, but not limited to, GRADE (strong, weak),[36] Centre for Evidence-Based Medicine (A through D),[20] US Preventive Services Task Force (A through D, and I = Insufficient),[37] and SIGN (A through D).[30] A comprehensive list of systems used for rating recommendations can be found in *Clinical Practice Guidelines We Can Trust* published by the IOM.[27]

Once complete, a group of recruited individuals with interest or knowledge in the topic area makes a guideline available for external review. All reviewers complete the Appraisal for Guidelines Research Evaluation (AGREE II) survey, which is a valid, reliable, and internationally used survey to assess the quality and reporting of guidelines.[38] Survey results are shared with the expert panel for final revisions.

Dissemination

The methodology and results of a systematic review can be disseminated in a variety of ways, including

---

Recommendation:

Diabetes Mellitus: Initial Series of Medical Nutrition Therapy Encounters

The registered dietitian nutritionist (RDN) should implement three to six medical nutrition therapy (MNT) encounters during the first 6 months, and determine if additional MNT encounters are needed. In studies reporting on the implementation of an initial series of RDN encounters (three to 11; total of 2 to 16 hours), MNT significantly lowered Hemoglobin A1c by 0.3% to 2.0% in adults with type 2 diabetes and by 1.0% to 1.9% in adults with type 1 diabetes during the first 6 months, as well as optimization of medication therapy and improved quality of life.

Rating: Strong
Imperative

Diabetes Mellitus: Medical Nutrition Therapy Follow-Up Encounters

The registered dietitian nutritionist (RDN) should implement a minimum of one annual medical nutrition therapy (MNT) follow-up encounter. Studies longer than 6 months report that continued MNT encounters resulted in maintenance and continued reductions of Hemoglobin A1C for up to 2 years in adults with type 2 diabetes and for up to 6.5 years in adults with type 1 diabetes.

Rating: Strong
Imperative

Figure 10.8 Sample recommendation statement

Adapted with permission from Academy of Nutrition and Dietetics, Evidence Analysis Library. Diabetes Type 1 and Type 2. www.andeal.org/template.cfm?template =guide_summary&key=4494. Accessed May 23, 2018.[35]

Strong

A **Strong** recommendation means the work group believes the benefits of the recommended approach clearly exceed the harms (or the harms clearly exceed the benefits in the case of a strong negative recommendation) and the quality of the supporting evidence is excellent/good (grade I or II). In some clearly identified circumstances, strong recommendations may be made based on lesser evidence when high-quality evidence is impossible to obtain and the anticipated benefits strongly outweigh the harms.

Practitioners should follow a **Strong** recommendation unless a clear and compelling rationale for an alternative approach is present.

Fair

A **Fair** recommendation means the work group believes the benefits exceed the harms (or the harms clearly exceed the benefits in the case of a negative recommendation), but the quality of evidence is not as strong (grade II or III). In some clearly identified circumstances, recommendations may be made based on lesser evidence when high-quality evidence is impossible to obtain and the anticipated benefits outweigh the harms.

Practitioners should generally follow a **Fair** recommendation but remain alert to new information and be sensitive to patient preferences.

Weak

A **Weak** recommendation means the quality of existing evidence is suspect or well-done studies (grade I, II, or III) show little clear advantage to one approach vs another.

Practitioners should be cautious in deciding whether to follow a recommendation classified as **Weak**, and should exercise judgment and be alert to emerging publications that report evidence. Patient preference should have a substantial influencing role.

Consensus

A **Consensus** recommendation means expert opinion (grade IV) supports the guideline recommendation even though the available scientific evidence did not present consistent results or controlled trials were lacking.

Practitioners should be flexible in deciding whether to follow a recommendation classified as **Consensus**, although they may set boundaries on alternatives. Patient preference should have a substantial influencing role.

Insufficient Evidence

An **Insufficient Evidence** recommendation means there is a lack of pertinent evidence (grade V) and/or an unclear balance between benefits and harms.

Practitioners should feel little constraint in deciding whether to follow a recommendation labeled as **Insufficient Evidence** and should exercise judgment and be alert to emerging publications that report evidence clarifying the balance of benefit vs harm. Patient preference should have a substantial influencing role.

Figure 10.9 Rating scheme for the strength of the recommendations, Academy of Nutrition and Dietetics[4]
See Figure 10.7 for definitions of grades.

peer-reviewed publications, online platforms, technical reports, professional presentations, and continuing education materials.

Results of EAL systematic reviews including evidence summary tables, narrative evidence summaries, conclusion statements and grading, and research protocol are the essential components for dissemination resources. An evidence-based guideline is usually presented in the publication produced by the same agency that developed the guideline. Academy guidelines are published on the EAL and published in the *Journal of the Academy of Nutrition and Dietetics*. Evidence tables may be included as attachments or included as online-only appendixes for published journal articles. For examples of guidelines, see the EAL website (www.andeal.org). The value of this work requires dissemination to users, including practitioners, researchers, and policy makers, so that findings can be incorporated into practice and lead to more effective and higher-quality care.

To achieve consistency in the reporting quality of systematic reviews, in 2005 the Quality of Reports of Meta-Analyses of Randomized Controlled Trials (QUOROM) was revised and expanded to meet the advances in systematic review methodology and renamed Preferred Reporting Items for Systematic Reviews and Meta-Analysis (PRISMA).[19] The PRISMA checklist and flow diagram are designed to help authors improve the reporting of systematic reviews and meta-analyses. Most journals recommend that authors use these documents to guide their systematic reports. In addition, there are some companion standards that suggest common evaluation criteria for studies: Consolidated Standards of Reporting Trials (CONSORT),[39] Strengthening the Reporting of Observational Studies in Epidemiology (STROBE),[40] Meta-Analysis of Observational Studies in Epidemiology (MOOSE),[41] and Standards for the Reporting of Diagnostic Accuracy Studies (STARD).[42]

STRENGTHS AND LIMITATIONS OF SYSTEMATIC REVIEWS AND EVIDENCE-BASED PRACTICE GUIDELINES

EBP, grounded in systematic reviews and consequent guidelines, is an ever-evolving process and,

like any research process, contains strengths and limitations. The systematic review process takes into consideration both the breadth and depth of available evidence. Systematic reviews enable an objective assessment of the quality and strength of available evidence, which enables development and rating of recommendations, when appropriate. It is an efficient and objective way to review best available evidence on a research topic. Another strength of systematic reviews is the transparency of each step of the process; each step is documented and reported. Also, when uncertainties are formulated into answerable questions, available data can be gathered and graded. When the level of evidence or the grade is low (III to V), additional research is warranted. The identification of unanswered problems and uncertainties can stimulate research to fill gaps in important areas. The Academy of Nutrition and Dietetics EAL provides a search function that clearly identifies all questions where uncertainties exist, those that are graded III, IV, and V.[13]

Stand-alone systematic reviews and systematic reviews used to support EBP guidelines are subject to many of the same limitations as other types of research, including publication bias, timeliness of data publication, and methodologic issues. Several limitations of systematic reviews are of particular concern: amount of time and resources required to complete a thorough evidence review, skills to conduct the search and evidence review, availability of relevant research, and applicability of randomized controlled trial results to routine clinical settings.[1,28] The methods by which researchers and analysts are involved in completing the work of a systematic review are extremely important in ensuring that the final results are valid and reproducible. Most groups that undertake a systematic review have a multidisciplinary composition with various roles to ensure that the work completed is objective and that the process has checks and balances. For example, Box 10.2 describes the various groups and roles for the process used by the Academy of Nutrition and Dietetics.

EBP guidelines bridge the gap between research and practice and promote standardization of effective practice.[4] The quality of health care improves as practitioners make decisions that are supported by empirical data and recognize where

Personnel Involved in Academy Evidence Analysis	Tasks Performed
Council on Research	Priortize topics with input from Academy members and stakeholders
	Appoint Evidence Analysis Library Workgroup members
Scientific Affairs and Research Staff	Manage evidence analysis process, work assignments, and timeline
	Provide evidence analysis training
	Publish in the Evidence Analysis Library
	Provide methodologic expertise in conducting systematic reviews and guideline development
Evidence Analysis Project Managers	Manage workflow in an individual project using Evidence Analysis Library software
	Coordinate and facilitate teleconferences to accomplish work
	Ensure that work is consistent with formatting and process requirements
Evidence Analysis Work Groups	Identify subtopics and develop research questions
	Review and approve search strategy, inclusion and exclusion criteria, sort lists, evidence summaries, evidence summary tables, conclusion statements, and recommendations
	Reach consensus on grade for conclusion statements and rating for recommendations
	Review and incorporate changes suggested by review process (from the Evidence-Based Practice Committee and reviewers)
Lead Analysts	Create proposed search strategy, search terms, inclusion and exclusion criteria
	Create sort lists from search results
	Prepare list of articles included and excluded and reason for exclusion
	Assign articles to analysts
	Review all work completed by analysts
	Perform a second quality rating for each research article
	Draft evidence summary, evidence summary tables, conclusion statements, and recommendations
	Propose grading for conclusion statements and rating for recommendations
	Review all work completed by individual analysts
	Mentor evidence analysts as they complete their work

Box 10.2 Roles in Academy of Nutrition and Dietetics Evidence Analysis   (*continued*)

Evidence Analysts	Complete data extraction from articles
	Complete quality rating for each research article
	Propose content of evidence summary tables
	Work with Lead Analyst to complete evidence summary documents
Librarians	Complete literature searches
	Document searches
	Provide training
	Serve as consultant to lead analysts
Editors	Edit documents to meet editorial style before publication on Evidence Analysis Library

Box 10.2 (cont.) Roles in Academy of Nutrition and Dietetics Evidence Analysis

uncertainties exist. Review of the evidence; consideration of potential harms, benefits, and costs; and stakeholder input are brought together to form clear and concise recommendations that aid practitioner decision-making. High-quality guidelines are developed using a systematic and transparent process applied by a multidisciplinary work group, thereby limiting bias.

Strong systematic reviews are essential for high quality EBP guidelines. The aforementioned limitations in systematic reviews—lack of transparency, lack of diversity in the work group, and unmanaged conflict of interest—are common downfalls of EBP guidelines. Numerous organizations from several countries are developing evidence-based guidelines. For example, the International Guidelines Library (www.g-i-n.net/library/international-guidelines-library/international-guidelines-library) has more than 6,300 guidelines from 96 organizations and 82 countries; however, lack of reconciliation between conflicting guidelines is another limitation, as it adds confusion for practitioners attempting to implement EBP.[27] Reviews, recommendations, and guidelines developed from these reviews can become obsolete as new research becomes available and new procedures and therapies are introduced. In most areas of dietetics practice, updates of reviews should be considered in at least 2-year intervals.

FUTURE RESEARCH

Questions for future research include comparing the various methodologies for determining quality of research articles, determining the best way to document the process to ensure reliability and validity of the findings, and determining the desirability and impact of automated evidence-based decision guides for practitioner implementation in daily practice.

Rigorous systematic reviews are still considered more trustworthy than other research designs. High-quality systematic reviews help provide high-quality evidence to help clinicians make practice-based decisions. Conducting high-quality systematic reviews requires adhering to gold standard methods, which can be very time consuming.[43] To tackle this issue of timeliness and to meet the demands of stakeholders, many organizations or independent researchers are discussing the possibility of conducting rapid systematic reviews. To date, there is no one standardized method to conduct rapid systematic reviews, and it is unclear whether they can replace in-depth systematic reviews.[44] The Academy of Nutrition and Dietetics conducts large systematic reviews with multiple questions, and this results in longer time to completion and publication. To tackle this, the Academy of Nutrition and Dietetics is evaluating the benefit of developing focused systematic reviews to address hot topics in the field (a rapid systematic review).

Another technique that can help manage the time issue is evidence mapping (or scoping review). Evidence mapping on topics included in previous guidelines or projects helps scan the landscape of the literature in broad topic areas and helps identify gaps in the literature. Experts recommend updating systematic reviews every 2 years, and updates require time and effort. Using the approach of scoping or evidence mapping helps to prioritize topics/areas where a sufficient update of evidence is available.

RESOURCES FOR DEVELOPING SYSTEMATIC REVIEWS AND EVIDENCE-BASED PRACTICE GUIDELINES

Numerous organizations provide resources for developing systematic reviews and guidelines (see Box 10.3).

CONCLUSION

Systematic reviews are a comprehensive synthesis of the best and most relevant available literature to answer research questions. Systematic reviews are the backbone of EBP guidelines. Systematic reviews identify the evidence and EBP guidelines help prac-

---

Resources for Developing Systematic Reviews

General Resources on Systematic Review Process and Methodology

Academy of Nutrition and Dietetics Evidence Analysis Manual (www.andeal.org/evidence-analysis-manual)

Academy of Nutrition and Dietetics Methodology for Conducting Systematic Reviews for the Evidence Analysis Library[4]

Agency for Healthcare Research and Quality (AHRQ) series paper 3: identifying, selecting, and refining topics for comparative effectiveness systematic reviews: AHRQ and the effective health-care program[45]

Cochrane Handbook for Systematic Reviews of Interventions[8]

Centers for Disease Control and Prevention: The Community Guide (www.thecommunityguide.org)

Finding What Works in Health Care: Standards for Systematic Reviews[9]

HuGENet™ Handbook of Systematic Reviews[46]

Methodological standards for the conduct of new Cochrane Intervention Reviews[47]

Centre for Reviews and Dissemination (CRD). *Systematic Reviews: CRD's Guidance for Undertaking Reviews in Health Care*[48]

Systematic reviews and meta-analyses: an illustrated, step-by-step guide[49]

The Campbell Collaboration (https://campbell collaboration.org)

The Joanna Briggs Institute (http://joannabriggs.org)

Quality Evaluation Tools

A Measurement Tool to Assess Systematic Reviews (AMSTAR) (https://amstar.ca/Amstar_Checklist.php)[4]

Academy of Nutrition and Dietetics' Quality Criteria Checklist (www.andeal.org/evidence-analysis-manual)

AHRQ series paper 5: grading the strength of a body of evidence when comparing medical interventions— Agency for Healthcare Research and Quality and the effective health-care program[50]

Box 10.3 Resources for Systematic Reviews and Guideline Development *(continued)*

Newcastle-Ottawa Scale (NOS) for Assessing the Quality of Nonrandomized Studies in Meta-Analysis[23]

QUADAS-2: a revised tool for the quality assessment of diagnostic accuracy studies[51]

Guides for Reporting Systematic Reviews

Consolidated Standards of Reporting Trials (CONSORT) (www.consort-statement.org)

Meta-analysis of Observational Studies in Epidemiology (MOOSE)[41]

Preferred Reporting Items for Systematic Reviews and Meta-Analyses (PRISMA) (http://prisma-statement.org)

Standards for the Reporting of Diagnostic Accuracy Studies (STARD)[42]

Strengthening the Reporting of Observational Studies in Epidemiology (STROBE) (www.strobe-statement.org/index.php?id=strobe-home)

Resources for Evidence-Based Practice Guidelines

Academy of Nutrition and Dietetics Evidence Analysis Manual (www.andeal.org/evidence-analysis-manual)

Clinical Practice Guidelines We Can Trust[27]

Developing NICE Guidelines: The Manual[29]

Guidelines International Network: toward international standards for clinical practice guidelines[32]

World Health Organization *Handbook for Guideline Development*[28]

SIGN 50: A Guideline Developers Handbook[30]

Procedures and requirements for meeting the 2011 National Health and Medical Research Council standard for clinical practice guidelines[31]

Tools for Guideline Development and Assessment

GRADEpro GDT (https://gradepro.org)

AGREE II (www.agreetrust.org)

Guideline Registries

International Guideline Library (www.g-i-n.net/library/international-guidelines-library/international-guidelines-library)

Australian Clinical Practice Guidelines (www.clinicalguidelines.gov.au)

Box 10.3 (cont.) Resources for Systematic Reviews and Guideline Development

titioners implement evidence into their daily practice. However, practitioners must exercise clinical decision-making skills to determine if and how these guidelines apply to individual clients or patients.

REFERENCES

1. Sackett D, Straus, SE, Richardson, WS, Rosenberg, W, Haynes RB. *Evidence-Based Medicine: How to Practice and Teach EBM*. St Louis, MO: Churchill Livingstone; 2000.

2. Academy of Nutrition and Dietetics. Definition of Terms List. www.eatrightpro.org/-/media/eatrightpro-files/practice/scope-standards-of-practice/academy definitionoftermslist.pdf . Accessed May 22, 2018.

3. Handu D, Moloney L, Wolfram T, Ziegler P, Acosta A, Steiber A. Academy of Nutrition and Dietetics methodology for conducting systematic reviews for the evidence analysis library. *J Acad Nutr Diet*. 2016;116(2):311-318.

4. Papoutsakis C, Moloney L, Sinley RC, Acosta A, Handu D, Steiber AL. Academy of Nutrition and Dietetics methodology for developing evidence-based nutrition practice guidelines. *J Acad Nutr Diet.* 2017;117(5): 794-804.

5. Cochrane Library. About Cochrane Reviews. www.cochranelibrary.com/about/about-cochrane -systematic-reviews.html. Accessed May 22, 2018.

6. Klassen TP, Jadad AR, Moher D. Guides for reading and interpreting systematic reviews: I. Getting started. *Arch Pediatr Adolesc Med.* 1998;152(7):700-704.

7. Evidence Based Medicine Toolkit. www.ebm.med.ualberta .ca/EbmIntro.html. Updated 2008. Accessed May 22, 2018.

8. Higgins J, Green S, eds. *Cochrane Handbook for Systematic Reviews of Interventions.* Version 5.1.0. The Cochrane Collaboration. http://handbook.cochrane.org. Updated March 2011. Accessed May 22, 2018.

9. Institute of Medicine. *Finding What Works in Health Care: Standards for Systematic Reviews.* Washington, DC: The National Academies Press; 2011.

10. Craig JC, Irwig LM, Stockler MR. Evidence-based medicine: useful tools for decision making. *Med J Aust.* 2001;174(5):248-253.

11. Academy of Nutrition and Dietetics. Nutrition Terminology Reference Manual (eNCPT): Dietetics Language for Nutrition Care. https://ncpt.webauthor.com. Accessed March 1, 2017.

12. Academy of Nutrition and Dietetics. Academy of Nutrition and Dietetics Evidence Analysis Manual: Steps in the Academy Evidence Analysis Process. www.andeal .org/evidence-analysis-manual. Published 2016. Accessed May 24, 2018.

13. Davies K. Formulating the evidence based practice question: a review of the frameworks. *Evid Based Libr Inf Pract.* 2011;6(2):75-80.

14. Academy of Nutrition and Dietetics. Diabetes Type 1 and 2 Systematic Review (2013–2015): Medical Nutrition Therapy (2015). www.andeal.org/topic.cfm?cat=5161&pcat =5491&menu=5305. Accessed May 22, 2018.

15. Althuis MD, Weed DL. Evidence mapping: methodologic foundations and application to intervention and observational research on sugar-sweetened beverages and health outcomes. *Am J Clin Nutr.* 2013;98(3):755-768.

16. Arksey H, O'Malley, L. Scoping studies: towards a methodological framework. *Int J Soc Res Methodol.* 2005;8(1):19-32.

17. Levac D, Colquhoun H, O'Brien KK. Scoping studies: advancing the methodology. *Implement Sci.* 2010;5:69.

18. Cooper MJ, Zlotkin SH. An evidence-based approach to the development of national dietary guidelines. *J Am Diet Assoc.* 2003;103(12 suppl 2):S28-S33.

19. Moher D, Liberati A, Tetzlaff J, Altman DG; PRISMA Group. Preferred reporting items for systematic reviews and meta-analyses: the PRISMA statement. *BMJ.* 2009;339:b2535.

20. Centre for Evidence-Based Medicine. Levels of Evidence. www.cebm.net/category/ebm-resources/loe. Accessed March 7, 2017.

21. West S, King V, Carey TS, et al. *Systems to Rate the Strength of Scientific Evidence*: AHRQ Evidence Report Summaries. No. 47. Rockville, MD: Agency for Healthcare Research and Quality; 2002. AHRQ Publication No. 02-E015.

22. Jadad AR, Moore RA, Carroll D, et al. Assessing the quality of reports of randomized clinical trials: is blinding necessary? *Control Clin Trials.* 1996;17(1):1-12.

23. Wells G, Shea B, O'Connell D, et al. The Newcastle-Ottawa Scale (NOS) for assessing the quality of nonrandomised studies in meta-analyses. www.ohri.ca/programs/clinical _epidemiology/oxford.asp. Accessed May 23, 2018.

24. Berkman ND, Lohr KN, Ansari M, et al. Grading the strength of a body of evidence when assessing health care interventions for the effective health care program of the Agency for Healthcare Research and Quality: an update. In: *Methods Guide for Effectiveness and Comparative Effectiveness Reviews.* Rockville, MD: Agency for Healthcare Research and Quality; 2013.

25. Shea BJ, Reeves BC, Wells G, et al. AMSTAR 2: a critical appraisal tool for systematic reviews that include randomised or non-randomised studies of healthcare interventions, or both. *BMJ.* 2017;358:j4008.

26. Langendam MW, Aki EA, Dahm P, Glasziou P, Guyatt G, Schunemann HJ. Assessing and presenting summaries of evidence in Cochrane Reviews. *Syst Rev.* 2013;2(1):81.

27. Institute of Medicine. *Clinical Practice Guidelines We Can Trust.* Washington, DC: The National Academies Press; 2011.

28. World Health Organization. *WHO Handbook for Guideline Development.* 2nd ed. Geneva, Swtizerland: WHO Press; 2014.

29. National Institute for Health and CareExcellence (NICE). *Developing NICE Guidelines: The Manual.* www.nice.org.uk /process/pmg20/chapter/about-this-manual. Published October 2014. Accessed March 10, 2017.

30. Scottish Intercollegiate Guidelines Network. *SIGN 50: A Guideline Developer's Handbook.* Edinburgh: Scottish Intercollegiate Guidelines Network; 2015.

31. National Health and Medical Research Council. Procedures and requirements for meeting the 2011 NHMRC standard for clinical practice guidelines. Version 1.1. www.nhmrc.gov.au/_files_nhmrc/publications /attachments/cp133_nhmrc_procedures_requirements _guidelines_v1.1_120125.pdf. Published May 2011. Accessed May 24, 2018.

32. Qaseem A, Forland F, Macbeth F, Ollenschlager G, Phillips S, van der Wees P; Board of Trustees of the Guidelines International Network. Guidelines International Network: toward international standards for clinical practice guidelines. *Ann Intern Med.* 2012;156(7):525-531.

33. Guyatt GH, Thorlund K, Oxman AD, et al. GRADE guidelines: 13. Preparing summary of findings tables and evidence profiles—continuous outcomes. *J Clin Epidemiol.* 2013;66(2):173-183.

34. Agency for Healthcare Research and Quality. National Guideline Clearinghouse. www.guideline.gov/. Accessed March 1, 2017.

35. Academy of Nutrition and Dietetics. Evidence Analysis Library Diabetes Type 1 and 2 Guideline: Medical Nutrition Therapy Recommendations Summary. 2015; www.andeal.org/template.cfm?template=guide _summary&key=4494. Accessed May 23, 2018.

36. Guyatt GH, Oxman AD, Vist GE, et al. GRADE: an emerging consensus on rating quality of evidence and strength of recommendations. *BMJ.* 2008;336(7650): 924-926.

37. US Preventive Services Task Force. Grade definitions. www.uspreventiveservicestaskforce.org/Page/Name /grade-definitions. Accessed May 23, 2018.

38. Brouwers MC, Kho ME, Browman GP, et al. AGREE II: advancing guideline development, reporting, and evaluation in health care. *Prev Med.* 2010;51(5):421-424.

39. Begg C, Cho M, Eastwood S, et al. Improving the quality of reporting of randomized controlled trials. The CONSORT statement. *JAMA.* 1996;276(8):637-639.

40. von Elm E, Altman DG, Egger M, Pocock SJ, Gotzsche PC, Vandenbroucke JP; STROBE Initiative. The Strengthening the Reporting of Observational Studies in Epidemiology (STROBE) statement: guidelines for reporting observational studies. *Lancet.* 2007;370(9596): 1453-1457.

41. Stroup DF, Berlin JA, Morton SC, et al. Meta-analysis of observational studies in epidemiology: a proposal for reporting. Meta-analysis of Observational Studies in Epidemiology (MOOSE) group. *JAMA.* 2000;283(15): 2008-2012.

42. Bossuyt PM, Reitsma JB, Bruns DE, et al; Standards for Reporting of Diagnostic Accuracy. Towards complete and accurate reporting of studies of diagnostic accuracy:the STARD Initiative. *Ann Intern Med.* 2003;138(1):40-44.

43. Schünemann HJ, Moja L. Reviews: Rapid! Rapid! Rapid! . . . and systematic. *Syst Rev.* 2015;4(1):4.

44. Ganann R, Ciliska D, Thomas H. Expediting systematic reviews: methods and implications of rapid reviews. *Implement Sci.* 2010;5(1):56.

45. Whitlock EP, Lopez SA, Chang S, Helfand M, Eder M, Floyd N. AHRQ series paper 3: identifying, selecting, and refining topics for comparative effectiveness systematic reviews: AHRQ and the effective health-care program. *J Clin Epidemiol.* 2010;63(5):491-501.

46. Little J, Higgins JPT. The HuGENet™ HuGE Review Handbook, version 1.0. 2006. www.cdc.gov/genomics /hugenet/participate.htm. Accessed May 24, 2018.

47. Higgins JPT, Lasserson T, Chandler J, Tovey D, Churchill R. Methodological Expectations of Cochrane Intervention Reviews (MECIR). Version 1.05. http://community .cochrane.org/mecir-manual. Updated January 2018. Accessed May 24, 2018.

48. Centre for Reviews and Dissemination (CRD). *Systematic Reviews: CRD's Guidance for Undertaking Reviews in Health Care.* York, United Kingdom: York Publishing Services; 2009.

49. Pai M, McCulloch M, Gorman JD, et al. Systematic reviews and meta-analyses: an illustrated, step-by-step guide. *Natl Med J India.* 2004;17(2):86-95.

50. Owens DK, Lohr KN, Atkins D, et al. AHRQ series paper 5: grading the strength of a body of evidence when comparing medical interventions—Agency for Healthcare Research and Quality and the effective health-care program. *J Clin Epidemiol.* 2010;63(5):513-523.

51. Whiting PF, Rutjes AW, Westwood ME, et al; QUADAS-2 Group. QUADAS-2: a revised tool for the quality assessment of diagnostic accuracy studies. *Ann Intern Med.* 2011;155(8):529-536.

Chapter 11

Bridging Disciplinary Boundaries

Madeleine Sigman-Grant, PhD, RD | *Sharon M. Donovan, PhD, RD*

LEARNING OBJECTIVES

1. Define interdisciplinary, multidisciplinary, and transdisciplinary research.

2. Describe the benefits and challenges of engaging in multidisciplinary research.

3. Describe the personal characteristics that contribute to an individual's ability to work effectively in a multidisciplinary research team.

Multidisciplinary research is best described by the old parable of the blind men and the elephant (see Figure 11.1 on page 218). Six men were led to different parts of an elephant. When asked, "What sort of a thing is an elephant?" they each provided a different answer. The one touching a leg said an elephant is a pillar, the one who touched the ear believed an elephant is a fan, the one who touched the tail was certain an elephant is a rope, and so on. The men argued vehemently about how to truly describe an elephant. In reality, they were each correct from their unique perspective, yet they were each incorrect because they only had one perspective. This tale has two morals: (1) it is only when all the pieces are put together that the complete picture can be revealed; and (2) it is important to be tolerant and accept other viewpoints in order to see the truth.

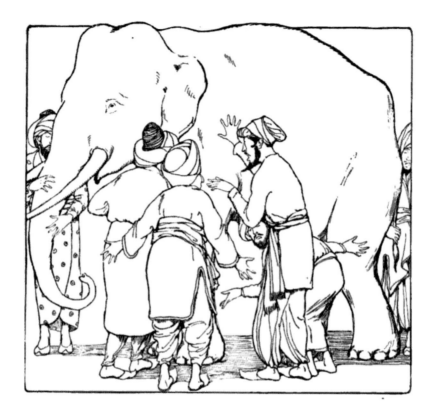

Figure 11.1 Illustration of the parable of the six blind men and the elephant

Reproduced from Martha Adelaide Holton & Charles Madison Curry, Holton-Curry readers, Rand McNally & Co. (Chicago), p. 108.

In a similar manner, one can ask, "What is nutrition research?" Some might respond that it examines how nutrients affect gene expression (biological and physiological research); others might say it describes what individuals eat and why they make their choices (behavioral and psychological research); others might indicate that it is about communication (humanities and consumer research); another might reply that it is about measuring the effect of food placement on supermarket shelves (environmental research); and still others might describe how taxing unhealthy food products affects sales (economic research). Each response is correct but is limited in perspective. However, as science becomes more specialized, it is easy to lose sight of the larger picture. Consider, for example, the translation of new information. A biological researcher might determine that consumers should eat more of a particular nutrient, a behavioral psychologist might track how

consumers respond to this new information, an economist might consider the financial impact of choosing a food containing the nutrient, and an agriculturalist might consider how growing that food affects the environment. When each discipline follows its own separate path without integrating findings, the result is a disjointed attempt at presenting a cohesive and coherent picture.

The complex interrelationships between an individual and his or her environment demand searching for answers in different ways and from different perspectives. Biomedical scientists working alongside social scientists can form teams from different disciplines to extend knowledge, promote innovation, and provide a holistic view of truth. These teams are essential to finding solutions to critical problems and can help bridge the gap between research and practice. Such teams allow researchers increased awareness of the social, moral, and ethical dimensions of their work.[1] A research team in place from the onset of a project could guarantee that appropriate attention is paid to the unintended consequences of the initial research.

DESCRIPTION OF MULTI-DISCIPLINARY, INTERDISCIPLINARY, AND TRANSDISCIPLINARY RESEARCH

Whether a team is considered multidisciplinary, interdisciplinary, or transdisciplinary depends on the level of integration.[2] Multidisciplinary research can be defined as research that integrates theories, methods, and knowledge from various disciplines while maintaining each discipline's distinctness (eg, a team composed of registered dietitian nutritionists, sociologists, and economists).[3] Interdisciplinary research integrates distinctly different academic areas (eg, nutrition, sociology, and economics) in such a way as to effectively form a new unified discipline (eg, women's health studies). Interdisciplinary teams often create a new identity, theoretical perspective, methodologic approach, or some combination of the three, whereas multidisciplinary teams tend to retain much of their separateness.[2] More recently, the concept of transdisciplinary research has gained popularity.

Transdisciplinary research is distinguishable from multidisciplinary and interdisciplinary research in that it compels researchers with diverse expertise to create new research concepts and approaches by exploring research questions that exist at the intersection of their respective fields through integrating and synthesizing content, theory, and methodology from those disciplines.[4,5] As such, research can be viewed as a continuum of increasing integration and blurring of disciplinary boundaries as it moves from multidisciplinary to interdisciplinary to ultimately transdisciplinary research (see Figure 11.2 on page 220). As Gray[6] noted, the distinctions between interdisciplinary and transdisciplinary research may be difficult to tease out in practice. McMichael's[7] concept that transdisciplinarity promotes "theoretical, conceptual, and methodological reorientation with respect to core concepts of the participating disciplines" is often quoted.

Rather than an alternative to other types of research, transdisciplinarity can be viewed as a complement to ongoing discipline-based scientific inquiry that "might lead to a different, higher, plane of inquiry"[7] and enable different questions to be asked.

Additionally, transdisciplinarity brings together researchers, practitioners, and stakeholders to collaborate in addressing complex societal problems[8] and promotes connections across intrapersonal, interpersonal, organizational, community, and societal levels of influence on social problems.[9,10] As will be elaborated upon later in the chapter, the reciprocal relationships between levels of analysis across the continuum from individual biology (eg, cell) to culture have been taken into account in research on childhood obesity in the 6-Cs model proposed by Harrison and colleagues.[11]

The Impetus for Research That Bridges Disciplinary Boundaries

Multidisciplinary and transdisciplinary research has become more compelling. As the availability of funding shrinks and becomes more competitive, the need for accountability rises, and the breadth of knowledge around a topic expands beyond disciplinary boundaries. The most pragmatic reason for establishing a multidisciplinary nutrition research team is financial—funding agencies often require proposals to take a multidisciplinary approach.[12] More than a decade ago, the National Institutes of Health (NIH) embraced the integration of basic social science concepts and constructs with health research to define the etiology of disease and wellness in order to apply these concepts to treatment and prevention services.[13-15] In 2010, the National Institute for Food and Agriculture promoted the application of transdisciplinary research and training in the area of childhood obesity.

Rewards of Multidisciplinary Research

Multidisciplinary research enhances understanding of complex issues, such as prevention of chronic disease, in ways that are not achievable by a single field of inquiry. Specialization leads to compartmentalization, which in turn limits knowledge of what is

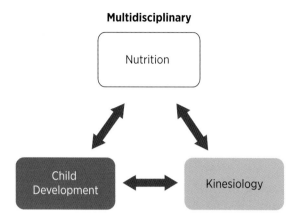

Multidisciplinary

Nutrition

Child Development

Kinesiology

- Separate bodies of knowledge
- Different languages

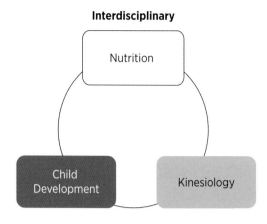

Interdisciplinary

Nutrition

Child Development

Kinesiology

- Shared bodies of knowledge
- Shared vocabulary

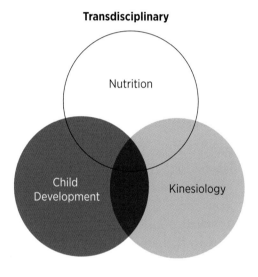

Transdisciplinary

Nutrition

Child Development

Kinesiology

- Integrated bodies of knowledge and theory
- Shared language
- Shared conceptual framework
- Jointly developed new approaches

Figure 11.2 Comparison of multidisciplinary, interdisciplinary, and transdisciplinary research

happening beyond the confines of a researcher's specific area. No longer can any one person or discipline be completely knowledgeable about a specific topic or method. Indeed, researchers can miss significant findings from other fields that share common interests but are asking different questions or using different methods.

On the professional level, multidisciplinary teams can increase personal creativity and inspire complex thinking. They also strengthen collegiality, enhance flexibility, and stimulate intellectual exchange.[12,16-19] Finally, multidisciplinary research can be the means to achieving goals that could not be achieved alone.[17,18]

Challenges to Research That Crosses Disciplinary Boundaries

The task of changing from having a single-discipline perspective to including multiple viewpoints does not come without inherent barriers.[12,19-22] Some of these are personal, whereas others are financial[20] and institutional.[21] Perceived personal risks of entering into multidisciplinary research include expectations about impacts on promotion and tenure, publication records, and the ability to secure new positions.[17] Multidisciplinary research can be more expensive, and it requires extensive coordination and surveillance. For biomedical research, the traditional top-down approach to tackling a problem needs to be set aside to allow for the free exchange of ideas and a willingness to overcome differences.[23,24]

Nutrition researchers might need to collaborate with researchers from departments across their institutions that have not traditionally worked together. Additionally, nutrition researchers may need to work with researchers from different universities, external organizations, and public-private enterprises. One way to mitigate differences is to find colleagues who share a similar worldview and are familiar with the basic concepts of each other's discipline. Establishing a clear conceptual framework at the beginning of the collaboration is essential.[25]

These interactions, in addition to the common frustrations that come from working with colleagues within one's own profession, create other challenges. Working with those who were trained in a different lexicon, follow a different set of values, or respond to different incentives requires a period of adjustment before research can begin. For example, scientists trained in quantitative biomedical methodologies may find it uncomfortable to accept qualitative methodologies when working with researchers trained in the social sciences. Conflict and loss of interest are two major barriers in creating and maintaining multidisciplinary research endeavors.[12,18] Many obstacles can be overcome with strategies that promote open communication and acceptance that all team members come to the table with a unique expertise and perspective.

Effective leadership is also critically important to the success of transdisciplinary research. Gray[6] described three types of leadership tasks: cognitive, structural, and processual. Cognitive leadership primarily consists of visioning and framing the transdisciplinary question, which is critical to moving the researchers to a new mindset that engages the transdisciplinary process. Frame change must also address the problem of differences in language between disciplines (see Figure 11.3 on page 222). Structural leadership primarily involves coordination and communication. The most successful leaders of transdisciplinary research are at the center of a social network linking the team of researchers. They often serve as brokers among the various groups of researchers and solve conflicts that may arise. Lastly, processual leadership includes a host of activities related to ensuring that interactions among team members are constructive and productive. This refers more to the nuts and bolts of day-to-day activities than to structural leadership but is critical to ensuring productive and constructive interactions among members of the research team.[26] In summary, to promote successful transdisciplinary research, leaders must "have the credibility to get the right individuals together to create visions, solve problems, and reach agreements about implementable actions."[27] These leadership tasks could be performed by a single leader or could be handled in a distributed fashion by multiple members of a transdisciplinary team.[28]

HOW TO SUCCESSFULLY CONDUCT RESEARCH THAT BRIDGES DISCIPLINES

Who Should Be Involved?

Frequently, nutrition researchers know which other disciplines to seek to include in a research project. As a first step into multidisciplinary research, nutrition researchers will often include someone from a discipline with expertise in analyzing data (eg, a biostatistician, epidemiologist, or economist) to help prepare the experimental design and data analysis aspects of the research proposal. Psychologists may be included for research into eating disorders, whereas sociologists may be invited to join studies involving cultural differences where an understanding of the processes underlying the relationships is needed.

Today, for example, cancer research encompasses diverse disciplines.[14,29] Though initial work on cancer was limited to biochemical and genetic research in animals and humans, it soon became apparent that epidemiologists and statisticians were required to further explain cancer incidence. Finally, cancer researchers acknowledged the need to understand environmental and social factors (eg, diet and lifestyle). The progression to including multiple disciplines has led to significant advances in understanding the treatment and prevention of many types of cancer. The NIH's *Collaboration and Team Science: A Field Guide* has recommendations on best practices for scientists and researchers who wish to form successful research teams.[30]

For research questions where the connections between disciplines are less obvious, Kostoff[22] suggests "text mining." This technique involves conducting a literature search in databases not normally used by the nutrition researcher, for example, social sciences, psychology, behavioral sciences, and humanities databases. The nutrition researcher interested in a particular issue (eg, obesity) enters key words to identify papers and authors who are investigating the same issues in other disciplines. A librarian can be an excellent resource for help in text mining.

Booth and colleagues[31] used a similar technique to generate a list of disciplines needed to create a conceptual framework for understanding the complex relationships between unhealthful eating and physical inactivity. Initially, experts from the fields of nutrition and exercise physiology were included, along with representatives from the food industry. After conducting literature reviews and brainstorming sessions, the researchers created a final list of disciplines that included sociology, anthropology, architecture and community building, economics, consumer research, food policy, transportation, geography, history, health care, and food and sensory sciences. The result was an intricate schema depicting the relationships between individuals and the environment as viewed through the lens of different disciplines (see Figure 11.3).[32] The factors high-

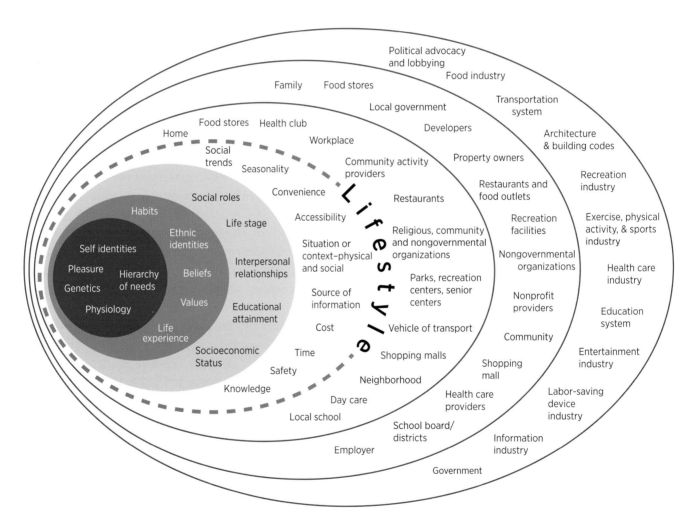

Figure 11.3 Schema depicting multiple disciplines for studying determinants of eating and physical activity[31]

Adapted with permission from Oxford University Press. Booth SL, Sallis JF, Ritenbaugh C, et al. Environmental and societal factors affect food choice and physical activity: rationale, influences, and leverage points. *Nutr Rev.* 2001;59 (3):S21-S39.

lighted provide a starting point for nutrition researchers to envision which other disciplines might be useful to include in research.

Personal Characteristics That Enhance Multidisciplinary Research

Crossing the established boundaries of disciplinary silos can pose challenges even for scientists who have well-developed interpersonal skills.[6] Those who are successful working as part of a multidisciplinary research team demonstrate strong, nonhierarchical mutual and personal respect for those with different opinions.[18] They possess self-awareness, are self-reflective, and are willing to have their ideas scrutinized.[25] Researchers who approach conflict as a learning experience are confident in their own discipline, value two-way communication and differences of opinion, and can synthesize various perspectives (including those of senior and junior investigators), and so make excellent partners. Trust, nurturance, understanding, tact, and thoughtfulness also provide stability to the research team. Individuals who are less comfortable with compromise, role blurring, and collective ownership of research may not be suited for multidisciplinary research.

Decisions to Make

Once specific disciplines and researchers are identified, roles must be defined. Will a researcher be a full member of the team or a consultant? Who will set the ground rules? How will differences be resolved? Answers to these and other questions are needed to establish a working relationship based on trust and mutual respect. While this is true for all collaborations, the time required for building multidisciplinary relationships may take longer. Collaborators from the same discipline share a uniformly understood language that allows them to immediately begin planning the project; for example, almost every nutritionist knows BMI means body mass index but an economist might not. With collaborators from distinctly different fields, team members should explain commonly used terms and jargon in informal conversations.[18] Developing a glossary of terms from the different disciplines might also be helpful.

For many research projects, however, proposal due dates often preclude lengthy preliminary interaction where differences can be identified, discussed, and negotiated. When time for mutual exploration is not possible, researchers may want to exchange basic readings that explain the problem at hand from the perspective of their discipline. After this exchange, researchers will be able to establish a common language, synergistic missions, and agreed-upon common goals. It is essential to continue to refer to these common goals throughout the project so researchers do not drift back toward their more familiar disciplinary work.

Some decisions—such as who is responsible for daily management, who makes which decisions, who makes the final decision, and who communicates with the funding agency—must be made initially and reviewed periodically as the research progresses. Continuity of leadership is essential. Investigators should also exchange information about available resources and time commitments; negotiate budgetary requirements (including indirect costs and in-person meetings); clarify contractual language (especially if working with external partners); work out intellectual property rights; compare human participants protocols; and coordinate statistical, referencing, and other software packages. Attending to these issues up front is critical at the proposal stage and throughout the research project. Certain issues, such as grant management, sharing of databases and analyses, and authorship, may be drastically different among disciplines. Rather than assuming similarities, those involved with multidisciplinary research should ask new colleagues to clarify how they handle each situation. This can be done as each portion of the grant application and study design is addressed but clearly must be established early in the collaboration.

Strategies for Working on a Multidisciplinary Team

Communication, negotiation, and mutual respect are the main strategies consistently mentioned when describing multidisciplinary research.[2,12,15,17-22,23,24] Face-to-face meetings are vital at all stages of the research,[12] and budgets should include sufficient funds to support them. Retreats, including social activities, establish a mechanism for providing the extended period of discussion and assimilation needed to create a common language, fuse methods, and nurture all team members.[12,24]

Additional communication tools are especially useful when more than one site is involved. These include a central website or depository, electronic chat rooms and bulletin boards, email lists, text messaging, web casting, newsletter and periodic updates, and conference calls. Other helpful technological tools include those that manage and track task trajectories over time, internet meeting sites, software to schedule meetings and calls, referencing packages, and videoconferencing workshops.[12] A single contact person should be appointed to coordinate these tools.

In addition to the aforementioned strategies, Morgan and colleagues[15] developed key elements for successful multidisciplinary research (see Box 11.1). Though they were developed to coordinate NIH centers, they are applicable to all multidisciplinary research endeavors.

Similarly, Brown and colleagues[23] identified five principles their team used to enhance collaborative efforts: (1) forge a shared mission to instill a sense of purpose; (2) develop "T-shaped" researchers who are able to extend the depth and breadth of the research in and beyond their own discipline; (3) nurture constructive dialogue; (4) give institutional support to ensure progress for academics; and (5) bridge research, policy, and practice with enduring connections. Furthermore, in response to concerns regarding acceptance, they suggest ways for funders, institutions, publishers, and researchers to make interdisciplinary research mainstream.

Two examples of transdisciplinary research and training have been implemented at the University of Illinois at Urbana-Champaign. The first is the Synergistic Theory and Research on Obesity and Nutrition Group (STRONG) Kids Program (SKP). This research program takes a comprehensive cross-disciplinary, theory-driven approach to examine the synergistic contribution of biological (genetics, microbiome) and environmental (nutrition, child development, and family) factors in the development of childhood weight imbalance, obesity, health behaviors, and health beliefs from birth to 5 years of age.[11] The SKP team comprises faculty from a variety of disciplines, including human development and family studies, food science, nutrition, kinesiology, community health, social work, agricultural and consumer economics, and communication. Faculty worked together to develop multidisciplinary questionnaires for participants to complete. A steering committee provides the leadership, and its primary roles are to obtain funding and institutional review board approval to support the longitudinal cohort, develop policies and procedures, and construct a data management plan. A sampling of articles illustrates the SKP team's collaborative, 6 Cs—cell to culture—approach.[32-48]

The SKP has provided an exceptional opportunity to educate undergraduate and graduate students in transdisciplinary approaches to research. The SKP faculty developed and taught a two-semester undergraduate course on applied research methods (HDFS 494). In addition to learning the theory underlying the SKP, students gain professional skills and participate in faculty-supervised research as a member of a transdisciplinary team investigating questions related to the health and well-being of children and families. Students propose their own research questions and present findings developed from data gathered by the team. Barbara Fiese, PhD, garnered a nearly $750,000 grant from the US Department of Agriculture (USDA) for the

Regular structured communications across disciplines

Respect for others' models and methods

Development of a common language

Institutional commitment and support

Funds to support infrastructure (especially communications and travel)

Emphasis on expanding to include other disciplines

Box 11.1 Elements for Successful Multidisciplinary Research[15]

Transdisciplinary Obesity Prevention Program–Undergraduate to modify and expand this course to work in a flip-the-classroom format to make modules available online for other programs to use. Hundreds of students from multiple departments and colleges have completed HDFS 494 and, in most cases, conduct research linked to SKP.

A second example relates to the $4.5 million USDA grant awarded to the University of Illinois to develop a transdisciplinary graduate program focused on childhood obesity prevention. The Illinois Transdisciplinary Obesity Prevention Program (I-TOPP) is a combined PhD/MPH program in which doctoral students can complete their degree in any of seven doctoral programs, but their research must focus on childhood (many conduct research focused on the SKP cohort). The MPH degree provides trainees with an in-the-trenches perspective that informs their research and academic coursework. I-TOPP and the training it provides illustrate how transdisciplinary research teams can address an important societal problem with a complex etiology and how transdisciplinary research and educational programs can be blended for mutual benefit. A recent publication from the I-TOPP team of investigators assessed the benefits and barriers to transdisciplinary training perceived by the faculty and students and made institutional recommendations.[49] Another publication compared the productivity, impact, and collaboration between students in the I-TOPP training program compared with traditionally trained doctoral students and found that I-TOPP students published works that were accepted into higher-impact journals, were more frequently cited, and had more cross-disciplinary collaborations than publications from students in traditional PhD programs.[50]

CONCLUSION

Bridging disciplinary boundaries in nutrition research provides an opportunity to expand beyond the professional constraints of insufficient knowledge, tunnel vision, and limited perspective. Despite the challenges that can arise when working across distinctly different disciplines, the findings of such research more closely approach the truth. New and established researchers might consider incorporating at least one other discipline into their next project to determine the value of expertise beyond nutrition.

REFERENCES

1. Robinson B, Vasko SE, Gonnerman C, et al. Human values and the value of humanities in interdisciplinary research. *Cogent Arts Human.* 2016;3(1):1-16. doi:10.1080/23311983 .2015.1123080.

2. Van den Besselaar P, Heimeriks G. Disciplinary, multidisciplinary, interdisciplinary: concepts and indicators. In: Davis M, Wilson CS, eds. *ISSI 2001, 8th International Conference of the Society for Scientometrics and Informetrics.* Sydney, Australia: UNSW; 2001:705-716.

3. Collins J. May you live in interesting times: using multidisciplinary and interdisciplinary programs to cope with change in the life sciences. *BioScience.* 2002;52(1): 75-83.

4. Rosenfield PL. The potential of transdisciplinary research for sustaining and extending linkages between the health and social sciences. *Soc Sci Med.* 1992;35(11): 1343-1357.

5. Sommerville MA, Rapport DJ, eds. *Transdisciplinarity: Recreating Integrated Knowledge.* Montreal, Canada: McGill-Queens University Press; 2002.

6. Gray B. Enhancing transdisciplinary research through collaborative leadership. *Am J Prev Med.* 2008;35 (2 suppl):S124-S132.

7. McMichael AJ. What makes transdisciplinarity succeed or fail? First Report. In: Somerville MA, Rapport DJ, eds. *Transdisciplinarity: Recreating Integrated Knowledge.* Oxford, United Kingdom: EOLSS Publishers Ltd; 2000.

8. Abrams DB. Applying transdisciplinary research strategies to understanding and eliminating health disparities. *Health Educ Behav.* 2006;33(4):515-531.

9. Emmons KM, Viswanath K, Colditz GA. The role of transdisciplinary collaboration in translating and disseminating health research. *Am J Prev Med.* 2008;35 (2 suppl):S204-S210.

10. Nash JM. Transdisciplinary training: key components and prerequisites for success. *Am J Prev Med.* 2008;35 (2 suppl):S133-S140.

11. Harrison K, Bost KK, McBride BA, et al. Toward a developmental conceptualization of contributors to overweight and obesity in childhood: the six-Cs model. *Child Devel Perspect.* 2011;5(1):50-58.

12. Cummings J, Kiesler S. Collaborative research across disciplinary and organizational boundaries. *Soc Stud Sci.* 2005;35(5):703-722.

13. Bachrach C, Abeles R. Social science and health research: growth at the National Institutes of Health. *Am J Public Health.* 2004;94(1):22-28.

14. Forman M, Hursting S, Umar A. Nutrition and cancer prevention: a multidisciplinary perspective on human trials. *Ann Rev Nutr.* 2004;24:223-254.

15. Morgan G, Kobus K, Gerlach K, et al. Facilitating transdisciplinary research: the experiences of the transdisciplinary tobacco use research centers. *Nicotine Tob Res.* 2003;5(suppl):S11-S19.

16. Bronstein L. Index of interdisciplinary collaboration. *Soc Work Res.* 2002;26(2):113-123.

17. Bronstein L. A model for interdisciplinary collaboration. *Soc Work.* 2003;48(3):297-306.

18. Creamer E. Collaborators' attitudes about differences of opinion. *J Higher Educ.* 2004;75:556-571.

19. Nissani M. Ten cheers for interdisciplinarity: the case for interdisciplinary knowledge and research. *Soc Sci J.* 1997;34(2):201-217.

20. Ellison P, Kopp C. A note on interdisciplinary research in developmental/behavioral pediatrics/psychology. *Pediatrics.* 1985;75(5):883-886.

21. Kezar A. Moving from I to we. *Change.* 2005;37(6):50-57.

22. Kostoff R. Overcoming specialization. *BioScience.* 2002;52(10):937-941.

23. Brown RR, Deletic A, Wong THF. Interdisciplinarity: how to catalyze collaboration. *Nature.* 2015;525(7569): 315-317.

24. Tracy MF, Chlan L. Interdisciplinary research teams. *Clin Nurse Spec.* 2014;28(1):12-14.

25. Oughton E, Bracken L. Interdisciplinary research: framing and reframing. *Area.* 2009;41(4):385-394.

26. Chrislip DE, Larson CE. *Collaborative Leadership: How Citizens and Civic Leaders Can Make a Difference.* San Francisco, CA: Jossey-Bass; 1994.

27. Stokols D, Harvey R, Gress J, Fuqua J, Phillips K. *In vivo* studies of transdisciplinary scientific collaboration: lessons learned and implications for active living research. *Am J Prev Med.* 2005;28(2 suppl 2):202-213.

28. Jevning R, Biedebach M, Anand R. Cruciferous vegetables and human breast cancer: an important interdisciplinary hypothesis in the field of diet and cancer. *Fam Econ Nutr Rev.* 1999;12(2):26-30.

29. Hill J, Goldberg J, Pate R, Peters J. Introduction. *Nutr Rev.* 2001;59(3):S4- S9.

30. Bennett LM, Gadlin H, Levine-Finley S. *Collaboration and Team Science: A Field Guide*. National Institutes of Health. NIH Publication No. 10-7660. August 2010. http://teamscience.nih.gov. Accessed September 16, 2017.

31. Booth SL, Sallis JF, Ritenbaugh C, et al. Environmental and societal factors affect food choice and physical activity: rationale, influences, and leverage points. *Nutr Rev.* 2001;59(3 part 2):S21-S39.

32. Shim JE, Kim J, Mathai RA; STRONG Kids Research Team. Associations of Infant feeding practices and picky eating behaviors of preschool children. *J Am Diet Assoc.* 2011; 111(9):1363-1368.

33. Grigsby-Toussaint DS, Chi SH, Fiese BH. Where they live, how they play: neighborhood greenness and outdoor physical activity among preschoolers. *Int J Health Geogr.* 2011;10(1):66.

34. Harrison K, Liechty JM; STRONG Kids Program. US preschoolers' media exposure and dietary habits: the primacy of television and the limits of parental mediation. *J Child Media.* 2012;6(1):18-36.

35. Dev DA, McBride BA; STRONG Kids Research Team. Academy of Nutrition and Dietetics benchmarks for nutrition in child care 2011: are child-care providers across contexts meeting recommendations? *J Acad Nutr Diet.* 2013; 113(10):1346-1353.

36. Fiese BH; STRONG Kids Team. Context matters in pediatric obesity: commentary on innovative treatment and prevention programs for pediatric overweight and obesity. *J Pediatr Psychol.* 2013;38(9):1037-1043.

37. Dev DA, McBride B, Fiese BH, Jones BL, Cho H; STRONG Kids Research Team. Risk factors for overweight/obesity in preschool children: an ecological approach. *Child Obes.* 2013;9(5):399-408.

38. Bost KK, Wiley AR, Fiese BH, Hammons A, McBride B; STRONG Kids Team. Associations between adult attachment style, emotion regulation, and preschool children's food consumption. *J Dev Behav Pediatr.* 2014;35(1):50-61.

39. Jones BL, Fiese BH; STRONG Kids Team. Parent routines, child routines, and family demographics associated with obesity in parents and preschool-aged children. *Front Psychol.* 2014; 5:374.

40. Speirs KE, Liechty JM, Wu CF; STRONG Kids Research Team. Sleep, but not other daily routines, mediates the association between maternal employment and BMI for preschool children. *Sleep Med.* 2014;15(12):1590-1593.

41. Liechty JM, Saltzman JA, Musaad SM; STRONG Kids Team. Health literacy and parent attitudes about weight control for children. *Appetite.* 2015;91:200-208.

42. Harrison K, Peralta M; STRONG Kids Research Team. Parent and child media exposure, preschooler dietary intake, and preschooler healthy-meal schemas in the context of food insecurity. *J Commun.* 2015;65:443-464.

43. Speirs KE, Fiese BH; STRONG Kids Research Team. The relationship between food insecurity and BMI for preschool children. *Matern Child Health J.* 2016;20: 925-933.

44. Harrison K, Peralta M, Costa Jacobsohn G, Grider D, Grider DT; STRONG Kids Research Team. The placemat protocol: measuring preschoolers' healthy-meal schemas with pretend meals. *Appetite.* 2016;96:209-218.

45. Shim JE, Kim J, Lee Y; STRONG Kids Team. Fruit and vegetable intakes of preschool children are associated with feeding practices facilitating internalization of extrinsic motivation. *J Nutr Educ Behav.* 2016;48:311-317.

46. Saltzman JA, Liechty JM, Bost KK, Fiese BH; STRONG Kids Program. Parent binge eating and restrictive feeding practices: indirect effects of parent's responses to child's negative emotion. *Eat Behav.* 2016;21:150-154.

47. Shim JE, Kim J, Lee Y; STRONG Kids Team. Fruit and vegetable intakes of preschool children are associated with feeding practices facilitating internalization of extrinsic motivation. *J Nutr Educ Behav.* 2016;48:311-317.

48. Musaad SMA, Donovan SM, Fiese BH. The independent and cumulative effect of early life risk factors on child growth: a preliminary report. *Child Obes.* 2016;12: 193-201.

49. Keck A-S, Sloane S, Liechty JM, et al. Longitudinal perspectives of faculty and students on benefits and barriers to transdisciplinary education: program assessment and institutional recommendations. *Palgrave Commun.* 2017;3:40.

50. Keck AS, Sloane S, Liechty JM, Fiese BH, Donovan SM. Productivity, impact, and collaboration differences between transdisciplinary and traditionally trained doctoral students: a comparison of publication patterns. *PLoS One.* 2017;12(12):e0189391.

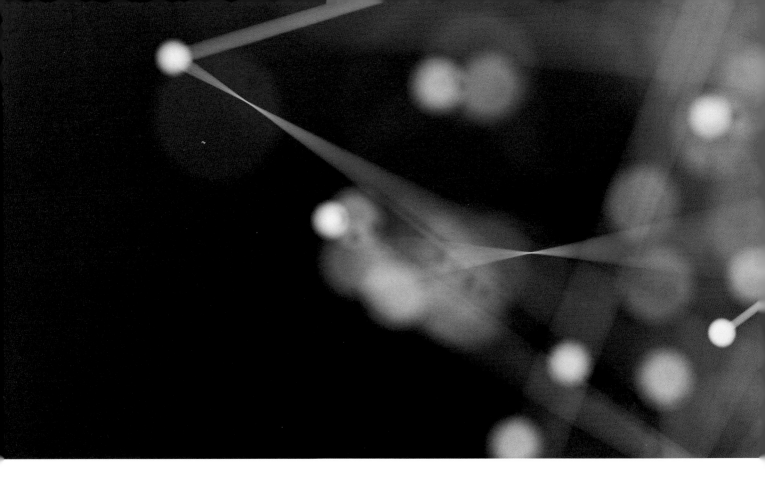

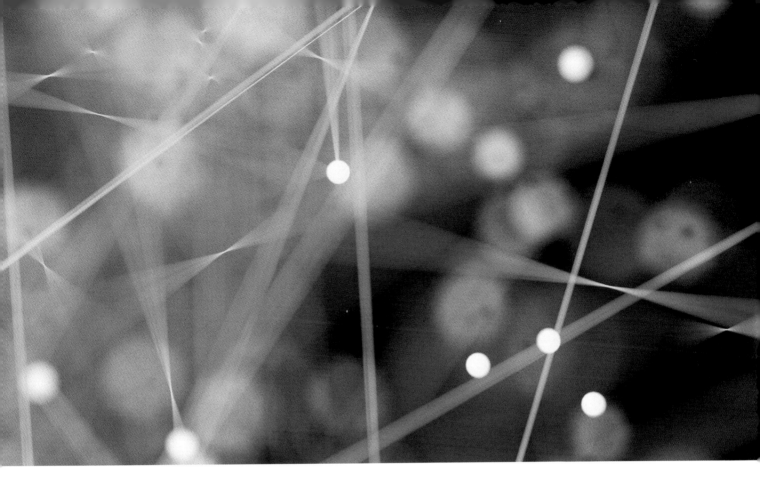

Survey Research Planning and Questionnaire Design

Jacqueline A. Vernarelli, PhD | *Barbara Millen, DrPH, RD, FADA*

LEARNING OBJECTIVES

1. Describe the steps in designing a survey.

2. Describe the ways in which nutrition surveys are conducted.

3. Identify the difference between effective and ineffective survey questions.

4. List and describe the strengths and weaknesses of survey research.

Survey research is among the most important and frequently utilized approaches in human nutrition investigations at both the individual and population-based levels. Survey research is central to the National Nutrition Monitoring and Related Research Program (NNMRRP), which includes the continuous National Health Interview Survey conducted by the Centers for Disease Control and Prevention and state health departments,[1] as well as the ongoing National Health and Nutrition Examination Surveys (NHANES) conducted by the Department of Health and Human Services (HHS).[2] Survey methods are broadly drawn upon in health-related research as they enable researchers to explore links between nutrition-related factors and a wide range of sociodemographic characteristics and health-related outcomes among individuals, communities, or populations. Survey research is also used to evaluate many dimensions of the national food, nutrition, and agricultural systems in both the public and private sectors. Surveys extend our understanding of the nature and quality of the food supply; the production, distribution, and sales of agricultural commodities; and the features and impact of nutrition-related programs and services.

Given the importance, scope, and widespread application of survey research in nutrition and related domains and practice, it is essential that nutrition practitioners develop relevant skills and expertise, particularly related to overall study design and questionnaire development. The following discussion provides an overview of the stages of survey research planning and implementation with particular emphasis on questionnaire and related protocol design.

SURVEY RESEARCH APPLICATIONS

One of the primary applications of survey research methods is the NNMRRP. The survey research elements of the NNMRRP provide the chief mechanisms for assessing the health and nutritional status of the US population and for determining progress toward national nutrition- and health-related policies and goals (such as Healthy People 2020).[3] In this context, survey methods are used to evaluate the diet- and health-related knowledge and attitudes of individuals or households and the environmental determinants of individual nutritional status (risk) or behaviors. Survey techniques are also applied to assess the nutrition-related health characteristics and behaviors of individuals (such as meal consumption patterns and food and nutrient intake); the data produced from these investigations can be linked to the individual's biological risk factors or relevant health- or disease-related characteristics or outcomes (such as nutrition-related acute, chronic, and infectious conditions and their comorbidities, complications, or consequences).

A second widespread application of survey methods in human nutrition research is in the field of nutrition epidemiology. This research domain has grown rapidly in recent years as validated survey questionnaire methodologies (such as food frequency questionnaires, telephone-administered dietary assessment techniques, and—more recently—web-based diet and health-risk appraisal platforms) have emerged for use in population-based investigations and prospective cohort studies. These new evidence-based approaches have become a standard of quality research. They are used in large federal surveys, such as the collaborative effort between the US Department of Agriculture and the HHS in the form of the What We Eat in America (WWEIA) dietary survey, which is the nutrition component of the NHANES.[4] Chapter 10 has a complete description of the NHANES. Briefly put, WWEIA survey data allow for the comprehensive evaluation of the nutritional intake of noninstitutionalized Americans. Using advanced statistical techniques to analyze data from WWEIA and other large nutrition surveys, researchers have developed innovative analytic and interpretive approaches to better understand the relationship between diet and disease.

Historically, single foods and nutrients were the most common nutrition exposures of interest in nutrition epidemiology; however, researchers increasingly acknowledged that analytic models using these exposure variables were inherently statistically confounded by colinearities in food and nutrient intake (see Box 12.1 on page 232 for definitions).[5]

Today, investigators often use potentially more informative measures of overall dietary quality to assess comprehensive dietary exposures, such as the Healthy Eating Index and other dietary quality indexes,[6,7] male and female dietary patterns,[5,8,9] and composite nutritional risk scores.[5,9,10] Experts believe evidence-based approaches examining overall dietary quality and dietary patterns offer promise to better inform our understanding of diet-disease risk relationships and may add new insights into intervention design strategies as they are translated into innovative, preventive nutrition programs and treatments.[5,6,10]

The domain of clinical nutrition research also often utilizes survey methods to assess the various dimensions of an individual's nutritional status, such as retrospective and current dietary exposures, the key behavioral and ecological or environmental determinants of nutritional risk, and related

Colinearity: When two or more predictor variables are closely related. For example, milk consumption is closely related to calcium consumption in children. As milk intake increases, calcium intake also increases.

Confounding variables: Variables that were not accounted for in data analysis, making causal associations difficult to determine. For example, a fictional study found that coffee drinkers were more likely to have lung cancer than non-coffee drinkers, causing researchers to declare that coffee consumption increased cancer risk. Years later it was determined that 95% of the coffee drinkers were also smokers—a hidden variable that contributed to the outcome (cancer) but was not accounted for in the results.

Box 12.1 Colinearity and Confounding Variables

health outcomes. Such information has proven essential to evidence-based practice and the design of effective preventive nutrition intervention strategies and medical nutrition therapies.

In addition, survey research can extend to investigations of programs, communities, or entire systems. In the area of program or services evaluation research, survey methods may be used to assess the type, quality, impact, and efficacy of nutrition programs or interventions at the individual, community, or population levels. Alternatively, surveys could be designed to evaluate the characteristics of organizations, communities, or entire business frameworks as they relate to individual or population nutrition. For example, the characteristics of communities or workplace settings (such as availability of healthy food options, food retail stores, or farmers markets) might be evaluated and used in assessing their relationships to population nutritional risk or to determine whether adequate resources exist to support population nutrition behavior change.

In the agricultural sector, survey methods can be used to monitor the nature and quality of the US food supply and the nation's food production systems. This research provides information on commodities

and the agricultural infrastructure, including domestic and international food production and distribution, food product imports and exports, food processing practices (eg, pesticide and chemical use, animal feeds and treatment, acreage in organic farming), and many other dimensions of the food, foodservice, and nutraceutical industries.

Clearly, the applications of survey methods are widespread in nutrition-related research and offer many opportunities for practitioners in the field. The following section delves into the survey research planning process and is followed by details relating to the methods of survey data collection and questionnaire design.

AN ECOLOGICAL FRAMEWORK FOR NUTRITION RESEARCH PLANNING

At the outset of survey planning, researchers carefully identify the research problem area, the different domains of research interest, and relationships between different aspects of the study; the specific research questions; and the variables needed to achieve the study aims and answer all research questions. Nutrition and health experts have used the ecological framework,[11] which can facilitate the conceptualization of the relationships between potential domains of research investigations, including human behaviors (such as diet), their determinants, and health-related outcomes. This model is designed to aid in various research planning processes (such as instrument design). Adapted for this discussion, the model considers the relationships between food intake, nutrient intake, or both food and nutrient intake and related dietary behaviors (including dietary patterns and composite dietary quality measures); other key lifestyle-related modifiable behaviors (such as physical activity and smoking); the personal, social, and other environmental influences on these behaviors; and potentially associated health outcomes (including chronic disease risks). See Figure 12.1.

The National Heart, Lung, and Blood Institute (NHLBI) used the ecological framework to inform a research planning process specifically relating to the examination of relationships between diet, physical activity, and obesity-related health outcomes; a

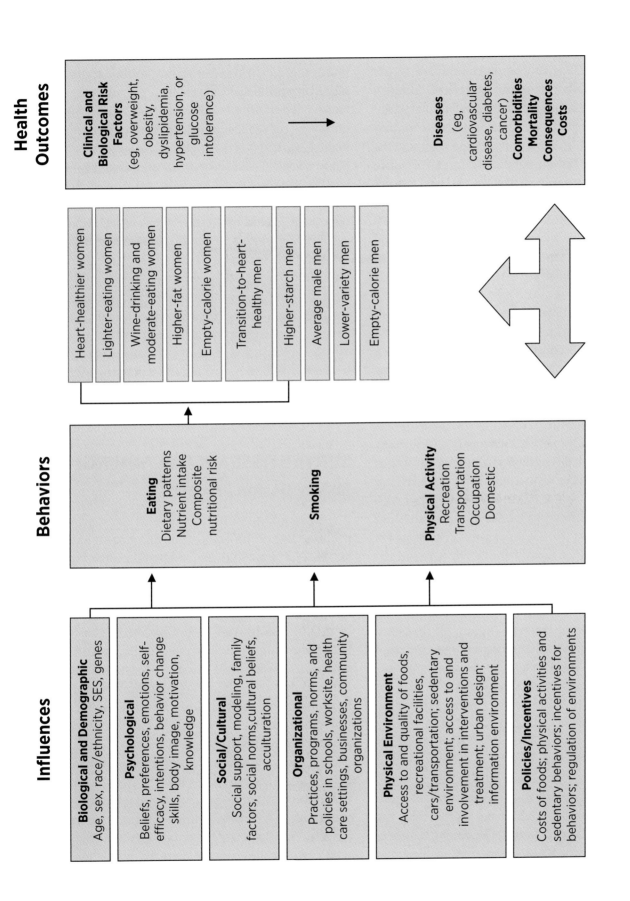

Figure 12.1 An ecological model of diet and health outcomes with dietary patterns

SES = socioeconomic status

"Heart-healthier women," "Average male men," and similar terms refer to subgroups of men and women defined in the Framingham Nutrition studies that display habitual dietary patterns characterized by food and nutrient intake and diet quality profiles that distinguish them from other subgroups.

summary of its expert workshop can be found at the NHLBI website.[12] The Framingham Nutrition Studies added to the ecological framework by identifying multiple dimensions of eating behaviors (dietary patterns, nutrient intake, and composite nutritional risk scores) and presenting the dietary patterns and behaviors of Framingham men and women, as shown in Figure 12.1 on page 233. In addition, the ecological framework was the conceptual model used by the 2015 Dietary Guidelines Advisory Committee (DGAC)[13] and is integrated into the 2015–2020 Dietary Guidelines for Americans.[14]

The ecological framework identifies diet, including the alternative ways of measuring this exposure noted earlier, as one of the primary modifiable human behaviors of research interest. The model acknowledges relationships between diet and other human behaviors, such as smoking and physical activity. It considers the complex array of environmental or ecological influences on these behaviors, including characteristics of the individual (knowledge, attitudes, and biological and demographic factors); the psychological, social/cultural, organizational, or physical environments in which the individual lives, functions, or is served or treated; and public and private policies, programs, and incentives that may influence diet and nutrition (eg, Supplemental Nutrition Assistance Program [SNAP], the Special Supplemental Nutrition Program for Women, Infants, and Children [WIC]; elder nutrition programs; or Medicare reimbursement of medical nutrition therapies). Any of these domains could become the topic of survey research. During survey planning and questionnaire design activities, consider whether these research domains and variable categories are applicable to the research. Other instrument design considerations are discussed in more detail later in this chapter.

Key in the ecological framework, particularly as interpreted and expanded by the DGAC, is the additional focus on the relationships between diet (and other lifestyle behaviors) and a wide range of nutrition and health-related outcomes across the life span, including growth and development, physical performance, as well as biological risk factors, diseases or health conditions and their comorbidities or consequences, and disease-specific or overall mor-

tality. The self-report of such health-related parameters or other sources of this information may be of interest in survey research planning and instrument or protocol development. Alternatively, relevant clinical data on nutrition-related health outcomes may be assessed independently using biological assays (such as plasma lipids, glucose, or blood pressure levels) or other techniques and may be linked analytically with survey research questionnaire data. Such approaches enable a more thorough exploration of diet–disease risk relationships and may provide information and insights of use in developing evidence-based interventions, therapies, and clinical practice guidelines.

Using the ecological framework can guide investigators in making careful decisions about broad domains or topics of research interest, focused research questions, and specific study variables. Investigators will use all of these considerations in the survey planning process, particularly in the development of instruments and other research protocols.

SURVEY RESEARCH PLANNING
Survey Design Process

The goal of human nutrition survey research is to produce data or information on a sample of individuals drawn from a well-defined population relating to one or more of the following: nutrition-related beliefs, attitudes, or behaviors (or any combination of the three); their environmental influences, contexts, or determinants; and their relationship to related health outcomes or consequences. Surveys may answer single or multiple research questions, test specific hypotheses, estimate population characteristics, formally model relationships between a set of nutrition characteristics and other variables, or accomplish other well-defined goals.[15] Survey research is carried out in a series of complex stages, including determining the research problem area and population of interest, creating a preliminary survey plan, formulating the final survey plan and operating guidelines, implementing data collection (including quality control activities), and managing and analyzing data sets and reporting.[16] Sound survey research uses a relatively systematic planning strategy, but experts acknowledge that the process unfolds dynamically during progressive stages of development and implementation. Researchers can refer to a number of helpful resources, full texts on survey research, and web-based resources for survey planning and instrument design.[15-24] The design and implementation of a survey follows a series of steps, illustrated in Figure 12.2.

The first step in survey design is to identify the goal of the survey and how the information collected helps to achieve the goal. The survey goal guides the research aims. Commonly, surveys are designed to describe the nutritional, economic, or social behaviors in a population of interest. Depending on the specific method of data collection, the information can allow the researcher to (1) characterize a specific population or interest; (2) compare nutritional, economic, or social behaviors between various sub-

groups within the population of interest; or (3) explore relationships between nutrition- and health-related factors and other characteristics of individuals (such as the individual's food beliefs or purchasing behaviors). The population of interest might include specific types of individuals, families, households, consumer or professional subgroups, communities or populations with unique characteristics, or other key groups or entities that may affect human nutrition. Identifying the population of interest requires unbiased participant selection, knowledge of participation likelihood, and use of valid and reliable survey research tools. Survey researchers commonly select the population using random or probability techniques rather than convenience sampling in order to identify their well-defined population.[15-17] Research goals and questions, budget realities, and desired study population characteristics guide the selection

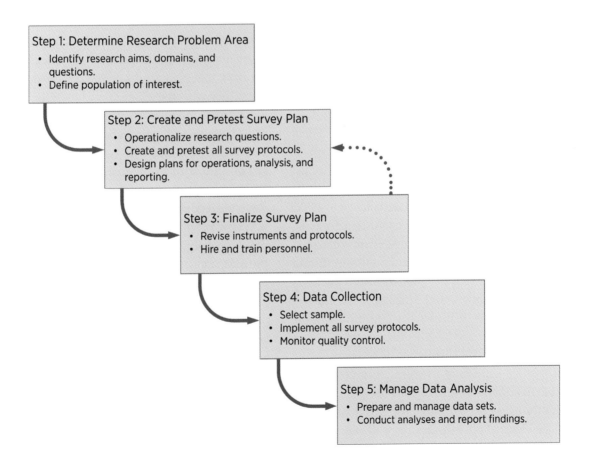

Figure 12.2 Steps for design and implementation of a survey

of the most appropriate and feasible survey methods, including respondent sampling strategies, questionnaire/instrument design, data collection protocols, and plans for analysis and reporting. Regardless of the final research strategy, researchers should monitor all operations to ensure that quality control is maintained throughout and that objective and ethical standards are followed in conducting research.

The next step is to create and pretest the survey plan. Survey research protocols, including questionnaires, are carefully constructed and pretested to establish that they are well-suited to achieve research study goals and to answer all research questions. Also, research instruments and protocols should be designed such that respondents can understand what is asked and are capable of providing the intended information or finishing the study protocols. Respondents should be able to complete questionnaires and other study components relatively easily, accurately, and according to established research methods. During the preliminary planning stages, researchers typically review the existing literature to explore alternative approaches to the research design and data collection strategies. Researchers also identify the availability of established protocols for data collection, including validated survey questionnaires. As researchers begin to assemble the design elements and instruments, it is important to ask experts to review and comment on the approach. Ideally, the researcher should conduct preliminary pretests of survey protocols and specific questionnaire items. All research protocols, including participant sampling strategies, full questionnaires, and other data collection devices should be more fully pretested. Staging multiple pretests with one or more samples of suitable respondents whose profiles closely resemble the population of research interest is optimal. This enables researchers to fully understand the suitability of their methods and approaches and may prevent difficulties that could arise in actual survey operations.

Instrument and protocol pretesting often results in revisions of questionnaires and refinements to plans of research operation, including data collection methods, staff training, quality control procedures, and analytic plans. The pretesting stages are important in devising a survey management plan

> Data collected in large studies, such as the National Health and Nutrition Examination Survey, are cleaned and checked for accuracy before data analysis. For example, if a participant reported more than one response to a "check one" answer (ie, checking the box for age 18–35 and the box for age 50–75), researchers would have to determine which answer is correct and which box should be checked before analyzing the data.

Box 12.2 Example of Data Cleaning

that facilitates the smooth, objective, and ethical implementation of research and the successful achievement of research aims.

Revisions made after pretesting are used to finalize the survey plan (step 3) and begin data collection (step 4). Using an organized and tested plan, researchers collect and compile the data into one or more data sets. Once data have been collected, careful data cleaning and editing are necessary before implementing data analysis (see Box 12.2 for an example).

The type of data cleaning and editing should be decided in advance, with consideration for the statistical implications of any data cleaning (eg, what will be done with incomplete survey data responses?). Researchers should recognize that all research surveys are subject to a variety of constraints (eg, budgetary constraints that may limit the sample size or the scope and methods of data collection). Potential limitations need to be considered carefully in the planning process to optimize study design. As data analysis is managed (step 5), researchers summarize the findings in keeping with the research questions and produce reports or publications for various audiences. As appropriate, study limitations should be acknowledged in research reporting.

Successful survey research is evidence based, and findings should add to the body of evidence on a given topic or domain. Thus, existing peer-reviewed literature is used to inform as many of the research planning stages as possible and is applied (as feasible and appropriate) to each study. Researchers rely on available literature not only to carefully articulate the research questions but also to identify options for instruments and protocols as well as data collection and statistical methods. Reviewing the current literature and drawing insights from experts in the field of interest help researchers make informed decisions about study population characteristics, sampling strategies, methods to promote respondent participation and survey completion rates, and how to enhance other features of the research. For example, one area where experts may be particularly helpful is population sampling. Given that it is unlikely that *all* members of a population of interest will be surveyed, researchers need to develop and document appropriate sampling strategies and incorporate methods to increase respondent participation. Researchers must summarize and report on nonresponse, noncompliance, and missing data, and they must consider these limitations in devising the statistical analyses and reporting plan.[15,17]

Statistical Considerations for Survey Design

Population Sampling

The research aims and available resources affect population sampling strategies. Box 12.3 defines key sampling terms.

Choices, such as whether to use random, probability, or cluster sampling strategies, should also be guided by published research and the current, state-of-the-art products in the field. Advanced technologies are now available to facilitate random sampling and can be applied to telephone or web-based surveys (such as random-digit dialing and random email access). Alternatively, increasingly complex probability or cluster sampling devices may be used to achieve efficiencies in research. These techniques facilitate the selection and inclusion of respondents with specific characteristics (eg, area/geography, age, or racial/ethnic characteristic), and the data can be statistically modeled to allow the research results to more fully reflect the population of interest. A more detailed explanation of statistical strategies used in nutrition research can be found in Chapters 25 and 26. Researchers may also want to

refer to other resources and references on these topics.[15,17-20]

Most of the previous discussion has pertained to single-population (sample) surveys. However, researchers may also be interested in comparing two or more populations (or subgroups) of research interest (eg, clinical case vs control participants, program/intervention participants compared with matched nonparticipants, majority populations in contrast to underrepresented minorities). In these situations, researchers carefully sample the various populations or subgroups of interest and ensure that they have sufficient numbers of participants in each category to enable meaningful comparisons between groups.

The definition of the population sampling strategy in conjunction with the methods of data collection are important research planning decisions that affect all aspects of survey operations; furthermore, they also affect decisions about the research project's analytic plan. As a result, plans for data management,

Random sampling: Selecting participants without a specific intended distribution so that each individual has an equal probability of being selected for the study.

Probability sampling: Selecting participants for a study in a way that makes the probability of being selected for the study equal based on certain characteristics. For example, if a researcher wanted to select 100 adults for a study but wanted an equal distribution of age across study participants, he or she would use probability sampling techniques to ensure that the 100 individuals are selected based on the probability of meeting the age spread.

Cluster sampling: Used to randomly select participants for a study where the overall list of potential study participants is very large (eg, selecting 100 adults from the entire US population).

Box 12.3 Key Terms in Sampling Methodology

statistical analysis, and reporting should be outlined in advance of data collection to ensure that budget and resources are appropriately allocated to meet the research goals.

Estimating Statistical Power

Another important planning consideration for researchers is to determine a study's statistical power. Within available resources, researchers need sufficient numbers of survey respondents (ie, adequate study power) to answer the research questions confidently. Depending on the stated research goals and aims, researchers need to be in a position to test the hypotheses; derive sound estimates of the characteristics or outcomes of interest; determine the effect of programs, treatments, or interventions; or explore relationships among research variables. Researchers need to become accustomed to thinking about the study power early in the research planning process in order to arrive at a sound survey research design.

The existing literature provides important information for establishing the power of a research study. Researchers need to review the literature pertaining to the specific research problem area to identify what might be expected for each research question. For example, researchers might be interested in estimating a population's rate of a nutrition-related problem, so they review the available literature to assess what the expected rate(s) might be, including the confidence intervals around the estimates. To accomplish this task, researchers should examine the literature for the following: What proportion of the population of interest might be expected to have a specific nutrition problem (ie, to be overweight and obese)? How do these rates vary in published population estimates? Alternatively, researchers may be interested in determining how a specified nutrition intervention affects some population characteristic of interest. For example, over the 3-week period of a nutrition intervention in which a motivational and a conventional counseling process are being compared, what level of dietary behavior change (changes in energy or other nutrient intakes) might be expected? In another study, researchers might also be interested in examining the strength of association between a dietary exposure (eg, food or nutrient intake, level of

dietary quality) and a potential set of behavioral determinants or certain health outcomes (eg, How strongly correlated is overall diet quality and body weight or body mass index? Is the observed relationship independent of other key macronutrients, micronutrients, or other characteristics of the individual?). In such cases, the literature helps researchers identify the expected study results and potential variation (confidence intervals) around the data estimates. To the extent possible, researchers need to identify and summarize published data on the research questions to make formal calculations of the research study's statistical power. See Chapters 24 and 25 for a more thorough discussion regarding sample size selection and statistical applications for nutrition research.

Final Planning Considerations

A final planning consideration encompasses recruiting, training, and monitoring qualified survey research personnel. All staff need to be suitably experienced and fully trained in the protocols for which they are responsible. Requirements for staff training are guided by the instrument and study protocol designs. Training should also focus on any problems or issues identified in the research pretesting process. Researchers need to apply quality control measures to all staff activities, including sampling, data collection, coding, statistical analyses, and reporting procedures. Quality control at all levels is essential to ensure that requisite research operational procedures are maintained and to achieve confidence in the research.

METHODS OF SURVEY DATA COLLECTION AND QUESTIONNAIRE DESIGN

One of the most important stages of survey research is selecting the mode(s) and method(s) of data collection, including the development of research questionnaires and other data collection protocols. The general options for human survey data collection include self-administered (print or electronic) instruments and interviewer-administered questionnaires (using face-to-face or telephone formats). Data may be collected on one or more individuals in solo or group settings. In-depth consideration of these topics is found in several classic and current texts[15,17-19] and web-based resources.[20] Nonetheless, selected key details of these processes are summarized here with applications to nutrition research.

The mode of data collection selected depends on a variety of factors, including the ease of identifying suitable and available study participants, characteristics of respondents, complexity and sensitivity of the desired survey data, difficulty of reporting or data collection activities, perceived optimal methods of data collection, staffing requirements, and budgetary and resource constraints.[15-17] To make coherent decisions, researchers consider each factor and select a mode or method that best suits the research interests and plan. Ideally, one or more strategies for data collection are selected that allow researchers to collect as complex a set of data as required from a desired sample of suitable respondents and to do this with the most efficient use of resources.

Among the things that researchers consider early in the research planning process is whether the research questions demand that researchers assess one or more domains of an individual's nutritional risk or status, including dietary behavior, anthropometric indexes, clinical characteristics, biomarkers or biological risk factors, and diseases or other health outcomes. It is also important to assess whether information is needed on the environmental determinants of dietary behavior or nutritional risk or other outcomes (such as hospital or long-term care admissions, costs of services). (To make such decisions, review the earlier discussion of Figure 12.1). Once the domains of interest and specific research variables are articulated, researchers can better determine the ideal mode(s) and method(s) of data collection.

The design of the actual survey instrument considers similar factors; researchers weigh the options and arrive at a methodology that best suits the study goals and research questions, characteristics of the participants and project staff, and available financial and related resources and constraints. Early in the planning process, researchers must clearly define each research question and break it into its discrete component variables.[15,17] Experts refer to this process as operationalizing the research questions and variables. Throughout this process, researchers seek to identify a final set of research domains and research questions and to determine the comprehensive list of variables needed to answer all research questions. Each variable is then linked to a method of measurement that will be incorporated into the data collection instrument(s) and protocol(s). In addition, researchers consider how each variable measurement strategy directs the data analysis plan.

A wide range of specific participant characteristics may affect research protocols and methods of data collection, including the respondents' location and researchers' access to them; primary language, literacy levels, level of cognitive function, and memory; functional capacity or disability; and conditions or characteristics that may affect responses or behaviors, such as willingness to participate in the research and likely compliance with protocols. If respondent characteristics pose serious limitations, research protocols must be adjusted. In some situations, proxy respondents may be used if available and as appropriate to the research. Proxy respondents are suitable substitutes if they adequately represent the intended research participant and are able to answer a sufficient number of the research questionnaire items or complete the specified study protocols. For example, food recalls in children often use proxy respondents, such as a parent or caregiver who is best suited to describe the food intake of a young child; obtaining the data from the child directly would be less accurate.

Variable measurement strategies and research protocols also affect research staffing requirements. Researchers conduct training and implement quality control procedures that are appropriate to the data collection activities. These research aspects need to be considered before finalizing the data collection methods and designing and implementing a coherent and suitable plan of research operation.

Ultimately, researchers should settle on data collection and measurement techniques and as complex an evidence-based study design as is feasible and appropriate to the research aims and questions, study population characteristics, and resources. Researchers will always be faced with a wide range of issues and options to consider in setting the research plan and operations. As needed, researchers weigh design complexity against what is suitable and manageable within resource constraints. During this process, data accuracy should not be sacrificed as it only undermines confidence in the research plan and data. Refer to important references on this topic.[15-24]

Data Collection Methods

Survey researchers consider a variety of data collection methods. The most common include qualitative, quantitative, or semiquantitative questionnaires that typically use one of four approaches:

- Self-administered mail protocols
- Self-administered electronic (computer or web-based) protocols
- Interviewer-administered telephone methodologies
- Interviewer-administered face-to-face (in-person) methodologies

In addition, researchers may consider design modifications to increase response rates. For example, researchers may use a group format to complete self-administered questionnaires. Alternatively, researchers might use research staff to hand deliver or pick up surveys. These data collection features may facilitate clarification of questions or responses and enable interactions with survey participants that might increase their participation and completion of protocols.

As noted, depending on the research questions of interest, survey instruments (questionnaires) may be qualitative, semiquantitative, or quantitative in nature. All of these methods are broadly used in survey research. For example, nutrition epidemiologists may assess nutritional exposures in a variety of ways. Qualitative questionnaires may evaluate dietary behaviors (eg, dietary supplement use, self-imposed or professionally recommended dieting). They might also be used to assess environmental factors (including personal characteristics; cultural influences; involvement in private and public nutrition programs, interventions, or treatments) that may influence dietary exposures and health-related

outcomes. Semiquantitative questionnaires, such as certain food frequency instruments, can be used to characterize food intake behavior or to rank-order participants' nutrient intake. Quantitative questionnaires might be used to determine an individual's level of food and nutrient intake or related characteristics and behaviors. The types of survey items and protocols affect the mode of data collection and other dimensions of the research and need to be carefully considered. Methods used to develop various types of questionnaires and specific survey items are discussed in greater detail in the following section.

All the procedures for survey questionnaire administration have strengths and have been used widely in survey research. However, a particular method may have certain advantages or disadvantages when used in a specific study population, in a certain area of research investigation, or with a particular study design. For example, respondents who live in distant locations may be best surveyed using telephone interviews or self-administered techniques (mail or electronic). However, the mail and electronic options may have lower response rates depending on survey content, participant incentives, and accuracy of respondent contact lists (phone numbers and email addresses). Survey research bias may be introduced if respondents do not have access to the mode of data collection (eg, unlisted phone numbers, no email address). Participants who are more readily accessible may provide the option for potentially more complex face-to-face interviewing or in-person survey data collection (as well as the collection of biological samples, anthropometric data, clinical testing, duplicate meals, and so on). The existence of a large and suitable respondent audience in one location may make group-level surveying by self-administered questionnaires another viable alternative. The particular site depends on the nature of the research but might include a mobile research unit, an intervention or clinical site, or a community location.

The mode of data collection also varies with the type of research question or variable. If domains of research interest are quite sensitive, they might be better suited to self-administered methods of data collection that offer higher levels of potential anonymity.[15,17] In contrast, biological, anthropometric, and clinical testing rely on direct respondent contact unless an accurate alternative method of data collection can be identified (such as mailed blood or urine samples for biological testing).

Researchers need to weigh further advantages and disadvantages related to each of the available modes of survey data collection. Interviewer-assisted methods have the advantages of providing a mechanism for personal contact, rapport building, and review of survey questions and responses as well as enabling trained staff to guide respondents through instruments and item sequences. They also allow facilitators to clarify instructions and questions and provide opportunities as needed for interviewer probing of respondent answers. The latter is particularly key if a questionnaire protocol includes complex items. This might include a questionnaire with a large number of items, questions with numerous response categories, or questions that only certain respondents answer. In this situation, instructions may be needed to help respondents successfully navigate the instrument (such as directions to skip certain items).[15-17]

Self-administered questionnaires may ease respondent burden by giving them time to think through responses and, depending on the location of administration, enabling participants to search for necessary data to complete diaries that may facilitate self-reporting or to check records for information that may influence responses. The disadvantages of self-administered protocols, however, are that they may lack a level of quality control seen with other data collection modes; furthermore, they may require higher respondent literacy levels or cognitive functioning and do not enable investigators to control who actually completes the questionnaire. Once again, computer technology can be applied, if feasible, to help maintain levels of quality control and to check for consistency or erroneous responses.

Computer-assisted personal or telephone interviews (termed "CAPI" or "CATI," respectively) may offer further advantages by increasing opportunities for research quality control and increasing anonymity among participants, which may reduce response bias and promote accuracy on survey responses. The system can guide interviewers through the logic and detail of the interview questionnaire and offer prompts, as needed, if they make any mistakes. The main disadvantages of interviewer-administered surveys, regardless of print or electronic administration, are that they tend to be more costly and time consuming.[15-17] They may also pose field management difficulties if respondents are accessible only in dangerous or potentially hazardous settings. Under these circumstances, telephone interviewing may offer economies of time and cost efficiencies and may provide better population access and response rates than mail or electronic methods. Another alternative to consider is the use of hand delivered and picked up instruments. This approach enables survey staff to introduce the instrument, provide instructions, and clarify protocols, as well as possibly provide opportunities to motivate respondents, increase response rates, and check surveys for completeness at pickup.[15-17,19]

Self-administered mailed or web-based surveys are advantageous and cost-efficient, particularly if respondents are not easily accessible or researchers want to increase response rates and provide ease of access. They also offer the aforementioned advantages of allowing respondents time to contemplate and complete instruments. However, they may have only limited capacity to personally guide respondents or offer clarification if needed; furthermore, there may be issues of potential response or nonresponse bias as noted earlier. Yet, web-based platforms and tools can integrate information to make self-administration easier (such as tips on how to measure height, weight, or waist circumference or how to assess food portion size); they can also offer electronic feedback or chat technology to assist respondents who may be having difficulties with platform use or specific survey questionnaire items. The use of evidence-based electronic platforms in nutrition survey research is expanding rapidly and offers tremendous new opportunities to enhance multiple dimensions of research and related practice.[25]

Researchers should carefully consider alternative modes of data collection and select one or more methods that meet the research aims. The domains of research interest may also dictate that questionnaires be combined with the collection of biological, clinical, anthropometric, and potentially other types of data. As noted previously, the goal of data collection methods, however simple or complex, is to achieve a strategy that accomplishes the research aims with the highest level of accuracy possible, the least respondent and staff burden, and resource allocations that enable all stages of the research planning process to be accomplished, including analyses and reporting.

Survey Protocol Design

The design of research instruments and protocols should follow a logical, systematic process that includes operationalizing the research questions and specifying all the information that is needed to achieve the research aims. Ideally, each question is translated into one or more specific research variables. Then, researchers can be more directed when reviewing published literature and web resources for suitable research protocols, instruments, or specific survey items and questions. Consider how variable measurement strategies might influence research operations and staffing. In addition, review how the variable measurement methods dictate the data analysis plan. The final approaches to data collection are those researchers deem to be most suitable, accurate, and feasible within the project's aims, resources, and budget.

Upon selecting data collection methods, researchers then conduct one or more rounds of pretesting that include evaluating the questionnaires, other study protocols if used, and the overall plan of operations. Revisions to instruments and protocols are guided by information gleaned from these activities.

During the instrument and protocol development process, it is important to clearly conceptualize what information is needed to answer each research question as completely as possible. Each research question needs to be formally operationalized such that the data collected are useful.[15] Survey questions can vary greatly in complexity and accuracy (eg, self-report vs observed or measured dietary intake). The complexity of the variable affects the mode of data collection (ie, staff measurement, interview, or self-report). Additionally, data collection can be done on various levels using qualitative,

quantitative, or semiquantitative strategies, each of which may vary in complexity (such as type and format of questions, number of items). As alternative data collection modes and techniques are considered, researchers narrow their selection to those strategies that allow an optimal level and complexity of variable measurement. Researchers should arrive at a set of instruments and protocols that enable them to answer the research questions as completely and accurately as possible after evaluating validity, reliability, and sensitivity to elicit the highest likelihood of respondent participation and completion rates.

Questionnaire Design

When constructing survey questionnaires, there are a number of particularly key considerations. Each research variable is translated into one or more survey items; each item should contain response categories that capture the variable meaningfully and completely.

Survey questions fall into two categories, open ended or closed ended, and are further discussed later in this chapter (page 246). Box 12.4 presents descriptions of these categories.

The items should also meet specific structural requirements Response categories should be mutually exclusive and exhaustive, as shown in Box 12.5.[14,15]

Variable measurement strategies also consider that the qualities and characteristics under investigation may have specific underlying attributes that determine how they are measured and affect subsequent data analyses. Variables can be measured using nominal, ordinal, interval, or ratio scales. Researchers should be aware that variable measurement terminology differs somewhat depending on the survey resources used. For example, variable measurement scales may also be described as discrete, categoric (binary or ranked), or continuous (normally distributed or skewed).[16,17,21] Relationships between this terminology are integrated here.

Nominal variables are also discrete (binary or multiple categoric variables) and meet the aforementioned properties of being exhaustive and

Closed-Ended Question

Limited number of possible responses

Responses can be numeric or categoric

Categoric responses can be ordinal (ranked) or nominal (unordered)

Example: What is your gender? Male or female

Open-Ended Question

Unrestricted response

Allows for more details from participant

Example: What is your usual weekday eating pattern?

Box 12.4 Closed-Ended vs Open-Ended Questions

Criteria	Example

Mutually exclusive	Gender:
	  a) Male
	  b) Female

Exhaustive	Which of the following tools do you use for daily meal planning?
	  a) Menu planning website
	  b) US Department of Agriculture MyPlate Checklists
	  c) Recipes from family/friends
	  d) All of the above
	  e) None of the above

Box 12.5 Question Criteria for Response Categories

mutually exclusive. However, these variables are qualitative and do not have specified or implied quantitative relationships between responses. Researchers might use nominal variable measurement techniques when evaluating a respondent's use of specific food items, types of diets, dietary supplements, or meals (eg, "Do you eat breakfast daily? Yes or No."). Response categories may also include lists of items for a respondent to consider (eg, "Check all that apply."). Researchers might use nominal measurement scales to assess the environmental characteristics that could influence a respondent's nutrition behavior or outcomes (such as the individual's cultural background and characteristics, exposure to nutrition services, family and household characteristics).

Ordinal (ranked, categoric) variables contain response categories that also achieve the structure of being mutually exclusive and exhaustive but generate responses that are logical and rank-ordered. Sample ordinal questions are shown in Figure 12.3 (page 244).

Interval measurement of variables provides ordered continuous response categories with a unique distance between the responses. For example, the difference in intake between 10 and 20 mg of calcium is the same as the difference between 50 and 60 mg of calcium.

Ratio measurement, statistically speaking, is similar to interval measurement, but it also contains a zero point. Many clinical or biological parameters of interest in nutrition research (such as plasma

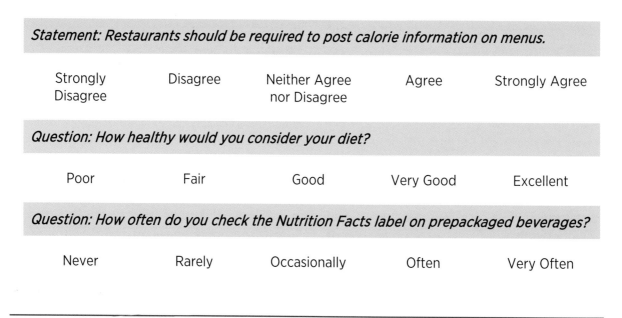

Figure 12.3 Sample statements and questions on an ordinal scale

lipid, glucose, or nutritional biomarkers levels) also use ratio measurement scales—an intake of 0 g of iron is equivalent to the absence of iron intake. Be aware that ratio data can be continuous and normally distributed or skewed. It may require statistical adjustment (such as log transformations) in order to be handled correctly in the analyses.

Depending on the research question, nominal scales may be the only available variable measurement strategy and can be used quite appropriately. If researchers have established the need for quantitative measurement of the research variables, however, appropriate interval or ratio (continuous) scales should be identified or developed to assess the relevant research variables. If the levels of desired variable measurement are not exactly clear at the outset, researchers would be advised to opt for higher levels of quantitative (continuous) measurement. This, of course, depends on whether suitable techniques are available or can be developed and tested within the research timetable.[16,17]

The approaches to variable measurement outlined previously have direct implications for the data analysis plan. Ratio (continuous) measurement, the most quantitative of techniques, is common in survey and nutrition research. Ratio scales meet the underlying assumptions of some of the most complex and informative statistical techniques; thus, they may be particularly useful in nutrition research.

To be successful, survey instruments need to contain suitable and unambiguous wording; researchers need to make certain that instructions, questions, and response categories are clear and understood by staff and respondents and that items cannot be misinterpreted. The terms and conditions used in specific questions need to be well-defined (eg, "Between midnight (day/date) and 8 AM (day/date), do you eat or drink anything other than water?"). Researchers should take care that responses have only single dimensions; double or multiple components (referred to as double-barreled items) should be avoided; for example "How often do you eat apples and peanut butter?" is confusing. It is unclear whether the respondent should answer how often they consume apples, how often they consume peanut butter, or how often they consume both together.

When designing questions for the survey, researchers may incorporate certain qualifying statements to clarify items (eg, "What is the specific time frame of interest?" or "Since midnight, can you describe everything you ate or drank?"). Qualifiers are designed to allow respondents to make a summary judgment (eg, "Considering all sources of influence on your eating behavior, what is most important?"

or "Overall, would you say you are satisfied or not with your experience?"); such items call for qualified adjectives (eg, "Identify your most important source of nutrition information."). These types of categoric survey responses are considered ordinal or ranked responses. See Box 12.4 on page 243 for a sample of ordinal responses for three different types of nutrition survey questions.

As noted earlier, items are constructed to include a set of responses (mutually exclusive and exhaustive) but may actually have a long or complex list that researchers want the respondent to consider. Be careful to make this task as easy as possible for the respondents. Alternatively, open-ended responses allow respondents to provide information in their own form. The process of formatting questionnaires is discussed in further detail in various resources and texts.[15-17,19,20]

Survey Layout

Once the level and complexity of variable measurement levels are established, questions can be carefully formatted and laid out in the survey instruments. Remember that the overall goal of survey research is to collect data in a manageable, defined manner from a carefully identified population using an appropriate array of statements, questions, and protocols. All are designed to achieve the intended level of research complexity, accomplish the study aims, and answer the research questions. A detailed discussion of these topics is found in key references and websites.[15-17,20]

Question ordering in a survey instrument is another consideration. Items can be laid out randomly, but layout is often determined by the method or format of instrument administration. Self-administered questionnaires often begin with the most interesting items in order to engage respondents. Interviewer-administered surveys might begin with the simplest items to gain rapport. Typically, all instruments begin with instructions and other details to set a context for the research.

As with the stages of survey planning, once researchers have drafted the instruments and protocols, they conduct one or more levels of pretesting. Experts may be used to review and comment on item content, format, and overall layout of questionnaires or aspects of the research protocols. Focus groups involving experts on the research topic or a small sample of respondents (similar to the study population of interest) might also react to the protocols. Researchers may also devise small-scale pretests to mimic the survey in operation. Subjecting the instruments and other study protocols to critical review and pretesting is an important step in detecting potential flaws or problems. Researchers continue to revise the research instruments and protocols as this process unfolds. During these procedures, researchers are likely to debrief on a number of occasions with staff and respondents who are involved in the pretests. Researchers may also want to observe staff behavior, participant behavior, or both during pretesting activities to confirm that the research methods work in practice.

The preceding discussion of instrument pretesting assumes that the protocols were previously tested formally for reliability and validity. Instrument reliability and validity are essential for successful survey research. The best survey instruments are both reliable and valid. Instrument validity is an indication of whether the question measures what it was intended to measure; survey reliability is a measure of whether asking the question multiple times yields the same result. Survey questions can be reliable but not valid, and vice versa. Figure 12.4 on page 246 gives a visual explanation of this principle. Reliable questions are those with a great deal of reproducibility—they produce the same answer time and time again (shown with all points to the left of the target). Valid questions are accurate—they correctly identify true information (ie, some points hit the target and some points miss). The best questions are both accurate and reproducible—they correctly identify true information time and time again, hitting the bull's-eye.

If researchers are actually developing new instruments or protocols, they need to be tested in advance of use. The methods of testing for instrument reliability and validity are important in survey research, and readers are guided to explore further in texts such as *A Primer on the Validity of Assessment Instruments*.[26] The development and testing of survey questionnaires and dietary instruments is an active area of research in the field of nutrition and in dietetics practice.

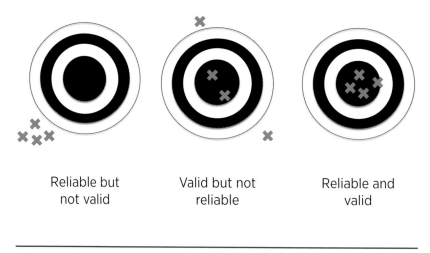

Figure 12.4 Reliability vs validity

Overall, the design of survey instruments should make their administration as easy as possible for respondents and staff; self-administered surveys should be self-explanatory unless researchers intend staff interaction with respondents. Questionnaire items should meet the following characteristics: clear (unambiguous), appropriate to the research, as short as possible, unbiased, and as positive in terminology as possible. Instruments should be clearly formatted and as short as possible. Related items should be clearly linked. All of these features are embedded in the instruments and protocols to make it easier for respondents and staff.

Data Analysis Considerations

Generally speaking, the application of statistical techniques in data analysis is defined by the research questions and variable measurement techniques. As summarized in Table 12.1, researchers can apply methods to compare data from two groups depending on the nature of the survey methods used. If the data were not measured on interval or ratio scales, researchers need to consider options for nonparametric testing.[27] Researchers should be aware that the assignment of numeric codes to nominal and ordinal scale response categories creates continuous data and should not be analyzed as such. Take, for example, the following question regarding tea consumption:

How often do you drink hot tea?

a. Never
b. Less than once a month
c. 1–3 times a month
d. 1–2 times a week
e. 3 times a week or more

If this ordinal list were converted to numeric codes for statistical analysis (never = 1, less than once a month = 2, and so on), the discrete numeric data would imply that the distance between each numeric response is equal, which simply is not correct (the distance between never and less than once a month is not the same as the distance between 1 to 2 times a week and 3 times a week or more) and is difficult to interpret. Instead, the more common approach is to create dummy variables to be used for analysis. These dummy variables recode the categoric data as "Never" or "Non-never" and so on, but again, researchers should be careful in applying and interpreting these variables.

Particularly in nutrition research, data measured using ratio or interval scales may be converted to qualitative or categoric scales for statistical analyses. This is appropriate and may be needed to answer certain research questions. For example, researchers may want to interpret data (such as total saturated fat intake, measured as a percent of total energy intake, or dietary energy density) in relation to expert guidelines (Does saturated fat in-

	Number of Samples			
Type of Data	**Two Paired**	**Two Independent**	**More than Two Paired**	**More than Two Independent**
Nominal	McNemar test	χ^2 or Fisher exact probability test	Cochran Q test	χ^2 test
Ordinal	Sign test or Mann-Whitney U test	Mann-Whitney U test	Friedman two-way ANOVA[a]	Kruskal-Wallis one-way ANOVA
Ratio	Paired t test	Independent t test	Repeated ANOVA	Factorial ANOVA

[a] ANOVA, analysis of variance

Table 12.1 Statistical Tests to Compare Groups

take fall below 7% of energy or not?), so the data are converted to binary or categoric scales. Descriptive analyses based on these newly derived variables might be used to compare study participants who meet expert criteria with those who do not in terms of another characteristic (such as biological risk factors like plasma cholesterol levels). Such variables might also be used in more complex modeling of health or disease outcomes.

A final consideration is the impact of variable measurement on respondents, study personnel, and project implementation. While it is imperative that research questionnaires are designed to achieve study aims using sound and suitably complex methods, they must also be feasible and manageable for research personnel, respondents, and available resources. Before finalizing the instruments and protocols, review and consider their impact on all individuals involved in conducting the research (including intended respondents—and their proxies, as appropriate—and research staff). Be certain that resources are adequate not only for data collection and management but also for analyses and reporting activities. Develop training and quality control activities that ensure the successful completion of all data collection and maintain confidence in the analyses and reporting.

CONCLUSION

The implementation of evidence-based survey research requires researchers to conduct careful systematic planning and adhere to valid, ethical, and strict protocols as discussed in this chapter. Survey research planning is a complex process that needs to be carried out thoughtfully and thoroughly to ensure that the investigation achieves its stated aims and that it adds meaningfully to the literature in a specified research domain. Researchers must consider many options for data collection and evaluate a wide array of factors before settling on the optimal study design, survey instruments, and research protocols.

This chapter has discussed the basic concepts involved in survey planning and questionnaire design. From a research perspective, investigators should better appreciate the importance of a staged planning process for survey research. Researchers should also have a thorough understanding of the methods of survey data collection, options for research variable measurement, and the relationships between data collection strategies and methods of statistical analysis. The hope is that readers will be able to more critically evaluate the survey research literature and will be increasingly comfortable in using survey methodology strategically to inform their own investigations. Among the key uses of the literature are the identification of valid and suitable survey research techniques and protocols as well as the data and information needed to calculate the statistical power of a proposed research study.

If the planning process is carefully accomplished, researchers should have confidence in the overall study design, including the respondent sampling procedures, methods of data collection, and other survey protocols and procedures. Researchers must lay out a sound plan of analysis and have resources allocated to complete all aspects of the work, including research reporting. Researchers must also comprehend the importance of conducting quality control of all survey activities, including staff training, and recognize that research should be carried out according to established protocols and acceptable standards.

Researchers have many opportunities to make professional contributions using survey research. The techniques have been applied to a wide range of nutrition-related areas. Among the most important are the assessment of a population's nutrition and health status and levels of disease risk; progress toward achieving the nation's nutrition and health objectives; development of new techniques of nutritional risk assessment; establishment of relationships between diet and lifestyle behaviors and health-related outcomes; and identification of effective and innovative nutrition services and programs, preventive intervention strategies, and medical nutrition therapies. Survey research methods are well suited to investigations at the individual and population levels. The techniques are also applicable to even broader realms that encompass the food and agriculture, foodservice, pharmaceutical, and health-related industries. Given these widespread applications, dietetics practitioners who develop sound survey research skills are positioned to make important contributions to the exciting and expanding field of nutrition.

REFERENCES

1. National Center for Health Statistics. National Health Interview Survey. www.cdc.gov/nchs/nhis/index.htm. Updated April 4, 2016. Accessed April 24, 2018.

2. Centers for Disease Control and Prevention, National Center for Health Statistics. National Health and Nutrition Examination Survey Questionnaire. www.cdc.gov/nchs/nhanes/nhanes_questionnaires.htm. Accessed May 11, 3018.

3. US Department of Health and Human Services, Office of Disease Prevention and Health Promotion. Healthy People 2020 Framework. www.healthypeople.gov/sites/default/files/HP2020Framework.pdf. Accessed January 22, 2017.

4. US Department of Agriculture, Agricultural Research Service, Food Surveys Research Group. *What We Eat in America, NHANES*. www.ars.usda.gov/northeast-area/beltsville-md-bhnrc/beltsville-human-nutrition-research-center/food-surveys-research-group/docs/wweianhanes-overview. Accessed January 2, 2017.

5. Hu FB. Dietary pattern analysis: a new direction in nutrition al epidemiology. *Curr Opin Lipidol*. 2002;1(1)3:3-9.

6. Kennedy ET, Ohls J, Carlson S, Fleming K. The Healthy Eating Index: design and applications. *J Am Diet Assoc*. 1995;95(10):1103-1108.

7. Haines PS, Siega-Riz AM, Popkin BM. The Dietary Quality Index revised: a measurement instrument for populations. *J Am Diet Assoc*. 1999;99(6):697-704.

8. Murabito JM, Garrison RJ, Millen BE. Lifestyle issues. In: Levy D, ed. *Fifty Years of Discovery: Medical Milestones from the National Heart, Lung and Blood Institute's Framingham Heart Study*. Hackensack, NJ: Center for Bio-Medical Communications; 1999:252-259.

9. Millen BE, Quatromoni PA, Copenhafer DL, Demissie S, O'Horo CE, D'Agostino RB. Validation of a dietary pattern approach for evaluating nutritional risk: the Framingham Nutrition Studies. *J Am Diet Assoc*. 2001;101(2):87-94.

10. Millen BE, Pencina MJ, Kimokoti RW, Meigs JB, Ordovas JM, D'Agostino RB. Nutritional risk and the metabolic syndrome in women: opportunities for preventive intervention from the Framingham Nutrition Study. *Am J Clin Nutr*. 2006;84(2):434-441.

11. Story M, Kaphingst KM, Robinson-O'Brien R, Glanz K. Creating healthy food and eating environments. Policy and environmental approaches. *Annu Rev Public Health*. 2008;29:253-272.

12. Millen BE, Pencina MJ, Kimokoti RW, D'Agostino RB. The Framingham Nutrition Studies: insights into weight history, dietary patterns, obesity prevention, and risk reduction (Abstract). Summary: Predictors of Obesity, Weight Gain, Diet, and Physical Activity Workshop; 2004. www.nhlbi.nih.gov/events/2004/predictors-obesity -weight-gain-diet-and-physical-activity-workshop-2004. Accessed May 10, 2018.

13. US Department of Agriculture, US Department of Health and Human Services. Scientific Report of the 2015 Dietary Guidelines Advisory Committee: Advisory Report to the Secretary of Health and Human Services and the Secretary of Agriculture. https://ods.od.nih.gov/pubs/2015_DGAC _Scientific_Report.pdf. Published February 2015. Accessed April 24, 2018.

14. US Department of Health and Human Services, US Department of Agriculture. 2015–2020 Dietary Guidelines for Americans. 8th ed. https://health.gov/dietaryguide lines/2015/resources/2015-2020_Dietary_Guidelines.pdf. Published December 2015. Accessed April 24, 2018.

15. Czaja RF, Blair J. *Designing Surveys: A Guide to Decisions and Procedures*. 3rd ed. Thousand Oaks, CA: Sage Publications; 2014.

16. Fowler FJ. *Survey Research Methods*. 5th ed. London: Sage Publications; 2003.

17. Babbie E. *The Practice of Social Research*. 13th ed. Belmont, CA: Wadsworth Publishing; 2013.

18. Czaja RF, Blair J. *Designing Surveys: A Guide to Decisions and Procedures*. 3rd ed. Thousand Oaks, CA: Sage Publications; 2014.

19. Fowler FJ, Mangione TW. *Standardized Survey Interviewing. Minimizing Interviewer-Related Error*. Newbury Park, CA: Sage Publications; 1990.

20. Kiernan NE. *Creating Valid Answer Categories*. Tipsheet #59. University Park, PA: Penn State Cooperative Extension; 2001.

21. Kiernan NE. *Crafting Questions With Less Bias*. Tipsheet #35. University Park, PA: Penn State Cooperative Extension; 2001.

22. Glanz K, Rimer B. *Theory at a Glance: A Guide to Health Promotion Practice*. 2nd ed. Rockville, MD: National Cancer Institute; 2012.

23. Glanz K, Rimer B, Viswanath K, eds. *Health Behavior: Theory, Research, and Practice*. 5th ed. San Francisco, CA: Jossey-Bass Publishers; 2015.

24. Green LW, Kreuter. *Health Promotion Planning. An Educational and Environmental Approach*. 4th ed. New York, NY: McGraw-Hill; 2004.

25. Kimokoti RW, Millen BE. Nutrition for the prevention of chronic diseases. *Med Clin North Am*. 2016;100(6):1185-1198.

26. Sullivan GM. A primer on the validity of assessment instruments. *J Grad Med Educ*. 2011;3(2):119-120.

27. Ajetunmobi O. *Making Sense of Critical Appraisal*. London, United Kingdom: Hodder Headline Group; 2002.

13

Dietary Assessment Methods and Validation

Linda Van Horn, PhD, RDN

LEARNING OBJECTIVES

1. Describe the purpose of diet assessment.

2. Contrast various methods and their uses.

3. Categorize the study design priorities requiring specific methods.

4. Distinguish appropriate validation methods for developing specific assessment tools.

5. Recognize diet assessment resources available for choosing validated methods.

Assessment of dietary intake is a complex process that requires consideration of several different elements before choosing the best approach. Diet is increasingly recognized as a primary determinant of health and disease at all ages, but a single, standardized, validated approach to diet assessment does not exist. Likewise, despite many advances in biostatistical analyses relevant to diet assessment, lingering questions remain regarding choice of one approach vs another that further complicate interpretation of results. This chapter reviews dietary assessment methods appropriate for research involving individual and group intakes of various nutrients, foods, food groups, or dietary patterns. Choosing the best assessment method requires researchers to consider the study purpose, level of precision, specific population, time period of interest, and available resources.

The chapter further addresses the importance of using validated dietary intake methodology. Dietary assessment and validation of dietary intakes are increasingly incorporated into the design of national and international nutrition status and epidemiologic studies.[1-4] Methods for estimating national food availability or disappearance data are described in other publications.[5-9] Their major use is to measure the adequacy of the food supply and to assess dietary trends among and within countries. Armstrong and Doll[8] correlated per capita food and nutrient intakes from selected countries with cancer incidence or mortality rates to illustrate associations of diet and disease, such as the hypothesized relationships of dietary fat and breast cancer and of meat and colon cancer. Such correlations provide leads for further research but cannot be used to demonstrate cause and effect or true associations, as discussed by Willett.[4] Chapter 14 of this book reviews the US Department of Agriculture (USDA) National Nutrition Monitoring System used in the United States to identify dietary intakes of Americans. This method has also been used in other selected countries.[10]

Several methods have been developed to assess dietary intake, including the 24-hour dietary recall (eg, the five-step, automated, multiple-pass method), food records or diaries, diet histories, and food frequency questionnaires (FFQs). Often more than one method is used in a particular study, and the methods should be tested for reproducibility, comparability, and validity of the reported dietary intake data. Increasingly, studies attempt to include an objective biomarker—such as doubly labeled water for energy intake; urinary measures of protein, potassium, or sodium; or blood levels of carotenoids—to enhance the validity and accuracy of certain measures.[11,12] Chapter 16 reviews the rationale and methodology involved with conducting biomarker studies. The opportunity to blend approaches to estimate intake has added considerably to our knowledge of nutrient needs and potential excesses and deficiencies.[13,14]

To augment this chapter, readers are also referred to extensive descriptions of existing assessment methods, illustrations of questionnaires, and validation studies described by Thompson and Subar.[1] Also the National Cancer Institute (NCI) website (https://dietassessmentprimer.cancer.gov) has a Dietary Assessment Primer that provides a comprehensive overview of the topic and available resources (see Figure 13.1 on page 252). The aim of this chapter is to briefly review the individual methods by discussing strengths and limitations and providing selected examples of their use. Reproducibility of methods and techniques for cross-comparisons and validation of dietary methods using biomarkers are also illustrated.

24-HOUR DIETARY RECALL: INTERVIEWER ADMINISTERED

In collecting a 24-hour dietary recall, the interviewer (ideally a registered dietitian nutritionist or a nonnutritionist trained in the use of the method) obtains information on all food items consumed during the previous 24 hours, the previous day, or a defined 24-hour period. Traditionally, diet information was recorded and coded by hand, and then the data were entered into analysis software. Increasingly today, data are recorded utilizing a computer programmed to achieve this function.[15,16] Interviewers benefit from knowledge of foods available in the community, usual eating and cooking practices, and probing methods to specify other relevant data. Once the respondent reports the food he or she consumed, interviewers typically follow computer-driven steps to collect further details. Recalls may be administered face-to-face or by telephone with similar results.[17] Visual aids, such as food models, geometric models, photographs, or household measuring utensils may be useful to help a respondent estimate the quantities he or she consumed.[18] The goal is to minimize errors and increase reliability of interviewing.[19] Standardized approaches among interviewers, including taped telephone interviews, can improve quality control and have been used in multiethnic population studies using 24-hour dietary recalls to calibrate a mailed quantitative FFQ.[20]

Historically, from 1965 to 1991, the USDA used the 24-hour dietary recall combined with 2

Diet Assessment Primer Roadmap

What would you like to do?	Visit this section	Components
Learn about self-report dietary assessment instruments.	Instrument Profiles	24-hour recall (24HR) Food record (FR) Food frequency questionnaire (FFQ) Screeners
	Comparing Dietary Assessment Instruments	Comparing instruments table
Learn about key concepts in dietary assessment.	Key Concepts	Measurement error Validation
Learn how to use self-report instruments to address different research questions.	Choosing an Approach for Dietary Assessment	Principles Underlying Recommendations Details of Recommendations and Further Considerations o Describing Dietary Intake o Examining the Association between Diet as an Independent Variable & a Dependent Variable o Examining the Association between an Independent Variable & Diet as a Dependent Variable Evaluating the Effect of an Intervention on Diet
	Choosing an Approach for Dietary Assessment Table	Comparing approaches table
Learn more about specific aspects of dietary assessment research.	Learn More	Biomarkers Calibration Combining Instruments Day-of-Week Effect Diet History Dietary Supplements and Estimating Total Nutrient Intakes Deriving Group-level Estimates from Individual-level Intakes Energy Adjustment Food Composition Databases for 24-hour Dietary Recalls and Food Records Food Composition Databases for Food Frequency Questionnaires and Screeners Misreporting Normal Distribution Observation and Feeding Studies Outliers Ratios and Proportions Reactivity Regression Calibration Scoring Algorithms for Screeners Season Effect Social Desirability Software for 24-Hour Dietary Recalls (24HR) and Food Records Software for Food Frequency Questionnaires and Screeners Statistical Modeling Surrogate Reporting Technology in Dietary Assessment Usual Dietary Intakes
Understand the terminology.	Glossary of Key Terms	Glossary
Find articles cited in the Primer and become familiar with related resources.	References & Resources	References Resources

Figure 13.1 National Cancer Institute Diet Assessment Primer Roadmap

Adapted from National Cancer Institute. Dieatry Assessment Primer Roadmap. https://dietassessmentprimer.cancer.gov/roadmap.html. Accessed May 26, 2018.

subsequent days of food records to derive average daily intakes of randomized samples of the US population in its nationwide food consumption surveys.[7] After 1991, the USDA began using 2 days of 24-hour dietary recalls in its nationwide surveys.[21] Similarly, the National Health and Nutrition Examination Survey (NHANES) used 24-hour recalls, as well as frequencies of various food items, in its surveys of stratified national probability samples of the population.[22,23] Since 1999, NHANES has been conducted as a continuous survey, and in 2002, it merged with USDA's Continuing Survey of Food Intake by Individuals, using the 24-hour dietary recall component, What We Eat in America Study.[17,24-26] Since 2003, NHANES has continued to collect two 24-hour recalls, one in person and one over the telephone 7 to 10 days later, sometimes coupled with targeted FFQs in some of the NHANES cycles.[27]

The major strength of the 24-hour dietary recall is its ability to compare groups of individuals. The landmark Ni-Hon-San study among men of Japanese ancestry living in San Francisco, Hawaii, and Japan demonstrated a stepwise increase in dietary fat intake and a similar decrease in carbohydrate intake going westward from Japan to Hawaii to San Francisco, that paralleled the increase in coronary heart disease mortality rates among these populations.[28] The NHANES continually collects biological, anthropometric, and physiological measurements on diverse individuals that then constitute the What We Eat in America database that is used in evaluating the US population's diet and informing the dietary guidelines development every 5 years.[29-31]

An advantage of the interviewer-administered 24-hour dietary recall is the minimal burden it places on participants. In addition, if unannounced, the recall is unlikely to alter eating behavior and general willingness to respond to the interviewer. Direct coding of the foods reported during the interview using automated software helps to further specify and clarify the information needed.[32,33]

USDA surveys are conducted on a continuous basis on a 2-year cycle. The Automated Multiple-Pass Method (AMPM) 24-hour dietary recall was designed specifically to limit underreporting of food intake by conducting five distinct passes to gather diet data from midnight to midnight of the preceding day and uses a computer-assisted interview[34:]

- **First pass—quick list:** The interviewer asks, "Please recall everything you ate and drank during previous day." This pass uses any recall strategy the respondent chooses without interruptions.

- **Second pass—forgotten foods:** The interviewer asks, "Please consider whether you may have eaten any other foods not mentioned in the quick list." For example, breakfast cereal, would trigger the interviewer to ask whether milk was consumed with the cereal and, if so, the type and amount.

- **Third pass—review:** The interviewer reviews the list of foods mentioned and probes for additional eating times and occasions (for example, "Did you eat anything between your 5:00 PM dinner and midnight?").

- **Fourth pass—detail cycle:** The interviewer asks more difficult, detail-oriented questions to elicit descriptions of foods, food preparation, additions, and portion sizes.

- **Fifth pass—final probe review:** The interviewer gives the respondent one last opportunity to remember any foods consumed.

Another limitation of 24-hour recalls, besides underreporting, is the large intraindividual variability in food and nutrient intakes of most individuals; thus, more than a single 24-hour recall is required to estimate the usual intakes of one individual.[1] Multiple 24-hour recalls obtained on random days over a 1-year interval are considered to provide a satisfactory picture of the usual diet estimates for group data analyses. A minimum of 2 days is typically considered satisfactory, but, preferably, more recalls are better the longer the time period. When group assessment is the objective, the interviews should be scheduled on various days of the week to account for daily variation in food choices, particularly between weekdays and weekends, as well as between weeks and seasons of the year. Individual data analyses require modeling to assess usual intake on the group level to correct for day-to-day variability but are considered inadequate for clinical purposes.

Automated Self-Assessed 24-Hour Recalls

A major breakthrough in diet assessment methodology over the past decade has been the technological advances made in computerized self-administration of 24-hour recalls.

The most widely used recall is the Automated Self-Administered Recall System (ASA24), a 24-hour dietary assessment tool developed at the NCI,[3,35,36] which allows researchers and clinicians to apply many elements of the USDA's AMPM 24-hour interviewer-administered recall with use of photographs and other detailed prompts to help individuals document their dietary intake over the previous 24 hours.[18] The system is a freely available web-based, self-administered recall or record based on recent USDA dietary data and can be accessed on desktop, notepad, and mobile phone technologies.[37-41] The ASA24 requires literacy and comfort with computers, but interviewer assistance can accommodate such concerns. For detailed information, instructions, and access to ASA24, including a very comprehensive literature review and training tools, go to the ASA24 website (https://asa24.nci.nih.gov).

FOOD RECORDS OR DIARIES

To complete a food record or diary, participants weigh, measure, or estimate and then record all foods consumed over a specified period of time, usually 3 to 7 consecutive days or multiple periods within a year. This method benefits from clear instructions, demonstrations, and—ideally—some observations. Generally, individuals who agree to participate are inherently dedicated, highly motivated, and literate and thus may not be representative of the general population. Although research participants are typically asked to follow their usual dietary patterns, they may modify their usual eating practices to reduce their workload (for example, substituting a frozen dinner or simple ingredients rather than preparing their usual recipe to prevent having to write down all of the details).

The greatest accuracy is achieved by weighing all ingredients in recipes, measuring the exact portion selected, and measuring plate waste. This is generally feasible only among individuals familiar with using scales calibrated in grams and kilograms in their own food preparation or in the work setting.[42] Household measuring utensils, such as cups and spoons, have been used more frequently than scales in food record studies in the United States[1]; however, weighed food records are more common in the United Kingdom and Europe, where kitchen scales are commonly used.[43,44] In both instances, directions should be included concerning methods of estimating and recording food items consumed away from home. Other methods of quantifying consumption have been reported. Methods involving photographic assessment of food intake and self-monitoring apps are now available and increasingly preferred over more traditional handwritten diaries.[45,46]

Food records do not rely on memory but are considered reactive and thus acceptable for assessing a individual's true usual intake for a day at a time. Multiple records (minimum of two but preferably more as time and budget permit) or recalls on nonconsecutive days can be used as a reference or standard for validating other dietary methods that rely on long-term recall.[1] With the advent of biomarkers, objective measures of nutrients derived from blood, urine, or other body fluids or tissues, validation of diet assessment methods can be more specific and accurate.[14,47] Indeed, none of the dietary intake methods (weighed food records, 24-hour recalls, FFQs, or diet history questionnaires) gives completely accurate estimates of usual energy (calorie) intakes of individuals, but careful documentation can help.[48,49] Low energy reporting is recognized as a major limitation in diet assessment, especially among individuals who are overweight or obese.[50,51] Regardless, food records and recalls are useful in developing structured FFQs, especially for a particular population of interest, such as children, the elderly, or a specific ethnic group.

Beyond reactivity, the necessary motivation, and the literacy required, limitations of food records include the inaccuracy associated with eating out, travel, illness, and the time period selected for collecting and recording intakes, among others.[42]

Intraindividual Variability of Diet

Neither single/multiple 24-hour dietary recalls nor food records are sufficient for identifying exact intakes. Day-to-day, week-to-week, or season-to-season intake variability cannot be captured with just a few days of intake. This is particularly true in developed countries, but it is increasingly true in developing countries as well.

Variability of diet within person (or intraindividual) and variation between persons (interindividual variation) represent major considerations in choosing the best assessment method. Intraindividual variation represents day-to-day differences in intake and is generally as large as or larger than interindividual variation.[52-57] Consequently, a longer time period is needed to characterize the individual's usual diet than the usual diet of a group of individuals. Several investigators have analyzed the variability in multiple 24-hour dietary recalls and food records and determined the number of days needed to achieve reliable estimates of average nutrient intakes of individuals.[1,4] For example, in a study of 29 adults who measured and recorded their food intakes for 1 year, Basiotis and colleagues[53] found that 57 days were needed to estimate the total fat intake within 10% of the true average individual intakes for men with 95% confidence, whereas 71 days were needed for women. For vitamin A, 390 days were needed for men and 474 days for women. When the objective was to estimate mean intakes of the group with precision, a smaller number of days of food records was needed—specifically, 6 days to estimate fat intakes of both men and women and approximately 40 days to estimate the vitamin A intakes with 95% confidence. Research needs can be met with multiple days for group data. Clinical assessment for individuals is much more challenging and requires careful consideration based on the diagnosis, medical concerns, and specific nutrient needs involved.

To learn more about measurement error, validation, and other key concepts related to selecting the best assessment tool, readers are encouraged to access the aforementioned NCI Dietary Assessment Primer[59] (https://dietassessmentprimer.cancer .gov), which offers readers extensive details and rationale for choosing a specific diet assessment instrument.

DIET HISTORIES

For research concerning the etiology of diseases, such as cancer and heart disease, investigators seek information on the usual diet consumed over a longer time frame. The first and classic diet history to assess the usual diet was conceived by Burke,[59] who developed a subjective interview administered by highly trained dietitians. This very comprehensive method included a 24-hour recall with typical variations (such as information on the different fruits that might be eaten at breakfast), a checklist of foods consumed over the preceding month (or the previous 3 to 6 months), and a 3-day record of foods weighed and measured by each participant. From these data, the dietitians calculated the average daily intake of energy and nutrients. This method was used in research concerning diet and child growth[60,61] and was subsequently modified for use in epidemiologic studies of diet and heart disease.[62,63]

More recently, a diet history was developed for use in the study of Coronary Artery Risk Development in Young Adults (CARDIA) that has been continued for more than 35 years.[64,65] However, the subjective diet history is time-consuming, is expensive, and involves a highly skilled professional to collect and process the data, thereby minimizing the number of studies that opt to use this diet assessment method.

FOOD FREQUENCY QUESTIONNAIRES

Burke's[59] checklist was the forerunner of the many structured FFQs in use today. The basic premise of FFQs is that the average long-term dietary intake reflects the conceptually important exposure relevant to the development of disease or risk of disease vs dietary intake over a few specific days. Precision is sacrificed, but simplicity, convenience, cost, and participant self-administration provide distinct advantages over other methods. Most FFQs are computerized or can be optically scanned for analysis. Examples of FFQs that currently remain in use include the Harvard University or Willett Food Frequency Questionnaire,[66] the Block Questionnaires,[67] the Fred Hutchinson Cancer Research Center Questionnaire,[68] and the NCI's Diet History Questionnaire (https://epi.grants.cancer.gov/dhq2). This objective method is based on lists of selected foods and groups of foods with similar nutrient values. The grouping of foods can simplify and abbreviate the data collection, but it confounds the results because of the loss of precision regarding the specific foods consumed in potentially variable amounts, especially among certain ethnic subgroups.[69,70]

Selection of Food Items for the FFQ

Selection of food items for the FFQ is appropriately based on the study population's eating patterns. General guidelines are to choose foods that are consumed by a sizable number of individuals, vary in frequency and quantity among the population, and provide significant amounts of all dietary components. These food items may be selected using various methods. For example, Tucker and colleagues[71] used 24-hour dietary recalls to describe the major food and nutrient contributors, recipes, and portion sizes commonly used from a representative sample of the study population. Others have used population data, such as 24-hour recalls of adults participating in national surveys,[72,73] to select representative food items for questionnaires. Due to ever-changing food supply, FFQs are modified or expanded periodically to account for additional or replacement foods on the market or to test particular hypotheses.[4,74]

Semiquantitative vs Quantitative FFQs

FFQs that solicit frequency responses only or that list a standard serving size are called semiquantitative FFQs. The questionnaires developed for the Nurses' Health Study[75] and the Male Health Professionals Follow-Up Study[76] exemplify this method. Frequencies are obtained by checking the appropriate column showing ranges per day, week, month, or year. The nutrient intakes are then computed by multiplying the midpoint of the frequency interval by the nutrients in the specified portion of the food. This method may be satisfactory when the respondents consume similar amounts—for example, 3 oz of meat or a half cup of vegetables—but not if the usual portions of some participants differ markedly from the portions specified and if the respondents do not adjust the frequencies accordingly. In general, studies have found that the frequency of eating particular foods was a greater determinant of nutrient intakes than quantity and that the use of a single serving size did not introduce a large systematic bias; but, of course, the accuracy of energy intake at the individual level is limited.[77]

Various techniques have been used to help participants estimate amounts consumed using an FFQ that includes visuals (eg, illustrations and photographs).[78] New innovations in automated diet assessment, such as ASA24, provide illustrations of portion sizes to accompany self-reported dietary intake. This can facilitate more accurate documentation of portion sizes.[58]

Before implementing any dietary research instrument, researchers should pretest it extensively among representative samples of the population.[1,4] Pretesting a food frequency instrument should include a write-in section for participants to list other items usually eaten. If the questionnaire will be self-administered by mail, administered by telephone interview, or completed online, trial runs should be conducted among representative samples of the study population. In some geographic areas it may be desirable to translate the instrument into other languages to ensure that participants will comprehend it. Likewise, if particular groups will be studied, such as the elderly, children, pregnant women, or other distinct populations, videotapes or observations may be needed to obtain an accurate estimate of individual intakes. Figure 13.2 compares the different assessment methods based on research needs and priorities.

Comparing Dietary Assessment Instruments

This table provides an at-a-glance comparison of the major features of self-report instruments for assessing diet. Further details on each instrument can be found in the Instrument Profiles. Considerations for the use of different instruments or combinations of instruments in different types of studies can be found in Choosing an Approach for Dietary Assessment.

		24-Hour Recall (24HR)	Food Record (FR)	Food Frequency Questionnaire (FFQ)	Screener (SCR)
Study Design	Cross-sectional	X	X	X	X
	Retrospective			X	X
	Prospective	X	X	X	X
	Intervention	X		X	X
Scope of interest	Total diet	X	X	X	
	One or a few components			X	X
Captures contextual details regarding food preparation, timing of meals, location of meals, etc.	Yes	X	X		
	No			X	X
Time frame of interest	Short term	X	X		
	Long term			X	X
Can be used to query diet in distant past	Yes			X	X
	No	X	X		
Allows cross-cultural comparisons	Yes	X	X		
	No			X	X
Major type of measurement error	Random	X	X		
	Systematic			X	X
Potential for reactivity	High		X		
	Low	X		X	X
Time required to complete	<15 min				X
	>20min	X	X	X	
Memory requirements	Specific	X			
	Generic			X	X
	Does not rely on memory		X		
Cognitive difficulty	High			X	X
	Low	X	X		

Figure 13.2 National Cancer Institute comparison of dietary assessment instruments

Adapted from National Cancer Institute. Comparing Dietary Assessment Instruments. https://dietassessmentprimer.cancer.gov/profiles/table.html. Accessed May 26, 2018.

BRIEF DIET ASSESSMENT INSTRUMENTS (SCREENERS)

As described by Thompson and Subar,[1] a variety of brief assessment tools have been developed to focus on specific foods, food groups, nutrients, or other targeted aspects of the diet.

Because comprehensive FFQs often include over 100 responses, this can be unnecessarily time-consuming as a self-reported instrument if the focus is more specific. Instead, brief assessment tools often focus on relatively fewer responses, for example, fruits and vegetables, fats and oils, sugar-sweetened beverages, or other categories of research interest. The NCI[79] has developed a registry of such brief assessment tools and targeted instruments that are available for review. Screeners have also been developed to assess diet adherence to recommended dietary guidelines, such as the Dietary Approaches to Stop Hypertension (DASH)[80] diet and the diet associated with the Healthy Eating Index (HEI).[81] There are numerous ways of augmenting or combining different assessment tools to better target key eating behaviors of interest. For example, a screener or other FFQ can be enhanced by a food propensity questionnaire (FPQ) that queries other foods beyond those listed to determine whether a particular individual might consume that food on certain days or occasions not captured by the assessment tool. These FPQs typically do not include portion sizes and are best suited to enhance data from recalls or food records.[79]

POTENTIAL ERRORS OF INDIVIDUAL DIETARY INTAKE METHODS

No individual methods of dietary assessment are free from error, but knowing the likely sources can facilitate approaches to minimize these problems. Briefly, in 24-hour dietary recalls, records, and diet histories, participants may fail to recall all foods and amounts consumed, partly because they were not involved in food preparation and may not be aware of the components, ingredients, preparation techniques, or amounts used. Due to issues of social desirability, they may want to please the interviewer by ignoring consumption of an alcoholic beverage or an excessive intake of candy, chips, or desserts. They may substitute a different food for the one actually consumed (substitution error) because they believe certain foods are good or bad for health. Also, large intakes tend to be underestimated and small intakes overestimated.[4]

The food composition databases are also not error free, but the values published by the USDA are carefully selected averages from various sources and are reviewed and revised periodically. Beginning in 1972, these reviews and revisions incorporated new dietary components and updated analyses to the existing database.[82] This database remains the relevant primary resource for studies in the United States, but it may need supplementation from other publications and sources, such as Pennington and Spungen[83] and the Minnesota Nutrition Data System,[84] as well as from subsequent additions, commercial tables, and laboratory analyses of local foods. Food composition tables may include imputed values for some nutrients. Other potential contributors to error include seasonality, old data (nutrients measured long ago), and use of averages from a food database to estimate exposure to certain nutrients/micronutrients. Although differences exist between calculated and analyzed values of food intake data,[85,86] these errors cannot be eliminated in large population studies.

Failure to identify a relationship between a dietary variable and a disease does not necessarily mean the absence of an association. For example, there has been inconsistent evidence from epidemiologic studies on the relationship of dietary fat and breast cancer.[87,88] This inconsistency may be due to the homogeneity of fat intakes within populations, substantial measurement error in dietary assessment,[89-91] large intraindividual variation in dietary fat intakes,[92] and selective underreporting of high-fat foods.[92]

Measurement error may be a significant problem in large population or cohort studies that include subgroups for whom a single FFQ may perform differently; this fact complicates comparisons between the groups.[20] A number of biomarkers are being used to both validate and calibrate dietary assessments instruments.[1,13]

Validity and Reproducibility of Dietary Intake Data

To promote confidence in dietary data and diet-disease findings, the dietary method should be tested for both validity and reproducibility (ie, reliability) in a representative sample of the study population. Although it would be expedient to use a method evaluated in another population, the instrument is appropriate only if the eating patterns of the reference and study populations are similar. Structured quantitative FFQs, in particular, should be tailored to the eating patterns of the study population. For example, a valid and reproducible questionnaire developed for nurses or health professionals in the United States would most likely not be appropriate for a multiethnic randomized population of Japanese Americans, Latinos, African Americans, Native Hawaiians, and whites living in Hawaii and Los Angeles.[93]

Several studies and reviews have been reported on the evaluation of particular dietary methods, including Thompson and Subar's[1] succinct and comprehensive review. The NCI also maintains a web-based register of validation and calibration studies.[94,95] This chapter includes only a brief review to illustrate the study objectives, general protocols, and relevant findings.

Dietary Validity or Comparability

Dietary validity is the ability of an instrument to measure what it purports to measure in regard to diet, such as the intake in a particular meal or day or the usual diet consumed during the past year. Validation requires comparison with the truth, and the truth is impossible to measure among free-living individuals for extended periods. Dietary validity studies during short time intervals have been assessed by surreptitiously weighing foods of individuals eating in an institutional setting and then asking the participants the following day to recall what they ate.[96-99] FFQs were validated by measuring the relative validity of the new instrument compared with a method, such as weighed/measured food records or multiple recalls, that had evidence of greater accu-

racy.[4,20,100,101] Currently, recovery biomarkers are now more commonly compared with dietary intake to validate food intake measurements.[47,102]

FFQs are being used in several large cohort studies on diet and disease in the United States, Europe, and elsewhere.[39,43,101,103] In these investigations, participants (preferably randomly selected among participants defined by age, gender, ethnicity, or profession) complete an FFQ at the start of the study. Several years later, the original dietary intakes are tested for associations with diseases that may have developed, such as cancer and heart disease. The aim is to identify dietary and other environmental or genetic factors that may be related to risk of disease. The findings, if confirmed among multiple populations and substantiated with biological research, may be used to identify potential risks and, it is hoped, to prevent these diseases. A major problem is that estimates of risk within cohorts can be substantially attenuated by measurement errors in assessing individual intakes.[20] These problems are increased in cohort studies that include subgroups in which the questionnaire may perform differently. Consequently, the use of calibration substudies, in which data from the questionnaires are compared with a second source that is assumed to provide an unbiased estimate, allows researchers to correct risk estimates for measurement error.[14] In these studies, investigators begin by assuming that there is error in FFQs. Thus, rather than trying to validate the frequency data, statistical methods, such as regression calibration and correlated measurement errors, are used to adjust the dietary intakes of each participant within the subgroup.[104-107]

USE OF BIOMARKERS TO VALIDATE DIETARY INTAKE METHODS

All the traditional dietary intake methods (24-hour dietary recalls, food records, diet histories, and FFQs) rely on information reported by the participants themselves. Because self-reported information is known to be error prone, results can only be verified by the use of external independent markers of intake.[108] A biomarker is defined as a variable measured in body fluids or tissues that independently reflects the intake of a food component.[109] Examples include 24-hour urinary measures of dietary sodium or potassium intake, serum levels of folate, or, more currently, fecal measure of microbes relevant to the gut microbiome.

Doubly Labeled Water

Doubly labeled water (DLW) remains the most widely used and well-accepted biomarker; it is used as an ideal measure of individuals' free-living total energy expenditure. Lifson and colleagues[110] originally described the DLW method for use in small animals in the 1940s. It is based on the principle that carbon dioxide production can be estimated by the difference in elimination rates of body hydrogen and oxygen. These researchers concluded that the oxygen in expired carbon dioxide was derived from total body water resulting from the equilibrium between the oxygen in body water and the oxygen in respiratory carbon dioxide.[111,112] Based on this finding, the researchers predicted that carbon dioxide production could be indirectly measured by separately labeling both the hydrogen and oxygen pool of the body water with naturally occurring, stable isotopes. In 1982, Schoeller and van Santen[112] first used this technique to measure total energy expenditure in free-living humans.

The DLW method provides an accurate measure of the total energy expenditure in free-living participants and is now well accepted as an unbiased instrument to assess the validity of tools designed to measure energy intake if individuals are in energy balance.[113] The DLW technique has numerous advantages, including ease of administration and the participant's ability to engage in free-living activities during the measurement period. This characteristic is extremely advantageous when the DLW method is used as an objective criterion measure to validate self-reported estimates of dietary intake because the participant is not confined to a clinical research setting (such as a whole-room calorimeter) where usual activities are restricted. Most important, the method is accurate and has a precision between 2% and 8%.[114] Unfortunately, the expense of the stable isotopes (well over $100 per dose for an adult of average weight) and the expertise required to operate the highly sophisticated and costly mass spectrometer

for analysis of the isotopes are the primary disadvantages to this method. Researchers used this approach in the classic European Prospective Study of Diet and Cancer (EPIC)[115] and the Observing Protein and Energy Nutrition (OPEN) study.[31,47]

Other Biomarkers

In recent years several other biomarkers, mostly derived from blood or urine, that reflect nutrient intake have attracted considerable attention in nutrition epidemiology and are being used to validate dietary assessment methods.[12,116] Chapter 16 reviews this topic much more extensively. Briefly, the origins of diet assessment involving biomarkers trace back to studies of fatty acids in the blood to provide objective evidence of intakes of eicosapentaenoic acid and docosahexaenoic acid, as well as fish, which is significantly related to concentrations of these fatty acids in plasma phospholipids.[117] In this study, dietary intake data generated from an FFQ were validated when both dietary and biomarker data classified individuals into similar groupings of intake. This type of analysis can increase confidence that the estimated intake actually reflects the intake of a nutrient or a food containing that nutrient.[118] For example, a biomarker confirming the quintile distributions of fat intake would have added substantially to the credibility of reports suggesting that a diet providing 30% of energy as fat was unlikely to result in a substantial reduction in the risk of breast cancer[119] or that total dietary fat was not associated with coronary heart disease in women.[120]

Blood biomarkers also provide objective measures of key nutrients found in certain foods or food groups. For example, vegetables and fruits are the primary source of carotenoids in the diet,[121] and circulating concentrations (as shown in feeding studies[122,123]) respond to dietary changes. Serum carotenoid concentrations, as well as ascorbic acid levels, are used as markers of fruit and vegetable consumption.[124-126] Similarly, relationships between reported dietary intakes of lutein, lycopene, and beta carotene compared with concentrations in blood confirmed that plasma carotenoid concentrations were indicative of dietary intakes of these carotenoids.[127] Bingham used plasma carotenoids and vitamin C to validate dietary assessments for the EPIC.[115] Serum carotenoids have also been shown to validate changes in fruit and vegetable consumption resulting from nutrition education intervention.[128] Although biomarkers offer valuable findings to help interpret results, it is important to remember that recovery biomarkers help to sort out errors in a report but that concentration biomarkers vary considerably based on personal characteristics such as body mass index or smoking status.

Urinary measures have also been used to provide objective measures of certain nutrients. Bingham and Cummings[129] pioneered the use of urinary nitrogen measurement to validate protein intake. For individuals in energy and nitrogen balance, urinary nitrogen level, as assessed from 8 days of complete 24-hour urine collections, is an independent measure of protein intake.[129] Since that time the 24-hour urinary nitrogen technique has been used to validate reported protein intakes in 24-hour recalls, FFQs, and food records.[108,115,130] Urinary potassium is considered as reliable as urinary nitrogen for use as a biomarker in dietary measurement studies.[131]

Urinary sodium assessment has been the topic of numerous discussions regarding its role in establishing population-wide sodium intake.[132] While there is general recognition of the usefulness of multiple 24-hour urine measures as the gold standard for assessing dietary sodium intake, it is limited in practicality and expense for widespread population use.[133] Efforts to validate spot urine collection[134-136] or to calibrate data based on self-reported intake have been generally limited and inconclusive. Sodium assessment remains challenging because the vast majority of sodium is consumed in processed foods and foods eaten in restaurants or other commercial establishments such that traditional dietary databases lack the specificity needed to accurately list valid amounts.[137] For these reasons, underreporting of sodium intake is common, and without an objective measure, self-reported diet, whether by recall, food frequency, or history method, is typically unreliable.[39]

More recently, urinary fructose and sucrose have been studied as a predictive marker to estimate total sugar and sucrose intake.[138-140]

As "omic" technology advances, the collection of biological samples to validate estimates of dietary intake will become routine in nutrition epidemiology and surveillance[13,141,142] Although objective methods of assessing dietary intake are valuable, researchers need to be aware of within-person variability in biomarkers just as with diet assessment. Ideally, multiple measurements per individual should be collected to reduce attenuation.[143] Regardless of the benefits of objective measures, it is important to recognize that biomarkers cannot substitute for assessment of dietary intake. Biomarkers can be used to validate and interpret dietary intake data, but the goal of diet assessment is to inform potential preventive and treatment efforts.

UNDERREPORTING DIETARY INTAKE AND MEASUREMENT ERROR

Underreporting occurs when individuals report food intakes much lower than their measured total energy expenditure such that the intakes are not biologically plausible. In other words, a individual could not support fundamental physiological processes or survive over the long term on intakes so low.[58] Underreporting errors can occur anywhere in the distribution, especially in data from FFQs and less so in recalls or records. Also, underreporting of energy, macronutirents, and micronutrients is common but may vary by type of nutrient. Care must be used in interpreting these results.

Likewise, another key concept identified in the Dietary Assessment Primer[58] is *measurement error*, defined as the difference between the true value of a parameter and the value obtained from the reported dietary intake. Validation studies are needed to address this problem.

Who Underreports?

Underreporters constitute anywhere from 10% to 45% of the total population reporting, with age, gender, and body composition influencing the results. Participants who are overweight or obese underreport more often and to a greater degree (30% to 45%) compared with participants who are lean.[144-146] Women underreport more often than men.[147-150] Individuals of low socioeconomic status also underreport energy intakes.[147-150] These characteristics are also risk factors for a number of chronic diseases, so simply eliminating data related to questionable energy intake values would seriously alter the nature of most studies.

Why Do Individuals Underreport?

Obesity itself does not cause individuals to underreport; rather, the psychological and behavioral characteristics associated with obesity likely lead individuals to underreport. A high need for social acceptability, high levels of body dissatisfaction, and attempts at dietary restraint have been associated with underreporting among both men and women, obese and nonobese.[151-153]

What Foods and Nutrients Are Prone to Underreporting?

Unfortunately, there is no simple solution to identifying foods that are universally underreported.[154] Foods most likely to be underreported in nationwide surveys include cake and pie, savory snacks, cheese, white potatoes, meat mixtures, regular soft drinks, fat-type spreads, and condiments.[155] Some research suggests that lower intakes of fat as a percentage of total energy are commonly underreported.[149,156] But other research suggests an underreporting bias not only toward fat but also carbohydrate and alcohol.[47]

EFFECT OF UNDERREPORTING ON CONCLUSIONS ABOUT DIET AND HEALTH

The possibility of misclassifying participants' nutrient intakes confers significant consequences in interpreting studies of diet and disease. This problem is exacerbated because the probability of underestimating food intake and differential reporting of foods and nutrients increases with other known factors of health risk, such as obesity and low socioeconomic status. For example, because obesity is a known risk factor for a number of chronic diseases, such as coronary heart disease, individuals at higher risk of these diseases are more likely to differentially report foods and macronutrients. Because bias in measuring dietary intake can both remove and create associations, it can generate seriously misleading conclusions about the impact of diet on disease.[93,157-159]

Identifying Underreporters

Ideally, all dietary studies should incorporate recovery biomarkers and DLW for measuring energy intake. Recovery biomarkers are unbiased reference instruments and include 24-hour urine collections to measure protein, sodium, and potassium intakes and DLW, which measures energy expenditure and is used as a measure of energy intake when individuals are in energy balance.[1] Unfortunately, no biomarkers are currently available for use in the field on a routine basis. DLW is expensive, and its use requires sophisticated laboratory technology. However, researchers can apply the Goldberg cutoff, which has been extensively described by Goldberg and colleagues[160] and Black and colleagues.[161] The Goldberg cutoff evaluates energy intake against estimated energy requirements and defines cutoff limits, which identify the most obviously implausible intake values. Briefly, height and weight measurements are used to predict basal metabolic rate (BMR) from a standard formula (Goldberg and colleagues[162] recommend the Schofield equation). A ratio of estimated energy intake (EI) to predicted BMR is calculated as EI divided by BMR. This ratio can then be compared with a study-specific cutoff value (using values suggested by Black[163] that represents the lowest value of EI divided by BMR that could, within defined bounds of statistical probability (± 2 standard deviation), reflect the habitual energy expenditure, given a sedentary lifestyle. In a large study of British adults, 39% of the women (344 of 873) and 27% of the men (264 of 983) were classified as low energy reporters using a cutoff 1.2 for EI divided by BMR.[148] In the NHANES III, Briefel and colleagues[149] used the Goldberg cutoff and classified 18% of the men and 28% of the women as underreporters. These examples illustrate how the Goldberg cutoff has provided some indication of whether estimates of dietary intake are biased.

Limitations of the Goldberg cutoff include underestimates of the incidence of underreporting because it assumes that all individuals have a sedentary physical activity level. Data collection, including lifestyle, occupation, and leisure physical activity, is required to estimate participant-specific physical activity levels and calculate more participant-specific cutoffs.[163,164]

McCrory and colleagues[159] have developed an alternative method for identifying underreporters to compensate for some of these limitations. They found that using ±1 standard deviation bounds, taking into account within-participant errors in the parameters of EI and predicted total energy expenditure (estimated using the Institute of Medicine's recently published prediction equations[165]), may be more effective in identifying implausible dietary intakes.

Epidemiologists recommend adjusting nutrient intakes for energy intake using the regression of nutrient vs energy,[104] but this is valid only when underreporting results from a systematic underestimation of portion sizes (across the board underestimation), even if actual foods are accurately reported. This is unlikely since certain foods are underreported more than others (systematic omissions); thus, energy adjustment could make matters worse.[166] For example, if fat-containing foods are more likely to be underreported or unreported and foods containing vitamin A are less likely to be underreported, energy adjustment would provide a lower than actual measure of fat intake and a higher than actual measure of vitamin A intake. Researchers have acknowledged that energy adjustment cannot eliminate bias caused by selective underreporting of certain foods, which is further complicated by correlation of errors when estimating nutrient intake.[147,167] Statistical adjustments have been further explored using data from the EPIC studies indicating that the effect of energy adjustment can vary widely when models of correlated measurement error are used.[106,107]

SPECIAL POPULATIONS: CHILDREN, THE ELDERLY, AND MINORITIES

Increasingly, studies of diet and health have included younger, older, and minority populations as awareness of specific nutrient needs emerge.[31] Each of these groups have assessment concerns that re-

quire careful consideration to match the needs of these groups. For example, the child's age dictates whether diet assessment can be self-reported (adolescents) or whether the parent/guardian or caregiver may need to serve as a surrogate (younger children). Likewise, if cognitive ability is compromised in an elderly participant, the caregiver may need to be involved, whereas self-reported dietary intake may be used in cognitively functional elderly. Ethnic subgroups may also represent an important consideration regarding diet and health among younger and older individuals. In all of these cases, the preferable assessment involves an interviewer of the same ethnic background, someone who is fluent in the native language, or someone both fluent and with the same ethnic background in order to best assess the diet in these groups. A thorough review is available.[1,168-170]

CONCLUSION

There are no perfect self-report dietary intake assessment methods for all dietary research. Traditional dietary assessment methods include 24-hour dietary recalls, food records or diaries, diet histories, and FFQs. Researchers must decide the best method to use for their study based on the data being collected, the purpose of the research, and the strengths and weaknesses of the different methods. The method selected should be tested for reliability and validity in a representative sample of the study population before the study begins.

The field of nutrition continues to advance substantially with the identification of a number of biomarkers that can be used to independently validate self-reports of dietary intake. These biomarkers have been used to identify the phenomenon of underreporting, and they have furthered an understanding of who might underreport and what foods are more likely to be underreported. There is a pressing need for more research to identify novel methods of collecting dietary intake data. Further analytic approaches that can account for underreporting in dietary databases are also needed. Researchers and practitioners are wise to interpret dietary intake data cautiously and with considerable effort to identify measurement error and offer well-documented diet and health hypotheses and associations.

REFERENCES

1. Thompson FE, Subar AF. Dietary assessment methodology. In: Coulston AM, Boushey CJ, Ferruzzi MG, Delahanty LM, eds. *Nutrition in the Prevention and Treatment of Disease.* 4th ed. London, United Kingdom: Academic Press; 2017: 5-48.

2. US Department of Agriculture. What We Eat in America (WWEIA). https://data.nal.usda.gov/dataset/what-we-eat-america-wweia-database/resource/7b0bad02-cb7d-4a8f-9d11-e19eeab682ba. Modified October 3, 2017. Accessed May 25, 2018.

3. National Cancer Institute. Automated Self-Administered 24-Hour (ASA24) Dietary Assessment Tool. https://epi.grants.cancer.gov/asa24/. Updated February 26, 2018. Accessed May 25, 2018.

4. Willett W. *Nutritional Epidemiology.* 3rd ed. New York, NY: Oxford University Press; 2012.

5. Anderson SA. Guidelines for use of dietary intake data. *J Am Diet Assoc.* 1988;88(10):1258-1260.

6. Peterkin B, Rizek R, Tippett K. Nationwide Food Consumption Survey, 1987. *Nutr Today.* 1988;23:18-27.

7. Pao EM, Sykes KE, Cypel YS. *USDA Methodological Research for Large-Scale Dietary Intake Surveys, 1975–88.* Washington, DC: US Dept. of Agriculture, Human Nutrition Information Service; 1989. Human Economics Research Report No. 49. www.ars.usda.gov/ARSUserFiles/80400530/pdf/meth/methods1989_herr49.pdf. Accessed May 25, 2018.

8. Armstrong B, Doll R. Environmental factors and cancer incidence and mortality in different countries, with special reference to dietary practices. *Int J Cancer.* 1975;15(4): 617-631.

9. Jolliffe N, Archer M. Statistical associations between international coronary heart disease death rates and certain environmental factors. *J Chronic Dis.* 1959;9(6): 636-652.

10. James WPT, Bingham SA, Cole TJ. Epidemiology and epidemiological methods. *Nutr Cancer.* 1981;2(4):203-212.

11. Bingham SA, Gill C, Welch A, et al. Validation of dietary assessment methods in the UK arm of EPIC using weighed records, and 24-hour urinary nitrogen and potassium and serum vitamin C and carotenoids as biomarkers. *Int J Epidemiol.* 1997;26(suppl 1):S137-S151.

12. Dragsted LO. Relying on biomarkers for intake assessment in nutrition. *Am J Clin Nutr.* 2017;105(1):8-9.

13. Hedrick VE, Dietrich AM, Estabrooks PA, Savla J, Serrano E, Davy BM. Dietary biomarkers: advances, limitations and future directions. *Nutr J.* 2012;11:109.

14. Neuhouser ML, Tinker L, Shaw PA, et al. Use of recovery biomarkers to calibrate nutrient consumption self-reports in the Women's Health Initiative. *Am J Epidemiol.* 2008; 167(10):1247-1259.

15. Buzzard IM, Faucett CL, Jeffery RW, et al. Monitoring dietary change in a low-fat diet intervention study: advantages of using 24-hour dietary recalls vs food records. *J Am Diet Assoc.* 1996;96(6):574-579.

16. Casey PH, Goolsby SL, Lensing SY, Perloff BP, Bogle ML. The use of telephone interview methodology to obtain 24-hour dietary recalls. *J Am Diet Assoc.* 1999;99(11): 1406-1411.

17. Moshfegh AJ, Rhodes DG, Baer DJ, et al. The US Department of Agriculture Automated Multiple-Pass Method reduces bias in the collection of energy intakes. *Am J Clin Nutr.* 2008;88(2):324-332.

18. Subar AF, Crafts J, Zimmerman TP, et al. Assessment of the accuracy of portion size reports using computer-based food photographs aids in the development of an automated self-administered 24-hour recall. *J Am Diet Assoc.* 2010; 110(1):55-64.

19. Poslusna K, Ruprich J, de Vries JH, Jakubikova M, van't Veer P. Misreporting of energy and micronutrient intake estimated by food records and 24 hour recalls, control and adjustment methods in practice. *Br J Nutr.* 2009;101(suppl 2):S73-S85.

20. Stram DO, Hankin JH, Wilkens LR, et al. Calibration of the dietary questionnaire for a multiethnic cohort in Hawaii and Los Angeles. *Am J Epidemiol.* 2000;151(4):358-370.

21. Moshfegh AJ, Borrud L, Perloff B, LaComb R. Improved method for the 24-hour dietary recall for use in national surveys. *FASEB J.* 1999;13:A603.

22. Woteki CE. Dietary survey data: sources and limits to interpretation. *Nutr Rev.* 1986;44:204-213.

23. Welch S. The Joint Nutrition Monitoring Evaluation Committee. In: Food and Nutrition Board, Commission on Life Sciences, National Research Council. *What Is America Eating?* Proceedings of a Symposium. Washington, DC: National Acedemy Press; 1986:7-20.

24. Conway JM, Ingwersen LA, Vinyard BT, Moshfegh AJ. Effectiveness of the US Department of Agriculture 5-step multiple-pass method in assessing food intake in obese and nonobese women. *Am J Clin Nutr.* 2003;77:1171-1178.

25. Raper N, Perloff B, Ingwersen L, Steinfeldt L, Anand J. An overview of USDA's Dietary Intake Data System. *J Food Compost Anal.* 2004;17:545-555.

26. US Department of Agriculture. AMPM - USDA Automated Multiple-Pass Method. What We Eat in America. https://data.nal.usda.gov/dataset/what-we-eat-america-wweia-database/resource/7b0bad02-cb7d-4a8f-9d11-e19eeab682ba. Modified October 3, 2017. Accessed June 2, 2018.

27. Zipf G, Chiappa M, Porter KS, Ostchega Y, Lewis BG, Dostal J. National health and nutrition examination survey: plan and operations, 1999-2010. *Vital Health Stat 1*. 2013;(56):1-37.

28. Kagan A, Harris BR, Winkelstein W, et al. Epidemiologic studies of coronary heart disease and stroke in Japanese men living in Japan, Hawaii and California: demographic, physical, dietary and biochemical characteristics. *J Chronic Dis*. 1974;27(7-9):345-364.

29. Archer E, Hand GA, Blair SN. Validity of U.S. nutritional surveillance: National Health and Nutrition Examination Survey caloric energy intake data, 1971–2010. *PloS One*. 2013;8:e76632.

30. Hebert JR, Hurley TG, Steck SE, et al. Considering the value of dietary assessment data in informing nutrition-related health policy. *Adv Nutr*. 2014;5(4):447-455.

31. Webb D, Leahy MM, Milner JA, et al. Strategies to optimize the impact of nutritional surveys and epidemiological studies. *Adv Nutr*. 2013;4(1):545-547.

32. Bliss RM. Researchers produce innovation in dietary recall. *Agric Res*. 2004;52(6):10-12.

33. Arab L, Tseng CH, Ang A, Jardack P. Validity of a multipass, web-based, 24-hour self-administered recall for assessment of total energy intake in blacks and whites. *Am J Epidemiol*. 2011;174(11):1256-1265.

34. US Department of Agriculture. AMPM - Features. AMPM - USDA Automated Multiple-Pass Method. What We Eat in America. https://data.nal.usda.gov/dataset/what-we-eat-america-wweia-database/resource/7b0bad02-cb7d-4a8f-9d11-e19eeab682ba. Modified October 3, 2017. Accessed June 2, 2018.

35. Vereecken CA, Covents M, Matthys C, Maes L. Young adolescents' nutrition assessment on computer (YANA-C). *Eur J Clin Nutr*. 2005;59(5):658-667.

36. Subar AF, Thompson FE, Potischman N, et al. Formative research of a quick list for an automated self-administered 24-hour dietary recall. *J Am Diet Assoc*. 2007;107(6):1002-10007.

37. Kirkpatrick SI, Subar AF, Douglass D, et al. Performance of the Automated Self-Administered 24-hour Recall relative to a measure of true intakes and to an interviewer-administered 24-h recall. *Am J Clin Nutr*. 2014;100(1):233-240.

38. Thompson FE, Dixit-Joshi S, Potischman N, et al. Comparison of interviewer-administered and automated self-administered 24-hour dietary recalls in 3 diverse integrated health systems. *Am J Epidemiol*. 2015;181(12):970-988.

39. Freedman LS, Commins JM, Moler JE, et al. Pooled results from 5 validation studies of dietary self-report instruments using recovery biomarkers for energy and protein intake. *Am J Epidemiol*. 2014;180(2):172-188.

40. Montgomery C, Reilly JJ, Jackson DM, et al. Validation of energy intake by 24-hour multiple pass recall: comparison with total energy expenditure in children aged 5–7 years. *Br J Nutr*. 2005;93(5):671-676.

41. Bokhof B, Buyken AE, Dogan C, et al. Validation of protein and potassium intakes assessed from 24 h recalls against levels estimated from 24 h urine samples in children and adolescents of Turkish descent living in Germany: results from the EVET! Study. *Public Health Nutr*. 2012;15(3):640-647.

42. Gibson RS. *Principles of Nutritional Assessment*: 2nd ed. New York, NY: Oxford University Press; 2005.

43. Bingham SA, Welch AA, McTaggart A, et al. Nutritional methods in the European Prospective Investigation of Cancer in Norfolk. *Public Health Nutr*. 2001;4(3):847-858.

44. Riboli E, Hunt K, Slimani N, et al. European Prospective Investigation into Cancer and Nutrition (EPIC): study populations and data collection. *Public Health Nutr*. 2002;5(6B):1113-1124.

45. He Y, Xu C, Khanna N, Boushey CJ, Delp EJ. Analysis of food images: features and classification. *Proc Int Conf Image Proc*. 2014;2014:2744-2748.

46. Chen HC, Jia W, Sun X, et al. Saliency-aware food image segmentation for personal dietary assessment using a wearable computer. *Meas Sci Technol*. 2015;26(2):025702.

47. Subar AF, Kipnis V, Troiano RP, et al. Using intake biomarkers to evaluate the extent of dietary misreporting in a large sample of adults: the OPEN study. *Am J Epidemiol*. 2003;158(1):1-13.

48. Hill RJ, Davies PS. The validity of self-reported energy intake as determined using the doubly labelled water technique. *Br J Nutr*. 2001;85(4):415-430.

49. Martin LJ, Su W, Jones PJ, Lockwood GA, Tritchler DL, Boyd NF. Comparison of energy intakes determined by food records and doubly labeled water in women participating in a dietary-intervention trial. *Am J Clin Nutr*. 1996;63(4):483-490.

50. Abbot JM, Thomson CA, Ranger-Moore J, et al. Psychosocial and behavioral profile and predictors of self-reported energy underreporting in obese middle-aged women. *J Am Diet Assoc*. 2008;108(1):114-119.

51. Seale JL. Predicting total energy expenditure from self-reported dietary records and physical characteristics in adult and elderly men and women. *Am J Clin Nutr*. 2002; 76(3):529-534.

52. Beaton GH, Milner J, Corey P, et al. Sources of variance in 24-hour dietary recall data: implications for nutrition study design and interpretation. *Am J Clin Nutr*. 1979; 32(12):2546-2559.

53. Basiotis PP, Welsh SO, Cronin FJ, Kelsay JL, Mertz W. Number of days of food intake records required to estimate individual and group nutrient intakes with defined confidence. *J Nutr*. 1987;117(9):1638-1641.

54. Hankin JH, Reynolds WE, Margen S. A short dietary method for epidemiologic studies. II. Variability of measured nutrient intakes. *Am J Clin Nutr*. 1967;20(9): 935-945.

55. Marr J, Heady J. Within-and between-person variation in dietary surveys: number of days needed to classify individuals. *Hum Nutr Appl Nutr*. 1986;40(5):347-364.

56. Nelson M, Black AE, Morris JA, Cole TJ. Between-and within-subject variation in nutrient intake from infancy to old age: estimating the number of days required to rank dietary intakes with desired precision. *Am J Clin Nutr*. 1989;50(1):155-167.

57. Sempos C, Johnson N, Smith E, Gilligan C. Effects of intraindividual and interindividual variation in repeated dietary records. *Am J Epidemiol*. 1985;121(1):120-130.

58. National Institutes of Health, National Cancer Institute. Dietary Assessment Primer. https://dietassessmentprimer .cancer.gov/. Accessed May 26, 2018.

59. Burke BS. The dietary history as a tool in research. *J Am Diet Assoc*. 1947;23:1041-1046.

60. Reed RB, Burke BS. Collection and analysis of dietary intake data. *Am J Public Health Nations Health*. 1954; 44(8):1015-1026.

61. Beal VA. The nutritional history in longitudinal research. *J Am Diet Assoc*. 1967;51(4):426-432.

62. Mann GV, Pearson G, Gordon T, Dawber TR, Lyell L, Shurtleff D. Diet and cardiovascular disease in the Framingham study. 1. Measurement of dietary intake. *Am J Clin Nutr*. 1962;11:200-225.

63. Paul O, Lepper MH, Phelan WH, et al. A longitudinal study of coronary heart disease. *Circulation*. 1963;28:20-31.

64. McDonald A, Van Horn L, Slattery M, et al. The CARDIA dietary history: development, implementation, and evaluation. *J Am Diet Assoc*. 1991;91(9):1104-1112.

65. Liu K, Slattery M, Jacobs D Jr, et al. A study of the reliability and comparative validity of the CARDIA dietary history. *Ethn Dis*. 1994;4(1):15-27.

66. Harvard T.H. Chan School of Public Health Nutrition Department's File Download Site. https://regepi.bwh .harvard.edu/health/nutrition.html. Accessed June 2, 2018.

67. Nutrition Quest. Questionnaires and Screeners. Block Questionnaires. www.nutritionquest.com/assessment/list -of-questionnaires-and-screeners. Accessed June 2, 2018.

68. Fred Hutchinson Cancer Research Center. Food Frequency Questionnaires (FFQ). https://sharedresources.fredhutch .org/services/food-frequency-questionnaires-ffq. Accessed June 2, 2018.

69. Flegal KM, Larkin FA. Partitioning macronutrient intake estimates from a food frequency questionnaire. *Am J Epidemiol*. 1990;131(6):1046-1058.

70. Kumanyika SK, Mauger D, Mitchell DC, Phillips B, Smiciklas-Wright H, Palmer JR. Relative validity of food frequency questionnaire nutrient estimates in the Black Women's Health Study. *Ann Epidemiol*. 2003;13(2):111-118.

71. Tucker KL. Assessment of usual dietary intake in population studies of gene–diet interaction. *Nutr Metab Cardiovasc Dis*. 2007;17(2):74-81.

72. Lassale C, Guilbert C, Keogh J, Syrette J, Lange K, Cox DN. Estimating food intakes in Australia: validation of the Commonwealth Scientific and Industrial Research Organisation (CSIRO) food frequency questionnaire against weighed dietary intakes. *J Hum Nutr Diet*. 2009;22(6):559-566.

73. Haftenberger M, Heuer T, Heidemann C, Kube F, Krems C, Mensink GB. Relative validation of a food frequency questionnaire for national health and nutrition monitoring. *Nutr J*. 2010;9:36.

74. Dodd KW, Guenther PM, Freedman LS, et al. Statistical methods for estimating usual intake of nutrients and foods: a review of the theory. *J Am Diet Assoc*. 2006;106(10): 1640-1650.

75. Willett WC, Sampson L, Stampfer MJ, et al. Reproducibility and validity of a semiquantitative food frequency questionnaire. *Am J Epidemiol*. 1985;122(1):51-65.

76. Rimm EB, Giovannucci EL, Stampfer MJ, Colditz GA, Litin LB, Willett WC. Reproducibility and validity of an expanded self-administered semiquantitative food frequency questionnaire among male health professionals. *Am J Epidemiol*. 1992;135(10):1114-1126.

77. Clapp JA, McPherson RS, Reed DB, Hsi BP. Comparison of a food frequency questionnaire using reported vs standard portion sizes for classifying individuals according to nutrient intake. *J Am Diet Assoc*. 1991;91(3):316-320.

78. Naska A, Lagiou A, Lagiou P. Dietary assessment methods in epidemiological research: current state of the art and future prospects. *F1000Research*. 2017;6:926.

79. National Cancer Institute. Food Frequency Questionnaire at a Glance. Dietary Assessment Primer. https://dietassessmentprimer.cancer.gov/profiles/questionnaire/. Accessed June 2, 2018.

80. Apovian CM, Murphy MC, Cullum-Dugan D, et al. Validation of a web-based dietary questionnaire designed for the DASH (Dietary Approaches to Stop Hypertension) diet: the DASH Online Questionnaire. *Public Health Nutr.* 2010;13(5):615-622.

81. Schwingshackl L, Bogensberger B, Hoffmann G. Diet Quality as assessed by the Healthy Eating Index, Alternate Healthy Eating Index, Dietary Approaches to Stop Hypertension Score, and Health Outcomes: an updated systematic review and meta-analysis of cohort studies. *J Acad Nutr Diet.* 2018;118(1):74-100.

82. US Department of Agriculture, Agricultural Research Service. USDA food composition databases. https://ndb.nal.usda.gov/ndb. Accessed June 2, 2018.

83. Pennington JAT, Spungen J. *Bowes & Church's Food Values of Portions Commonly Used.* 19th ed. Philadelphia, PA: Lippincott, Williams and Wilkins; 2010.

84. University of Minnesota Nutrition Coordinating Center. Food and Nutrient Database. www.ncc.umn.edu/food-and-nutrient-database. Accessed June 2, 2018.

85. Block G. A review of validations of dietary assessment methods. *Am J Epidemiol.* 1982;115(4):492-505.

86. Marr JW. Individual dietary surveys: purposes and methods *World Rev Nutr Diet.* 1971;13:105-164.

87. Willett W, Reynolds R, Cottrell-Hoehner S, Sampson L, Browne M. Validation of a semi-quantitative food frequency questionnaire: comparison with a 1-year diet record. *J Am Diet Assoc.* 1987;87(1):43-47.

88. Hankin JH. Role of nutrition in women's health: diet and breast cancer. *J Am Diet Assoc.* 1993;93(9):994-999.

89. Prentice RL, Pepe M, Self SG. Dietary fat and breast cancer: a quantitative assessment of the epidemiological literature and a discussion of methodological issues. *Cancer Res.* 1989;49(12):3147-3156.

90. Bingham SA, Luben R, Welch A, Wareham N, Khaw K-T, Day N. Are imprecise methods obscuring a relation between fat and breast cancer? *Lancet.* 2003;362(9379):212-214.

91. Freedman LS, Potischman N, Kipnis V, et al. A comparison of two dietary instruments for evaluating the fat–breast cancer relationship. *Int J Epidemiol.* 2006;35:1011-1021.

92. Freedman L, Schatzkin A, Kipnis V. Dealing with dietary measurement error in nutritional cohort studies. *J Natl Cancer Inst.* 2011;103(14):1086-1092,

93. Kolonel LN, Henderson BE, Hankin JH, et al. A multiethnic cohort in Hawaii and Los Angeles: baseline characteristics. *Am J Epidemiol.* 2000;151(4):346-357.

94. Thompson FE, Moler JE, Freedman LS, Clifford C, Stables G, Willett W. Register of dietary assessment calibration-validation studies: a status report. *Am J Clin Nutr.* 1997;65(4 suppl):1142S-1147S.

95. National Cancer Institute. Dietary Assessment Calibration/Validation (DACV) Register: Studies and Their Associated Publications. https://epi.grants.cancer.gov/dacv. Updated June 28, 2017. Accessed May 26, 2017.

96. Madden JP, Goodman SJ, Guthrie HA. Validity of the 24-hr. recall. Analysis of data obtained from elderly subjects. *J Am Diet Assoc.* 1976;68(2):143-147.

97. Gersovitz M, Madden JP, Smiciklas-Wright H. Validity of the 24-hr. dietary recall and seven-day record for group comparisons. *J Am Diet Assoc.* 1978;73(1):48-55.

98. Karvetti R, Knuts L. Validity of the estimated food diary: comparison of 2-day recorded and observed food and nutrient intakes. *J Am Diet Assoc.* 1992;92(5):580-584.

99. Linusson EE. Validating the 24-hour recall method as a dietary survey stool. *Latinoam Nutr.* 1974;24:277-294.

100. Subar AF, Thompson FE, Kipnis V, et al. Comparative validation of the Block, Willett, and National Cancer Institute food frequency questionnaires: the Eating at America's Table Study. *Am J Epidemiol.* 2001;154(12):1089-1099.

101. Bingham S, Riboli E. Diet and cancer—the European Prospective Investigation into Cancer and Nutrition. *Nat Rev Cancer.* 2004;4(3):206-215.

102. Preis SR, Spiegelman D, Zhao BB, Moshfegh A, Baer DJ, Willett WC. Application of a repeat-measure biomarker measurement error model to 2 validation studies: examination of the effect of within-person variation in biomarker measurements. *Am J Epidemiol.* 2011;173(6):683-694.

103. Schatzkin A, Subar AF, Moore S, et al. Observational epidemiologic studies of nutrition and cancer: the next generation (with better observation). *Cancer Epidemiol Biomarkers Prev.* 2009;18(4):1026-1032.

104. Willett WC, Howe GR, Kushi LH. Adjustment for total energy intake in epidemiologic studies. *Am J Clin Nutr.* 1997;65(4 suppl):1220S-1228S.

105. Fraser GE. A search for truth in dietary epidemiology. *Am J Clin Nutr.* 2003;78(3 suppl):521S-525S.

106. Michels KB, Bingham SA, Luben R, Welch AA, Day NE. The effect of correlated measurement error in multivariate models of diet. *Am J Epidemiol.* 2004;160(1):59-67.

107. Day N, Wong M, Bingham S, et al. Correlated measurement error—implications for nutritional epidemiology. *Int J Epidemiol*. 2004;33(5):1373-1381.

108. Bingham S, Cassidy A, Cole T, et al. Validation of weighed records and other methods of dietary assessment using the 24 h urine nitrogen technique and other biological markers. *Br J Nutr*. 1995;73(4):531-550.

109. Katan M. Biochemical indicators of dietary intake [abstract]. *Eur J Clin Nutr*. 1998;52(suppl):S5.

110. Lifson N, Gordon GB, Visscher M, Nier A. The fate of utilized molecular oxygen and the source of the oxygen of respiratory carbon dioxide, studied with the aid of heavy oxygen. *J Biol Chem*. 1949;180(2):803-811.

111. Lifson N, Gordon GB, McClintock R. Measurement of total carbon dioxide production by means of D_2O^{18}. *J Appl Physiol*. 1955;7:704-710.

112. Schoeller D, Van Santen E. Measurement of energy expenditure in humans by doubly labeled water method. *J Appl Physiol Respir Environ Exerc Physiol*. 1982;53(4): 955-959.

113. Black AE, Prentice AM, Goldberg GR, et al. Measurements of total energy expenditure provide insights into the validity of dietary measurements of energy intake. *J Am Diet Assoc*. 1993;93(5):572-579.

114. Schoeller DA. Measurement of energy expenditure in free-living humans by using doubly labeled water. *J Nutr*. 1988;118(11):1278-1289.

115. Bingham S. Dietary assessments in the European prospective study of diet and cancer (EPIC). *Eur J Cancer Prev*. 1997;6(2):118-124.

116. Combs GF, Trumbo PR, McKinley MC, et al. Biomarkers in nutrition: new frontiers in research and application. *Ann N Y Acad Sci*. 2013;1278:1-10.

117. Andersen LF, Solvoll, Drevon CA. Very-long-chain n-3 fatty acids as biomarkers for intake of fish and n-3 fatty acid concentrates. *Am J Clin Nutr*. 1996;64(3):305-311.

118. Connor SL. Biomarkers and dietary intake data are mutually beneficial. *Am J Clin Nutr*. 1996;64(3):379-380.

119. Willett WC, Stampfer MJ, Colditz GA, Rosner BA, Hennekens CH, Speizer FE. Dietary fat and the risk of breast cancer. *N Engl J Med*. 1987;316(1):22-28.

120. Hu FB, Stampfer MJ, Manson JE, et al. Dietary fat intake and the risk of coronary heart disease in women. *N Engl J Med*. 1997;337(21):1491-1499.

121. Chug-Ahuja JK, Holden JM, Forman MR, Mangels AR, Beecher GR, Lanza E. The development and application of a carotenoid database for fruits, vegetables, and selected multicomponent foods. *J Am Diet Assoc*. 1993;93(3): 318-323.

122. Yeum K-J, Booth SL, Sadowski JA, et al. Human plasma carotenoid response to the ingestion of controlled diets high in fruits and vegetables. *Am J Clin Nutr*. 1996;64(4): 594-602.

124. Martini M, Campbell D, Gross M, Grandits G, Potter J, Slavin J. Plasma carotenoids as biomarkers of vegetable intake: the University of Minnesota Cancer Prevention Research Unit Feeding Studies. *Cancer Epidemiol Biomarkers Prev*. 1995;4(5):491-496.

124. Bogers RP, Van Assema P, Kester AD, Westerterp KR, Dagnelie PC. Reproducibility, validity, and responsiveness to change of a short questionnaire for measuring fruit and vegetable intake. *Am J Epidemiol*. 2004;159(9):900-909.

125. Le Marchand L, Hankin JH, Carter FS, et al. A pilot study on the use of plasma carotenoids and ascorbic acid as markers of compliance to a high fruit and vegetable dietary intervention. *Cancer Epidemiol Biomarkers Prev*. 1994;3(3):245-251.

126. Al-Delaimy W, Slimani N, Ferrari P, et al. Plasma carotenoids as biomarkers of intake of fruits and vegetables: ecological-level correlations in the European Prospective Investigation into Cancer and Nutrition (EPIC). *Eur J Clin Nutr*. 2005;59(12):1397-1408.

127. Scott KJ, Thurnham DI, Hart DJ, Bingham SA, Day K. The correlation between the intake of lutein, lycopene and β-carotene from vegetables and fruits, and blood plasma concentrations in a group of women aged 50–65 years in the UK. *Br J Nutr*. 1996;75(3):409-418.

128. Murphy SP, Kaiser LL, Townsend MS, Allen LH. Evaluation of validity of items for a food behavior checklist. *J Am Diet Assoc*. 2001;101(7):751-761.

129. Bingham SA, Cummings JH. Urine nitrogen as an independent validatory measure of dietary intake: a study of nitrogen balance in individuals consuming their normal diet. *Am J Clin Nutr*. 1985;42(5):1276-1289.

130. Prentice RL, Mossavar-Rahmani Y, Huang Y, et al. Evaluation and comparison of food records, recalls, and frequencies for energy and protein assessment by using recovery biomarkers. *Am J Epidemiol*. 2011;174(5): 591-603.

131. Tasevska N, Runswick SA, Bingham SA. Urinary potassium is as reliable as urinary nitrogen for use as a recovery biomarker in dietary studies of free living individuals. *J Nutr*. 2006;136(5):1334-1340.

132. Cogswell ME, Maalouf J, Elliott P, Loria CM, Patel S, Bowman BA. Use of urine biomarkers to assess sodium intake: challenges and opportunities. *Annu Rev Nutr*. 2015;35:349-387.

133. Cogswell ME, Mugavero K, Bowman BA, Frieden TR. Dietary sodium and cardiovascular disease risk—measurement matters. *N Engl J Med.* 2016;375(6): 580-586.

134. Cogswell ME, Elliott P, Wang C-Y, Rhodes DG, Pfeiffer CM, Loria CM. Assessing US sodium intake through dietary data and urine biomarkers. *Adv Nutr.* 2013;4(5): 560-562.

135. Brown IJ, Dyer AR, Chan Q, et al; INTERSALT Co-operative Research Group. Estimating 24-hour urinary sodium excretion from casual urinary sodium concentrations in Western populations: the INTERSALT study. *Am J Epidemiol.* 2013;177(11):1180-1192.

136. Huang Y, Van Horn L, Tinker LF, et al. Measurement error corrected sodium and potassium intake estimation using 24-hour urinary excretion. *Hypertension.* 2014;63(2): 238-244.

137. Freedman LS, Midthune D, Carroll RJ, et al. Adjustments to improve the estimation of usual dietary intake distributions in the population. *J Nutr.* 2004;134(7): 1836-1843.

138. Tasevska N, Runswick SA, McTaggart A, Bingham SA. Urinary sucrose and fructose as biomarkers for sugar consumption. *Cancer Epidemiol Biomarkers Prev.* 2005; 14(5):1287-1294.

139. Tasevska NA, Midthune D, Potischman N, et al. Use of the predictive sugars biomarker to evaluate self-reported total sugars intake in the Observing Protein and Energy Nutrition (OPEN) study. *Cancer Epidemiol Biomarkers Prev.* 2011;20(3):490-500.

140. Beasley J, Jung M, Tasevska N, et al. Biomarker-predicted sugars intake compared with self-reported measures in US Hispanics/Latinos: results from the HCHS/SOL SOLNAS study. *Public Health Nutr.* 2016;19(18): 3256-3264.

141. Trujillo E, Davis C, Milner J. Nutrigenomics, proteomics, metabolomics, and the practice of dietetics. *J Am Diet Assoc.* 2006;106(3):403-413.

142. Garcia-Perez I, Posma JM, Gibson R, et al. Objective assessment of dietary patterns by use of metabolic phenotyping: a randomised, controlled, crossover trial. *Lancet Diabetes Endocrinol.* 2017;5(3):184-195.

143. Block G, Dietrich M, Norkus E, et al. Intraindividual variability of plasma antioxidants, markers of oxidative stress, C-reactive protein, cotinine, and other biomarkers. *Epidemiology.* 2006;17(4):404-412.

144. Prentice A, Black A, Coward W, et al. High levels of energy expenditure in obese women. *Br Med J (Clin Res Ed).* 1986;292(6526):983-987.

145. Lichtman SW, Pisarska K, Berman ER, et al. Discrepancy between self-reported and actual caloric intake and exercise in obese subjects. *N Engl J Med.* 1992;327(27): 1893-1898.

146. Bandini LG, Schoeller DA, Cyr HN, Dietz WH. Validity of reported energy intake in obese and nonobese adolescents. *Am J Clin Nutr.* 1990;52:421-425.

147. Price G, Paul A, Cole T, Wadsworth MJ. Characteristics of the low-energy reporters in a longitudinal national dietary survey. *Br J Nutr.* 1997;77(6):833-851.

148. Pryer JA, Vrijheid M, Nichols R, Kiggins M, Elliott P. Who are the 'low energy reporters' in the dietary and nutritional survey of British adults? *Int J Epidemiol.* 1997;26(1):146-154.

149. Briefel R, Sempos C, McDowell M, Chien S, Alaimo K. Dietary methods research in the third National Health and Nutrition Examination Survey: underreporting of energy intake. *Am J Clin Nutr.* 1997;65(4 suppl): 1203S-1209S.

150. Prentice RL, Mossavar-Rahmani Y, Huang Y, et al. Evaluation and comparison of food records, recalls, and frequencies for energy and protein assessment by using recovery biomarkers. *Am J Epidemiol.* 2011;174(5): 591-603.

151. Taren DL, Tobar M, Hill A, et al. The association of energy intake bias with psychological scores of women. *Eur J Clin Nutr.* 1999;53(7):570-578.

152. Johnson RK, Friedman AB, Harvey-Berino J, Gold BC, McKenzie D. Participation in a behavioral weight-loss program worsens the prevalence and severity of underreporting among obese and overweight women. *J Am Diet Assoc.* 2005;105(12):1948-1951.

153. Novotny JA, Rumpler WV, Riddick H, et al. Personality characteristics as predictors of underreporting of energy intake on 24-hour dietary recall interviews. *J Am Diet Assoc.* 2003;103(9):1146-1151.

154. Mertz W. Food intake measurements: is there a "gold standard"? *J Am Diet Assoc.* 1992;92(12):1463-1465.

155. Krebs-Smith S, Graubard B, Kahle L, Subar A. Low energy reporters vs others: a comparison of reported food intakes. *Eur J Clin Nutr.* 2000;54(4):281-287.

156. Voss S, Kroke A, Klipstein-Grobusch K, Boeing H. Is macronutrient composition of dietary intake data affected by underreporting? Results from the EPIC-Potsdam study. European Prospective Investigation into Cancer and Nutrition. *Eur J Clin Nutr.* 1998;52(2): 119-126.

157. Livingstone M, Prentice A, Strain J, et al. Accuracy of weighed dietary records in studies of diet and health. *BMJ.* 1990;300(6726):708-712.

158. Heitmann BL, Lissner L. Can adverse effects of dietary fat intake be overestimated as a consequence of dietary fat underreporting? *Public Health Nutr.* 2005;8(8):1322-1327.

159. McCrory MA, Hajduk CL, Roberts SB. Procedures for screening out inaccurate reports of dietary energy intake. *Public Health Nutr.* 2002;5(6A):873-882.

160. Goldberg G, Black A, Jebb S, et al. Critical evaluation of energy intake data using fundamental principles of energy physiology: 1. Derivation of cut-off limits to identify under-recording. *Eur J Clin Nutr.* 1991;45(12):569-581.

161. Black A, Goldberg G, Jebb S, Livingstone M, Cole T, Prentice A. Critical evaluation of energy intake data using fundamental principles of energy physiology: 2. Evaluating the results of published surveys. *Eur J Clin Nutr.* 1991;45(12):583-599.

162. Livingstone MB, Black AE. Markers of the validity of reported energy intake. *J Nutr.* 2003;133(suppl 3): 895S-920S.

163. Black AE. Critical evaluation of energy intake using the Goldberg cut-off for energy intake: basal metabolic rate. A practical guide to its calculation, use and limitations. *Int J Obes Relat Metab Disord.* 2000;24(9):1119-1130.

164. Black A. The sensitivity and specificity of the Goldberg cut-off for EI: BMR for identifying diet reports of poor validity. *Eur J Clin Nutr.* 2000;54(5):395-404.

165. Trumbo P, Schlicker S, Yates AA, Poos M; Food and Nutrition Board of the Institute of Medicine, The National Academies. Dietary reference intakes for energy, carbohydrate, fiber, fat, fatty acids, cholesterol, protein and amino acids. *J Am Diet Assoc.* 2002;102(11):1621-1630.

166. Carter LM, Whiting SJ. Underreporting of energy intake, socioeconomic status, and expression of nutrient intake. *Nutr Rev.* 1998;56(6):179-182.

167. Stallone D, Brunner E, Bingham S, Marmot M. Dietary assessment in Whitehall II: the influence of reporting bias on apparent socioeconomic variation in nutrient intakes. *Eur J Clin Nutr.* 1997;51(12):815-825.

168. Smith AF. Validation studies of diets of children and adolescents. *J Am Diet Assoc.* 2011;111(8):1124-1125.

169. Lu AS, Baranowski J, Islam N, Baranowski T. How to engage children in self-administered dietary assessment programmes. *J Hum Nutr Diet.* 2014;27:5-9.

170. Pfrimer K, Sartorelli DS, Rosa FT, et al. Calibration of the food list and portion sizes of a food frequency questionnaire applied to free-living elderly people. *Nutrition.* 2013;29(5)760-764.

Chapter 1

Food Composition Data and Databases

Catherine M. Champagne, PhD, RDN, LDN, FTOS, FAHA, FADA, FAND |
Pamela R. Pehrsson, PhD | David Haytowitz, MSc

LEARNING OBJECTIVES

1. Describe types of food composition databases and their uses.

2. Recognize the strengths and limitations of databases.

3. Describe how the available food composition files and databases can assist registered dietitian nutritionists involved in research.

Food composition databases are used for a variety of purposes relating to nutrition and dietetics, including nutrition monitoring, research, nutrition and health policy, and education. In addition, the food industry provides data for and uses data from these databases. Databases are also used to provide dietary advice to clients, assess dietary intake of populations, and design meal plans for patients as part of a health care environment. In the early 2000s, the World Health Organization (WHO) reported that up to 90% of diabetes, 80% of coronary heart disease, and one-third of all cancers could be prevented through physical activity and dietary behaviors.[1] An update issued in 2015 suggested that cardiovascular diseases, cancers, respiratory diseases, and diabetes still accounted for 82% of noncommunicable disease deaths worldwide.[2] While the distribution of diseases may vary globally, it is clear that understanding the composition of foods in the diet, along with recommending increases in physical activity, is important in monitoring and reducing noncommunicable diseases.

Agriculture, food production, and monitoring and research in nutrition/health outcomes encompass the processes behind the raw materials and processing and the food science that connects raw commodities to the wide spectrum of different foods available in the food supply.[3] These processes affect the chemical composition of foods and the determination of the amounts of individual components included in food composition databases or tables. These databases are the foundation for other food composition databases (both nationally and abroad), research, nutrition education, and nutrition monitoring and policies. Uses of food composition databases are multidimensional, serving not only the aforementioned but also a wide consumer base. Food composition databases are important in national and world trade, especially considering the diversity of foods now available globally. In addition, commodity-level foods are sold based on specific components, and, in some cases, these components may yield information about contamination or adulteration. In many countries, use of dietary supplements has increased significantly, and, since this contributes to nutrient intake, supplements become an important complement to food composition databases. Many standards for acceptance of foods into national and international food supplies are established on a national basis, for example, foods from the US Department of Agriculture (USDA) School Lunch Program (www.fns.usda.gov/nslp/national-school-lunch-program-nslp) and many from the Food and Agricultural Organization's (FAO) Codex Alimentarius (www.fao.org/fao-who-codexalimentarius/en), a set of international food standards, guidelines, and codes of practice for globally traded foods.

Food composition databases can be a valuable tool for these applications; however, there are limitations that should be observed for a food composition database to be used properly. Today, food composition databases are usually published electronically, although historically they were published in a hard-copy format as food composition tables. For many applications, the food composition databases, coupled with a well-designed nutrient analysis program, provide increased flexibility and ease of use.

The USDA has maintained tables of food composition for more than 115 years, since the pioneering work of W.O. Atwater.[4] Published in 1892, the Atwater table of 178 food items contained data on five proximate (macronutrient) components (water, protein, fat, total carbohydrates, and ash), kilocalories (called fuel in the Atwater table), and refuse. Atwater's data sheets are currently maintained in the Special Collections Section of the National Agricultural Library in Beltsville, MD. Historical tables are similar in content to the electronic spreadsheets used today for many aspects of the work. A similar system of index cards, although for many more nutrients, was maintained until the early 1970s and was used to compile data for the 1950 and 1963 editions of *Agriculture Handbook No. 8: The Composition of Foods: Raw, Processed, Prepared.*

Today, food composition data are processed using large relational databases to manage all the data needed to properly describe foods, nutrients, and other components found in foods, as well as certain ancillary information, such as household weights and refuse. The USDA's current database system was written in the late 1990s. A new system to better automate the processing of large amounts of data and to track and report all the diverse factors that affect the composition of foods is underway. Expected to launch 2019, the new, modernized, automated USDA FoodData Central (FDC) will allow for data submission from many sources and will house new USDA analytic data, the Food and Nutrient Database for Dietary Studies, Nutrition Facts panels from hundreds of thousands of food labels, Special Interest Databases (SIDs), legacy data (formerly the USDA National Nutrient Database for Standard Reference), links to relevant information on consumption of specific foods and food groups, and detailed descriptive information on food samples. The automation, expansion, and modernization through portals will allow for more efficient submission (by providers) and extraction (by users) of a larger and more current pool of research data.

This chapter provides an overview of the features and uses of food composition databases and emphasizes the care that should be taken in using the data for various purposes. Food composition data refer to the variety of food components (nutrients, contaminants, and other constituents) per specified unit of foods (usually per 100 g or per specified serving size/portion). The data are results of chemical analysis (eg, individual fatty acids or amino acids, macronutrients, vitamins, minerals, and bioactive compounds), calculations (eg, protein estimated from nitrogen, energy from calorie equivalents, summing values from recipe ingredients), or imputations/estimations. A food composition database refers to a collection of data, usually from various sources, on the levels of components in foods. Most food composition databases contain multiple foods and multiple food components, though some databases, such as those for newly analyzed components or those for components that are not widespread in the food supply, may contain only one or several food components. However, a well-designed food composition database contains much more information than just nutrient values, such as food descriptions, household weights, and refuse (or inedible portion). It is critical that the food items be properly described. Species or cultivar, processing, and preparation can affect the nutrient content of a food, so it is also critical that this information be incorporated into the food description so that it can be accurately matched to the food items being examined.[5] Similarly, precise nutrient names are essential as investigators use a number of analytic methods to measure the content of a nutrient in a food item, and the choice of a specific method depends on which definition of that nutrient is being used and, ultimately, the values obtained. The importance of variability estimates surrounding means of nutrients in foods will be a predominant theme throughout the chapter; in addition, the challenges and limitations of food composition databases will be discussed.

AVAILABLE DATABASES
Major US Databases

One compilation of food composition data in the United States is the International Nutrient Databank Directory (NDBC Directory]) this useful resource, developed by the Nutrient Database Conference, lists most US databases and consists of voluntary submissions from database developers.[6] Other examples of specific US composition databases include the US Food and Drug Administration (FDA) Total Diet Study database[7] and a host of commercial composition databases that use the USDA food composition databases as their foundation. The FAO/International Network of Food Data Systems (INFOODS) maintains a useful international compilation of food composition databases developed in other countries.[8] Most food composition databases are stored and maintained as computer files, and they may be available to users as hard copy, electronic files, or both hard copy and electronic. The national database developed for use in the United States is the Nutrient Database for Standard Reference (SR) developed by the Agricultural Research Service (ARS) of the USDA.[9] SR Legacy, the final version of SR, contains approximately 8,800 food items and includes data for up to 150 components. R had historically been updated about once a year; SR Legacy will be included in the new FDC, which will be updated routinely with new analytical data during the year. The SR serves as the foundation for many of the food composition databases that have been developed by US colleges, universities, hospitals, clinics, and private companies. The SR also serves as the foundation for databases in several other countries where resources for analyzing local foods are limited or not available. International food composition databases may contain data on foods consumed by immigrants to the United States who can still obtain foods imported from their native country and may be helpful in providing dietary guidance to growing number of immigrant clients.

The USDA Branded Food Products Database is the result of a public-private partnership.[10] With subsequent releases, this database now contains food labels for more than 240,000 foods; these data are publicly available, updated continuously, and include data from the Nutrition Facts label and ingredient listings available on food packaging.[11] This database will become part of FDC and will use common search programs to access the data. Data received from the manufacturer or retailer have been included on a serving-size basis (references amount customarily consumed or RACC) and converted to a 100-g basis, if not directly received from the manufacturer or retailer. Manufacturers or retailers determine the nutritional value of foods in various ways, ranging from laboratory analysis for large manufacturers to perhaps computer-generated nutrient profiles based on ingredient proportions and database ingredient values for smaller manufacturers. The USDA Branded Food Products Database is hosted by USDA's National Agricultural Library and is accessed through the same search program as the USDA National Nutrient Database for SR, but it is clearly identified as a distinctive but connected database. However, label rounding, as permitted in Nutrition Labeling Education Act regulations, especially from food products with small serving sizes, may introduce additional variability in the 100-g values. Therefore, while these data can be a useful tool for researchers and consumers, values may be different from those obtained through analytic measurements. This type of database is gaining momentum around the world as, especially in developed countries, foods in the food supply are commercially packaged or consumed in restaurants.

In addition to the SR, the ARS also maintains the Food and Nutrient Database for Dietary Studies (FNDDS),[12] which is used to assess the food and nutrient intakes of participants in the National Health and Nutrition Examination Survey (NHANES) conducted by the National Center for Health Statistics.[13] The FNDDS currently contains more than 8,000 food items; it will become part of FDC and will use the common search program to access the data. The database has no missing values; nutrient values that were not available from laboratory analysis or other sources were calculated from recipes or imputed by ARS. The foods in this database are generally in the "as consumed" state. It is routinely updated to keep pace with trends and changes in American eating patterns.

Information about the development of food composition databases in the United States and other countries is available on the INFOODS website. INFOODS was founded in 1984 to help improve the quality and quantity of food composition data worldwide and to serve as a vehicle allowing users to have access to the data. INFOODS has developed resources for data users and compilers and has held many regional meetings to facilitate communication and exchange of information regarding food composition databases.[14]

Features of food composition databases that may distinguish one database from another include the foods and food components contained, the electronic form of the database, periodicity of update (eg, time-stamped for day and time of release), format on the page or computer screen, intended use(s) (eg, reference, diet analyses, or product development), food and food component search capabilities, and associated software functions. Some databases are updated routinely as new data become available; others are updated at specific intervals, such as every year or every few years. Foods in databases may appear alphabetically by name or by food group. One common format for listing foods and nutrients is to list the foods in the left-hand column and the nutrient values in columns across the page or screen. An alternative format is listing one food per page or screen, with the nutrients in the left-hand column and the values per several serving portions in the columns across the page or screen. The computer system for a database may allow the user to select several alternative formats for data display and presentation. Software features may allow for assessment of dietary intake, comparison of dietary intake with country standards, and calculation of the composition of recipe items from ingredients. Figure 14.1 illustrates a typical display format.

Special Interest Databases

For new or emerging food components, the ARS often will first compile data in SIDs and then, when and if appropriate, incorporate the data into the SR. For

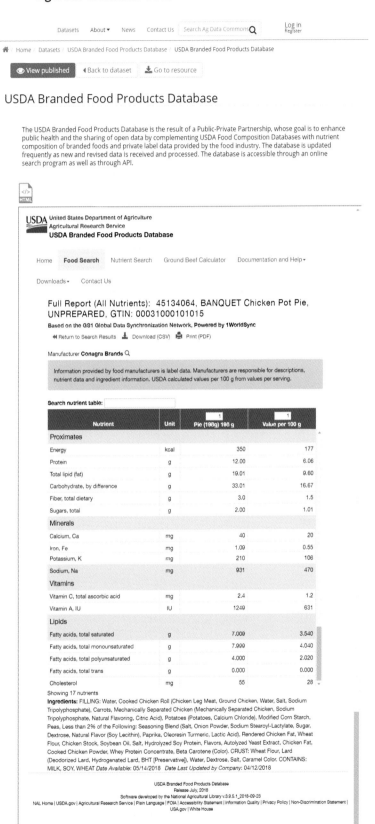

Figure 14.1 Screenshot of the US Department of Agriculture's Branded Food Products Database, a typical food composition database

example, the previously existing SID on carotenoids (beta carotene, alpha carotene, lutein plus zeaxanthin, and lycopene) was merged into SR release 16 (2003). Data from a separate vitamin K publication, as well as newly obtained data, were also added to SR. Later, vitamin D was added to SR. At the same time, any missing values for these foods in the FNDDS were calculated.

Because of increasing interest in the relationships of flavonoids and other polyphenols to various health outcomes and to diseases such as cancer, cardiovascular disease, and immune system diseases, databases on these compounds are of interest to various researchers.[15] There are about 5,000 flavonoid compounds; though only about 30 are commonly found in human foods—primarily in vegetables, fruits, cereals, nuts, tea, coffee, and wine, which are the major contributors of polyphenols and other antioxidants to the diet. Currently, the ARS has produced a number of SIDs (see Table 14.1).

Although they are separate databases, values for foods in the flavonoid, isoflavone, and proanthocyanidin databases that match the foods in SR are accessible through the Nutrient Data Library's online search program (https://ndb.nal.usda.gov/ndb). While some of the data in the choline and fluoride SIDs have been moved into SR, other data, such as the individual choline metabolites, can only be found in the SID.[16]

Because data for some food components, such as oxalic acid or other components, are only available for a limited number of foods,[22] these food components are sometimes listed as separate tables in hard-copy databases. In some cases, the food component may only occur in a small number of foods (eg, vitamins D and K), or costly or difficult analytic methods may prohibit data from being generated for many foods (eg, chromium).

Data are also available for other nutrients of public health importance, for example, fluoride in the drinking water supply and foods that are gaining importance in the US food supply, such as American Indian/Alaska Native foods and foods consumed by Hispanic populations. The latter foods may be highly specific to the different tribes and subpopulations that make up these communities. As demographics change and new immigrant populations

Database	Year	No. of Foods	Compounds
Isoflavones[16]	1999	128	Genistein, daidzein, and glycitein
	2008	549	
	2015	560	
Choline[17]	2004	434	Total choline, betaine, free choline,
	2008	630	glycerophosphocholine, phosphocholine, phosphatidylcholine, and sphingomyelin
Flavonoids[18]	2003, 2007	220	Flavonols, flavones, flavanones, flavan-3-ols, and anthocyanidins
	2011	385	
	2015[a]	506	
Fluoride[19]	2004	400	Fluoride
	2005	427	
Flavonoids expanded[20,bc]	2014, 2015	2926	Flavonoids and isoflavones
Proanthocyanidins[21]	2004	205	Oligomers and polymers of flavan-3-ols
	2015	283	
Glucosinolates	2017		In progress

Table 14.1 History of Special Interest Databases Released by the US Department of Agriculture

[a] Release 3.2 (2015) includes individual data points used to calculate mean values as well as individual glycosides.
[b] Includes 29 compounds for six subclasses
[c] Includes calculated values and assumed zeros

reflect the foods of their homeland, food composition databases must contain these foods.

As national and international food supplies become more complex, global trade increases, and the diversity of commodity and commercially packaged foods of more interest arise, commercial ingredient databases tracking ingredient sources are emerging. In addition, information about diet and health outcomes, import-export standards in global trade, interactions with other compounds, and so on become just as important as the nutrient estimates. Ontology on crop information (eg, cultivar, fertilizer, harvest date), and changes in animal feeding and breeding are also tracked in part to explain diversity in the food supplies and individual nutrients within foods.

Dietary Supplement Databases

Databases on dietary supplements are essential to fully capture intakes of food components and other constituents in nutrition surveys, in dietary research studies, and for patient care. Dietary supplements (capsules/pills, herbal preparations, and other dietary preparations) include thousands of different products with different brand names and potencies. In the Supplement Facts panels of dietary supplements, label information about the content of many vitamins and minerals is required, in a manner similar to the Nutrition Facts panels for foods. A recent study of nationally representative adult multivitamin/mineral supplements concluded that the analytic content varied by ingredient; some vitamins and minerals are close to labeled levels with low variability, and some are significantly higher than labeled levels with high variability.[23]

Labeling requirements are less stringent for other ingredients in dietary supplements (especially phytochemicals), which are, in many cases, extracts. Some products voluntarily report the level of concentration of these other ingredients and extracts, but many do not.

Data for dietary supplements are usually kept in separate databases rather than merged with food composition databases. The National Center for Health Statistics developed a dietary supplement database for use with the NHANES dietary intake data to track dietary supplements reported by survey participants.[24,25] The Office of Dietary Supplements at the National Institutes of Health (NIH) has developed a label-based dietary supplement database and is also collaborating with ARS to develop an analytically based dietary supplement database.[26-28] These and other databases for dietary supplements will likely evolve over the next decade as they contribute to research on the relationship of dietary supplements to health maintenance and disease prevention.[29]

Food Contaminant Databases

Data on the levels of contaminants in foods are usually not included in the databases that contain nutrient values. The development of food composition databases for food contaminants poses special challenges because average levels are not generally reported and could be misleading if they were reported. The presence of pesticide residues, industrial chemicals, microbial toxins, toxic elements (mercury, lead, arsenic, cadmium), and other contaminants in foods is often a matter of chance. Experts in these areas speak of the number of detections, rather than average levels, and the residue levels are usually quite low compared with accepted standards. For example, an analysis of 200 samples of a food may reveal a pesticide residue in only 10 of the samples. The average level for these 10 samples may be measurable; however, the average for the 200 samples may have no significant figures. In addition, levels of contaminants may be considerably reduced in foods during rinsing, peeling, and processing.

Although much work has been done to determine pesticide residues and other contaminants in foods, it has been done to monitor the food supply (to assess safety by confirming that levels are below acceptable daily intakes) rather than to provide average values for databases. It might be more informative for contaminant databases to provide a ratio of detected to nondetected contaminants and to provide reported values for the detected contaminants only, as well as for all samples analyzed. The databases for food contaminants are developing, and the accepted format and standards for these databases will likely evolve as the users and uses of these databases are made known. As an example, the European community has developed a database on contaminant levels of concern in seafood because of potential risks to the population.[30] Examples of contaminant databases developed in Europe for foods containing nitrosamines, heterocyclic amines, and polycyclic aromatic hydrocarbons[31] and used in the European Prospective Investigation into Cancer and Nutrition (EPIC) study were cited by Jakszyn and colleagues[32] for assessing the relationship of cancer to dietary intake. Indeed, the EPIC investigations have focused greatly on the associations between some of these contaminants and cancer in their European cohorts.[33,34]

In the United States, one of the primary sources of information on pesticide residues, industrial chemicals, radionuclides, toxic elements, and other contaminants in commonly consumed foods is the FDA Total Diet Study. This study collects 280 foods four times per year from various US locations and ships them to the Total Diet Laboratory for analysis; the results of this study are posted on the FDA website.[7]

DATA USERS AND DATA USES

Food composition databases are used to assess the dietary status of patients, clients, and students; to assess dietary intakes of population groups with defined demographic characteristics; to plan and evaluate the dietary adequacy of meals and diets; and to discern relationships among diet, health, and disease from the results of national, clinical, and epidemiologic studies. Food composition databases may be used to assess the nutrient content of individual foods or a group of similar foods for the purpose of developing food standards, formulating new food products, determining the potential use of foods in therapeutic diets, establishing definitions for dietary claims, or determining whether foods meet such claims. Databases are also used to develop nutrition education materials and programs for students, foodservice workers, caregivers, homemakers, and the general public.

Registered dietitian nutritionists (RDNs) may have a specific need or range of needs for food composition data, depending on their place of employment and job responsibilities. RDNs working in hospitals, schools, prisons, and other institutions, along with those in private practice, may use databases to plan and evaluate meals and daily diets, develop therapeutic diets, and provide nutrition

education. Within hospitals and clinics, databases may also be used to counsel patients and design diets for clinical trials. Academic nutritionists use databases for diet-disease epidemiologic research and for student education in nutrition, food science, and health courses. Government nutritionists at the federal level use databases to develop policies concerning nutrient fortification, food standards, and label claims; to assess the safety and adequacy of the food supply; to design and evaluate the results of epidemiologic studies and clinical trials; and to develop nutrition education materials for the general public and targeted population groups. RDNs who work in the food industry use databases for product development, nutrition labeling, and dietary claims. Grocery stores may use databases for shelf-labeling programs, and restaurants may use them to make nutrition claims about foods on their menus and to develop nutrition brochures for consumers. Food composition data offer a useful tool for nutrition and public health and, as Elmadfa and Meyer[35] point out, should be carefully prepared and maintained.

FOOD ANALYSTS AND FOOD ANALYSIS

Food composition data originate from the work of chemists in government, industry, academia, and private laboratories who analyze individual or composite samples (mixtures of individual samples) of foods to determine the levels of food components. The procedures and accepted methods for collecting and analyzing foods for various food components are discussed in detail in *Food Composition Data: Production, Management and Use*.[5] It is important for analysts to document how the foods are sampled, selected, collected, prepared, and analyzed, as well as how the results are verified and evaluated. If calculations are required to determine nutrient levels (such as protein calculated from nitrogen content), they should be explained and documented. The USDA uses the Key Foods approach to prioritize foods and nutrients for analysis.[36] Foods are then sampled, prepared, and analyzed using USDA's National Food and Nutrient Analysis Program (NFNAP).[37] The resulting data have been incorporated in to SR in the past and will now be incorporated into the FDC.

Each food that is analyzed requires a unique sampling design to ensure that the analyzed samples are representative of the foods typically consumed. The sampling design should include the variables that affect the composition of each food. Nationwide food sampling involves different variables than does local food sampling. The variables for raw fruits and vegetables may include season, geography, and cultivar (genetic strain or variety), whereas variables for processed foods may include the location of the processing plant and the market share of the brand-name products. If compositing methods are used for the foods, they should be appropriate for the intended purposes of the resulting data. It is critical that the description of the food sample accurately reflect all of these factors.

The Association of Official Analytical Chemists provides information on the analytic methods and sample preparations that laboratories should use to determine the levels of each food component.[38] Laboratories use such quality control procedures as duplicate analyses, recoveries of reference standards, recoveries of spiked/fortified samples, and standard reference materials. Spiked/fortified samples contain a known added amount of the food component and are used to determine if the analytic method accurately measures the amount present. Standard reference materials contain a government-certified amount of a component in a food; laboratories purchase and analyze them to ascertain the accuracy of their analytic methods. When sending food samples for analysis, researchers will find it useful to include various quality control materials to ensure that the lab is obtaining accurate results. While running duplicate analyses at the same time by the same analyst or the same equipment rarely identifies problems, introducing blind duplicates into the sample stream can be useful. Similarly, in-house control composites matched to the food matrix can also help researchers develop accurate data.[39]

When many samples of the same food are analyzed individually to determine the concentration of a food component, the distribution of those concentrations is rarely normal (Gaussian function). Statistical treatment of analytic data typically includes the calculation of means, standard deviations, coefficients of variation, and medians when appropriate. Means may be weighted by variety, cultivar, species, market share, or year-round availability of the individual foods.

Much can be learned by evaluating the distribution of the analytic data points for each food component. Outliers can be identified, and their treatment (ie, inclusion or omission from the evaluation) can be determined and documented. If bimodal or other modal distributions occur, it might be necessary to separate the samples into groups to obtain more useful data. For example, the distribution of the iron content of wheat flake breakfast cereals might show a bimodal distribution reflecting two different levels of iron fortification (eg, 4.5 mg/oz and 18 mg/oz). Perhaps two different brands or different products within the same company have different fortification levels. The overall mean concentration of iron would be an intermediate value (between 4.5 and 18 mg/oz) that would not reflect either type of cereal. It would be best to list both types of cereal separately in a database, even if all the other nutrient values for the two types of cereal are similar. In cases like this, it is probably best to report two unique breakfast cereals reflecting the different fortification levels.

DATA COMPILERS AND DATA COMPILATIONS

Data compilers must prioritize foods/nutrients to be included in the food composition database. Prioritization depends greatly on shifts from deficiency to excess that are identified in nutrition policy reports, such as the Dietary Guidelines for Americans,[40] for nutrients of public health importance—and which foods supply these nutrients. Data compilers must also consider new foods introduced by immigrant populations and, in general, must reflect the dynamic and expanding food supply. The example of iodine is a good illustration of the ever-changing priorities in food composition databases. Initially, the nutrient deficit was addressed with fortification—iodized salt. However, iodine deficiency later resurfaced with increased consumption of commercially prepared and restaurant foods (which typically do not use iodized salt). Frequent reformulations of commercially packaged foods require frequent updates. Changes in fortification practices, for example, adding folic acid to grain products, also require accurate updates.

The data compiler gathers data from the available sources, organizes the food names into groups and subgroups, and evaluates and aggregates the data into a useful database.[41] Compilers of food composition data might be employed by government agencies, food companies, academic institutions, private businesses, hospitals, clinics, foodservice institutions, or private companies. They might be independent contractors hired by these organizations or be self-employed. Compilers should hold degrees in nutrition, dietetics, or food science and should be knowledgeable about food sampling, analysis, descriptions, and processing; culinary terms; and cuisines. Knowledge about computerized database systems and the retrieval of information from databases is also very important. It is best to have the compiler work directly with the individual who designs the computer system so that the system performs the necessary operations accurately and efficiently. Paramount in effective food composition databases is transparency and drill-down capability for the users; all compiled data should also be available in the raw form.

Those who compile national databases usually have direct access to results from government or contract laboratories and supplement this with data from the scientific literature and the food industry. Other database compilers usually gather data from national data sets (such as the SR, FNDDS, or both), scientific papers, food companies, the internet, and other previous compilations. Data compilers in academia or clinical research may also obtain food component data directly from in-house or contract laboratories. The compiler should always document the sources of data used to determine an estimate in the database. Users of the database should also be able to access this information.

Compilers who use the SR or FNDDS as the foundation for their databases select the foods and nutrients they need from these sources and then add other foods and components obtained from the literature, food companies, restaurants, and other sources. The SR contains analytic values and imputed or calculated values, assumed zeros, and Nutrition Facts panel data from food labels. Imputed values may be derived using label and ingredients in descending order with target nutrients from the panel; a best-fit analysis using a linear programming tool allows a most likely set of ingredient proportions. A full nutrient profile based on estimated proportions and nutrient compositions of the ingredients may be generated. Alternatively, profiles are calculated from similar foods, adjusting for differences in food moisture or another key nutrient. In some cases where a specific nutrient was not expected to be found (eg, cholesterol in plant products), an assumed zero is defined. Database compilers may fill in missing SR values by imputation or calculation, and they may add foods that have nutrient values determined by imputation or calculation. Some compilers may include nutrition labeling values for some foods if the original data are not available from food companies.

The data generated by food companies for the purpose of nutrition labeling is not of the same accuracy as data generated directly from food composition laboratories, because the nutrition labeling data have been adjusted by using formulas and by rounding so that the resulting values are in compliance with FDA and USDA regulations. The USDA's Food Safety and Inspection Service regulates the nutrition labeling of meat, poultry, and products containing more than certain levels of meat and poultry; the FDA regulates the nutrition labeling of all other foods. Most individuals have difficulty keeping accurate food records, so the information on the label not only provides dietary guidance but also helps consumers estimate their nutrient intake. In May 2016, the FDA published new labeling regulations that required large companies to include potassium, vitamin D, and added sugars on the Nutrition Facts panel beginning July 2018 and to remove vitamins A and C.[42] The Daily Values have been updated to reflect new Dietary Reference Intakes developed by the National Academy of Medicine. In addition to the Daily Values, manufacturers are also required to report actual amounts for vitamin D, calcium, iron, and potassium. Other changes in the label were made to improve usability.

Data from the various sources are collected by database compilers and incorporated into their files along with appropriate source documentation.

Compilers cannot check the documentation for every component value for every food with regard to sampling, number of samples, analytic method, and laboratory quality control. However, any data that appear to be clearly out of line should be questioned and either verified or omitted. Often, the food item may just need a better food description.

DATA AGGREGATION

Database compilers standardize food names and descriptions and aggregate the data for foods with the same name to prevent duplicate listings. Aggregation allows the data for the same food (or very similar foods) to be summarized and thus prevents multiple repetitions of food items in the database. However, more sophisticated databases could offer a drill-down capability that allows users to see values for all the individual data sources. This aggregation requires that the data for foods that appear to have the same or similar name and descriptors be closely scrutinized to determine which foods and their corresponding nutrient values may be consolidated into a single food entry in the database. The compiler may also combine data for foods with similar descriptions that have identical (or nearly identical) composition data, such as different flavors for a brand name of reduced-fat yogurts or different cultivars of apples. However, as the database expands to cover more components, more unique food items may be required. For example, proximates, minerals, and vitamins in different cultivars of potatoes could be combined. However, if compilers add flavonoids to the database, purple or blue potatoes would need a separate entry because of their increased anthocyanidin content.

Aggregation of data from various sources has the potential benefit of enlarging or completing the nutrient profile for a food because some sources may provide food components that are not provided by other sources. For example, one source might have extensive trace mineral values for a food, another source might provide individual carotenoid values for the same food, and another might have macronutrients along with the more common vitamins and minerals. Before combining data from different sources, however, it is important to be sure the food names and descriptions indicate that the foods are the same and to check for comparability of common data provided by the sources. Similarity of common nutrient values (eg, water, energy, protein, and fat) for information from several sources provides some basis for data aggregation. In addition, evaluating major and minor nutrients might indicate that foods with slightly different names are basically the same food.

When data for the same food are aggregated from various sources, the challenge is usually calculating representative values for the various food components using statistical models that weight the important factors contributing to variability. Data for aggregated foods may be averaged (ie, each data point carries the same value), or they may be weighted and averaged (eg, data for four brands of canned corn might be weighted and averaged by market share or averaged by the number of samples from each source to produce data for generic canned corn). Due to the nature of the data, such as multiple sources with different sampling designs, more specialized statistical routines may be required to properly calculate the various statistical parameters, and the canned routines that are built into commercially available database programs may not be suitable. Data sources and data manipulation should be documented, but it is not usually possible to provide this documentation within the database; the information usually remains in the files of the data compiler.

DATABASE FEATURES

In order to develop a comprehensive database, multiple types of data may be needed. Due to limited resources, it is not always feasible to analyze every food sample for all nutrients. Furthermore, it would not be a good use of funds to analyze some foods for certain nutrients. The types of data sources can be categorized as follows:

● Analytic data: Analytic programs are supported by government agencies, the food industry, and academic/research institutions. They are generally the highest-quality data and are often representative of the US food supply; good analytic data should include measures of variability, comply with a rigorous quality control program, and be updated frequently. At the USDA, the National Food and Nutrient Analysis Program meets these criteria.

- Calculated data: Missing values may be calculated or imputed from similar foods[43] or use linear programming tools to generate nutrient profiles from the nutrients and ingredients listed on the Nutrition Facts panel or food label. Quality of the estimations is associated with the quality of data on the individual ingredients.

- Assumed zero: In many cases, a nutrient is expected to be zero in foods; for example, an assumption of zero is made for cholesterol in plant-based foods.

- Manufacturer's data/food labels (Nutrition Facts panel): Label data are sometimes used to complete nutrient profiles, but with commercially packaged foods often reformulating frequently, it is challenging to keep nutrient values current in the database. In addition, thousands of foods are removed from the US market every year, and keeping the database inventory current is also a challenge.

Food Names and Descriptions

Database compilers must give accurate and appropriate names to each food and sufficient descriptive terms to distinguish each food from all the other foods in the database. Foods that are vaguely named or that have inconsistent or ambiguous descriptive terms will confuse the user and may lead to improper use of the data. Similarly, when food composition data are published in journals, the data should be accompanied by complete and accurate food descriptions. For various computer applications where screen size is limited, it is important not to truncate useful information that would enable the user to differentiate two entries. Often the term distinguishing the two records may be near the end of the name, and truncating the description would remove this information. Abbreviated names can be useful in this situation, but the abbreviations must be clear and easy to understand.

Guidelines and methods for describing foods have been developed, and issues related to food descriptions and to the development of descriptive terms have been discussed.[44] Various coding systems, such as LanguaL[45] and CODEX,[46] have been developed to facilitate data retrieval worldwide, particularly when multiple languages are involved. To properly identify many agricultural products such as fruits and vegetables, particularly when dealing with regional or international names, including the scientific name of the item is essential. One compilation of plant-based foods and their scientific names is the systematic taxonomy database established by USDA's Germplasm Resource Information Network (GRIN).[47]

The luxuries of unlimited space for food names and open-ended food descriptors (as might be found in computer applications using large monitors, analytic reports, or scientific papers) are not usually possible when a database is used to develop a printed version for users who do not have access to a computer. Although electronic files are more flexible with regard to space than hard copies, the need for concise and accurate descriptions cannot be underestimated. Therefore, it is necessary to provide, within the allotted space, the food names and descriptive terms that will be most useful for the data user. The compiler should strive for uniformity in describing foods in a database by using a selected order of descriptors and standardized terms and abbreviations. For example, the compiler might use the order of descriptors shown in Box 14.1.

Not all of the descriptors shown in Box 14.1 are applicable or useful for each food. The information for "part of plant or animal" would also indicate if peel or seeds are present for fruits and vegetables, if fat is present on meat cuts or has been trimmed away, if rind is included or not for cheese, and so on. Redundant or commonly assumed information is not usually included (eg, that fruits and vegetables are rinsed before use, that ice cream is frozen, or that frozen or canned entrées are heated before serving). Footnotes might be added to provide ingredients for mixed dishes (eg, a footnote might say that a tuna-noodle-vegetable casserole contains tuna canned in water and drained; egg noodles; chopped, frozen broccoli; and condensed mushroom soup)

Type of Term	Food with Descriptive Terms
Color	Apple, *green*, Granny Smith, peeled, without core, steamed
Flavor	Pudding, *chocolate*, prepared from instant mix, JELL-O
Cultivar	Potatoes, *russet*, flesh and skin, baked
Breed	Beef, *American Angus*, loin, tenderloin steak/roast, boneless, separable lean only, choice, raw
Part of plant or animal	Turnips, *greens and root*, diced, boiled
Accompaniments	Ice cream, vanilla *with caramel syrup*
Preservation, treatment methods, and containers	Fruit cocktail *in heavy syrup, canned*, Del Monte
Preparation or cooking method	Frankfurter, beef, *boiled*
Brand name	Peas, green, and pearl onions in lightly seasoned sauce, frozen, *Birds Eye*

Box 14.1 Example of Order of Food Description Terms in a Database[a,36]

but are not usually necessary for well-known items with quality control (eg, a brand-name fast food sandwich).

A thorough index with cross-references is useful to locate foods in a hard-copy database because of the many synonyms for some foods (see Box 14.2) and the many ways of describing and placing foods in alphabetical listings and within food groups (eg, corn may be a vegetable or a cereal grain). Computerized systems, now the norm, usually have search functions that will bring up all foods with identified terms (eg, all foods called "sugar cookie" or all foods containing the words "soy" or "stir-fried"). These searches allow for very broad or narrow searching depending on the specificity of the terms and the number of terms used in the search. Some computerized systems also have built-in food name synonyms so that a search on a less familiar term (eg, aubergine, broad bean, and frankfurter) would bring up the preferred terms in the database (eg, eggplant, lima beans, hot dog, respectively).

The challenge in using the FNDDS[12] and other databases for assessing diets is to appropriately

Fries	French fries; fried potatoes; home fries; chips (UK)
Green beans	snap beans; string beans
Hamburger	ground beef; minced beef; ground round; ground chuck
Milkshake	malt; shake (may or may not contain dairy)
Pancakes	hotcakes; flapjacks

Box 14.2 Examples of Food Name Synonyms[36]

match the foods described by study participants, students, patients, or clients to the foods listed in the databases (ie, to select the best fit). This challenge is one reason why food descriptions are so important. Because survey participants are not always able to provide accurate descriptions of the foods they eat, the FNDDS includes generic foods with the descriptor "not further specified" (or NFS). The nutrient data for NFS foods are based on data for similar or representative foods. For example, "sandwich, NFS" might reflect the most commonly consumed sandwich in the survey (perhaps a cheese sandwich on white bread with mayonnaise), or it might be a composite sandwich with nutrient values calculated from weighted data from other sandwiches in the database. FAO/INFOODS has prepared Guidelines for Food Matching,[48] which provides tips on how to best match foods listed in a food composition database with foods reported in various studies, such as food intake or food consumption. It highlights the importance of good food descriptions and identification.

Food Groupings

Food groups are established for a number of reasons. These include promoting public health, such as MyPlate,[49] which was developed by USDA and based on the Dietary Guidelines for Americans 2015–2020.[40] Food composition database compilers often use these groupings as a starting point but may find them insufficient depending on the complexity of the food supply. For example, the MyPlate groups of fruits, vegetables, grains, proteins, and dairy do not clearly indicate where the plethora of mixed dishes should be included as many cross several food groups. The USDA developed the Food Pattern Equivalents Database to address this issue.[50] Therefore, additional food groups or subgroups, beyond those required for public health purposes, may be required to adequately categorize all the foods in a food composition database.

Foods are often organized into groups based on food source (eg, grains, fruits, nuts, or vegetables) or food use (eg, beverages, breakfast cereals, condiments, desserts, entrées, or snacks). Food groups may then be further organized into subgroup hierarchies. Food groups and subgroups in databases help users locate items and prevent redundancy in terms, such as "ready-to-eat cereal" or "candy bar." Food-use groupings have cultural significance that might make a database useful in its country or region of origin but less useful internationally. Therefore, databases designed specifically for international use may

need an alphabetical organizational structure or food groups that are based on food source rather than food use. Various tools, such as LanguaL or CODEX classification systems, can assist in data retrieval across languages or regional nomenclature within a country. In addition, individual foods may be linked or searched using Universal Product Codes. Given the improved search capabilities found within online food composition databases, rigid hierarchical naming conventions may not be as useful as they once were. Also, multiple hierarchies are possible for a particular food depending on which attribute is important for a particular use.

Basis of Data

Data for foods in databases are presented on a wet-weight basis (ie, as consumed), so data reported on a dry-weight basis (as may be done for literature papers on trace elements or contaminants) should be converted to wet weight before being added to a database. Dry-weight basis means that all the water in the food has been removed by a dehydration process and that the food is in a powdered state. Dry-weight data should not be included in a food composition database unless the product is available as a powder. It is important for analysts to include the percent water with the other food components for each food when they publish data in the scientific literature to allow food component values to be converted from a dry-weight to a wet-weight basis.

It should be clear in the database whether the data are presented as purchased (ie, with waste or refuse) or as edible portion and if the weight of the food includes or excludes possible waste or refuse (bone, peel, core, husk, or shell). For example, the data for an apple presented on a 100-g basis may or may not include the weight of the core and the peel, or the data for a baked chicken breast may or may not include the weight of the bones and skin. It should be clear whether the foods are in a raw, cooked, or processed state, and the specific methods of cooking and processing should be indicated. Also, if ingredients are added during the cooking or processing, that should be made clear; for example, a fried chicken leg may have been battered or floured, and salt may have been added.

RDNs are most likely to need nutrient values per weight of edible portion of foods as consumed (eg, cooked meat without bones, popped popcorn, or apples without cores). The food weight in the database may be per typical serving portion or per 100 g. If a serving portion is given, it should be unambiguously described, and a corresponding gram weight for the serving size should be included. Consistency in listing serving portions within each food group of a database is useful for comparative purposes so users can compare nutrient values for similar quantities of foods, for example, 8 fl oz of milks, 6 fl oz of fruit juices, 1 oz or 1 cup of ready-to-eat cereals, 3 oz of meats, 1 cup of cooked vegetables, 1 cup of canned fruits, 1 oz of nuts or seeds, and 1 oz of cheeses. In food composition databases, it is extremely important to have current and accurate serving sizes. For example, on a 100-g basis, an analysis of children's macaroni and cheese from several restaurant chains had very similar nutrient profiles; however, the serving size for one chain was 2.5 times that of a competing chain.[9] Units of measure for serving sizes must be current—not just an artifact of food labels—and be understood by users.

Aggregation of nutrient data for the same food from various sources requires that food components have the same specificity and units for measurements. For example, two different sources of vitamin E for the same food may have one expressed as international units and the other as milligrams of individual tocopherols.

Missing Values

Obviously, it would be cost prohibitive to analyze all of the foods in the food supply; when data are missing from a database, it is usually because the analyses have not been performed or because the manufacturers are unable to release the data. Currently, data for many multi-ingredient foods are not available for inclusion in food composition databases, especially some homemade, frozen, and shelf-stable entrées and desserts; fast foods and carryout foods; other restaurant foods; and ethnic foods. Unfortunately, a common mistake database users make is to assume that missing values are zeros. This can lead to underestimation of daily food component intakes

or to inappropriate foods being allowed on restricted diets. True zeros in a database are indicated with zeros.

Reference databases contain data gathered from available sources and generally do not contain imputed or calculated data for missing values, whereas databases used to analyze dietary information from food consumption surveys and studies (such as the FNDDS) should have as few missing values as possible.

Procedures used to impute food composition values are found in chapter 5 of *Guidelines for Compiling Data for Food Composition Databases*[41] and Schakel and colleagues.[43] Some blanks may be filled in with zeros (eg, cholesterol and vitamin B-12 for plant materials or dietary fiber for animal-based foods). Other data may be imputed from a different form of the same food; for example, some data for canned corn might be used for frozen corn (except for the sodium content), or data may be imputed from similar foods; for example, data for pinto beans might be used for navy beans. Missing values for multi-ingredient foods may be filled in with data calculated from recipes. These calculations usually require corrections for refuse (eg, bone, shell, peel, or trimmed fat), loss or gain of moisture or fat with cooking, and nutrient loss or retention with cooking. Chapter 6 of *Guidelines for Compiling Data for Food Composition Databases*[41] provides information on how to estimate nutrients for multi-ingredient foods. Imputed or calculated values in databases should be identified as such, and the process used for imputation should be documented.

DATABASE CHECKS

FAO/INFOODS has prepared Guidelines for Checking Food Composition Data Prior to the Publication of a User Table/Database.[51] When developing a database management system for producing food composition databases, it is critical to include various computerized tools to assess the validity and integrity of the compiled database.[52,53] These tools can help the compiler produce a high-quality food composition database and include checks for weights of major nutrients compared with the total weight of the food, caloric sums of energy-yielding nutrients compared with the caloric value of the food, and limits of nutrient concentrations in various food groups. For example, 1 cup of boiled mashed pumpkin weighs 245 g, and the sum of the weights of the values for water (229.54 g), protein (1.76 g), fat (0.17 g), and carbohydrate (12.01 g) is 243.48 g, which rounds to 243 g. The energy value of this food is 49 kcal/cup, and the sum of the energy equivalents of the protein (7.04 kcal), fat (1.53 kcal), and carbohydrate (with a correction for 2.7 g of dietary fiber; 37.24 kcal) is 45.81 kcal, which rounds to 46 kcal. These checks indicate data comparability, that is, 243 g is close enough to 245 g, and 46 kcal is close enough to 49 kcal.[8] The computer system can identify foods and nutrients with potential problems to allow the database compiler to evaluate them. Foods with missing values will generally be flagged with the database checks unless the system is designed to exclude them. Computer systems can also check for outliers by asking for the highest and lowest values for each food component or by setting threshold high and low values for each food component and asking for foods that are below or above these thresholds.

FOOD COMPONENT VARIABILITY

Except perhaps for carefully formulated products (such as medical formulas and infant formulas), the food component levels in databases should be expected to have inherent and acquired variability. For example, the average vitamin C content of a 131 g orange (2 5⁄8″ diameter) as listed in SR is 69.7 mg,[8] but the actual vitamin C content of an orange depends on factors such as season, sunlight exposure, cultivar, species, variety, time of day of harvest, storage length and temperature, and ripeness at harvest. Average values for individual food components may have large standard deviations. It is useful if the food composition database is able to provide standard deviations and the number of samples analyzed so that users get a better feel for the basis for the data.

The many causes of food component and nutrient variability are compounded in food composition databases because the data are aggregated from various sources. Variables within any one food include genetics; environmental conditions (climate,

temperature, and soil type); and methods of preservation, processing, and preparation. Because multi-ingredient foods are made from mixtures of different foods, they have mixtures of these variables. Contributing further to nutrient variation are different analytic methods and techniques, use of different recipes to calculate nutrient values for a mixed dish, and the compiler's unique methods of aggregating foods and nutrient values. Other factors—the use of international ingredients with unknown nutrient profiles, the difference between analytic and estimated or rounded (labels) values—contribute to the uncertainty of the composition of foods; in some cases, data are recycled from source to source. However, where resources are limited, this is unavoidable.

One example that demonstrates how variability can be significant when using food composition data shows that different brands of a pickle spear could vary widely in sodium, a nutrient of public health importance because many individuals in the United States consume too much salt and sodium. An average of the three brands may not give a true picture of the variability, so the data user should be aware of product to product differences (see Figure 14.2).

An extensive amount of literature on food component variation has been published and includes the evaluation of such variables as variety/cultivar and

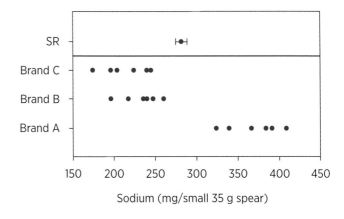

Figure 14.2 Sodium variability among brands of kosher dill pickles available in the United States

Values are given as mean and standard deviation. Brands A and B are national brands of kosher dill pickle, while C is made up of store brands (N=6 for each of the brands). The mean value from the US Department of Agriculture Database for Standard Reference (SR) is a weighted mean based on market share.

cultivation/growing conditions; geography; fertilization and season; crop yield; germination; feed composition and food cooking, processing, and storage; brewing techniques (for tea); brand names; and analytic/calculation issues.[54-71] In addition, the practice of fortification of commercially packaged foods sometimes shows overfortification for volatile nutrients in products with extended shelf life, for example, vitamin C in infant formulas.

Considering the extent of food component variation, diet recommendations for patients and clients should not be rigid. One food should not be recommended over another as a better or lower source of a food component unless the difference between the foods will be of practical importance for the patient or client. Small differences in average values for nutrients should not be used to make comparative selections of foods. Rigid dietary recommendations by RDNs may override the dietary variety that is necessary to ensure adequate nutrient intake. The case of immigrants not consuming their traditional foods has been documented because they decrease home meal preparation and rely on convenience foods in the United States.[72] On the other hand, immigrants who may try to consume their traditional foods may not find them available; if they are available, then these foods need to be better featured in US food composition tables.[73]

Some inconsistencies in food component values may be identified during database checks and may then be verified or corrected. Other inconsistencies may become apparent only when one compares nutrient values for foods with a group or subgroup. For example, one might expect higher values for a raw fruit or vegetable than one that has been canned or frozen, but the aggregated data from different varieties, regions, and seasons show somewhat higher average levels in the canned or frozen product. Such apparent inconsistencies might reflect the fact that the data for the raw and processed foods came from different sources and might be the result of differences in food storage, sampling, or laboratory analytic methods and techniques.

One example of an apparent inconsistency is that the cholesterol content of drained tuna canned in vegetable oil is 15 mg cholesterol per 3-oz serving; this is less than that for tuna canned in water, which is 26 mg cholesterol per 3-oz serving.[8,74] Cholesterol is lipid soluble, so some of it could migrate from the canned tuna into the vegetable oil and thereby reduce the amount of cholesterol in the drained tuna. Tuna in vegetable oil therefore might appear to be a better choice for cholesterol-conscious individuals; however, the cholesterol difference (9 mg per 3 oz of tuna) is not of practical significance. Tuna canned in water is still a better choice for individuals following diets low in total fat and energy because it contains 99 kcal and 0.7 g fat per 3 oz, whereas tuna canned in oil contains 168 kcal and 7.0 g fat per 3 oz.[8]

IMPLICATIONS FOR PRACTITIONERS

Some basic tips to help RDNs use databases are listed here:

- Be diligent in searching for the best match between the food of interest and the foods listed in the database. Consider food name synonyms (refer to Table 14.3) and appropriate descriptive terms.
- Never assume that missing values are zeros. If a food component value is missing, look for the level of that component in a similar food to provide a reasonable estimate of the potential content.
- Adjust the serving size to what was or will be consumed (ie, do not assume that the serving portion listed in the database is the amount consumed by the client).

Try not to extend the uses of food composition databases beyond their limitations. Databases may be used for multiday individual dietary assessments or 1-day group dietary assessments, but they probably should not be used to assess the dietary adequacy or deficiency of 1-day diets of individuals because of intraindividual variation. Databases may not be sufficiently accurate for use in planning or assessing diets for metabolic research or balance studies, nor for planning diets for patients on very restricted diets. Specific information from food manufacturers about the composition of some foods should be used in research studies or for planning restricted diets. If biological measures of body fluids are to be made after specific foods are consumed (eg, serum carotenoids measured after eating tomatoes), then samples of the consumed foods need to be analyzed, and the exact portions consumed by the study participant need to be measured.

Use databases knowledgeably and do not become unduly alarmed about uneven quality (eg, more detailed descriptions and more nutrient data for some foods than others) or inconsistencies. However, unreasonable data should not be accepted, and reasons for values that appear to be out of line compared with values for similar foods should be explored for accuracy. Several sources are available to address concerns or questions about the food component content of foods in databases. The ARS and food trade associations are good sources of information regarding the composition of basic and traditional foods. The ARS should be contacted for concerns about data in the SR[8] and the FNDDS.[12] Food companies could be contacted regarding data for brand-name products; and most food labels or websites provide addresses, telephone numbers, and company contact information. The headquarters of fast-food chains or other restaurants could be contacted via telephone, mail, or email for information on the nutrient content of restaurant foods. Growing interest in improving the quality of foods consumed away from home has resulted in regulations requiring restaurants to post nutrition information for health conscious consumers.[75,76]

The selection of a nutrient database or database system for use in a dietary department, educational facility, or research clinic requires consideration of the specific needs of the users and the features and limitations of the various database systems.[77-79] The users should consider such factors as the number and types of foods included, the food components included and their units of measure, the sources of the data, the quality of the data, availability of data updates, food search capabilities, and desired software features, along with considerations for such factors as initial cost, maintenance costs, and hardware concerns. It may be useful to talk with other professionals who use different database systems and to ask specific questions of the database system developers. The choices are many and varied. Experimentation with database systems at conference exhibits, such as the Academy of Nutrition and Di-

etetics Food & Nutrition Conference & Expo may be helpful in making decisions.

OUTLOOK FOR FOOD COMPOSITION DATABASES

Until newer technology becomes available, it will be necessary to analyze food samples and maintain food composition databases. However, the day when individuals can scan their foods and get an exact nutrient profile is foreseeable in the near future; of course, these devices have to take sampling issues into consideration. For example, they need to exclude refuse, such as skin on a piece of fruit or bones in a chicken wing. Often the density of a food will change from the external surface to the interior, such as the bark on a barbecued brisket compared with the interior or the outside of a doughnut compared with the jelly filling.

Food composition databases will continue to improve over time as work continues to improve and researchers develop new analytic methods, quality assurance techniques, and statistical analysis of results. The emphasis with regard to methodology will be on improved accuracy and identification of more compounds, increased speed, greater efficiency, lower cost, and greater output. More food samples analyzed by better analytic techniques and monitored by better quality control procedures produce more and better results. Current databases need to fill in the missing values for food components with analytic values and to analyze foods for which data are most needed (eg, prepared entrées and restaurant foods). As new data become available, they replace the older or missing values. Several publications indicate that when databases are updated, changes in dietary intake of nutrients are observed (in other words, changes to the database affect the results from food consumption surveys).[80-82] Thus, maintaining and improving food composition data are important to obtain reliable information about dietary status and diet-health relationships.

Improvements in food composition data quality do not result in decreased data variability because food component variability is inherent in the food materials. However, improved data quality does allow variability to be more readily measured.

As more data become available for the same food, outlying values are more clearly identified and can be omitted when averages are determined. For the future, better ways of determining and expressing nutrient variability as well as validating nutrient data in compiled databases should be found so that nutrition professionals can more easily evaluate the results of their nutrition surveys and studies, help patients and clients with dietary instruction, and educate students about the composition of foods.

Several activities are underway to continue to enhance the quality and quantity of food composition data. The ARS is collaborating with NIH on the NFNAP, which allows support money from NIH and other agencies within the US Department of Health and Human Services to be transferred to ARS for the analysis of foods.[37] The ARS sets the priorities for both the foods and food components to be analyzed under NFNAP. The data that result from these efforts are the foundation for most academic and commercial databases available in the United States. As cost of analysis is always an issue, collaboration among the government, the food industry, and academia is becoming essential to the advancement of food composition research.

The *Journal of Food Composition and Analysis* is devoted specifically to the publication of research dealing with the composition of foods and is a venue for sharing data (available at the Science Direct website, www.sciencedirect.com/science/journal/08891575). The US National Nutrient Databank Conference is a forum for presentations relating to food composition (www.nutrientdataconf.org), and the FAO's International Food Data Conference (www.fao.org/infoods/infoods/conferences/en) is another forum for sharing information and data on foods on an international basis. To learn more about food composition, visit FAO/INFOODS for eLearning courses (www.fao.org/infoods/infoods/training/en).

CONCLUSION

With more sophisticated technology, an expanding, dynamic food supply increasing in complexity, and improvements in analytic techniques, the chal-

lenges and limitations of developing current food composition databases also increase. The cost of analysis, uncertainty in calculations for frequently reformulated foods and missing nutrients, the representativeness of the foods sampled, new or modified analytic methods that may be costly, and frequency of reformulations are among the considerations for food composition database compilers and users. Above all, the sustainability of all of the aforementioned requires planning and scientific and monetary support. Factors such as inadequate food descriptions in data exchange among collaborators and data users are key; nutrient retention information in processing and cooking is also essential to more accurately represent foods as consumed. On a larger scale, constantly changing practices in animal feeds and breeding/raising practices and crop changes—for example, fertilizers, organic vs conventional, and new cultivars—are changing the composition of the food supply. The food composition database really represents a snapshot in time, and without constant sampling and analysis, it will not necessarily be representative over time. For example, new technology, such as apps for phones, present useful tools for planning personal interventions; nevertheless, no matter how consumer friendly or useful these apps may be in planning studies, the data they capture from food composition databases are limited. Limitations include truncation of food descriptions so as to change the actual food in a way that results in a profile that does not make sense. The only accurate way to assess intake in a more formal setting is to analyze the foods actually consumed by study participants.

In regards to the future of food composition databases, as national and global food supplies grow and change with an increase in imported and exported foods, food composition database compilers have a responsibility to reflect the changes in mainstream diets. The inclusion of immigrant and imported foods and information on nutrients of ongoing or emerging public health importance is essential. This is critical in the development of sound nutrition policy, which may vary from country to country and population to population. This includes secondary metabolites, such as bioactive compounds found in plants, iodine in foods (as the food industry generally does not use iodized salt in commercially packaged foods, which is important to women of reproductive age), and fluoride in the drinking water supplies around the country. Tracking detailed information on ingredients in foods through database ontology, linkages to internal and external databases (eg, CODEX), automation or increased usability by consumers and professionals, automated quality control checks, time-stamped updates (continuous), and better use of data through research will continue to improve food composition databases as tools for monitoring and improving health in the United States.

REFERENCES

1. World Health Organization (WHO), Food and Agricultural Organization (FAO). Diet, nutrition and the prevention of chronic diseases: Report of a joint WHO/FAO expert consultation. WHO Technical Report Series 916. http://apps.who.int/iris/bitstream/10665/42665/1/WHO _TRS_916.pdf. Published 2003. Accessed April 13, 2018.

2. World Health Organization. Noncommunicable diseases fact Sheet. www.who.int/mediacentre/factsheets/fs355 /en. Updated June 2017. Accessed April 13, 2018.

3. Pehrsson PR, Haytowitz DB. Food composition databases. In: Cavallero B, Finglas P, Toldra F, eds. *The Encyclopedia of Food and Health*. Vol 3. Cambridge, MA: Academic Press; 2016:16-21. doi:10.1016/B978-0-12-384947-2.00308-1. Accessed April 13, 2018.

4. Atwater WO, Woods CD. *Investigations Upon the Chemistry and Economy of Foods*. Report Connecticut (Storrs) Agricultural Experiment Staion for 1891. 1892.

5. Greenfield H, Southgate DAT. *Food Composition Data: Production, Management, and Use*. London, United Kingdom: Elsevier Applied Science; 1992.

6. National Nutrient Databank Conference. International Nutrient Databank Directory. Version 3.10. www.nutrientdataconf.org/indd. Accessed April 13, 2018.

7. Food and Drug Administration. Total Diet Study. www.fda .gov/Food/FoodScienceResearch/TotalDietStudy/default .htm. Updated February 23, 2018. Accessed April 13, 2018.

8. International Network of Food Data Systems. International food composition table and database directory. www.fao.org /infoods/infoods/tables-and-databases/en. Updated March 1, 2017. Accessed April 13, 2018.

9. US Department of Agriculture, Agricultural Research Service. USDA National Nutrient Database for Standard Reference. Release 28. Released September 2015; slightly revised May 2016. https://ndb.nal.usda.gov/ndb. Accessed April 13, 2018.

10. US Department of Agriculture, Agricultural Research Service. 2016. USDA Branded Food Products Database. https://ndb.nal.usda.gov/ndb. Accessed April 13, 2018.

11. US Department of Agriculture, Agricultural Research Service. USDA Branded Food Products Database, Release 2. https://ndb.nal.usda.gov/ndb. Published 2017. Accessed April 13, 2018.

12. US Department of Agriculture, Agricultural Research Service. 2016. USDA Food and Nutrient Database for Dietary Studies 2013–2014. Food Surveys Research Group home page. www.ars.usda.gov/nea/bhnrc/fsrg. Accessed April 13, 2018.

13. National Center for Health Statistics, Centers for Disease Control and Prevention. National Health and Nutrition Examination Survey. www.cdc.gov/nchs/nhanes/about _nhanes.htm. Accessed April 13, 2018.

14. International Network of Food Data Systems (INFOODS). Structure and roles of INFOODS. www.fao.org/infoods /infoods/structure-and-tasks-of-infoods/en. Accessed April 13, 2018.

15. Bravo L. Polyphenols: chemistry, dietary sources, metabolism, and nutritional significance. *Nutr Rev*. 1998; 56(11):317-333.

16. Bhagwat SA, Haytowitz DB. USDA database for the isoflavone content of selected foods. Release 2.1. www.ars .usda.gov/ARSUserFiles/80400525/Data/isoflav/Isoflav _R2-1.pdf. Published November 2015. Accessed April 13, 2018.

17. Patterson KY, Bhagwat SA, Williams JR, Howe JC. Holden JM. USDA database for the choline content of common foods. Release 2. www.ars.usda.gov/ARSUserFiles /80400525/Data/Choline/Choln02.pdf. Published January 2008. Accessed April 13, 2018.

18. Bhagwat S, Haytowitz DB. USDA database for the flavonoid content of selected foods. Release 3.2. www.ars.usda.gov /ARSUserFiles/80400525/Data/Flav/Flav3.2.pdf. Published September 2015. Slightly revised November 2015. Accessed April 13, 2018.

19. National Data Laboratory. USDA national fluoride database of selected beverages and foods. Release 2. www.ars.usda.gov/ARSUserFiles/80400525/Data /Fluoride/F02.pdf. Published December 2015. Accessed April 13, 2018.

20. Bhagwat S, Haytowitz DB, Wasswa-Kintu S. USDA's expanded flavonoid database for the assessment of dietary intakes. Release 1.1. Documentation and User Guide. www.ars.usda.gov/ARSUserFiles/80400525/Data/Flav /FDB-EXP_R01-1_Doc.pdf. Published December 2015. April 13, 2018.

21. Bhagwat SA, Haytowitz DB. 2015. USDA database for the proanthocyanidin content of selected foods. Release 2.0. www.ars.usda.gov/ARSUserFiles/80400525/Data/PA /PA02.pdf. Published September 2015. Slightly revised December 2015. Accessed April 13, 2018.

22. Agricultural Research Service (ARS), USDA. Products & Services, Data sets prepared by USDA-ARS's Nutrient Data laboratory. www.ars.usda.gov/Services/docs.htm?docid =5121. Accessed April 13, 2018.

23. Andrews KW, Roseland JM, Gusev PA, et al. Analytical ingredient content and variability of adult multivitamin/ mineral products: national estimates for the Dietary Supplement Ingredient Database. *Am J Clin Nutr*. 2017; 105(2):526-539.

24. Ervin RB, Wright JD, Kennedy-Stephenson J. Use of dietary supplements in the United States, 1988–94. *Vital Health Stat 11*. 1999;(244):i-iii, 1-14.

25. Dwyer JT, Picciano MF, Raiten DJ. Food and dietary supplement databases for What We Eat in America– NHANES. *J Nutr*. 2003;133(2):624S-634S.

26. Dwyer JT, MF Picciano MF, Betz JM, Coates PM. Mission and activities of the NIH Office of Dietary Supplements. *J Food Compost Anal*. 2004;17:493-500.

27. Dwyer JT, Picciano MF, Betz JM, et al. Progress in development of an integrated dietary supplement ingredient database at the NIH Office of Dietary supplements. *J Food Compost Anal*. 2008;21:S83-S93.

28. Office of Dietary Supplements, National Institutes of Health, Department of Health and Human Services, Dietary Supplement Label Database (DSLD). http://dietary -supplements.info.nih.gov/Health_Information/Dietary _Supplement_Ingredient_and_Labeling_Databases.aspx. Accessed April 13, 2018.

29. Costello RB, Saldanha LG. *Annual Bibliography of Significant Advances in Dietary Supplement Research 1999*. Bethesda, MD: National Institutes of Health Office of Dietary Supplements. http://dietary-supplements.info.nih .gov/publications/publications.html. Published 1999. Accessed April 13, 2018.

30. Vandermeersch G, Lourenço HM, Alvarez-Muñoz D, et al. Environmental contaminants of emerging concern in seafood—European database on contaminant levels. *Environ Res*. 2015;143(part B):29-45.

31. Jakszyn P, Ibanez R, Pera G, et al. Food content of potential carcinogens. Barcelona, Spain: Catalan Institute of Oncology; 2004. http://epic-spain.com/libro.html. Accessed April 13, 2018.

32. Jakszyn P, Agudo A, Ibanez R, et al. Development of a food database of nitrosamines, heterocyclic amines, and polycyclic aromatic hydrocarbons. *J Nutr*. 2004;134(8): 2011-2014.

33. Jakszyn PG, Allen NE, Lujan-Barroso L, et al. Nitrosamines and heme iron and risk of prostate cancer in the European prospective investigation into cancer and nutrition. *Cancer Epidemiol Biomarkers Prev*. 2012;21(3):547-551.

34. Keszei AP, Goldbohm RA, Schouten LJ, Jakszyn P, van den Brandt PA. Dietary N-nitroso compounds, endogenous nitrosation, and the risk of esophageal and gastric cancer subtypes in the Netherlands Cohort Study. *Am J Clin Nutr*. 2013;97(1):135-146.

35. Elmadfa I, Meyer AL. Importance of food composition data to nutrition and public health. *Eur J Clin Nutr*. 2010;64 (suppl 3):S4-S7.

36. Haytowitz DB. Updating USDA's Key Foods List for What We Eat in America, NHANES 2011–2012. *Procedia Food Sci*. 2015;4:71-78. www.sciencedirect.com/science/article /pii/S2211601X15000735?via%3Dihub. Accessed April 13, 2018.

37. Haytowitz DB, Pehrsson PR. USDA's National Food and Nutrient Analysis Program (NFNAP) produces high-quality data for USDA food composition databases: two decades of collaboration. *Food Chem*. 2018;238:134-136. www.sciencedirect.com/science/article/pii/S0308814 616319331. Accessed April 13, 2018.

38. AOAC. *Official Methods of Analysis of AOAC International*. 20th ed. Gaithersburg, MD: AOAC International; 2016.

39. Phillips KM, Patterson KY, Wolf WR, Sharpless KE, Holden JM. Reference materials to evaluate measurement systems for the nutrient composition of foods: results from USDA's National Food and Nutrient Analysis Program. *Anal Bioanal Chem*. 2008;389(1):219-229.

40. US Department of Health and Human Services, US Department of Agriculture. *Dietary Guidelines for Americans 2015–2020*. 8th ed. https://health.gov/dietary guidelines/2015/guidelines. Published December 2015. Accessed April 13, 2018.

41. Rand WM, Pennington JAT, Murphy SP, Klensin JC. *Guidelines for Compiling Data for Food Composition Databases*. Hong Kong: UNU Press; 1991.

42. US Food and Drug Administration. Changes to the Nutrition Facts Panel. www.fda.gov/Food/Guidance Regulation/GuidanceDocumentsRegulatory Information/LabelingNutrition/ucm385663.htm. Published 2016. Accessed April 13, 2018.

43. Schakel SF, Buzzard IM, Gebhardt SE. Procedures for estimating nutrient values for food composition databases. *J Food Compost Anal* 1997;10:102-114.

44. Truswell AS, Bateson DJ, Madafiglio KC, Pennington JAT, Rand WM, Klensin JC. INFOODS guidelines for describing foods: a systematic approach to facilitate international exchange of food composition data. *J Food Compost Anal*. 1991;4:18-38.

45. Pennington JAT, Smith EC, Chatfield MR, Hendricks TC. LANGUAL: a food description language. *Terminology*. 1995; 1:277-289.

46. Food and Agriculture Organization/World Health Organization. CODEX Classification of Foods and Animal Feeds. ftp://ftp.fao.org/codex/Meetings/CCPR/ccpr38/pr38CxCl .pdf. Published 2006. Accessed April 13, 2018.

47. US Department of Agriculture, US National Plant Germplasm System. https://npgsweb.ars-grin.gov /gringlobal/taxon/taxonomysimple.aspx. Accessed April 13, 2018.

48. International Network of Food Data Systems. FAO/ INFOODS Guidelines for Food Matching, Version 1.2. www.fao.org/infoods/infoods/standards-guidelines/en. Published 2012. Accessed April 13, 2018.

49. US Department of Agriculture. MyPlate. www.choosemyplate.gov. Accessed April 13, 2018.

50. US Department of Agriculture. Food Pattern Equivalents Database. www.ars.usda.gov/Services/docs.htm?docid =23871. Accessed April 13, 2018.

51. FAO/INFOODS. FAO/INFOODS Guidelines for Checking Food Composition Data prior to the Publication of a User Table/Database. Version 1.0. Rome: Food and Agriculture Organization; 2012.

52. Murphy SP. Integrity checks for nutrient databases. In: Stumbo PJ, ed. *Proceedings of the Fourteenth National Nutrient Databank Conference*. Ithaca, NY: CBORO Group; 1990:89-91.

53. Ahuja JKC, Perloff BP. Quality control procedures for the USDA Food and Nutrient Database for Dietary Studies nutrient values. *J Food Composit Anal*. 2008;21:S119-S124.

54. Baslam M, Morales F, Garmendia I, Goicoechea N. Nutritional quality of outer and inner leaves of green and red pigmented lettuces (Lactuca sativa L.) consumed as salads. *Sci Hortic*. 2013;151:103-111.

55. Farnham MW, Lester GE, Hassell R. Collard, mustard and turnip greens: effects of genotypes and leaf position on concentrations of ascorbic acid, folate, β-carotene, lutein and phylloquinone. *J Food Compost Anal*. 2012;27:1-7.

56. Lee SK, Kader AA. Preharvest and postharvest factors influencing vitamin C content of horticultural crops. *Postharvest Biol Technol*. 2000;20:207-220.

57. Leong SY, Oey I. Effects of processing on anthocyanins, carotenoids and vitamin C in summer fruits and vegetables. *Food Chem*. 2012;133:1577-1587.

58. Samuoliené G, Sirtautas R, Brazaitytė A, Duchovskis P. LED lighting and seasonality effects antioxidant properties of baby leaf lettuce. *Food Chem*. 2012;134:1494-1499.

59. Lubertzky R, Littner Y, Mimouni FB, Dollberg S, Mandel D. Circadian variations in fat content of expressed breast milk from mothers of preterm infants. *J Am Coll Nutr* 2006; 25:151-154.

60. Skupien K, Oszmian J. Comparison of six cultivars of strawberries (Fragaria x ananassa Duch.) grown in northwest Poland. *Eur Food Res Technol.* 2004;219:66-70.

61. Peterson J, Dwyer J, Jacques P, Rand W, Prior R, Chui K. Tea variety and brewing techniques influence flavonoid content of black tea. *J Food Compost Anal.* 2004;17: 397-406.

62. Kuman V, Rani A, Solanki S, Hussain SM. Influence of growing environment on the biochemical composition and physical characteristics of soybean seed. *J Food Compost Anal.* 2006;19:188-195.

63. Kim H-K, Ye S-H, Lim T-S, Ha T-Y, Kwon J-H. Physiological activities of garlic extracts as affected by habitat and solvents. *J Med Food.* 2005;8:476-481.

64. Nikkarinen M, Mertanen E. Impact of geological origin on trace element composition of edible mushrooms. *J Food Compost Anal.* 2004;17:301-310.

65. Davis DR, Epp M, Riordan H. Changes in USDA food composition data for 43 garden crops, 1950 to 1999. *J Am Coll Nutr.* 2004;23:669-682.

66. Milinsh MC, das Gracas Padre R, Hayashi C, et al. Effects of feed protein and lipid contents on fatty acid profile of snail (*Helix aspersa maxima*) meat. *J Food Compost Anal.* 2006; 19:212-216.

67. Judprasong K, Charoenkiatkul S, Sungpuag P, Vasanachitt K, Nakjamanong Y. Total and soluble oxalate contents in Thai vegetables, cereal grains and legume seeds and their changes after cooking. *J Food Compost Anal.* 2006;19: 340-347.

68. Gallaher RN, Gallaher K, Marshall AJ, Marshall AC. Mineral analysis of ten types of commercially available tea. *J Food Compost Anal.* 2006;19:S53-S57.

69. Menezes EW, de Melo AT, Lima GH, Lajolo FM. Measurement of carbohydrate components and their impact on energy value of foods. *J Food Compost Anal.* 2004;17: 331-338.

70. Smit LE, Schönfeldt HC, de Beer WHJ. Comparison of the energy values of different dairy products obtained by various methods. *J Food Compost Anal.* 2004;17: 361-370.

71. Leskova E, Jubikova J, Kovacikova E, Kosicka M, Porubska J, Holcikova K. Vitamin losses: retention during heat treatment and continual changes expressed by mathematical models. *J Food Compost Anal.* 2006;19: 252-276.

72. Langellier BA, Brookmeyer R, Wang MC, Glik D. Language use affects food behaviours and food values among Mexican-origin adults in the USA. *Public Health Nutr.* 2015;18(2):264-274.

73. Jiang S, Quave CL. A comparison of traditional food and health strategies among Taiwanese and Chinese immigrants in Atlanta, Georgia, USA. *J Ethnobiol Ethnomed.* 2013;9(1):61.

74. Mai J, Shimp J, Weihrauch J, Kinsella JE. Lipids of fish fillets: changes following cooking by different methods. *J Food Sci.* 1978;43:1669-1674.

75. Sinclair SE, Cooper M, Mansfield ED. The influence of menu labeling on calories selected or consumed: a systematic review and meta-analysis. *J Acad Nutr Diet.* 2014;114(9):1375.e15-1388.e15.

76. Long MW, Tobias DK, Cradock AL, Batchelder H, Gortmaker SL. Systematic review and meta-analysis of the impact of restaurant menu calorie labeling. *Am J Public Health.* 2015;105(5):e11-e24.

77. Buzzard IM, Price KS, Warren RA. Considerations for selecting nutrient-calculation software: evaluation of the nutrient database. *Am J Clin Nutr.* 1991;54:7-9.

78. Stumbo P. Considerations for selecting a dietary assessment system. *J Food Compost Anal.* 2008;21(suppl 1):S13-S19.

79. Probst YC, Tapsell LC. Overview of computerized dietary assessment programs for research and practice in nutrition education. *J Nutr Educ Behav.* 2005;37(1):20-26.

80. Guenther PM, Perloff BP, Vizioli TL Jr. Separating fact from artifact in changes in nutrient intake over time. *J Am Diet Assoc.* 1994;94(3):270-275.

81. Guilland JC, Aubert R, Lhuissier M, et al. Computerized analysis of food records: role of coding and food composition database. *Eur J Clin Nutr.* 1993;47:445-453.

82. Ahuja JKC, Goldman JD, Perloff,B. The effect of improved food composition data on national intake estimates. *J Food Compost Anal.* 2006;19:S7-S13.

Using the Dietary Reference Intakes to Assess Intakes

Regan L. Bailey, PhD, MPH, RD | *Connie Weaver, PhD* | *Suzanne P. Murphy, PhD*

LEARNING OBJECTIVES

1. Interpret the Dietary Reference Intake Framework for nutrition practice.

2. Select the appropriate Dietary Reference Intakes method to apply at the individual and group levels.

3. Understand the strengths, limitations, and appropriate applications of the Dietary Reference Intakes.

The Dietary Reference Intakes (DRIs) reflect a broad group of nutrient intake recommendations that may be used to estimate the risk of inadequacy, probability of adequacy, and risk of excessive intakes (see Box 15.1 for key DRI definitions).[1-9] The nutrient standards used for the different DRIs are based on a distribution of human requirements, when possible, and the risk of nutrient excess, when such information is known. The DRIs are fundamental for assessing adequacy of dietary intakes for individuals and groups and informing nutrition policy.

A comprehensive summary of the multiple uses of the DRIs and the many stakeholders involved with the DRIs was previously published.[10] It is important to note the DRIs reflect nutrient recommendations for healthy populations; a primary goal of the DRIs is to provide reference ranges that promote optimal health rather than simply prevent frank nutrient deficiency. The DRI framework is based on a U-shaped risk curve whereby nutrient intakes that are too low or too high may have adverse health consequences (see Figure 15.1 on page 298).

All dietary recommendations are intended to be met over time. In using the DRIs for research or clinical applications, before diet is characterized as at risk for being inadequate or excessive, researchers recommend using long-term usual or habitual intakes. This is because nutrients can be stored in the body, making it unnecessary to achieve nutrient and food intake recommendations every day. Typically, what individuals eat varies from day to day, making it impractical to achieve recommendations on a daily basis.

The first section of this chapter discusses each of the DRIs—how they were set, and how they may be used. Methods for using the DRIs to assess intakes for individuals are presented in the next section, and the final section covers methods for using the DRIs to assess intakes of population groups.

HOW DIETARY REFERENCE INTAKES ARE ESTABLISHED

The DRIs are established by a panel of scientific experts convened by the Food and Nutrition Board, part of the National Academy of Medicine, and represent recommendations for 22 age, sex, and life-stage categories: two for infants; two for young children; six for boys and men; six for girls and non-pregnant, nonlactating women; three for pregnant women (depending on age group); and three for lactating women (also depending on age group).

Most of the available DRIs were set between 1997 and 2005 as a series of six reports. Only two nutrients have been updated since; in 2011, calcium and vitamin D were updated.[9] In 2006, a summary report covering the DRIs through 2005 was published,[8] and two reports on the applications of the DRIs

Estimated Average Requirement (EAR): The average daily nutrient intake that is estimated to meet the requirement of half the healthy individuals in a particular life stage and gender group.

Recommended Dietary Allowance (RDA): The average daily dietary nutrient intake that is sufficient to meet the nutrient requirements of nearly all (97% to 98%) healthy individuals in a particular life stage and gender group.

Adequate Intake (AI): The recommended average daily intake level based on observed or experimentally determined approximations or estimates of nutrient intake by a group (or groups) of apparently healthy individuals that are assumed to be adequate, The AI is used when an RDA cannot be determined.

Tolerable Upper Intake Level (UL): The highest average daily nutrient intake level that is likely to pose no risk of adverse health effects to almost all individuals in the general population. As intake increases above the UL, the risk of adverse effects may increase.

Box 15.1 Dietary Reference Intake Definitions[1-9]

have also been published: one on using the DRIs to assess dietary intakes[11] and the other on using the DRIs to plan diets.[6] The DRI tables may also be accessed through the National Academies of Sciences, Engineering and Medicine website (www.national academies.org/hmd/~/media/Files/Activity%20Files /Nutrition/DRI-Tables/5Summary%20TableTables %2014.pdf?la=en).

The federal government has determined that it is not feasible to produce regular updates of nutrient requirements for all 51 nutrients that have a DRI. Updating calcium and vitamin D cost more than $2 million. This was a substantial increase in cost relative to previous efforts because an evidence-based process was adopted, including an a priori systematic review.[12] Nevertheless, it is negligent to not prioritize updating nutrient recommendations more frequently given their importance worldwide.

Recently, a subcommittee of the Food and Nutrition Board began to develop a streamlined process, an evidence scan, to identify DRI nutrients in most need of a new or updated systematic review.[13] Two nutrients, thiamin and phosphorus, were used as case studies to develop the process, which involves creating an analytic framework to identify relevant clinical outcomes and indicator markers, to systematically scan the literature published since the previous update of the selected nutrient, to review abstracts for relevance and then review full publications from those identified by a panel of experts, and finally to recommend priority for a comprehensive systematic evidence review. Researchers and practitioners hope that a standing committee will be charged with regularly reviewing all nutrients using the evidence scan and that those identified as a high priority be nominated for a full review. This streamlined approach provides a systematic, evidence-based, data-driven assessment that can be used to inform the prioritization of nutrients that are in need of a DRI update.

THE DIETARY REFERENCE INTAKES FRAMEWORK

Estimated Average Requirement and the Recommended Dietary Allowance

Ideally, the starting point for establishing a DRI is to garner a sense of the average human requirement for the nutrient of interest. This is designated as the Estimated Average Requirement (EAR). For each nutrient with an EAR, panel members determined a health indicator or biomarker criterion of the average amount of a nutrient required for adequacy. Because the EAR is the level of usual intake that would be adequate for half of the individuals in a population or group, the probability of inadequacy would be 0.5 (or 50%) if an individual's usual intake is equal to the EAR. Among a group of individuals with intakes exactly equal to the EAR, 50% of the group would be expected to have intakes that are at risk for inadequacy for the criterion that was chosen—for example, near-maximal maintenance of neutrophil vitamin C concentrations with minimal urinary loss.

Because the EAR is only adequate for half of the population, it is not an appropriate target for an individual's intake.

After determining the mean (or median) requirement for a nutrient, the panel members estimated the distribution of human requirements around the average. For all nutrients except iron, the distribution was assumed to be normal (or, in the case of protein, the logarithms of the requirements were distributed normally). Because the data are sparse on the standard deviation (SD) of human requirements, a coefficient of variation (CV) of 10% was assumed for most nutrients $[CV = (SD/Mean) \times 100]$. Other estimates of the CV were used for protein (12.5%), niacin (15%), vitamin D (15%), calcium (15%), and vitamin A (20%). Because the distribution of iron requirements is skewed, especially for menstruating women, the components of iron requirements were modeled to determine the risk of inadequacy at various levels of intake.

The Recommended Dietary Allowance (RDA) is calculated as two SDs above the EAR. For nutrients with a CV of 10% of the requirement, the RDA is 20% above the EAR (ie, $RDA = EAR \times 1.2$). The RDA is often used to plan diets for individuals because intake at the RDA for a nutrient has a low risk of being inadequate (approximately 2% to 3%). It is possible to calculate other nutrient standards that may be used instead of the RDA. For example, if a 15% probability of inadequacy were considered acceptable for an individual (instead of the 2% to 3% inherent in the RDA), a number lower than the RDA could be used as a target (approximately the EAR plus one SD, rather than the EAR plus two SDs). The RDA is not useful when calculating the prevalence of inadequacy for population groups.

Adequate Intake

When the scientific and experimental data are insufficient to estimate the average requirement and set an EAR and RDA, an Adequate Intake (AI) is set. Ideally, an AI is the mean intake of a healthy population (ie, one with a low prevalence of inadequacy based on a defined criterion). However, other methods have been used to derive an AI, such as experimentally determined intake. An AI is expected to exceed the RDA for a nutrient, if an RDA could be determined, because the mean intake of a healthy population could be well above the RDA. Thus, in applying the AI, the proportion of a group that exceeds the AI should have adequate intakes, but there is no scientific basis to state that the proportion of intakes lower than the AI is an estimate of the prevalence of inadequacy.

An AI is used as the nutrient standard for almost all nutrients for infants and is based on the mean intake supplied by human milk for healthy, exclusively breastfed infants. An exception is vitamin D. Vitamin D content of breastmilk reflects maternal exposure rather than a regulated level to meet the infant's needs. The panel determined that 400 IU vitamin D per day is sufficient to maintain serum 25-hydroxy vitamin D concentrations >50 nmol/L for most infants.[7]

Tolerable Upper Intake Level

Although intakes at or above the RDA have a very low risk of inadequacy, at some point intake can become high enough to increase the risk of consuming an excessive amount of the nutrient, particularly when nutrients from dietary supplements are consumed. The risk of excessive intake begins to increase at levels above the Tolerable Upper Intake Level (UL). For each nutrient with a UL, a specific adverse effect was identified. In setting the UL, consideration is given to selecting the adverse effect that would first appear as intake became excessive, so the initial adverse effect might be relatively mild. For example, the adverse effects for excessive vitamin C intake are osmotic diarrhea and related gastrointestinal disturbances. If usual intake exceeds this level, the risk of diarrhea increases. At even higher levels, other adverse effects might occur. For many nutrients, the data were insufficient to set a UL. The lack of a UL does not mean that intake at any level is considered safe, however, only that data were lacking. In the future, distributions of adverse effects around a mean may be available for some nutrients, thus enabling an estimated average UL comparable to the EAR. Such an approach would allow scientists to estimate the prevalence of adverse effects within a population.[14]

Figure 15.1 on page 298 is a graph of the risk (or probability) of inadequacy and excess as intake increases for a hypothetical nutrient, assuming a normally distributed requirement distribution. When intake is zero, the risk of inadequacy is 1.0 (or 100%).

As intake increases, the risk of inadequacy decreases until it is essentially zero. In Figure 15.1, the EAR is the point on the curve where the risk of inadequacy is 50%.[10] When intake is equal to the RDA, the risk of inadequacy is low, about 2.5%. No such quantitative risk estimates can be made from the AI or the UL. It is important to note that the figure suggests a wide range of intakes between adequacy and excess; this is the case for some nutrients, but other nutrients have a much narrower range; this is especially true for young children.

Estimated Energy Requirement and Acceptable Macronutrient Distribution Range

The nutrient standard for energy intake is the Estimated Energy Requirement (EER), that is, the average energy intake needed to maintain energy balance in an adult. For children, the EER also includes the energy needed for growth; for pregnant women, it includes the energy to sustain growth of fetal and maternal tissues; and for lactating women, it includes the energy needed to produce milk. For adults, the EER is estimated using equations that consider the individual's sex, age, weight, height, and level of physical activity. As such, the EER may be used at the individual level to plan energy intakes that will maintain or alter body weight.

For macronutrients, the standard is the Acceptable Macronutrient Distribution Range (AMDR), which is expressed as a range of recommended percent of energy intake from five macronutrients: total fat, n-6 polyunsaturated fatty acids (linoleic acid), n-3 polyunsaturated fatty acids (alpha-linolenic acid), carbohydrate, and protein. The AMDRs represent intakes that minimize the risk of chronic disease and permit an adequate intake of essential nutrients. Protein and carbohydrate also have EARs and RDAs that are expressed as grams per day.

Considerations with the Dietary Reference Intakes

Some of the DRIs are expressed to encompass different forms and units of nutrients, some of which are not traditionally included in food composition tables.[14,15]

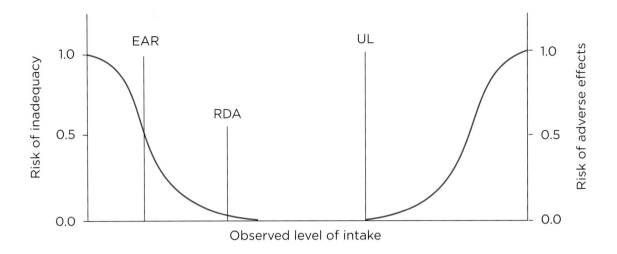

Figure 15.1 Relationship among Dietary Reference Intakes

This figure shows that the Estimated Average Requirement (EAR) is the intake at which the risk of inadequacy is 0.5 (50%) to an individual. The Recommended Dietary Allowance (RDA) is the intake at which the risk of inadequacy is very small—only 0.02 to 0.03 (2% to 3%). The Adequate Intake does not have a consistent relationship to the EAR or the RDA because it is set without estimating the requirement. At intakes between the RDA and the Tolerable Upper Intake Level (UL), the risks of inadequacy and excess are both close to zero. At intakes above the UL, the risk of adverse effects may increase.

Adapted from Institute of Medicine. *Dietary Reference Intakes: The Essential Guide to Nutrient Requirements.* Washington, DC: National Academies Press; 2006.[12] Used with permission of the National Academies Press.

As a result, it can be challenging to evaluate nutrient intakes by comparing them to the DRIs, and researchers need to exercise caution. Bioequivalence is a metric used to standardize different forms of nutrients to account for different biological activity, and it varies from nutrient to nutrient. For example, vitamin A activity can come from provitamin A carotenoids from plant sources in the diet (eg, beta carotene) and can be converted, along with retinol from animal sources in the diet, to a standardized bioequivalence metric, the retinol activity equivalent (RAE). Similarly, folic acid from fortification and dietary supplements is more bioavailable than naturally occurring folate; thus, the dietary folate equivalent (DFE) has been established to account for this differential potency.

Table 15.1 lists special case nutrients with regard to the DRIs. Some ULs apply only to nutrients added through dietary supplements (eg, magnesium salts), whereas other ULs specify synthetic or added forms of a nutrient through fortification and supplementation but not naturally occurring forms. For example, folic acid from all synthetic sources counts toward the UL, but naturally occurring folate in foods does not. Unless the food composition table disaggregates the sources of these micronutrients, it

is not possible to make such comparisons to the DRIs. The Fortification Committee of the International Life Sciences Institute North America has developed a special database that disaggregates nutrients according to whether they are intrinsic to foods or added through fortification or enrichment.

The USDA food composition database was recently substantially expanded with a branded–food products database. This large effort was the result of a public–private partnership launched by the Secretary of Agriculture on September 16, 2016. Another recent and ongoing development is the database addition of 25-hydroxy vitamin D values in animal flesh.[16] Adding this vitamin D metabolite to databases helps users more accurately estimate vitamin D exposures and reduces the discrepancy between estimated insufficiency of vitamin D from dietary and serum measures. For more on food composition tables, see Chapter 14.

The units often provided on dietary supplement labels can differ from the units provided in food composition databases, adding an extra challenge when estimating intakes. For example, dietary supplement labels may list international units (IUs) for vitamin A, including both retinol and carotenoids,

Nutrient	Estimated Average Requirement	Tolerable Upper Intake Level	Notes
Vitamin A	Retinol activity equivalent (RAE); includes activity from alpha and beta carotene and beta-cryptoxanthin (all at different equivalence)	Preformed retinol and its ester forms from all sources; measured in RAEs	Supplement labels list vitamin A in terms of international unit (IUs) of retinol; retinyl esters (such as palmitate), and carotenoids; each has different conversion factors to match an RAE to an IU.
Vitamin E	For alpha-tocopherol alone (the one form that occurs naturally in foods and the four stereoisomeric forms that occur in fortified foods and supplements)	Applies to all forms of alpha-tocopherol, including the eight stereoisomers present in synthetic vitamin E	Supplement labels list vitamin E in terms of IUs of alpha-tocopherol and its ester forms; supplement labels list vitamin E in IUs.
Folate/folic acid	Dietary folate equivalents	Only synthetic form (folic acid); metric is micrograms	Added folic acid through fortification and supplementation counts toward the UL; supplement labels list folate/folic acid in terms of micrograms of folic acid/folate; generally, folic acid is separated out in most databases.
Niacin	All forms	Only synthetic form; listed in milligrams, not niacin equivalents	Can be prescription medication to treat hyperlipidemia; the synthetic form is not often separated out in databases.
Magnesium	All forms	Only from dietary supplements	Magnesium salts
Calcium	All forms	All forms	Can be found in over-the-counter antacids; ensure that the database has standardized to elemental calcium

Table 15.1 Nutrients That Have Special Considerations When Applying the Dietary Reference Intake Framework

an estimate of biological activity rather than the discrete quantity used in food databases. Starting in 2018, the Food and Drug Administration issued labeling requirements to change the IUs to the traditional metric used for foods.[17]

Usual and Total Intakes

Dietary recommendations are intended to be met over time. Daily intakes of nutrients can vary and be stored in the body; therefore, it is unnecessary to achieve nutrient and food intake recommendations every day.[18] Before comparing the diet of an individual or a group to a DRI, it is necessary to have a sense of usual intakes. The concept of usual intake means a long-term estimate about what an individual or group typically consumes. See Chapter 13 for a full description of the time frame used for different methods. In short, most dietary assessment methods attempt to capture a short time frame,

with the exception of food frequency questionnaires. The remainder of this chapter will sidestep the question of how well dietary assessment methods perform in capturing what they purport to capture and simply assume that 24-hour recalls capture a single day's diet, food frequency questionnaires capture usual intake, and multiday diaries or records capture average daily intake over their purported time frame.

Conceptual difficulties arise when attempting to use short-term assessments to inform decisions about long-term usual intake. Due to day-to-day variation in intakes, a single day's intake, even if captured perfectly, is unlikely to reflect habitual or usual intake. So, conceptually, a researcher would want to average many 24-hour recalls per individual before making assessments about individual or group usual intake. At the group level, this is not always practical, and statistical adjustment procedures have been developed to use a small number of 24-hour recalls per individual to estimate the distribution of usual intakes.[19-23] All of these methods share a similar approach and require at least 2 days of intake data in at least a subsample, though they do vary considerably in their complexity, strengths, limitations, and fitness for purpose.

For some clinical and research applications, it is also important to include the use of dietary supplements, given their widespread use and large contribution to nutrient exposures in the United States, before evaluating the quality of the diet using the DRIs. Not including nutrients derived from supplements overestimates the prevalence of inadequacy and underestimates the prevalence of intakes above the UL when assessing intakes of population groups.[24-28] To estimate total usual intakes at the group level, model observed intakes from food sources using one of the methods referenced earlier, and then incorporate the estimated usual intakes of supplements to produce a distribution of usual total nutrient intake.[29] If supplement-based nutrient amounts are first added to single-day diet-based nutrient amounts, and the resulting numbers are run through usual intake software, there is the potential for erroneous estimates, particularly at the tails of the distribution (ie, less than the EAR, more than the UL). The next sections describe assessment with the DRIs at the individual and the group level.

ASSESSING INTAKES OF INDIVIDUALS

Does an individual's diet meet his or her nutrient requirements? Is he or she at risk of adverse effects from excessive intakes? The way in which these seemingly simple questions are addressed may vary considerably between what is practical and feasible in the practice setting and what is appropriate in a research context. In the practice setting, registered dietitian nutritionists (RDNs) may use relatively informal methods to assess their clients' nutrient intakes. For example, an RDN might compare a client's intake on a typical day to serving recommendations from MyPlate[30] or use an overall screening tool.[31] Inferences about potentially low nutrient intakes are often made on this basis of professional judgment (eg, it might be inferred that calcium intake is low if no servings of dairy products or calcium supplements were consumed). Rarely, if ever, should a clinician assume dietary adequacy based on self-reported intake alone because information about requirements is only specified up to an assumed normal distribution and is not tailored to a specific individual. Thus, clinicians hoping to evaluate nutritional status should do so by incorporating self-reported diet along with anthropometry, biomarkers, and clinical status.[11] The remainder of this section includes a description of an approach to help clinicians incorporate self-reported diet information into their judgment.

In contrast, in a research setting a higher degree of rigor may be needed, and it is important to obtain an accurate estimate of usual intake so that associations with outcome measures are not attenuated.[32] As in the clinical setting, reliance on other markers of nutrient status may be appropriate. The remainder of this section also describes how the DRIs may be used to assess usual intakes of individuals. In all cases, it is essential to begin with accurately measured food intake data; all self-reported dietary intake data are subject to measurement error and should be given full consideration before making judgments and recommendations relative to the DRI.[33]

Nutrients with an Estimated Average Requirement and Recommended Dietary Allowance

At the individual level, the EAR is used is used to determine the probability of inadequacy. Intakes that exceed the RDA can be generally assumed to be adequate, but intakes below the RDA are not necessarily inadequate. Although an individual's requirement for a nutrient is generally not known, knowledge of the EAR and CV of the requirement distribution provides information on the range within which the requirement likely falls. As described earlier, the requirement distribution for most nutrients is assumed to be normal, with a mean at the EAR and a CV of 10%. Figure 15.2 shows an example of a requirement distribution, in this case magnesium, for women aged 19 to 30 years. The EAR is 255 mg/d, and the SD is 25.5 mg/d (based on an assumed CV of 10%). The figure shows that most individuals have requirements that are relatively close to the EAR, whereas

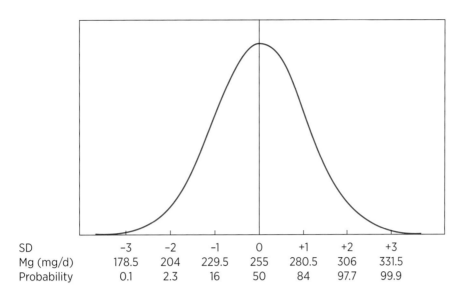

SD	−3	−2	−1	0	+1	+2	+3
Mg (mg/d)	178.5	204	229.5	255	280.5	306	331.5
Probability	0.1	2.3	16	50	84	97.7	99.9

Figure 15.2 Example of a requirement distribution: magnesium requirements for women aged 19 to 30 years

The Estimated Average Requirement (EAR) is 255 mg/d, and the standard deviation (SD) is 25.5 mg/d (based on an assumed coefficient of variation [CV] of 10%). Also shown are the probabilities of adequacy for usual intakes at the EAR, and one, two, or three SDs above or below the EAR.

smaller proportions have requirements that are considerably higher or lower.

Figure 15.2 also shows the probability that a given usual intake is adequate. Based on characteristics of the normal curve, the probability ranges from near zero (at intakes more than 2 SDs below the EAR) to nearly 100% (at intakes more than 2 SDs above the EAR). The probability is calculated by subtracting the EAR from the usual intake and dividing by the SD of the requirement distribution to yield a z score (a difference divided by its SD) and then consulting a table of z scores to determine the associated probability.

For example, the probability that a usual magnesium intake of 280 mg/d is adequate would be estimated as follows: $z=$ (Usual intake − EAR)/SD = (280 − 255)/25.5 = 0.98. A z score of 0.98 (about 1.0) is associated with a probability of about 84%. In other words, a usual intake of 280 mg/d meets or exceeds the magnesium requirements of about 84 of 100 women aged 19 to 30 years. These probability calculations assume that an individual's long-term usual intake has been measured. However, because intakes vary from day to day, it is difficult to obtain true usual intake measures. Therefore, additional calculations can be performed to estimate the level of confidence that intake is adequate for an individual (described in detail in *Dietary Reference Intakes: Applications in Dietary Assessment*[11]). The extent of uncertainty about an individual's true usual intake is a function of both the number of days for which records or recalls are kept (collecting intake data over a larger number of days leads to less uncertainty) and the specific nutrient being assessed. Consider once again the example of magnesium, in which there was an 84% probability that a usual intake of 280 mg/d was adequate. Suppose that the within-person or day-to-day variability in magnesium intake is 86 mg. If usual intake was estimated as the mean of four single-day measurements, the level of confidence that the usual intake is adequate is computed to be 69%. Therefore, the level of confidence that usual intake is adequate is lower taking into consideration the uncertainty associated with estimating usual intake from a small number of short-term measurements.

Day-to-day or within-person variability (and therefore uncertainty) is much greater in intakes of nutrients found in high concentrations in a small number of foods compared with those nutrients widely distributed throughout the food supply. Thus, the assumption of normally distributed within-person fluctuations seems to be violated to a great degree by certain nutrients, including vitamin A, carotene, vitamin C, and vitamin B-12. Practically, however, advice to individuals regarding nutrient intake adequacy depends on the quality of the intake measure (ie, how it reflects an individual's usual long-term intake) and on the level of intake relative to the EAR and RDA. Because of the difficulty of measuring true usual intake, a conservative qualitative assessment may be more appropriate. As noted in the report on dietary assessment,[11] one could consider that usual intakes below the EAR need improvement, intakes between the EAR and the RDA probably need improvement, and those above the RDA are likely to be adequate if the intake measure includes a large number of days.

Nutrients with an Adequate Intake

By definition, the EAR is unknown for nutrients that have an AI. If an individual's usual intake equals or exceeds the AI, researchers can conclude that the diet is almost certainly adequate, as the AI is thought to exceed the requirements of almost everyone. If, however, intake falls below the AI, no quantitative (or qualitative) estimate can be made of the probability of nutrient inadequacy because the requirement is not known and cannot be estimated from the AI. Nutrition professionals should use their judgment, after considering additional types of information about the individual, when interpreting intakes below the AI.

Nutrients with a Tolerable Upper Intake Level

The UL may be used to assess whether an individual's usual nutrient intake is so high that it poses a potential risk of adverse health effects. For some nutrients, the UL applies only to intake from supplements, fortificants, or medications, whereas for other nutrients, total intake from all sources is considered. Many uncertainties exist with regard to the

UL, so clinical expertise and careful evaluation are needed.

Macronutrients with an Acceptable Macronutrient Distribution Range

Because the AMDRs have both lower and upper boundaries, the goal for an individual is to consume a diet with macronutrient intakes that fall within the AMDR. Thus, assessment using the AMDRs involves determining whether usual intakes are above or below the recommended ranges.

Evaluating Energy Intake Using the Estimated Energy Requirement

In most cases, it is not appropriate to use the EER to evaluate the adequacy of an individual's energy intake—an EER that has a high probability of being adequate for an individual (eg, an intake two SDs above the mean) would have an equally high probability of leading to weight gain. Furthermore, energy intake is subject to a systematic bias in self-reported energy-related intakes.[34,35] Unlike other nutrients, energy has a valid, reliable, and accessible indicator of whether requirements are being met: stability or change in body weight.

Assessing Individual Diets Using the Dietary Reference Intakes: An Example

A hypothetical example of a dietary assessment for a man aged 74 years is shown in Table 15.2. This man reports 7 days of dietary data that he says is a typical week's diet. Nutrient intake has been calculated for five nutrients (riboflavin, folate, calcium, potassium, and zinc) and assumes that the dietary data collected represent a usual diet. The researcher wishes to provide feedback to this man and, thus, chooses a qualitative assessment, as shown in Table 15.2.

Several points are apparent from this example:

● Although riboflavin intake is above the EAR, it is below the RDA of 1.3 mg/d, leading to an assessment of possible inadequacy because the probability of inadequacy is greater than 2% to

Nutrient	Mean Intake	EAR[b] or AI[c]	RDA[d]	UL[e]	Qualitative Assessment
Riboflavin, mg	1.2	(1.1 (EAR)	1.3	Not established	Possibly inadequate
Folate, µg DFE[f]	200	(320 (EAR)	400	1,000 (synthetic folate only)	High probability of inadequacy
Calcium, mg	1,250	(1,000 (EAR)	1,200	4,000	Likely adequate but not excessive
Potassium, mg	2,300	(4,700 (AI)	Not established	Not established	Unable to assess adequacy
Zinc, mg	11	(9.4 (EAR)	11	40	Likely adequate but not excessive

Table 15.2 Evaluation of a 74-Year-Old Man's Diet Based on Usual Intake[a] from Food and Supplements

[a] Assumes that usual nutrient intake from both food and supplements has been measured using a comprehensive method that reflects typical long-term intake.
[b] EAR = Estimated Average Requirement
[c] AI = Adequate Intake
[d] RDA = Recommended Dietary Allowance
[e] UL = Tolerable Upper Intake Level.
[f] DFE = dietary folate equivalent

3%. A slightly different situation exists for zinc, where the man's intake equals the RDA of 11 mg, leading to an assessment of likely adequacy, assuming usual intake was captured.

- Folate intake is well below the EAR, so inadequacy is likely.
- Calcium intake exceeds the EAR and the RDA and, therefore, is likely adequate if true long-term intake was accurately captured.
- Potassium does not have an EAR or RDA, only an AI of 4,000 mg/d. The man's intake is 2,300 mg/d. It is not possible to determine whether the intake is sufficient to maintain clinically normal blood pressure and health, and it would be inappropriate to state that he is deficient in potassium intake. Nevertheless, it would be appropriate to recommend that he increase his intake to meet the AI so that adequacy could be ensured.
- Three of the analyzed nutrients have a UL (folate, calcium, and zinc), but the reported nutrient intakes are well below these ULs, so there are no concerns about a risk of adverse effects from excessive intakes.

ASSESSING INTAKES OF POPULATIONS

Using the DRIs to assess the prevalence of inadequacy or excess poses challenges. Rarely, if ever, is it feasible to monitor dietary intake exactly over a long enough period of time to calculate usual intake for an individual directly, and doing so for a large group is even more difficult. However, under some assumptions about the measurement properties of dietary assessment instruments, it is possible to estimate the distribution of usual intakes using data collected as part of population surveys or studies. Once this estimated distribution is obtained, further assumptions about the distribution of requirements allows researchers to estimate the prevalence of inadequacy as the percentage of the group with usual intakes below the EAR. Thus, the EAR, rather than the RDA, is the DRI that is used in assessing the intakes of populations.

Statistical Procedures for Estimating Intake Distributions from Short-Term Measurements

The distribution of single-day intakes, or of the within-person means of 2 days of intake, is not the same as the distribution of usual intakes because the former includes both between-person variability (some individuals habitually have higher nutrient intakes than others) and within-person variability (on the day of the recall, a given individual's intake might be much higher or much lower than his or her usual intake). As shown in Figure 15.3, the mean is the same, but the variance (or spread) of nutrient intakes in the distribution of 1-day intakes is much greater than the variance in a distribution of usual intakes that reflects only between-person variabil-

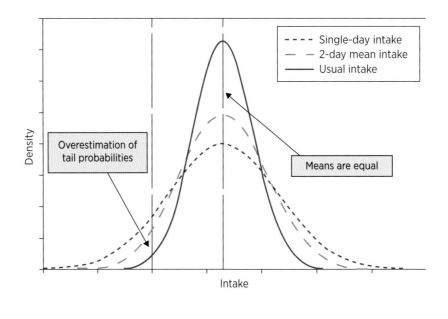

Figure 15.3 Hypothetical nutrient distribution with and without usual intake methods applied

ity. Such differences in the variance would usually be seen even for multiple days of intake for each individual. Only a very large number of days per individual would approach a usual intake distribution. The prevalence of nutrient inadequacy in a group can often be estimated from the proportion of individuals in the group with intakes below the EAR for the nutrient, as discussed later in this chapter. Figure 15.3 shows that the prevalence of inadequacy (intakes below the EAR) would be overestimated if the distribution of 1-day or 2-day intake was used.

In population-level nutrition surveys, a large number of days of intake data is never available. Instead, such surveys typically collect at most one or two 24-hour recalls per individual. Several statistical methods have been developed to estimate usual nutrient intake distributions from such sparse data, though the methods can be applied to other short-term assessments, such as food records/diaries or recovery biomarkers.[19-23] The goal of all of these methods is to approximate the distribution one would obtain by averaging many 24-hour recalls per individual. All of these methods have a similar underlying framework, and make several assumptions that are beyond the scope of this chapter but are reviewed elsewhere.[23] This method, originally proposed in 1986 by the National Research Council, is called the NRC method. Future independent iterations enhanced the approach and include the bias-corrected best power method (BCBP), the Iowa State University (ISU) method, and the National Cancer Institute (NCI) method.

Currently, researchers use the ISU and NCI methods most frequently. The ISU method is implemented as a stand-alone program that can run on Linux or Windows operating systems, whereas the NCI method is implemented in sets of macros that require the SAS software. All of the approaches require at least two repeat measurements for at least a representative subsample of the population group of interest to allow computation of both variance components. Although it is possible to use external estimates of these variance components from a different but similar group, it is preferable to calculate this variability directly from the group being evaluated unless, for example, no individuals have repeated measures.

Calculating Prevalence of Adequacy/ Inadequacy

Researchers and public health officials are often interested in estimating the prevalence of nutrient inadequacy in a group or population. This information may be required for a variety of reasons, including monitoring the health status or designing interventions to improve intakes for a given group. An individual does not consume an adequate amount of a nutrient when the usual intake of the nutrient does not meet his or her requirement for the nutrient. Similarly, the proportion of individuals in a group with inadequate intakes is given by the proportion whose intakes do not meet their requirements. In principle, therefore, in order to estimate the prevalence of nutrient inadequacy in a group, researchers would need to know—for each individual in the group—both the usual intake and requirement for the nutrient. Because researchers never know each individual's requirement for a nutrient and can only estimate each individual's usual intake, estimating prevalence seems, at first glance, to be an impossible task. However, under some assumptions, and with knowledge about the distribution of requirements and usual intakes in the group, it is possible to estimate the prevalence of inadequacy. Two approaches that have been proposed are the probability approach and the EAR cut-point method.

The Probability Approach

The probability approach for estimating the prevalence of nutrient inadequacy was first proposed by the National Research Council[19] and is not commonly used, with the exception of iron (discussed later). The idea is straightforward: Using the distribution of requirements in a group, first compute the risk curve, which indicates the risk of inadequacy at each usual intake level. For example, if the distribution of requirements in a group is normal, with an EAR (mean) equal to 100 units of the nutrient and an SD equal to 10 units, then from a normal probability table a researcher can find the risks associated with any level of intake. Figure 15.2 shows that the risk associated with any level of usual intake depends on how far the intake is from the mean (ie, the number of SDs between the intake and the mean). If estimates of usual intake for each individual in the group have been obtained, risk of inadequacy can be computed for each individual in the group. The risks

associated with each intake (illustrated in Figure 15.2 on page 301) can be calculated using statistical software, such as the PROBNORM function in SAS. Using the mean (EAR) and the SD of the requirement, the program will calculate the probability (risk) of inadequacy for each individual. The prevalence of inadequacy would then be computed as the simple average of the individual-level risks.

The probability approach for estimating the prevalence of inadequacy relies on a few assumptions. The distribution of requirements does not need to be normal or symmetric. Usual intake distributions can have any shape and, in particular, can be skewed. The method cannot be applied, however, when intakes and requirements are not independent, as is the case with energy. Finally, it is not possible to apply the probability approach for estimating prevalence of inadequacy unless the requirements distribution is known. This mean that the researcher must at least know the mean and SD (or the CV) of requirements in the group and be willing to make some assumptions regarding the shape of the distribution of requirements before implementing this method. Thus, the probability approach cannot be applied to nutrients for which an AI but not an EAR has been established. The probability approach (rather than the EAR cut-point method) must be used for iron because the requirement distribution is known to be skewed. Percentiles of the requirement distributions for iron are available by age and sex group in DRIs for vitamin A, vitamin K, arsenic, boron, chromium, copper, iodine, iron, manganese, molybdenum, nickel, silicon, vanadium, and zinc.[4]

The Cut-Point Approach

Carriquiry[36] proposed a shortcut to the probability approach for estimating the prevalence of nutrient inadequacy in a group—the EAR cut-point method, which is commonly used. The method is simple to implement if an estimate of the usual intake distribution in the group is available. Essentially, the EAR cut-point method consists of estimating the prevalence of nutrient inadequacy as the proportion of individuals in a group whose usual intakes of the nutrient are below the EAR for the nutrient. The theoretical underpinnings of the EAR cut-point method can be found in Carriquiry,[36] and *Dietary Reference Intakes: Applications in Dietary Assessment*[11] provides an extensive discussion of the approach, including a derivation of the method. It is crucial that estimated intake distributions reflect usual intake before the EAR cut-point method is applied. For example, the prevalence of inadequacy of vitamin B-6 intakes for women was examined using a single recall and using usual intake distributions obtained using a usual intake method.[11] The prevalence estimate based on 1 day of intake was approximately 32%, whereas the prevalence computed using the usual intake method was approximately 18%. This example illustrates the impact of accounting for within-person variance in short-term measures of intake. If such incorrect estimates are made at the national level, it could result in inappropriate nutrition policies.

Although the EAR cut-point method is relatively simple to implement, it relies on more assumptions than the probability approach does and thus cannot be applied as widely. As with the probability approach, the EAR cut-point method works well only when intakes and requirements can be assumed to be independent. Therefore, the EAR cut-point method cannot be used with energy. Further, this method requires that the distribution of requirements be normal or at least symmetric around the EAR. As a consequence, it cannot be used to estimate the prevalence of iron inadequacy in a group (the probability approach, however, can be applied to iron intake). In addition, the EAR cut-point method works well when the variance of requirements is less than the variance of usual intakes, an assumption that is likely to hold for most nutrients, at least in free-living populations. On the positive side, it is not necessary to know the exact SD of the requirement (ie, the variance of the requirement) when applying the EAR cut-point method, as long as this variance is relatively small compared with the variance of intakes. The EAR cut-point method provides a closer approximation to the prevalence than that estimated by the probability approach when the true prevalence of inadequacy in the population is neither too low nor too high. Clearly, as is the case with the probability approach, the method cannot be applied when an EAR for the nutrient has not been established.

Limitations of Adequate Intakes

The approaches addressed thus far cannot be used for nutrients with an AI because the requirement distribution is not known for these nutrients. For this reason, the AI is of limited use in assessing the adequacy of nutrient intake for groups. Nevertheless, the following statements can be made:

- If a group has a mean or median intake at or above the AI, it is likely that there is a low prevalence of inadequate intakes. However, because the AIs are set using different criteria, confidence in this assessment varies and is high only if the AI represents the mean or median intake of an apparently healthy group of individuals. The derivation of each AI is described in the individual DRI reports.
- It is not possible to make any assumptions about the prevalence of inadequacy when the mean intake of a group is below the AI: it is possible that the prevalence of inadequate intake could be extremely low. For example, pantothenic acid deficiency is virtually unknown in North America, so even among a group with a mean intake below the AI, it is probable that pantothenic acid status is satisfactory.
- Although the percentage of individuals with usual intakes less than the AI can be estimated, this proportion cannot be interpreted as having inadequate intakes.

Calculating the Prevalence of Potentially Excessive Intakes

The prevalence of potentially excessive intakes is estimated by determining the proportion of the usual intake distribution that falls above the UL for the age and sex group. It is important to ensure that usual intakes of the appropriate form of the nutrient are being assessed. For example, for vitamin A, one would determine the prevalence of usual intake of preformed retinol above the UL rather than of the total vitamin A intake from both retinol and carotenoids. Nutrients from dietary supplements are not easily incorporated into existing statistical software to produce usual intakes.

Assessing Energy and Macronutrients with the Estimated Energy Requirement and Acceptable Macronutrient Distribution Range

The mean energy intake of a group that is weight stable (or, in the case of children or pregnant women, gaining weight at an appropriate rate) should be equal to the group's mean energy requirement. This means that the adequacy of a group's energy intake could theoretically be assessed by comparing the mean energy intake to the mean predicted EER for the group: a mean intake approximating the EER would reflect an adequate energy intake, whereas a mean intake below or above the mean EER would reflect an inadequate or excessive intake, respectively. However, as was also the case for individuals, it is more appropriate to assess the adequacy of a group's energy intake by assessing group members' relative weights, most commonly using body mass index. For each macronutrient with an AMDR, the proportion of the usual (adjusted) intake distribution that falls within the AMDR would be assessed as intakes consistent with minimizing the risk of chronic disease and permitting adequate intakes of essential nutrients.

What to Do with Small Groups

Most statistical methods have been established for large groups. Practitioners often ask how many individuals constitute a group. The answer, unfortunately, is not always a specific number, such as 30, 50, or 100. Rather, whether individuals are just individuals or form a group depends in great measure on the objectives of the investigation. If the final objective is to provide nutrition counseling to each individual, then even a sample of 1,000 individuals should be treated as 1,000 individuals, and their nutrient intakes should be assessed as described in the chapter section on assessing intakes of individuals. If, however, the goal of the study is to characterize the intake distribution in a population or perhaps to estimate the prevalence of inadequate intakes of a nutrient, those individuals should be treated as a group—although it is still difficult to give a specific number because the appropriate sample size depends on several factors.

When applying statistical modeling to short-term measurements of intake, one important consideration is the number of individuals in the group with at least one replicate observation. It may be better to have 100 individuals in a group when 2 days of daily intakes have been collected from each than to have a sample of 500 individuals for whom a replicate observation is available for only 25.

The size of the group will determine the precision with which percentiles of the usual nutrient intake distribution can be estimated. If only a rough estimate of the usual intake distribution is required, then a small group with 30 or 40 individuals might suffice. In this case, the practitioner might be able to reliably estimate the mean, variance, and skewness of the usual intake distribution but will be surrendering the capability of estimating percentiles at the tails with any degree of accuracy.

Finally, those nutrients with large (and perhaps heterogeneous) day-to-day variance in intake require larger sample sizes for reliable estimation. It is easier (in terms of group size) to estimate the usual intake distribution of, for example, protein than to estimate the usual intake distribution of, for example, vitamin A.

A group of 100, in which at least half of the individuals have a replicate observation, is probably almost always large enough to implement any of the three methods described earlier to estimate usual nutrient intake distributions. At the other end, a group with 30 or fewer individuals, even if all have a replicate intake observation, is probably too small to implement any of the three approaches.

Statistical Tests of Differences Between Groups

Nutrition researchers often want to know whether the difference in nutrient intakes between two groups is significant. A relevant question that can be addressed using the DRIs is as follows: Do the two groups differ in the prevalence of dietary nutrient inadequacy (or adequacy)?

The dietary adequacy of two groups can be compared with relatively simple statistical tests. For example, suppose the adequacy of vitamin C intakes is compared for adolescent boys and adolescent girls. The first step would be to determine the prevalence of adequate vitamin C intakes for each group, after appropriately adjusting the intake distributions for the effect of day-to-day variation (as described earlier). Then, the prevalence of adequate intakes for each group would be estimated as the percentage of the group with intakes above the EAR. Finally, a statistical test, such as a *t* test, can be used to determine whether the prevalence for boys is statistically different from the prevalence for girls. When comparing the nutrient adequacy of two groups, it is often desirable to consider covariates—such as age, income, and education level—that might affect nutrient intakes. For example, when comparing adolescent boys and girls, one might wish to adjust for age. One possible approach is to estimate the usual intake distributions as if all children had the same age, then estimate prevalence in the two sex groups. In some circumstances, it may be of interest to estimate the association between an individual-level covariate and adequacy. For example, a researcher might be interested in comparing different food assistance packages by testing whether individuals enrolled in the different programs have different probabilities of inadequacy. Many possible approaches could be used to carry out this type of analysis. An approach relying on multivariate analysis has been proposed but has not been widely used to date.[37]

EXAMPLES AT THE GROUP LEVEL

The National Health and Nutrition Examination Survey (NHANES), conducted by the Centers for Disease Control and Prevention's National Center for Health Statistics, is a nationally representative, cross-sectional survey that samples noninstitutionalized, civilian US residents using a complex, stratified, multistage probability cluster design.[38] The NHANES protocol includes an in-person 24-hour dietary recall and a telephone 24-hour recall as part of the What We Eat in America survey.[39] NHANES researchers place emphasis on collecting both week and weekend days to ensure representativeness of the diet. Dietary supplement use is measured through a 30-day food frequency questionnaire and as part of the 24-hour diet recall.

Usual dietary intakes of Americans by sex and age group have been assessed from diet alone and from all sources (including dietary supplements and nutrients from medications) using the ISU method,[40] the BCBP method,[41] and the NCI method.[42] These types of analyses can be used to help identify nutrients of public health concern when prevalence of risk for inadequate or potentially excessive intakes is large; for example, among US adults, <3% exceed the AI for potassium (ie, low probability for adequacy) and 90% exceed the UL for sodium.[43]

Dietary supplements help users to meet the EAR across almost all nutrients but do increase the risk of usual intakes above the UL.[25,44,45] Some children exceed the UL for folic acid, zinc, vitamin A, and copper from the diet alone with much higher proportions when dietary supplement use is considered.[26,46] To estimate total usual nutrient intake, researchers recommend adding nutrient intakes from dietary supplements to the adjusted usual nutrient intake from foods.[47]

CONCLUSION

Researchers face many challenges when assessing intakes using the DRIs. However, most of these can be addressed by understanding the underlying concepts and using appropriate software. For individuals, it is possible to estimate the probability that usual intake is inadequate and whether usual intake is potentially at risk of being excessive. For population groups, the prevalence of inadequacy can be estimated from a usual intake distribution, as can the prevalence of intakes at risk of being excessive. Ultimately, the DRIs give researchers the ability to assess intakes with far more detail and accuracy than is possible when the RDA is the only available nutrient intake standard.

REFERENCES

1. Food and Nutrition Board. *Dietary Reference Intakes for Calcium, Phosphorus, Magnesium, Vitamin D and Fluoride.* Washington, DC: National Academy Press; 1997.

2. Food and Nutrition Board. D*ietary Reference Intakes for Thiamin, Riboflavin, Niacin, Vitamin B6, Folate, Vitamin B12, Pantothenic Acid, Biotin, and Choline.* Washington, DC: National Academy Press; 1998.

3. Food and Nutrition Board. *Dietary Reference Intakes for Vitamin C, Vitamin E, Selenium, and Carotenoids.* Washington, DC: National Academy Press; 2000.

4. Food and Nutrition Board. *Dietary Reference Intakes for Vitamin A, Vitamin K, Arsenic, Boron, Chromium, Copper, Iodine, Iron, Molybdenum, Nickel, Silicon, Vanadium and Zinc.* Washington, DC: National Academy Press; 2001.

5. Food and Nutrition Board. *Dietary Reference Intakes for Energy, Carbohydrate, Fiber, Fat, Fatty Acids, Cholesterol, Protein, and Amino Acids (Macronutrients).* Washington, DC: Institute of Medicine; 2002/2005.

6. Food and Nutrition Board. *Dietary Reference Intakes: Applications in Dietary Planning.* Washington, DC: Institute of Medicine; 2003.

7. Food and Nutrition Board. *Dietary Reference Intakes for Water, Potassium, Sodium, Chloride, and Sulfate.* Washington, DC: Institute of Medicine; 2004.

8. Food and Nutrition Board. *Dietary Reference Intakes: The Essential Guide to Nutrient Requirements.* Washington, DC: Institute of Medicine; 2006.

9. Food and Nutrition Board. *Dietary Reference Intakes for Calcium and Vitamin D.* Washington, DC: National Academy Press; 2011.

10. Weaver C, Murphy SP. Food scientists & Dietary Reference Intakes: an important alliance. *Food Technol.* 2014;68(11): 46-54.

11. Food and Nutrition Board. *Dietary Reference Intakes Applications in Dietary Assessment.* Washington, DC: National Academy Press; 2000.

12. Chung M, Balk EM, Brendel M, et al. V*itamin D and Calcium: Systematic Review of Health Outcomes.* Evidence Report/Technology Assessment No. 183. Rockville, MD: Agency for Healthcare Research and Quality; 2009.

13. Brannon PM, Weaver CM, Anderson CA, Donovan SM, Murphy SP, Yaktine AL. Scanning for new evidence to prioritize updates to the Dietary Reference Intakes: case studies for thiamin and phosphorus. *Am J Clin Nutr.* 2016; 104(5):1366-1377.

14. Murphy SP. Changes in dietary guidance: implications for food and nutrient databases. *J Food Comp Anal.* 2001;14: 269-278.

15. Murphy SP. Dietary Reference Intakes for the U.S. and Canada: update on implications for nutrient databases. *J Food Comp Anal.* 2002;15(4):411-417.

16. Taylor CL, Patterson KY, Roseland JM, et al. Including food 25-hydroxyvitamin D in intake estimates may reduce the discrepancy between dietary and serum measures of vitamin D status. *J Nutr.* 2014;144(5):654-659.

17. Food and Drug Administration. Food labeling: revision of the Nutrition and Supplement Facts labels. *Fed Regist.* 2016; 381(103):33741-33999. Codified at 21 CFR §101.

18. National Cancer Institute. The Measurement Error Webinar Series. http://riskfactor.cancer.gov /measurementerror. Published 2011. Last updated January 9, 2018. Accessed April 10, 2018.

19. National Research Council. *Nutrient Adequacy.* Washington, DC: National Academy Press; 1986.

20. Nusser SM, Carriquiry AL, Dodd KW, Fuller WA. A semiparametric transformation approach to estimating usual daily intake distributions. *J Am Stat Assoc.* 1996; 91(436): 1440-1449.

21. Subar AF, Dodd KW, Guenther PM, et al. The food propensity questionnaire: concept, development, and validation for use as a covariate in a model to estimate usual food intake. *J Am Diet Assoc.* 2006;106(10): 1556-1563.

22. Tooze JA, Midthune D, Dodd KW, et al. A new statistical method for estimating the usual intake of episodically consumed foods with application to their distribution. *J Am Diet Assoc.* 2006;106(10):1575-1587.

23. Dodd KW, Guenther PM, Friedman LS, et al. Statistical methods for estimating usual intake of nutrients and foods: a review of the theory. *J Am Diet Assoc.* 2006;106(10): 1640-1650.

24. Bailey RL, Fulgoni VL, Keast DR, Lentino CV, Dwyer JT. Do dietary supplements improve micronutrient sufficiency in children and adolescents? *J Pediatr.* 2012;161(5):837-842.

25. Bailey RL, Fulgoni VL III, Keast DR, Dwyer JT. Examination of vitamin intakes among US adults by dietary supplement use. *J Acad Nutr Diet.* 2012;112(5):657. e4-663.e4.

26. Bailey RL, Gahche JJ, Lentino CV, et al. Dietary supplement use in the United States, 2003–2006. *J Nutr.* 2011;141(2):261-266.

27. Bailey RL, Gahche JJ, Miller PE, Thomas PR, Dwyer JT. Why US adults use dietary supplements. *JAMA Intern Med.* 2013;173(5):355-361.

28. Bailey RL, Gahche JJ, Miller PE, Thomas PR, Dwyer JT. Why US children use dietary supplements. *Pediatr Res.* 2013;74(6):737-741.

29. Carriquiry AL. Estimation of usual intake distributions of nutrients and foods. *J Nutr*. 2003;133(2): 601S-608S.

30. US Department of Agriculture. MyPlate. z www.choosemyplate.gov. Accessed January 25, 2017.

31. Bailey RL, Miller PF, Mitchell DC, et al. Dietary screening tool identifies nutritional risk in older adults. *Am J Clin Nutr*. 2009;90(1):177-283.

32. Kipnis V, Midthune D, Freedman L, et al. Bias in dietary-report instruments and its implications for nutritional epidemiology. *Public Health Nutr*. 2002;5(6A):915-923.

33. Kipnis V, Subar AF, Midthune D, et al. Structure of dietary measurement error: results of the OPEN biomarker study. *Am J Epidemiol*. 2003;158(1):14-21; discussion 22-26.

34. Schoeller DA, Bandini LG, Dietz WH. Inaccuracies in self-reported intake identified by comparison with the doubly labelled water method. *Can J Physiol Pharmacol*. 1990; 68(7): 941-949.

35. Subar AF, Kipnis V, Troiana RP, et al. Using intake biomarkers to evaluate the extent of dietary misreporting in a large sample of adults: the OPEN study. *Am J Epidemiol*. 2003;158(1):1-13.

36. Carriquiry AL. Assessing the prevalence of nutrient inadequacy. *Public Health Nutr*. 1999;2(1):23-33.

37. Food and Nutrition Board. *Dietary Reference Intakes: Applications in Dietary Assessment*. Washington, DC: Institute of Medicine; 2000.

38. National Center for Health Statistics. About the National Health and Nutrition Examination Survey. www.cdc.gov /nchs/nhanes/about_nhanes.htm. Updated September 15, 2017. Accessed April 10, 2018.

39. USDA Agricultural Research Service. WWEIA Documentation and Data Sets. www.ars.usda.gov/Services /docs.htm?docid=18354. Update October 13, 2016. Accessed April 10, 2018.

40. Sebastian RS, Cleveland LE, Goldman JD, Moshfegh AJ. Older adults who use vitamin/mineral supplements differ from nonusers in nutrient intake adequacy and dietary attitudes. *J Am Diet Assoc*. 2007;107(8):1322-1332.

41. Bailey RL, Dodd KW, Gahche JJ, et al. Total folate and folic acid intake from foods and dietary supplements in the United States: 2003–2006. *Am J Clin Nutr*. 2010;91(1): 231-237.

42. Bailey RL, Dodd KW, Goldman JA, et al. Estimation of total usual calcium and vitamin D intakes in the United States. *J Nutr*. 2010;140(4):817-822.

43. Bailey RL, Parker EA, Rhodes DG, et al. Estimating sodium and potassium intakes and their ratio in the American diet: data from the 2011–2012 NHANES. *J Nutr*. 2016; pii: jn221184. Epub ahead of print.

44. Bailey RL, Fulgoni VL III, Keast DR, Dwyer JT. Dietary supplement use is associated with higher intakes of minerals from food sources. *Am J Clin Nutr*. 2011;94(5): 1376-1381.

45. Murphy SP, White KK, Park SY, Sharma S. Multivitamin-multimineral supplements' effect on total nutrient intake. *Am J Clin Nutr*. 2007;85(1):280S-284S.

46. Bailey RL, McDowell MA, Dodd KW, Gahche JJ, Dwyer JT, Piccian MF. Total folate and folic acid intakes from foods and dietary supplements of US children aged 1–13 y. *Am J Clin Nutr*. 2010;92(2):353-358.

47. Garriguet D. Combining nutrient intake from food/ beverages and vitamin/mineral supplements. *Health Rep*. 2010;21(4):71-84.

Chapter 16

Biomarkers in Nutrition Research

Yasmin Mossavar-Rahmani, PhD, RD

LEARNING OBJECTIVES

1. Describe how key biomarkers are used in nutrition assessment and intervention.

2. Identify biomarkers related to key macronutrients, micronutrients, and food components.

3. Illustrate use of biomarker-calibrated data as a strategy to reduce measurement error and strengthen diet-disease associations.

4. Describe how metabolomics can be used to identify granular-level biomarkers.

5. Describe practical considerations in collecting and processing biospecimens.

A biomarker is most simply defined as a biological marker or indicator. As used in nutrition research, this term encompasses diverse biological markers that differ in conceptual basis, interpretation, and use. For example, biomarkers of particular interest in nutrition research include biological markers or indicators of dietary intake, which are useful in validating dietary intake measures or as a way of quantifying exposure to various foods or dietary factors.[1,2] Another type of biomarker reflects the biological or cellular activity of dietary constituents (or pharmacologic agents), although the activity may not be the primary mechanism by which the constituent or agent affects the disease process.[3] Other biological markers that are useful in nutrition research as surrogate end-point biomarkers are the molecular or cellular markers that reliably predict disease risk,[4] typically reflecting a specific molecular mechanism that appears to play a role in promoting or inhibiting the disease process. As the focus of this chapter is on biomarkers that indicate dietary intake, the focus of this chapter will be on nutritional biomarkers useful in assessment and intervention.

Modern metabolomics technologies have initiated an unprecedented potential for generating biomarkers for various physiological states.[5] Microbiome measures are also biomarkers; however, there are limitations to use of biomarkers relating to quality, reliability, validity, and usefulness.[6] These biomarkers are cellular, biochemical, microbial, molecular, or genetic alterations by which a normal or abnormal biological process can be identified or monitored, and they are measurable in tissues, cells, or body fluids. Microbiome measures are also biomarkers. Nutrient biomarkers identifying biochemical, functional, or clinical indicators of nutrient intake, status, or functional effects are needed to support evidence-based guidelines for nutrition and health.[5,6] An example of a direct biochemical measure of plasma or serum is pyridoxal 5′-phosphate (PLP), while the functional indicator of vitamin B-6 could be examining activities of erythrocyte transaminase and, more recently, plasma levels of metabolites involved in PLP-dependent reactions, such as one-carbon metabolism. In the case of vitamin B-6, nutritional status is best assessed by using a combination of biomarkers because of the influence of potential confounders, such as inflammation, alkaline phosphatase activity, low serum albumin, renal function, and inorganic phosphate. The clinical indicator would be the level of nutrient at a biochemical or functional level that is associated with a health outcome. Metabolomics based on mass spectrometry allows the simultaneous quantification of a large number of metabolites, which are currently evaluated as functional biomarkers.[7]

Using biomarkers in nutrition research involves measuring biological materials, such as blood, urine, or fecal samples; surgical specimens; or tissue biopsies. Blood collection enables investigators to measure several different components or circulating pools, such as serum (the fluid portion remaining when blood has been allowed to clot and the clotted material is discarded), plasma (the fluid portion remaining when clotting has been inhibited and the formed elements [red and white blood cells] are removed), and red and white blood cell fractions. Although blood and the various components of blood are liquid at ambient temperature, blood should be considered (and described) as tissue, as one would consider and describe peripheral or solid tissue, such as cervix or skin. Urine collection allows investigators to measure excretory products and urinary metabolites that may reflect dietary intake or be responsive to interventions. Urine collections used in nutrition research are typically timed collections (eg, urine collected over a 24-hour period). With the health of the microbiome, especially gut microbiome, emerging as an important area of research, collection of fecal samples may become more commonplace. Gut microbiota are very sensitive to drugs, diet, and even environmental pollutants.[8]

Biological samples are considered biohazardous materials because exposure to microorganisms while collecting and processing these samples presents a potential health risk. Health care facilities and research units or institutions at which biological materials are collected, handled, or measured must adhere to strict guidelines for handling the samples, and careful monitoring and documentation of these procedures are necessary. Universal precautions that must be employed to safely handle biological materials are described in detail elsewhere.[9]

The factors measured in biological samples are likely to be present in very small concentrations and are usually vulnerable to degradation once outside their normal environment—the biological system. Thus, scrupulous collection and handling procedures are necessary to obtain quality data on biomarkers. Collection and processing procedures are nearly always specific to the biomarker of interest, so one should determine the measurements desired before beginning the sample collection and processing so that appropriate procedures and supplies are used from the beginning of the study.

This chapter is not intended to be a comprehensive review; instead, it presents the basic concepts and key issues involved in the use of biomarkers in nutrition research. It focuses on the concepts and principles, as well as some areas of current interest, with an emphasis on clinical and community-based research applications. Examples related to research on cancer and cardiometabolic outcomes are presented; however, the basic principles and key issues are uniformly applicable to any aspect of nutrition research in which biomarkers would enhance the ability to answer a research question.

BIOMARKERS: NUTRITION ASSESSMENT AND DIETARY INDICATORS

Biomarkers are used in nutrition assessment for several reasons. One basic reason is to provide biochemical data on nutritional status by generating objective evidence that enables researchers to evaluate dietary adequacy or rank individuals on exposure to particular nutrients or dietary constituents. Biochemical or biological measurements may also be collected to provide objective evidence of a dietary pattern, such as overall fruit and vegetable consumption, or to validate dietary assessment instruments. For example, biomarkers could be used to support self-reported dietary data, which may be used to generate a dietary pattern score, such as the Alternative Healthy Eating Index.[10] This score can be used to assess the degree to which individuals adhere to the US Dietary Guidelines. Another possible purpose for obtaining these biological measures is to establish the biological link between the nutritional factor and a physiological or biochemical process when the concentration of the micronutrient or dietary constituent in the target peripheral tissue is measured.

Biological Measures in Nutrition Assessment

Because of the well-known limitations in the use of self-reported dietary intake data, the development and increased availability of dietary biomarkers is of critical importance in research on nutrition and disease risk.[5,6,11] Biochemical measures of nutrients or other dietary constituents can be a valuable component of nutrition assessment and monitoring. Overall, the usefulness of biochemical indicators of nutritional status or exposure is based on knowledge of the physiological and other determinants of the measure. For several micronutrients, the concentration of the nutrient in the circulating body pool (eg, serum) appears to be a reasonably accurate reflection of overall status for the nutrient. Selenium is an example where plasma selenium increases in expected linear fashion with intake.[12] In contrast, the amount of some micronutrients in the circulating pool may be homeostatically regulated when the storage pool is adequate, or it may be unrelated to intake and, thus, has little relationship to total body reserves or overall status. For example, serum calcium is homeostatically maintained the same over the range of usual calcium intakes. Estimating body calcium requires measurements of bone mineral.[12] Plasma retinol also stays the same over most vitamin A intakes, but it does decrease at very low intakes, so this test is useful in low-resource communities. Vitamin C concentration plateaus at intakes of about 150 mg/day, so it is no higher in individuals who take megadoses than in those who eat a moderate amount of fruit.[12] Biochemical indicators of nutritional status range from the gut microbiota to lipodome, metabolome, and proteome as well as genetic factors.[13]

Knowledge of influencing nondietary factors is particularly important for accurate interpretation of biomarkers of nutrient concentration in tissues. For example, tocopherols and carotenoids are transported in circulation nonspecifically by the cholesterol-rich lipoproteins,[14] so higher concentrations of these lipoproteins are predictive of higher concentrations of the associated micronutrients in circulation, independent of dietary intake or total body pool. Smoking and alcohol consumption need to be considered when interpreting serum and other tissue concentrations of several micronutrients, particularly compounds that may be subject to oxidation (eg, vitamin C, tocopherols, carotenoids, and folate). Knowledge of the relationship between the indicator and the risk of nutrient depletion, in addition to knowledge of the responsiveness of the indicator to interventions or change, is also necessary.[15] For some nutrients, such as calcium and zinc, a specific sensitive biomarker of diet or a biochemical status indicator has not yet been identified.

Practical considerations in the use of a biochemical measure of status include the ability to conveniently access the body compartment for measurement, the procedures necessary to collect and process the sample, participant burden, and the resources for laboratory analysis. For example, accurate quantification of vitamin C or folate in a circulating body pool requires processing steps that must be conducted immediately after blood collection to preserve the sample appropriately and prevent degradation that would otherwise make the resulting measurement inaccurate. These extra steps can add time and effort to the labor of blood processing, making these measurements more difficult to obtain in a large study in which resources are limited.

Technological challenges (and capabilities) are also often linked with biochemical measurement capabilities. For example, the development of high-performance liquid chromatography (HPLC), gas chromatography-mass spectrometry (GC-MS), liquid chromatography-mass spectrometry (LC-MS), and improved detection technologies that are currently emerging allow investigators to separate and quantify many micronutrients and other dietary constituents that are present in very low concentrations in biological samples. These technologies enable metabolomics, lipidomics, and proteomics, that is, assessment of the unique chemical fingerprints that specific cellular processes leave behind related to metabolism, lipids, or protein. Depending on the biomarker, assessment can occur over a short-, medium-, or long-term period (see Box 16.1).[16]

The development of specialized cell separation tubes for blood collection now permits easier separation of the leukocyte pool, allowing much easier measurement of micronutrients in this pool; vitamin C and zinc are notable examples.

Tables 16.1 and 16.2 (see page 316) list several examples of biochemical measures of macronutrients that may be useful in nutrition assessment or monitoring dietary intake. An important concept is that a static measurement (eg, a tissue concentration) is typically not as sensitive as a functional marker in assessing status. Also, functional measures, such as the in vitro activity of an erythrocyte-derived enzyme with and without the micronutrient cofactor, will more directly reflect the body function. However, a good functional measure is still lacking in many instances, or the extra labor involved in the procedures limits researchers' ability to use the functional measures in large-scale studies. In-depth reviews of biological status indicators for the various macronutrients and macronutrients give more details.[19-25] In considering which biomarkers to select, investigators need to determine time period assessed (short- vs long- term), quality, reliability, validity, and usefulness of biomarkers.[16]

Short-term biomarkers: These biomarkers reflect only recent consumption (hours or days). Examples include urinary sucrose and fructose, which serve as biomarkers for sugars intake. These biomarkers are based on 24-hour urine collections and, as such, only reflect recent consumption.[17,18]

Medium-term biomarkers: These biomarkers assess intake over weeks or months. An example is a fingerstick serum carbon-13 (^{13}C) measure of cane sugar/high-fructose corn syrup, which appears to assess medium-term intake, in contrast to a plasma ^{13}C measure of cane sugar/high-fructose corn syrup,[16] which only assesses extremely recent meal intake (last meal). More research is needed to ascertain the time period, however.

Long-term biomarkers: These biomarkers assess longer time periods for consumption of the related food component, relating to months or years. Examples include the plasma biomarkers for n-3 fatty acids (eicosapentaenoic acid and docosahexaenoic acid) or plasma, serum, or tissue levels of essential fatty acids.[16]

Box 16.1 Examples of Short-, Medium-, and Long-Term Biomarkers

Macronutrient	Biological Sample	Biomarker	Type
Energy	Spot urine collection	Doubly labeled water	True gold standard: Recovery biomarker
Protein	Hair or 24-hour urine collection	Protein: Urinary nitrogen	Recovery
Animal protein		Animal protein: carbon-13; nitrogen-15 from hair; and creatinine, taurine, 1-methylhistidine, and 3-methylhistidine from 24-hour urine collection	
Vegetable protein		Carbon and nitrogen isotope ratios from hair and urine to detect ratio of animal to vegetable protein	
Carbohydrate	Fasting serum or fingerstick analysis for carbon-13 Urinary fructose or sucrose from 24-hour urine collection	Carbon-13 (for cane sugar and high-fructose corn syrup)[a] Fructose Sucrose Carbon isotope ratios from fingerstick for detecting added sugars	Predictive
Fat	Hair or blood	Fatty acids: polyunsaturated fatty acid, monosaturated fatty acid, and saturated fatty acid Essential fatty acids: alpha-linolenic acid, linoleic acid, eicosapentaenoic acid, and docosahexaenoic acid	Concentration
Sodium	Spot or 24-hour urine collection	Urinary sodium from 24-hour urine collection	Replacement/databases are not available or incomplete; salt at table difficult to quantify (other examples: phytoestrogens); can be considered recovery
Potassium	2-hour urine collection	Urinary potassium from 24-hour urine collection	Recovery

Table 16.1 Biomarkers for Dietary Assessment of Macronutrients[16]

[a] Corn, corn derivatives, and meat from animals consuming corn are reflected in this measurement.

Biomarkers as General Dietary Indicators

Monitoring overall dietary patterns or changes in patterns in response to dietary interventions present additional challenges. The goal is to assess and monitor the intake of certain types of foods or food groups, rather than specific nutrients; therefore, these dietary indicators ideally should be distributed generally within certain types of foods. Table 16.3 (page 317) provides examples of several biochemical indicators that are useful as biomarkers of plant-based diets, illustrating the use of biomarkers as objective evidence of an overall dietary pattern.

Plasma carotenoids provide a good example of the use of biomarkers as a dietary indicator when the goal is to assess and monitor dietary patterns. Vegetables and fruits contribute the vast majority of carotenoids in the diet, and plasma carotenoid concentrations have been shown to be useful biomarkers of vegetable and fruit intakes in cross-sectional descriptive studies, controlled feeding studies, and clinical trials.[26-29] The consistency of this relationship across diverse groups and involving various

Nutrient	Characteristics	Comments[a]
Tocopherols, plasma or serum	Vary directly with vitamin E (tocopherol) intake; slow tissue turnover, and relatively large body pool	Influenced by cholesterol-carrying lipoprotein levels and smoking status
Carotenoids, plasma or serum or skin (beta carotene, alpha carotene, lycopene, lutein, beta-cryptoxanthin, zeaxanthin)	Vary directly with carotenoid intakes, although relationship with specific calculated intakes is usually modest; generally reflects total vegetable and fruit intake; skin levels detected using resonance Raman spectroscopy is noninvasive and may better detect long-term levels than blood levels[26]	Serum levels influenced by cholesterol-carrying lipoprotein levels, smoking status, body mass, and alcohol intake
25-hydroxy vitamin D, plasma or serum	Good biochemical indicator of overall vitamin D status (intake plus what is endogenously synthesized in response to sun exposure)	Effect of skin pigmentation can be great and should be considered in interpretation of results; seasonal changes can also be notable
Vitamin C, plasma or serum	Varies directly with vitamin C intake only up to a threshold level	A preservative must be incorporated into the sample immediately after blood collection and separation and before preparing aliquots and freezing; influenced by smoking status
Folate, whole blood or erythrocyte	Acceptable biochemical indicator of long-term folate status	A preservative must be incorporated into the sample immediately after blood collection and before freezing; influenced by smoking status; hemoglobin (which must be conducted with fresh blood) is necessary to interpret results
Pyridoxal 5'-phosphate, plasma	Acceptable biochemical indicator of vitamin B-6 status	Influenced by circulating albumin concentration, exercise, and protein and carbohydrate intakes
Vitamin B-12, plasma or serum	Not the first biochemical change that occurs in response to dietary vitamin B-12 deficiency but a definitive indicator of prolonged vitamin B-12 inadequacy	Low concentrations can result from several physiological abnormalities (eg, pernicious anemia, atrophic gastritis, hypochlorhydria, and gastric surgery), in addition to dietary inadequacy
Ferritin, serum	Considered the most sensitive and specific indicator of overall iron status; increased concentration in response to excess iron uptake and body stores	Reference (normal) ranges vary depending on the method used; increased in several physiological abnormalities in which normal uptake regulation is overridden (eg, hereditary hemochromatosis), resulting in excessive accumulation of iron
Fatty acids, serum phospholipids or plasma	Modified in response to inadequate fat intake and in response to substantial changes in n-6 and n-3 fatty acid ingestion	Used as a biomarker of compliance with supplementation in fish oil supplement studies

Table 16.2 Blood Concentration Biomarkers Useful in Nutrition Assessment or Monitoring Dietary Intakes[22-25,b]

[a] Comments includes additional measures that must be obtained concurrently for interpretation, as well as other factors crucial in the usefulness of values obtained. Notably, demographic characteristics (eg, age, sex, and racial/ethnic group) are also useful for interpreting all of these measures.
[b] Good or acceptable biochemical indicators of status have been established for several nutrients not on this list, but the effort involved in the analytic procedures precludes their usefulness in large clinical or community-based nutrition research studies. Also not listed are several nutrients (eg, zinc, copper, and calcium) for which serum or plasma concentrations are easily measured and may contribute to the evaluation of status, but the values produced need substantial additional information for accurate interpretation.

concurrent diet manipulations (with differences in amounts of dietary factors that could alter carotenoid bioavailability) is notable, although considerable interindividual variation in the degree of response is typically observed. Also, nondietary factors that are among the determinants of plasma carotenoid concentrations (eg, body mass and plasma cholesterol concentration) influence the absolute concentration that is observed in response to dietary intake.

Measured in	Biochemical Indicators							
	Beta-Cryptoxanthin (Plasma)	Alpha and Beta Carotene (Plasma)	Lycopene (Plasma)	Lutein (Plasma)	Isoflavones (Plasma/Urine)	Lignans (Plasma/Urine)	Dithiocarbamate (Urine)	Alkylresorcinol (Plasma/Serum/Urine)
Vegetables		X		X				
Soy					X			
Cruciferous vegetables							X	
Tomatoes and tomato products			X					
Green leafy vegetables				X				
Fruit	X	X				X		
Grains (whole)						X		X

Table 16.3 Biochemical Indicators Useful as Biomarkers of Plant-Based Diets

Although vitamin C is also provided predominantly by fruits and vegetables in the diet, this measure is much less useful as a biomarker of this dietary pattern because the relationship between vitamin C intake and plasma concentration is linear only up to a certain threshold.[12] The use of vitamin C supplements (which is common) often increases the intake level beyond the range in which linearity between intake and plasma concentration occurs, and it also obscures the relationship between food choices and tissue concentrations.

Polyphenols or plant-based nonnutritive metabolites vary in their distribution in foods. Over 500 polyphenols have been identified and consist of four classes: flavonoids, phenolic acids, lignans, and stilbenes.[30] These are also constituents of herbs and spices, such as saffron and turmeric. Once absorbed, polyphenols are rapidly excreted into the urine. Polyphenols have recently been considered important in preventing and treating oxidative stress-related disease, such as cardiovascular disease and type 2 diabetes.[31]

Polyphenols that are not absorbed, in addition to those excreted in bile, are extensively metabolized by the gut microbiota to produce a range of simple phenolic compounds.[32] For example, enterolactone and enterodiol are enterolignans formed by intestinal microbiota from lignan precursors, which are contained mainly in vegetables, whole-grain products, berries, and flaxseeds.[33]

Lignans are a group of compounds that are present in high-fiber foods, particularly cereals and fruits.[34] These compounds are not found in animal products and, like carotenoids, are useful markers of a plant-based diet.[35] Lignans provide an example of how using dietary constituents as biomarkers requires an understanding of the metabolism of the compounds. Lignans in plant foods are altered by intestinal microflora, so the specific compounds monitored in plasma or urine are actually bacterial metabolites. Generally, enterolactone and enterodiol are measured. Because of this bacterial conversion, lignan concentrations in urine or plasma in response to a similar dietary dose will vary significantly among individuals. In addition, nondietary factors (eg, orally administered antibiotics) reduce enterolactone and enterodiol production.[36]

As another example, the fatty acid composition of membrane phospholipids is in part determined by the n-6 and n-3 fatty acid composition of the diet. Thus, the fatty acid pattern of serum phospholipids or plasma aliquots has been used as a biomarker of compliance with n-3 fatty acid supplementation in clinical trials.[37,38] Although enzyme selectivity and other physiological factors are also important determinants of the fatty acid composition of phospholipids, a diet high in n-3 polyunsaturated fats results in increased amounts of eicosapentaenoic and docosahexaenoic acids in circulating tissue pools.

Specific fatty acids can also be associated with certain types of foods. Pentadecanoic acid (15:0) and heptadecanoic acid (17:0) are fatty acids produced by bacteria in the rumen of ruminants. These fatty acids, with uneven numbers of carbon atoms, are not synthesized by humans; therefore, their presence in human biological samples can be indicative of dietary exposure to milk fat. Proportions of 15:0 and 17:0 in adipose tissue and concentrations of 15:0 in serum have been found to correlate with milk-fat intake in men and women.[39,40] In summary, there are a variety of ways of assessing a plant-based diet ranging from plasma carotenoids and vitamin C to polyphenols. Other helpful biomarkers include fatty acids in adipose tissue and serum, which provide information about n-6 and n-3 fatty acid composition of the diet.

Biomarkers of Polyphenol Intakes

Although not recognized as essential for life, numerous dietary components—particularly of plant origin—have demonstrated biological activity and are thought to play an important role in preventing chronic disease. These polyphenols or phytochemicals are absorbed, often metabolized in the intestinal epithelium and liver, and excreted; thus, the metabolites can be monitored in urine, serum, or plasma.

Dietary exposure to flavonoids and other polyphenols can be monitored in urine or plasma.[41] The isoflavones daidzein and genistein are highly concentrated in soybeans and soy products. Much remains to be learned about their metabolism in human beings.[42,43] These compounds can be measured in urine and plasma by immunoassay or HPLC with diode array, coulometric array detection, or mass spectrometry. Urinary isoflavone excretion is associated strongly and directly with soy protein intake under controlled dietary conditions.[44] In observational studies of populations that usually consume soy, soy food intake and urinary isoflavonoid excretion are also positively correlated.[45-47] Because the plasma half-lives of the isoflavones genistein and daidzein are short (6 to 8 hours),[48] intermittent soy consumption may be severely underestimated or overesti-

mated if isoflavone exposure is monitored in plasma or spot urine specimens. The metabolism of isoflavones is also inextricably linked to the health of colonic bacterial populations, and plasma and urinary levels may be influenced by the effects of diet and drugs on the colonic environment.

Other compounds that have been utilized as biomarkers of dietary intake, such as sulforaphane and other isothiocyanates in cruciferous vegetables, have been of interest because of putative chemopreventive effects. Dithiocarbamates (metabolites of isothiocyanates) can be quantified in urine after extraction and measurement by HPLC; they provide an estimate of cruciferous vegetable exposure.[49]

Biomarkers of Energy

To date, few biological measures objectively monitor energy intake, and available measures are cumbersome to perform in free-living populations, expensive, or both. Under steady-state conditions, as in the case of weight-stable participants, indirect calorimetry provides an estimate of energy expenditure and some insight about intake. Indirect calorimetry estimates the rate of oxidation or energy expenditure from the rate of oxygen consumption (VO_2) and the rate of carbon dioxide production (VCO_2). This technique is relatively inexpensive and portable, although some participant effort is required. These traits lend the technique to clinical applications.[50]

The chief premise behind indirect calorimetry is that VO_2 and energy metabolism are proportional. All energy-dependent metabolic processes depend on energy liberated from adenosine triphosphate hydrolysis. The adenosine triphosphate utilization rate dictates substrate oxidation.[51] Total body oxygen storage is very small compared with oxygen consumption. Given the first law of thermodynamics, energy from oxidative metabolism is converted into heat and work. If the participant is resting in a thermoneutral environment, heat released by oxidation and measurable by indirect calorimetry is equal to heat lost to the environment and measurable by direct calorimetry.

Indirect calorimetry produces two types of information: resting energy expenditure (REE) and respiratory quotient (RQ). The REE estimates fasting energy expenditure in an awake, resting individuals and is approximately 10% greater than basal energy requirements. The REE correlates with lean body mass.[52] The RQ is the ratio of carbon dioxide produced divided by oxygen consumed (VCO_2/VO_2), and the ratio indicates contributions from each substrate. An RQ of 1.0 suggests 100% glucose utilization, whereas an RQ of 0.7 corresponds to oxidation of 100% fat. Protein utilization results in an RQ near 0.8. However, urinary nitrogen excretion is used to determine what portion of the VCO_2 and VO_2 are contributed by protein utilization. Excluding the effects of protein produces the nonprotein RQ. Thus, for nonprotein RQ between 0.7 and 1.0, proportions of fat and carbohydrate oxidation can be identified.[53,54] It is important to note that the RQ represents substrate oxidation, which may or may not equal exogenous macronutrient intakes. In using the RQ to determine substrate oxidation, two assumptions are made: the participant is in a metabolically steady-state condition, and all expired carbon dioxide measured represents substrate oxidation.[50]

Various types of equipment are used in indirect calorimetry, and both open-circuit and closed-circuit systems are available. A closed-circuit system allows the participant to breathe from a pure-oxygen reservoir and calculates oxygen consumption from disappearance data. The more sophisticated open-circuit system, in which participants breathe room air and detectors calculate the difference in gases inhaled versus those exhaled, is more widely available in the United States. The apparatus used to collect respiratory gases may be a tent-like canopy, a fitted face mask, or a mouthpiece with nose clips directing all inhalation and expiration through the mouth. The canopy system may be best suited to clinical and research applications because it is comfortable and requires no fitting,[55] whereas the face mask system has been tested in healthy adults restricted to bed.[56] Despite validation in healthy participants, indirect calorimetry is generally applied to critically ill individuals due to the availability of instruments and the greater precision for prescribing nutrition support in those instances.[57]

In whole-room calorimetry or whole-body chamber the participant remains in a closed room with a constant and measured supply of fresh air for one or more days compared with the canopy system, which is used for short-term studies. Gas analyzers attached to the unit measure oxygen consumed and carbon dioxide produced. The whole-body chamber can be used for determining 24-hour energy expenditure.[58]

The limitations of indirect calorimetry in a community-based setting are significant. If the REE is measured, participants must provide accurate typical activity records; in addition, the thermic effect of food needs to be calculated in order to derive total energy expenditure. Such records introduce reporting bias and general inaccuracy. Indirect calorimetry can be used to measure total energy expenditure, but long data collection periods are necessary to control for error associated with extrapolation, and it is likely that usual activity would be hindered by even the most mobile system. Even measuring energy expenditure for a full day does not account for day-to-day variability.[59]

Energy expenditure can also be measured using a doubly labeled water (DLW) technique.[60] This method uses nonradioactive isotopes of hydrogen (^2H) and oxygen (^{18}O) to measure total energy expenditure in free-living participants by monitoring urinary isotope excretion. Energy expenditures determined by room calorimetry, indirect calorimetry, and DLW are not significantly different within the calorimeter environment; however, in free-living participants, DLW energy expenditures have been found to be 13% to 15% higher than energy expenditures from other methods.[59] The DLW method has the distinct advantage of allowing participants to go about their usual activities, with energy expenditure calculated after a study period of 7 to 14 days. Unfortunately, the ^{18}O isotope required to conduct DLW studies is expensive and often in short supply. Although DLW studies are suited to nutrition research aimed at quantifying total energy expenditure for specific groups, the cost for large samples limits its broad use.

One of the most important and relevant uses of DLW methodology in community-based nutrition research has been to produce an estimate of energy requirements, which can then be compared with the reported energy intakes obtained from various dietary assessment methodologies.[61] Underreporting is a recognized problem in dietary assessment, and DLW may be used to validate (or calibrate) assessment methods, such as dietary recalls and food frequency questionnaires. Although the data produced are objective and the approach is less disruptive to normal life activities than indirect calorimetry, measurement error does occur and can be compounded by estimates of various physiological factors and the assumptions used in the calculations. Furthermore, one of the most notable findings from the use of DLW methodology is that total daily energy expenditure varies dramatically among healthy, free-living human beings.[62]

Biomarkers for Protein, Sodium, Potassium, and Sugars Intake and Other Nutrients

Urinary nitrogen is a recovery biomarker for protein; protein intake (g/day) = $6.25 \times$ (24-hour urinary nitrogen/0.81).[63] Recovery biomarkers include DLW, urinary protein, and potassium, which are based on a known recovered proportion of intake over a certain period of time. Biomarkers that replace estimates for food components that are difficult to measure can be used as recovery biomarkers (such as 24-hour urinary sodium).

Twenty-four hour urinary excretion of sodium and potassium has been the traditional biomarker of intake because about 86% of sodium and 80% of potassium are excreted in the urine.[64-67] Intakes at the population level have been remarkably consistent across time and place and have regularly provided a basis for determining associations with physiological and health outcomes. This is almost certainly due to the fact that large sample sizes are robust to the random daily variation of individual intakes. For population estimates, a subsample with multiple measures suffices. Multiple collections of 24-hour urine are usually a better measure of usual intake among individuals. However, the use of 24-hour urinary excretion to assess individual (as opposed to population) intake is not without limitations. Consistency of intake, physical activity, ambient heat, humidity, and circadian rhythms affect the excretion of sodium and potassium,[68] and there may be more variability in potassium than sodium excretion related to racial differences.[69] More recently, spot urine collections that take into account timing of collection and race/ethnicity have also been used, but this is reported

to be a less accurate estimate than 24-hour urine collections.[68,70]

Controlled human feeding studies provide the opportunity for robust nutritional biomarker development and validation. Based on controlled feeding studies, 24-hour urinary sucrose plus fructose is a predictive biomarker for total sugars intake. Predictive biomarkers predict intake after being calibrated to account for a certain level of bias that is estimated from a feeding study.[17] Assessment of sugar biomarkers is not without its challenges. The type of assay used can affect the quality of assessment. Enzymatic assays may not work as well as LC-MS to assess total sugars, and several additional 24-hour urine collections may be necessary. In the Hispanic Community Health Study/Study of Latinos, this sugar biomarker did not correlate with intake, possibly because of measurement error in self-reported diet, high intraindividual variability in total sugars intake, urinary sucrose and fructose, or a combination of high intraindividual variability in total sugars intake and urinary sucrose and fructose, so it may not be a suitable proxy for total sugars intake in this study population.[18]

Concentration biomarkers are yet another class of biomarkers. These correlate rather than provide a direct measure of intake,[71] and with self-reported intake and pertinent participant characteristics, such as body size, concentration biomarkers can improve reliability of risk estimates and increase statistical power to detect an association with intake and health outcomes. In a Women's Health Initiative (WHI) feeding study of postmenopausal women, usual foods consumed by participants were provided, and serum concentration biomarkers of several vitamins and carotenoids performed similarly to established energy and protein urinary recovery biomarkers in representing nutrient intake variation.[72.]

Biomarker Calibration of Self-Reported Intake to Reduce Measurement Error in Energy, Protein, Sodium, and Potassium Intake and in Association with Health Outcomes

Although self-report measures of diet, such as dietary recalls, dietary records, and food frequency questionnaires, have been refined in the past decades, they are nevertheless confounded by subjectivity.[6] Accurate dietary assessment is critical and, as such, biomarkers can be indispensable as an objective measure to correct or add information about error-prone measures of self-report.[73] For example, in the Hispanic Community Health Study/Study of Latinos, systematic underreporting of energy (overall 25.3%) and protein intake (overall 18.5%) as well as overreporting of protein density (overall 10.7%) were found to vary significantly by Hispanic/Latino background.[74] These self-report measures may include systematic and random errors that can distort associations between diet and disease (see Box 16.2).[75-77] Recovery biomarkers, such as energy or protein, adhere to a classic measurement error model and generate unbiased estimates of intake.[74]

Calibration equations that adjust for systematic and random aspects of self-report measurement error provide a methodology for correcting diet and disease association estimates. Given the high cost of biomarkers, a representative subsample of a larger cohort provides biomarker data; regression calibration equations can be developed to apply biomarker results from the substudy to the larger cohort.

In the WHI, 24-hour urinary excretion in two subsamples of approximately 500 women each was used to develop calibration equations that corrected the self-report data for random and systematic bias aspects of measurement error.[73,79] The equations were used to develop calibrated intake estimates, which adjusted for the error in the self-reported intake, in the WHI study cohorts for use in disease association studies; these included pertinent participant characteristics associated with the biases in the self-reported intake. A recent study that compared calibration equations for self-reported potassium and sodium intakes across five cohorts found heterogeneity across the cohorts in the calibration coefficients.[80] In this study, the cohorts were predominantly white and college educated (81% in the one study that had the most racial diversity), and calibration equations only allowed for an effect of African American race; the absence of calibration equations based on Hispanic/Latino cohorts highlighted the need to focus on this population.

Therefore, in the Study of Latinos: Nutrition and Physical Activity Assessment Study, biomarker and self-report measures of dietary intake were collected in 447 participants from the multicenter Hispanic Community Health Study/Study of Latinos cohort (n=16,415) to calibrate self-reported sodium and potassium dietary intake. Results indicated that self-report underestimated sodium intake by 19.8% and 20.8% in men and women, respectively.[81] Calibration equations showed calibration coefficients specific to this diverse cohort of Latinos. Using this approach, Prentice and colleagues report that biomarker-calibrated (but not uncalibrated) energy was positively correlated with total and site-specific cancer incidence[75] and coronary heart disease incidence,[76] while Tinker and colleagues[77] note corresponding findings for calibrated (but not uncalibrated) protein intake in relation to diabetes risk. Figure 16.1 on page 322 illustrates measurement properties of three diet assessment instruments (food frequency questionnaire, 4-day food record, and 24-hour dietary recall) used in the WHI. Additionally, it depicts how the biomarker for energy (DLW) can explain the contribution of self-reported energy and participant characteristics, especially psychosocial and diet behavior factors (eg, eating at home), to accuracy in reporting energy. In this example, self-reported energy via food records explains more of the variation (R^2=8.7%) than either the 24-hour recall or food frequency questionnaire (R^2=3% and 3.6%, respectively). However, body mass contributes most to the variance (R^2=27% to 29% depending on diet assessment method used),

Systematic error: a source of error in which measurements consistently depart from the true value in the same direction; affects the sample mean or median and can result in incorrect estimates and conclusions

Random error: a source of error that contributes variability (ie, reduces precision) but does not influence the sample mean or median; a type of measurement error and contrasts with systematic error

Box 16.2 Definitions of Systematic and Random Error[78]

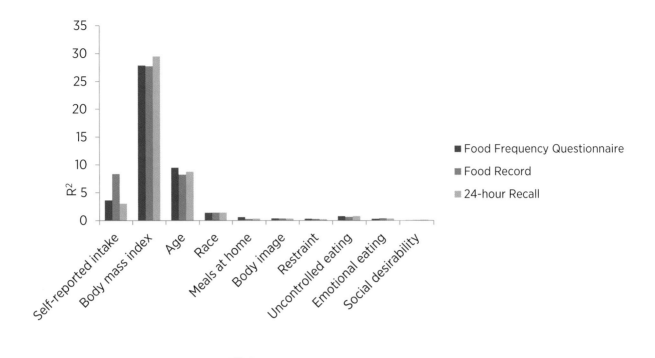

Figure 16.1 Fraction of biomarker (doubly labeled water) variance explained by dietary self-report in energy and participant characteristics[82]

with participants who are obese or overweight more likely to underestimate energy intake.

Metabolomics and Dietary Biomarkers

Metabolomics studies the small-molecular-weight molecules or metabolites that are present in biological samples with an aim to identify perturbations in metabolism under different conditions and can reflect activities at a functional level, that is, biochemical or biological effects.[83] This technology allows for assessment of dietary constituents with biochemical activity. For example, studying the metabolome could provide an early indicator of response to nutrients or disease.[84] Metabolomic analyses are done in a targeted or nontargeted fashion; the type of approach depends on the research question at hand. The nontargeted approach is designed to find a broad range of metabolites and, although time consuming, provides an opportunity for novel discoveries; targeted approaches work when compounds of interest are known a priori.

Technologies to assess metabolomics include nuclear magnetic resonance (NMR) spectroscopy,

mass spectrometry -MS) based technologies that use gas chromatography (GC) or liquid chromatography (LC). The chromatographic step allows metabolites to be separated before detection, which enhances resolution, sensitivity, and selectivity.[85] NMR spectroscopy is a most selective analytic technique that provides unambiguous information about a molecule; however, it has limited sensitivity compared with MS-based methods.[86] Metabolites assessed by this method include amino acids, organic acids, keto acids, sugars, alcohols, lipids (high-density lipoproteins, low-density lipoproteins, lipoprotein particles), and nucleotides. GC-MS has high selectivity and sensitivity and is suitable for volatile metabolites and metabolites that become volatile after chemical derivatization.[84] LC-MS does not need chemical derivatization of metabolites, which is an advantage of GC-MS.

Following are the three current approaches to identify novel biomarkers of dietary intake:

● Conduct specific intervention studies to identify specific biomarkers of intake.
● Search for biomarkers in cohort studies by

correlating them to self-reported intake of specific foods.

- Analyze dietary patterns in conjunction with metabolomics profiles to identify nutrient components and biomarkers using untargeted approaches.

In the case of intervention or feeding studies, a number of biomarkers have been identified.[87-90] These consist of participants consuming specific foods followed by collection of biofluids, such as urine. For example metabolic phenotyping in a randomized, controlled, crossover trial indicated four different metabolic signatures using proton NMR for the four different dietary interventions.[88]

In the case of biomarkers, metabolomics profiles are compared between consumers and nonconsumers of specific food based on self-report, which can be prone to error. Confirmation of these results are needed in an intervention study.

In the case of analysis of dietary patterns, the approach involves applying a multivariate statistical strategy, such as principal component analysis, to dietary data and then linking these metabolomics profiles to identify dietary biomarkers. These new technologies have enabled biomarkers to be identified for citrus, cruciferous vegetables, red meat, fish, walnuts, cocoa, coffee, tea, wine, beer, sugar-sweetened beverages, and olive oil among others.[16,88]

Biomarkers of Nutrition for Development

Supported by the Bill and Melinda Gates Foundation and managed by the National Institute of Child Health and Human Development, Biomarkers of Nutrition for Development (BOND) aims to harmonize the discovery, development, and distribution of biomarkers of nutritional status and advise researchers, clinicians, and policy makers on how best to use nutritional biomarkers.[5] The idea is to clarify confusion on how biomarkers can be used to distinguish among the following:

- exposure
- status
- function
- health effect

As an example, selenium status can be evaluated in light of its metabolism. Assessment of selenium intake/exposure relies on a different set of end points than assessment of nutritional selenium deficiency or adequacy for cancer risk reduction or risk of toxicity.[5] This approach focuses on fine-tuning the end points for each situation. Additionally, food components interact with each other and with an individuals's genomic profile. Genetics (eg, polymorphisms, deletions), epigenetics (eg, DNA methylation), and transcriptome regulation affect the response to foods and their components, making proteomics and metabolomics important technologies to assess the impact of foods at the granular level.

BIOMARKERS IN NUTRITION RESEARCH: PRACTICAL CONSIDERATIONS

Practical considerations in using biomarkers in nutrition research involve all the details related to study setting, population, equipment, and available resources as well as issues that are necessary for the appropriate collection, handling, processing, and storage of biological samples. Before selecting the biomarkers to examine, the nutrition researcher must know what is reflected in the pool or compartment to be measured and the various factors that might influence the interpretation of results.

Collection of Blood and Other Tissues

Although the risk involved in blood collection may be minimal, it is an invasive procedure, and participants must be informed of all inherent risks. Trained and certified personnel must be responsible for the procedure. Requirements for training and certification vary somewhat across institutions, but a key factor to consider for participant comfort is the experience of the individuals responsible for phlebotomy and how frequently he or she performs the procedure. Experienced phlebotomists should have the knowledge and skills to cope with the challenges that can arise. For example, collecting blood from a healthy adult can be very difficult if the participant is somewhat dehydrated. Most research studies specify a protocol (eg, how many attempts are to be made before allowing another phlebotomist to try or before a participant may be dismissed to return for another attempt at a later time). When blood collections are very frequent over a very short period (say, 12 hours), an indwelling catheter enabling access without repeated venipuncture may be necessary.

The choice of the tube for blood collection is determined by the compartment to be measured (eg, serum, plasma, erythrocytes, or leukocytes). Tubes for plasma collection contain various anticlotting chemicals, which may have positive or negative effects on the constituents being measured, so the choice will be driven by the effect on the measurement. If white blood cells are needed to extract cellular constituents, such as DNA, the heterogeneous buffy coat mixture of blood cells (the whitish layer of cells between the red blood cells and the plasma after centrifugation) is an appropriate fraction to remove and collect. If the leukocyte compartment is specifically desired, specialized cell separation tubes must be used. For many constituents of interest, especially constituents subject to oxidation by light exposure, the tube with collected blood may need to be immediately protected from light using an amber sample bag or aluminum foil during the processing steps when the tube is not in the centrifuge. If the erythrocyte pool is to be measured, the red blood cells remaining after the plasma has been removed typically need to be washed, which involves twice adding an equal volume of normal saline, centrifuging, and discarding the supernatant so that the plasma material adhering to the red blood cells is rinsed away.

Blood sample processing is often quite specific to the constituent to be measured. For example, extra processing steps to better preserve the constituent may need to be performed immediately after the blood has been collected and before the sample is placed in cryovials for storage or analysis. Additional considerations relevant to blood sample collection involve nonfasting vs fasting samples (and how many hours postprandial are considered acceptable) and timing of sample collection (which would be important if diurnal variations were known to occur). In planning the study design and protocol, researchers may need to consider seasonal effects on biochemical measurement.

When solid tissue samples, such as hair, fingernails, fat, or muscle tissue, are examined or measured, the exact tissue type (ie, histology of the tissue) needs to be considered before collection and processing, For example, a surgical biopsy sample of clinically normal tissue from breast or fat depots will often include connective tissue, adipose tissue, and glandular tissue (if the sample is from the breast). Different distributions of micronutrients or other dietary constituents are usually present in these tissue types, so dissection and examination is necessary before taking static measures of the sample. Before storage, solid tissue samples must be rinsed of blood with normal saline, and, depending on the measurement to be made, a chemical preservative may need to be added before storage. If the biopsy is a surgical sample of a possible or known lesion, the first priority is to ensure that there is sufficient tissue for histopathological examination for diagnosis and medical care; tissue for research purposes is considered a lower priority.

Urine Collection

Urine is an easily accessible pool for measuring numerous biomarkers; however, urinary markers of diet generally reflect recent intake. Timing and length of collection, as well as handling and processing methods, are determined by the biomarkers being measured. Collections may vary from a spot urine (a convenience sample, usually <100 mL, collected during a clinic visit) to days of complete urine collection (24-hour or 72-hour urine collections). Additional collection strategies include overnight collection (approximately a 10-hour collection) or first-voided fasting morning collection (collected upon waking in the morning). A first-voided morning specimen is usually the most concentrated sample of the day and is least affected by recent dietary intake.

Collecting 24-hour and 72-hour urine samples in free-living individuals is difficult. The collection procedure involves significant participant burden and can impair participant recruitment, retention, and compliance. Nonetheless, these total urine collections are often necessary to provide a useful measure of dietary exposure. Participants must be provided with an adequate supply of easy-to-use, leak-proof collection containers; clear instructions for collection, labeling, and handling; and, if necessary, commode specimen systems and transport coolers. Sometimes urine collection containers need to be pretreated with additives. For example, some biomarkers that undergo oxidation require the use of collection containers with ascorbic acid (1 g per 1-L bottle) added before collection. Boric acid (2.0 g or 0.5 level measuring teaspoon per 3-L bottle) is another component added as a preservative during urine collection. However, it can interfere with measurement of such metals as arsenic. Usually two 3-L bottles are provided to adults for 24-hour urine collection. A label stating "leave powder preservative inside the bottle" can remind participants not to throw out the preservative. To monitor the completeness of a 24-hour collection, para-aminobenzoic acid (PABA) can be used. This compound is ingested with meals (80 mg, three times per day) and is rapidly and completely excreted in the urine.[91] A urine collection containing less than 85% of the administered dose of PABA is considered incomplete. Analysis of PABA is costly and may not be necessary for assessing completion of urine collection.[92] Depending on the context, detailed records of how urine was collected (eg, how often it was spilled or missed) could suffice. For population studies, spot, overnight, and first-voided urine collections are more feasible than 24-hour collections. These collections are especially useful when a ratio of markers is determined (eg, drug metabolites to parent drug or one hormone metabolite to another). Urinary excretion of a marker can also be normalized to the creatinine content of the sample (milligrams of the marker per milligrams of creatinine) to correct for diurnal variation and urine volume.

Fecal Collection

Fecal collection is less frequently used than urine and blood collection in nutrition research, in part because of the logistics of, and aversion to, collection. However with the increasing importance of the gut microbiome, fecal collection is becoming more widespread in research studies. Absorption studies, as well as dietary interventions with outcomes related to gut function, bile acid metabolism, and colonic microbial changes, rely on fecal samples for biomarkers. As with urine collections, minimizing participant burden is an important consideration for fecal collections. This includes devising the least offensive method of sample collection that still meets the study's needs, identifying the shortest time over which samples need to be collected, and carefully arranging sample storage and transport.

Sample handling is specific to the measurements planned. Various additives may need to be provided to participants to add directly to the specimen at the time of collection. Often, samples must be frozen immediately to prevent continued microbial degradation of dietary fiber and preserve the bacterial community structure. Samples used for microbiological cultures may need to be collected with minimal exposure to air and processed immediately to minimize alterations in microbial populations. A careful understanding of the biology involved and testing of the collection protocol by the researchers are necessary to ensure that the samples are collected appropriately for the biomarker under investigation.

General Considerations

Unless the biological measurement is conducted immediately after sample collection, storage issues must be considered. Thawing and refreezing may degrade the constituents, so it is usually best to divide the sample into several aliquots for storage so that only portions of the material collected are removed for analysis at any one time. Regular laboratory refrigeration (eg, a refrigerated centrifuge) is typically at a temperature of 4°C, and biological samples nearly always must be stored at −20°C, or preferably at −70°C to −80°C, for best preservation. The ultralow freezers necessary for the lower temperature range and better preservation have an additional compressor unit and so are considerably more expensive. Additionally, samples must be stored in liquid nitrogen for some types of cellular measurements. Stability of the biological markers to be measured should be verified when planning the time span between collection and analysis.

Needless to say, freezers used to store biological samples for biomarker measurements should have an emergency backup power source and an alarm notification for when power is lost or the temperature rises above a preset level. Freezer space needs can be substantial in a study in which numerous aliquots are produced, and early planning can prevent future problems.

Quality Assurance

All compounds measured in biological samples have a certain amount of biological variability; this reflects the inherent fluctuation that is normal in the biological system because the constituents are not static but continuously influenced by rates of metabolism and flux across body pools. For that reason, biochemical measurements may need to be replicated (if possible) or measured in duplicate or triplicate (if the cost and effort of the measurement permit) to accurately characterize the situation. More important, knowledge of biological variability (eg, variability due to circadian rhythms) is an important consideration when interpreting actual values obtained from the measurements; the researcher must recognize that quantified values are not absolutes but estimates, even when the best procedures and methods are in place.

Although biological variability is to be expected, other sources of variation are ideally anticipated and minimized in the measurement methodologies used.[93] Biochemical methods used in measuring biological samples should always be tested for reliability before use in a research study. This aspect of quality assurance (QA) typically involves repeated measurements at several levels of set concentrations using various matrixes so that procedural sources of variation can be identified. Concentrations used to test the accuracy of the method should be in the range of the concentrations expected in the biological samples. For example, coefficients of variation obtained from QA procedures for HPLC methods produce figures for both run-to-run and day-to-day variability. External assistance with QA may be possible through the National Institute of Standards and Technology, from which samples with known concentrations of micronutrients and some other dietary constituents may be purchased for comparative testing of the validity of the methods in use in the researcher's laboratory. For micronutrients, the institute conducts a round-robin QA program in which samples with unknown concentrations are sent to participating laboratories for measurement as a type of blinded evaluation of laboratory performance.[94]

Several other strategies can be used to improve the quality of biochemical measurement data produced, as well as the interpretations and conclusions based on these data. For example, analyzing samples from a given participant collected at baseline and after intervention in the same batch may help minimize the potential effect of some sources of methodologic variation. However, with large numbers of samples from intervention studies that are conducted over years, it may be impossible to measure baseline and end-point samples within the time span of the research project, especially if cost is an issue. In this case, measurements from a pooled generic sample (eg, aliquots of pooled plasma samples from several participants that have been combined and stored) are obtained with each batch of samples measured. This allows researchers to examine the values produced for possible shifts or errors over time so that the methods and instrumentation can be adjusted accordingly. If the nutrition researcher is considering sending samples to a service or clinical laboratory for biochemical measurements, information about these types of QA procedures should be requested and evaluated before committing to use the service or laboratory.

CONCLUSION

Much can be gained by using biomarkers in nutrition research. Advancements in scientific knowledge and available technologies make this an area of imminent importance in nutrition research if the field is to function at a level equivalent to other areas of biomedical science. Even the biochemical measures of nutrient status, or those that provide objective evidence for an overall dietary pattern, provide powerful support for associations based on reported dietary intakes. Also, much remains to be learned about the relationship between diet and the disease process, especially at the cellular and molecular levels, which requires the use of biological markers in nutrition intervention studies. Crucial information for establishing the biological link is obtained by incorporating biochemical, cellular, and molecular markers in nutrition research. Although challenges can be anticipated, a thorough knowledge of the biological markers of interest, combined with advance planning, will prevent or overcome problems and barriers.

REFERENCES

1. Rock CL, Flatt SW, Thomson C, et al. Plasma triacylglycerol and HDL cholesterol concentrations confirm self-reported changes in carbohydrate and fat intakes in women in a diet intervention trial. *J Nutr.* 2004;134(2):342-347.

2. Polsinelli ML, Rock CL, Henderson SA, Drewnowski A. Plasma carotenoids as biomarkers of fruit and vegetable servings in women. *J Am Diet Assoc.* 1998;98(2):194-196.

3. Thomson CA, Giuliano AR, Shaw JW, et al. Diet and biomarkers of oxidative damage in women previously treated for breast cancer. *Nutr Cancer.* 2005;51(2):146-154.

4. Meyskens FL. Principles of human chemoprevention. *Hematol Oncol Clin North Am.* 1998;12(50):935-941.

5. Combs GF, Trumbo PR, McKinley MC, et al. Biomarkers in nutrition: new frontiers in research and application. *Ann N Y Acad Sci.* 2013;1278:1-10.

6. Dragsted LO. Relying on biomarkers for intake assessment in nutrition. *Am J Clin Nutr.* 2017:105(1):8-9.

7. Ueland PM, Ulvik A, Rios-Avila L, Midttun Ø, Gregory JF. Direct and functional biomarkers of vitamin B6 status, *Annu Rev Nutr.* 2015:35:33-70.

8. Jin Y, Wu S, Zeng Z, Fu Z. Effects of environmental pollutants on gut microbiota. *Environ Pollut.* 2017;222:1-9.

9. *Biosafety in Microbial and Biomedical Laboratories.* Washington, DC: US Department of Health and Human Services, Centers for Disease Control and Prevention, and National Institutes of Health; 2009. HHS publication no. (CDC) 21-112.

10. Chiuve SE, Fung TT, Rimm EB, et al. Alternative dietary indices both strongly predict risk of chronic disease. *J Nutr.* 2012;142(6):1009-1018.

11. Prentice RL. Dietary assessment and the reliability of nutritional epidemiology reports. *Lancet.* 2003;362(9379): 182-183.

12. Truswell S. Assessment of nutritional status and biomarkers. In: Mann J, Truswell S, eds. *Essentials of Human Nutrition.* Oxford. United Kingdom: Oxford University Press; 2012:505-519.

13. Ferguson JF, Allayee H, Gerszten RE, et al; American Heart Association Council on Functional Genomics and Translational Biology, Council on Epidemiology and Prevention, and Stroke Council. Nutrigenomics, the microbiome, and gene-environment interactions: new directions in cardiovascular disease research, prevention, and treatment. A scientific statement from the American Heart Association, *Circ Cardiovasc Genet.* 2016;9(3):291-313.

14. Clevidence BA, Bieri JG. Association of carotenoids with human plasma lipoproteins. *Methods Enzymol.* 1993;214: 33-46.

15. Prentice RL, Willett WC, Greenwald P, et al. Nutrition and physical activity and chronic disease prevention: research strategies and recommendations. *J Natl Cancer Inst.* 2004; 96(17):1276-1287.

16. Hedrick VE, Dietrick AM, Estabrooks PA, Savla J, Serrano E, Davy BM. Dietary biomarkers: advances, limitations and future directions. *Nutr J.* 2012;11:109.

17. Tasevska N. Midtune D, Potischman N, et al. Use of the predictive sugars biomarker to evaluate self-reported total sugars intake in the Observing Protein and Energy Nutrition (OPEN) study. *Cancer Epidemiol Biomarkers Prev.* 2011;20(3):490-500.

18. Beasley JM, Jung M, Tasevska N, et al. Biomarker-predicted sugars intake compared with self-reported measures in US Hispanics/Latinos: results from the HCHS/SOL SOLNAS Study. *Public Health Nutr.* 2016;19(18):3256-3264.

19. Blatt DH, Leonard SW, Traber MG. Vitamin E kinetics and the function of tocopherol regulatory proteins. *Nutrition.* 2001;17(10):799-805.

20. Shils ME, Olson JA, Shike M, Ross AC, eds. *Modern Nutrition in Health and Disease.* 9th ed. Philadelphia, PA: Williams & Wilkins; 1999.

21. Bowman BA, Russell R, eds. *Present Knowledge in Nutrition.* 9th ed. Washington, DC: ILSI Press; 2006.

22. Food and Nutrition Board, Institute of Medicine. *Dietary Reference Intakes for Calcium, Phosphorus, Magnesium, Vitamin D, and Fluoride.* Washington, DC: National Academy Press; 1997.

23. Food and Nutrition Board, Institute of Medicine. *Dietary Reference Intakes for Thiamin, Riboflavin, Niacin, Vitamin B6, Folate, Vitamin B12, Pantothenic Acid, Biotin, and Choline.* Washington, DC: National Academy Press; 1998.

24. Food and Nutrition Board, Institute of Medicine. *Dietary Reference Intakes for Vitamin C, Vitamin E, Selenium, and Carotenoids.* Washington, DC: National Academy Press; 2000.

25. Food and Nutrition Board, Institute of Medicine. *Dietary Reference Intakes for Energy, Carbohydrate, Fiber, Fat, Fatty Acids, Cholesterol, Protein, and Amino Acids.* Washington, DC: National Academy Press, 2002.

26. Aguilar SS, Wengreen HJ, Lefevre M, Madden GJ, Gast J. Skin carotenoids: a biomarker of fruit and vegetable intake in children. *J Acad Nutr Diet.* 2014;114(8):1174-1180.

27. Campbell DR, Gross MD, Martini MC, Grandits GA, Slavin JL, Potter JD. Plasma carotenoids as biomarkers of vegetable and fruit intake. *Cancer Epidemiol Biomarkers Prev.* 1994;3(6):493-500.

28. Rock CL, Flatt SW, Wright FA, et al. Responsiveness of carotenoids to a high vegetable diet intervention designed to prevent breast cancer recurrence. *Cancer Epidemiol Biomarkers Prev.* 1997;6:617-623.

29. Le Marchand L, Hankin JH, Carter FS, et al. A pilot study on the use of plasma carotenoids and ascorbic acid as markers of compliance to a high fruit and vegetable diet intervention. *Cancer Epidemiol Biomarkers Prev.* 1994;3(3):245-251.

30. Perez-Jimenez J, Hubert J, Hooper L, Cassidy A, Manach C, Williamson G. Urinary metabolites as biomarkers of polyphenol intake in humans: a systematic review. *Am J Clin Nutr.* 2010; 92(4):801-809.

31. Li AN, Li S, Zhang YJ, Xu XR, Chen YM, Li HB. Resources and biological activities of natural polyphenols. *Nutrients.* 2014;6(12):6020-6047.

32. Manach C, Williamson G, Morand C, Scalbert A, Rémésy C. Bioavailability and bioefficacy of polyphenols in humans. Review of 97 bioavailability studies. *Am J Clin Nutr.* 2005; 81(suppl 1):230S-242S.

33. Sun Q, Wedick NM, Pan A, et al. Gut microbiota metabolites of dietary lignans and risk of type 2 diabetes: a prospective investigation in two cohorts of US women. *Diabetes Care.* 2014;37(5):1287-1295.

34. Mazur W, Fotsis T, Wähälä K, Ojala S, Salakka A, Adlercreutz H. Isotope dilution gas chromatographic-mass spectrophotometric method for the determination of isoflavonoids, coumestrol, and lignans in food samples. *Anal Biochem.* 1996;233(2):169-180.

35. Lampe JW, Campbell DR, Hutchins AM, et al. Urinary isoflavonoid and lignan excretion on a Western diet: relation to soy, vegetable, and fruit intake. *Cancer Epidemiol Biomarkers Prev.* 1999;8(8):699-707.

36. Kilkkinen A, Stumpf K, Pietinen P, Valsta LM, Tapanainen H, Adlercreutz H. Determinants of serum enterolactone concentration. *Am J Clin Nutr.* 2001;73(6):1094-1100.

37. Meydani SN, Endres S, Woods MM, et al. Oral (n-3) fatty acid supplementation suppresses cytokine production and lymphocyte proliferation: comparison between young and older women. *J Nutr.* 1991;121(4):547-555.

38. Arab L. Biomarkers of fat and fatty acid intake. *J Nutr.* 2003;133(suppl 3):925S-932S.

39. Wolk A, Vessby B, Ljung H, Barrefors P. Evaluation of a biologic marker for dairy fat intake. *Am J Clin Nutr.* 1998; 68(2):291-295.

40. Smedman AEM, Gustafsson I-B, Berglund LGT, Vessby BOH. Pentadecanoic acid in serum as a marker for intake of milk fat: relations between intake of milk fat and metabolic risk factors. *Am J Clin Nutr.* 1999;69:22-29.

41. Gross MD, Pfeiffer M, Martini M, Campbell D, Slavin J, Potter J. The quantitation of metabolites of quercetin flavonols in human urine. *Cancer Epidemiol Biomarkers Prev.* 1996;5:711-720.

42. Coward L, Barnes NC, Setchell KDR, Barnes S. Genistein, daidzein and their β-glycoside conjugates: antitumor

isoflavones in soybean foods from American and Asian diets. *J Agric Food Chem.* 1993;41(11):1961-1967.

43. Franke AA, Custer LJ, Cerna CM, Narala K. Quantitation of phytoestrogens in legumes by HPLC. *J Agric Food Chem.* 1994;42(9):1905-1913.

44. Karr SC, Lampe JW, Hutchins AM, Slavin JL. Urinary isoflavonoid excretion in humans is dose-dependent at low to moderate levels of soy protein consumption. *Am J Clin Nutr.* 1997;66:46-51.

45. Adlercreutz H, Honjo H, Higashi A, et al. Urinary excretion of lignans and isoflavonoid phytoestrogens in Japanese men and women consuming a traditional Japanese diet. *Am J Clin Nutr.* 1991;54(6):1093-1100.

46. Franke AA, Custer LJ. High-performance liquid chromatography assay of isoflavonoids and coumestrol from human urine. *J Chromatogr B Biomed Appl.* 1994;662: 47-60.

47. Maskarinec G, Singh S, Meng L, Franke AA. Dietary soy intake and urinary isoflavonoid excretion among women from a multiethnic population. *Cancer Epidemiol Biomarkers Prev.* 1998;7:613-619.

48. Watanabe S, Yamaguchi M, Sobue T, et al. Pharmacokinetics of soybean isoflavones in plasma, urine, and feces of men after ingestion of 60 g baked soybean powder (kinako). *J Nutr.* 1998;128(10):1710-1715.

49. Shapiro TA, Fahey JW, Wade KL, Stephenson KK, Talalay P. Human metabolism and excretion of cancer chemoprotective glucosinolates and isothiocyanates of cruciferous vegetables. *Cancer Epidemiol Biomarkers Prev.* 1998;7(12):1091-1100.

50. McClave SA, Snider HL. Use of indirect calorimetry in clinical nutrition. *Nutr Clin Pract.* 1992;7(5):207-221.

51. Jequier E, Felber JP. Indirect calorimetry. *Baillieres Clin Endocrinol Metab.* 1987;1(4):911-935.

52. Owen OE. Resting metabolic requirements of men and women. *Mayo Clin Proc.* 1988;63(5):503-510.

53. Lusk G. Animal calorimetry: analysis of the oxidation of mixtures of carbohydrate and fat [a correction]. *J Biol Chem.* 1994;59:41-42.

54. Peronnet F, Massicotte D. Table of nonprotein respiratory quotient: an update. *Can J Sport Sci.* 1991:16(1):23-29.

55. Isbell TR, Klesges RC, Meyers AW, Klesges LM. Measurement reliability and reactivity using repeated measurements of resting energy expenditure with a face mask, mouthpiece, and ventilated canopy. *JPEN J Parenter Enteral Nutr.* 1991; 15(2):165-168.

56. Leff ML, Hill JO, Yates AA, Cotsonis GA, Heymsfield SB. Resting metabolic rate: measurement reliability. *JPEN J Parenter Enteral Nutr.* 1987;11:354-359.

57. Academy of Nutrition and Dietetics Evidence Analysis Library. EE: Evidence analysis: measuring RMR with indirect calorimetry (IC) (2006). www.andeal.org/topic .cfm?cat=2695&highlight=indirect%20calorimetry&home =1. Accessed July 27, 2017:

58. Prentice AM. Energy. In: Mann J, Truswell S, eds. *Essentials of Human Nutrition.* Oxford, United Kingdom: Oxford University Press; 2012:92-108.

59. Seale J. Energy expenditure measurements in relation to energy requirements. *Am J Clin Nutr.* 1995;62(suppl): 1042-1046.

60. Speakman JR. The history and theory of the doubly labeled water technique. *Am J Clin Nutr.* 1998;68(suppl): 932-938.

61. Sawaya AL, Tucker K, Tsay R, et al. Evaluation of four methods for determining energy intake in young and older women: comparison with doubly labeled water measurements of total energy expenditure. *Am J Clin Nutr.* 1996; 63(4):491-499.

62. Schultz LA, Schoeller DA. A compilation of total daily energy expenditures and body weights in healthy adults. *Am J Clin Nutr.* 1994;60(5):676-681.

63. Bingham S. The use of 24 hour urine samples and energy expenditure to validate dietary assessments. *Am J Clin Nutr.* 1994;59(suppl);227S-231S.

64. Freedman LS, Midthune D, Carroll RJ, et al. Adjustments to improve the estimation of usual dietary intake distributions in the population. *J Nutr.* 2004;134(7):1836-1843.

65. Holbrook JT, Patterson KY, Bodner JE, et al. Sodium and potassium intake and balance in adults consuming self-selected diets. *Am J Clin Nutr.* 1984;40(4):786-793.

66. McCullough ML, Swain JF, Malarick C, Moore TJ. Feasibility of outpatient electrolyte balance studies. *J Am Coll Nutr.* 1991;10(2):140-148.

67. Clark AJ, Mossholder S. Sodium and potassium intake measurements: dietary methodology problems. *Am J Clin Nutr.* 1986;43(3):470-476.

68. Cogswell ME, Elliott P, Wang CY, Rhodes DG, Pfeiffer CM, Loria CM. Assessing U.S. sodium intake through dietary data and urine biomarkers. *Adv Nutr.* 2013;4(5):560-562.

69. Turban S, Miller ER 3rd, Ange B, Appel LJ. Racial differences in urinary potassium excretion. *J Am Soc Nephrol.* 2008;19:1396-1402.

70. Brown IJ, Dyer AR, Chan Q, et al. Estimating 24-hour urinary sodium excretion from casual urinary sodium concentrations in Western populations: the INTERSALT study. *Am J Epidemiol.* 2013;177(11):1180-1192.

71. Freedman LS, Midthune D, Carroll RJ, et al. Using regression calibration equations that combine self-reported intake and biomarkers measures to obtain

unbiased estimates and more powerful tests of dietary associations. *Am J Epidemiol*. 2011;174:1238-1245.

72. Lampe JW, Huang Y, Neuhouser ML, et al. Dietary biomarker evaluation in a controlled feeding study in women from the Women's Health Initiative cohort. *Am J Clin Nutr*. 2017;105(2):466-475.

73. Prentice RL, Mossavar-Rahmani Y, Huang Y, et al. Evaluation and comparison of food records, recalls and frequencies for energy and protein assessment by using recovery biomarkers. *Am J Epidemiol*. 2011;174(5): 591-603.

74. Mossavar-Rahmani Y, Shaw PA, Wong WW, et al. Applying recovery biomarkers to calibrate self-report measures of energy and protein in the Hispanic Community Health Study/Study of Latinos. *Am J Epidemiol*. 2015;181(12): 996-1007.

75. Prentice RL, Shaw PA, Bingham SA, et al. Biomarker-calibrated energy and protein consumption and increased cancer risk among postmenopausal women. *Am J Epidemiol*. 2009;169(8):977-989.

76. Prentice RL, Huang Y, Kuller LH, et al. Biomarker-calibrated energy and protein consumption and cardiovascular disease risk among postmenopausal women. *Epidemiology*. 2011, 22:170-179.

77. Tinker L, Sarto G, Howard BV, et al. Biomarker-calibrated dietary energy and protein intake associations with diabetes risk among postmenopausal women from the Women's Health Initiative. *Am J Clin Nutr*. 2011;94(6): 1600-1506.

78. National Cancer Institute. Glossary of key terms and notation. https://epi.grants.cancer.gov/events /measurement-error/mews_glossary.pdf. Revised September 15, 2011. Accessed April 24, 2018.

79. Huang Y, Van Horn L, Tinker LF, et al. Measurement error corrected sodium and potassium intake estimation using 24-hour urinary excretion. *Hypertension*. 2014;63(2):238-244.

80. Freedman LS, Commins JM, Moler JE, et al. Pooled results from 5 validation studies of dietary self-report instruments using recovery biomarkers for potassium and sodium intake. *Am J Epidemiol*. 2015;181(7):473-487.

81. Mossavar-Rahmani Y, Sotres-Alvarez D, Wong WW, et al. Applying recovery biomarkers to calibrate self-report measures of sodium and potassium in the Hispanic Community Health Study/Study of Latinos. *J Hum Hypertens*. 2017; 31(7):462-473.

82. Mossavar-Rahmani Y, Tinker LF, Huang Y, et al. Factors relating to eating style, social desirability, body image and eating meals at home increase the precision of calibration equations correcting self-report measures of diet using recovery biomarkers: findings from the Women's Health Initiative. *Nutr J*. 2013;12:63.

83. Brennan L. Metabolomics in nutrition research: current status and perspectives. *Biochem Soc Trans*. 2013;41(part 1):670-673.

84. Putri SP, Nakayama Y, Matsuda F, et al. Current metabolomics: practical applications. *J Biosci Bioeng*. 2013; 115(6):579-589.

85. Wang Y, Liu Sy, Hu YG, et al. Current state of the art of mass spectrometry-based metabolomics studies—a review focusing on wide coverage, high throughput and easy identification. *RSC Adv*. 2015;5:78728-78737.

86. Ramautar R, Demirci A, de Jong GJ. Capillary electro-phoresis in metabolomics. *Trac Trends Anal Chem*. 2006; 25:455-466.

87. Garcia-Perez I, Posma JM, Gibson R, et al. Objective assessment of dietary patterns by use of metabolic phenotyping: a randomized, controlled, crossover trial. *Lancet Diabetes Endocrinol*. 2017;5(3):184-195

88. Gibbons H, Brennan L. Metabolomics as a tool in the identification of dietary biomarkers. *Proc Nutr Soc*. 2017; 76(1):42-53.

89. Gibbons H, Carr E, McNulty BA, et al. Metabolomic-based identification of clusters that reflect dietary patterns. *Mol Nutr Food Res*. 2017;61(10). doi: 10.1002/ mnfr.201601050.

90. Cheung W, Keski-Rahkonen P, Assi N, et al. A metabolomic study of biomarkers of meat and fish intake. *Am J Clin Nutr*. 2017;105(3):600-608.

91. Bingham S, Cummings JH. The use of 4-aminobenzoic acid as a marker to validate the completeness of 24 hr urine collections in man. *Clin Sci*. 1983;64(6): 629-635.

92. Subar AF, Midthune D, Tasevska N, et al. Checking for completeness of 24-h urine collection using para-amino benzoic acid not necessary in the Observing Protein and Energy Nutrition study. *Eur J Clin Nutr*. 2013;67(8): 863-867.

93. Guilliano AR, Matzner MB, Canfield LM. Assessing variability in quantitation of carotenoids in human plasma: variance component model. *Methods Enzymol*. 1993;214: 94-101.

94. Duewer DL, Thomas JB, Kline MC, MacCrehan WA, Schaffer R, Sharpless KE. NIST/NCI Micronutrients Quality Assurance Program: measurement repeatabilities and reproducibilities for fat-soluble vitamin-related compounds in human sera. *Ann Chem*. 1997;69: 1406-1413.

Chapter 17

Research Methods in Appetite Assessment

James H. Hollis, PhD, BSc (Hons),

LEARNING OBJECTIVES

1. Understand the relevance of appetite research to address public health problems related to energy intake.

2. Understand the influence of participant characteristics and environmental context on appetite measurement.

3. Describe the standard approaches to measuring appetite and their strengths and limitations.

4. Describe how hormones influence appetite and eating behavior.

In humans, eating is episodic and meals are separated by intervals of abstinence from eating. Consequently, total daily energy intake is influenced by meal size and frequency of eating. As several leading public health issues are related to aberrant energy intake (eg, obesity and the anorexia of aging), a better understanding of the factors that influence meal size or eating frequency may contribute to the development of new strategies to reduce the number of overweight or underweight individuals and improve the population's health. Box 17.1 on page 332 lists applications of appetite research.

Develop new or reformulated products to increase fullness.

Develop meal strategies to reduce energy intake.

Develop eating behaviors (eg, reducing eating rate or bite size) that reduce meal size.

Identify individuals who experience low satiety or identify characteristics that may be related to low satiety.

Identify dietary strategies that aid weight management, such as those based on foods or behaviors that augment satiety.

Box 17.1 Applications of Appetite Research Methods for Weight Management

To date, considerable effort has been spent to identify the physiological, psychological, environmental, and socioeconomic factors that influence appetite. These efforts have resulted in a large and growing number of publications related to appetite. Unfortunately, the appetite literature is inconsistent, and considerable uncertainty remains regarding what factors influence appetite, the magnitude of their effect on appetite, and how the various factors interact. The lack of consistency is due to differences in experimental design; the use of small samples, which increase the risk of false negatives and are inadequate to detect small effect sizes[1]; or difficulties replicating behavioral research.[2] A more standardized approach to measuring appetite may increase the consistency between studies and contribute to more robust knowledge regarding appetite.

This chapter will provide a brief and critical description of the current, widely used methodologies for measuring satiation and satiety in humans. The limitations of these approaches will be highlighted and discussed, and the chapter concludes with a discussion of potential new approaches to appetite research.

DESCRIPTION OF TERMINOLOGY

A terminology to provide a framework for appetite research has been proposed and will be used in this chapter.[3] While this terminology has not been universally agreed upon, it provides a framework for discussing appetite methodology. Blundell and colleagues[3] stated that two definitions of appetite are in use. The first is that appetite "covers the whole field of food intake, selection, motivation and preference." The second is that appetite "refers specifically to qualitative aspects of eating, sensory aspects or responsiveness to environmental stimulation, which can be contrasted with the homeostatic view based on eating in response to physiological stimuli, energy deficit etc."[3] Hunger was defined as (1) a "construct or intervening variable that connotes the drive to eat. Not directly measurable but can be inferred from objective conditions" or (2) a "conscious sensation reflecting a mental urge to eat. Can be traced to changes in physical sensations in parts of the body, stomach, limbs or head. In its strong form may include feelings of light-headedness, weakness or emptiness in stomach."[3] Satiation was defined as the "process that leads to the termination of eating; therefore controls meal size. Also known as inter-meal satiety."[3] Satiety was defined as the "process that leads to inhibition of further eating, decline in hunger, increase in fullness after a meal has finished. Also known as post-ingestive satiety or inter-meal satiety."[3]

RECRUITING PARTICIPANTS

When recruiting participants, it is important that the characteristics of the study group reflect the population in which the intervention will be used. This is particularly true for food products that promote satiety, which should be tested using a study population that is representative of the consumers of that product. This is not always the case, and it has been suggested that those who take part in behavioral studies are WEIRD (ie, drawn from Western, educated, industrialized, rich, and democratic societies).[4] Consequently, the results from such studies may not be applicable to the general population. Efforts should be made to identify the target demographics of the intervention and to recruit individuals representative of this group into the study. However, the results from such a study cannot be extrapolated to the general population.

LENGTH OF THE STUDY

Appetite studies are generally short in duration, lasting from less than 1 hour to several hours. A large number of studies use the preload paradigm to study appetite. In a preload study, a precisely prepared meal that is matched for all variables, except for the one of interest, is provided to the study participants, and they are asked to eat this preload meal in its entirety. After a predetermined period of time, the participant is then provided with a test meal and asked to eat until comfortably full. This allows researchers to determine how the preload affects food intake. Typically, preload studies last 3 to 4 hours but can be as short as 15 minutes. It is imperative that the time between the preload and test meal is realistic with regard to how the intervention would be used in normal situations. These short-term studies allow for relatively rapid data collection, but any changes in appetite may be transient and may not persist over the longer term to cause a reduction in body weight. For instance, while a change in food intake may be observed at one meal, the body may compensate by increasing food intake at subsequent meals.[5] This is because appetite may be a dynamic process influenced by the body's energetic state.

Scientists have hypothesized that appetite is part of a physiological system that regulates body fat.[6] While this system only weakly defends against weight gain, it defends strongly against weight loss. Consequently, loss of fat mass results in reduced plasma leptin,[7] which reduces the body's sensitivity to satiation/satiety signals and thus a greater amount of food must be consumed to reach the same level of satiation/satiety.[8] Consequently, while a short-term study may find that an intervention reduces food intake, its effectiveness may diminish over time.

Consuming a food with a high satiation value may lead to reduced meal size, which could be measured using a short-term study, but it may also lead to a new eating pattern (ie, increased eating fre-

quency) so that there is no change in daily energy intake. An example of this phenomenon is a study in which cholecystokinin (CCK) was infused into rodents immediately before feeding, which persistently reduced meal size.[9] However, total daily energy intake remained unchanged as feeding frequency increased to compensate for the reduced meal size.

While short-term appetite studies can provide information regarding the factors that influence energy intake, it is not clear that this will be predictive of changes in body weight due to physiological compensatory measures. A greater focus should be placed on longer-term studies (potentially several months) to determine how interventions that reduce meal size influence eating patterns and ultimately body weight. Moreover, researchers should determine if reducing meal size leads to unintended deleterious consequences (eg, increased snacking of low-nutrient-density foods).

ENVIRONMENTAL CONTEXT AND APPETITE STUDIES

Most appetite studies are conducted in a laboratory environment. This approach has a number of strengths. Laboratory studies provide the opportunity for strong experimental control. This means that an individual factor of interest could potentially be isolated and its influence on appetite unambiguously determined. Laboratory studies also provide the potential to collect physiological samples (eg, blood samples, chewing muscle activity, or electro-encephalogram activity) that may contribute to a mechanistic explanation for effects on appetite.

A substantial drawback to laboratory studies is that food is not typically consumed in a laboratory environment. In other words, study participants are not consuming food in their usual daily settings, such as their homes or workplace. Food is generally consumed in environments where multiple stimuli, both noticed and unnoticed, act to subtly or strongly influence food intake. For instance, meal size has also been influenced by the label on a bottle of wine,[10] number of individuals present,[11] or proximity of food. In addition, nutrition labeling has also been shown to influence energy intake.[12]

Internal validity	Internal validity relates to the extent to which a study minimizes systematic errors or bias so that causal inferences can be made.
External validity	External validity relates to the extent to which the results of a study can be generalized to other situations or populations.

Box 17.2 Internal vs External Validity

The palatability of a meal has a marked influence on food intake.[13] Therefore, it is noteworthy that seemingly trivial factors such as the weight of the cutlery, background music, or room color influence the rated palatability of a meal and therefore may influence food intake.[14] While laboratory studies offer strong internal validity, they are poor on external validity (see Box 17.2).

An alternative approach is to conduct field studies that examine eating behavior in real-life situations. While this has the advantage of strong external validity, this approach has several disadvantages. First, in free-living situations, there is a lack of strong control over experimental procedures. Consequently, extraneous factors may contaminate the relationship between the intervention under study and food intake. Second, replication of field studies may be difficult. Eating behavior is influenced by the environment it is expressed in, and mirroring all the environmental factors (many of which may be seen as irrelevant) to allow direct replication of the study is not feasible. Third, measuring food intake in free-living individuals is difficult and may provide inaccurate results.[15,16] Fourth, while subjective appetite questionnaires can be administered outside the laboratory using electronic devices, there may be issues with compliance (eg, poor response rate). Finally, it is also not generally feasible to collect physiological samples that may provide a mechanistic explanation for the observed results.

DECEPTION OF PARTICIPANTS

Participants in appetite studies are often deceived about the true purpose of the study. Strategies include asking participants to perform tasks that are unrelated to the study aims; manipulating the energy density of a food; or using devices, such as soup bowls that refill, that remove the cues that frequently bring eating to an end. These procedures are used to remove a demand bias where participants form an impression of the study's purpose and alter their behavior to fit that interpretation. While deception has had a prominent role in behavioral studies for more than a century, there is an argument that this approach has ethical implications and may infringe on the participant's rights and dignity.[17] Moreover, it is not clear how well these deceptive practices work, and appetite studies that employ ruses rarely present data to demonstrate that the ruse was successful. Investigators can conduct post-study interviews to inform participants about the true purpose of the study and to ask whether they were aware of the study purpose. Another consideration is that institutional review boards may not always approve protocols that deceive participants. Alternatively, they may allow deception if it is scientifically justified and a debriefing session is provided after the study to inform participants about the true purpose of the study. Participants may then withdraw their consent, and, if someone does, the data from that participant cannot be used.

In addition, ruses may contaminate normal eating behavior and further reduce the relevance of the collected data to normal eating situations. Humans may base eating decisions on a number of factors according to the information available to them (eg, energy or macronutrient content). Manipulating foods to alter these characteristics, and hiding this from participants, may remove the normal cognitive processes that contribute to eating decisions. However, the relevance to eating decisions in typical eating situations is reduced.

Another difficulty with appetite studies is hiding the experimental manipulation from both the researcher and the participant so that a double-blind study can be conducted. For instance, changing the macronutrient content of a food would likely also influence other factors, such as the taste, texture, or appearance of the food, which may provide clues regarding the experimental manipulation being tested and the purpose of the study. Consequently, true double-blind studies are difficult to conduct.

STATISTICAL PLAN

Currently, there are no generally accepted specific guidelines for the statistical analysis of data collected for studies of appetite or food intake. However, the statistical analysis should comply with good practice as used in clinical trials (eg, Pocock and colleagues[18] and Assmann and colleagues[19]). Good scientific practice demands that the study hypothesis and the statistical analysis plan to test this hypothesis are specified before the study begins. In particular, decisions regarding the chosen end points (eg appetite ratings, food intake, biomarkers of appetite), outliers, and missing data should be decided before the study begins. Moreover, before the study begins, researchers should determine how data will be presented (eg, area under the curve, mean at each time point, or average hunger over the study duration). These decisions should be reported in the methods. A power calculation should be conducted to determine an adequate sample size and reported in the methods. As studies often use several different scales or appetite measures, the experiment-wide error rate should be controlled for multiple analysis.

STUDY DESIGN

Where possible, appetite studies should be double-blinded, although this is frequently difficult when using foods. In addition, the study should be fully balanced and randomized to avoid bias. This can be achieved using a Latin square design. Studies of appetite often use within-subjects designs. Consequently, an adequate period between test sessions is required to reduce the risk of a carryover effect. This will depend on the nature of the intervention. The number of treatments used in a within-subject study can vary, but issues such as participant fatigue, participant attrition, or the time available for the experiment typically limit the number of test sessions to less than six. Box 17.3 on page 336 presents study design terminology.

MEASURING SATIATION

As satiation is considered to be equivalent to meal size, it is typically determined by measuring food intake at an ad libitum meal. In the laboratory, satiation is measured by measuring food consumption (by weight or energy intake) at an ad libitum meal under standardized conditions. While conducting a study of satiation appears straightforward, several methodologic choices need to be made when designing the study. These choices will be determined by the objective of the study. Inappropriate choices will lead to a study in which results are confounded and difficult to interpret.

First, the investigators need to determine if a single meal will be presented at the same time as the factor under investigation (concurrent evaluation paradigm) or if the factor of interest will be presented in a meal eaten shortly before another test meal (the preload paradigm). For the preload paradigm, the presentation of the test meal should be within a realistic time after the preload (typically up to 15 minutes). A longer period of time will not fall within the normal time frame of a meal, which may diminish its relevance to satiation. The approach used will be determined by the objectives of the study and the nature of the intervention.

Second, the characteristics of the test meal need to be determined. Two approaches are typically used in satiation research: a buffet-style meal or a single meal. The buffet meal approach provides several food options (often a mixture of savory and sweet foods), and the participants can select what they wish to eat. This approach potentially allows researchers to determine how an intervention affects food choices concurrent with a measure of the amount eaten (satiation). However, this approach has several drawbacks. First, a buffet meal consisting of a large number of foods is atypical and potentially promotes food intake due to increased sensory variety.[20,21] Moreover, unless the foods in a buffet meal are matched for macronutrient content, energy density, palatability, or physical characteristics (eg, texture, viscosity, or physical form), differences in food

Crossover study (within subjects)	This is a repeated measures design where each participant serves as his or her own control and receives different treatments spaced by a period of time; that is, the participants cross over from one treatment to another during the course of the trial.
Parallel-arm study (between subjects)	A parallel study is a clinical study where two treatments, A and B, are provided so that one group receives only A while another group receives only B.
Latin square	A table is filled with different symbols in such a way that each symbol occurs once in each row and once in each column.
Carryover effect	This is an effect that "carries over" from one experimental condition to another. Whenever participants perform in more than one condition (ie, a crossover study), there is a possibility of carryover effects. This effect is reduced by an adequate time period between test sessions
Randomly assigned	This technique assigns human participants to different groups in an experiment using randomization (eg, a random number generator).
Control condition	This serves as the basis of comparison for the experimental condition.

Box 17.3 Study Design Terminology

choices from the buffet meal may influence satiation independent of the intervention. The buffet meal approach is possibly more suited for investigating food choices after an intervention. However, researchers must consider the number of food choices made available to participants so as not to artificially increase food intake.

Because of the limitations of the buffet meal, the single-meal approach is more typically used. However, investigators must still decide how many foods to present in this single meal. Meals typically consist of a few different foods that provide sensory variety, may complement each other, and may have a synergistic effect on palatability. Again, unless all components of the meal are matched for macronutrient content, energy density, palatability, or physical characteristics, any differences in the amount of each component eaten may confound interpretation of the results. An alternative approach is to provide a meal that offers variety but is more homogeneous (eg, pizza or pasta mixed with tomato sauce). The type of test meal used will depend on the objective of the study.

A buffet-style meal is useful if the primary objective of the study relates to food choices, while a single meal is more useful for determining energy intake.

Third, the size of the test meal warrants consideration. Typically, the test meal provided is larger than could reasonably be expected to be eaten. Participants are then invited to eat until comfortably full. This approach reduces the risk that participants will have to request more food to reach satiation, which they may not be willing to do because of embarrassment or social norms. However, this approach may artificially inflate the amount eaten as studies have shown that increasing portion sizes increases food intake.[22,23] While the size of the test meal may be consistent between test sessions so as not to systematically bias the results, providing meals that are larger than typically eaten does not reflect typical eating conditions.

Fourth, a participant's past experiences of the test food may influence how much he or she eats. A participant who has experience of the test food may have learned how much is needed to eat to reach satiation.[24]

Moreover, participants may only eat an amount that they believe meets social norms to avoid embarrassment. Some studies have tried to avoid these issues by cutting portions of foods into unusual shapes to confuse participants by removing a visual cue of how much they have eaten. In a study demonstrating the importance of visual cues in satiation, Wansink and colleagues[25] removed the visual cue of how much was eaten by using a bowl that automatically refilled with soup; participants consumed 73% more but did not perceive that they had eaten more.

Fifth, other cognitive factors may be important in determining the amount eaten. Participants may not eat to be comfortably full but eat to excess if they will not have access to food for several hours after the test session. For instance, de Graaf and colleagues[26] found that participants ate more when they were told they would have no access to foods for 2 hours compared with 20 minutes. Moreover, participants may eat to excess so they can skip a meal. Conversely, participants may purposefully undereat so they can leave the laboratory more quickly and eat a food they desire. The participant's appetitive state should also be considered. Hunger is a predictor of meal size, and if the participant attends test sessions with different sensations of hunger this could contribute to differences in food intake. Some of these issues could be eliminated or their effect reduced by requiring participants to report to the laboratory at the same time, thereby keeping eating behavior consistent in the hours before a test session. For example, for a study that is conducted at lunch, participants may be asked to report to the laboratory first thing in the morning after an overnight fast and then be provided with a standardized breakfast. This would reduce the risk of previous food consumption contaminating the study. Keeping all the participants in the laboratory for a fixed amount of time after completing a meal may prevent their cutting the meal short.

While satiation studies appear relatively straightforward, there are fundamental questions about what is actually being measured. Why are participants eating the amount they do? Is it merely to satisfy hunger or to satisfy other goals unrelated to satisfying energy needs? Does measuring the food intake of participants who eat to excess because they are given a large portion of free food provide any meaningful information? Is satiation context specific (ie, can eating behavior in one context be extrapolated to other contexts?), or can participants use heuristics to aid eating decision-making based on prior experiences to achieve their goals?

MEASURING SATIETY

Many studies conducted to understand satiety use a preload study design. Typically, a participant will be required to report to the laboratory first thing in the morning after an overnight fast, although this design has been used at other times of the day. However, it should be recognized that many foods are only eaten at certain times of the day, and test foods should be appropriate for the time they are eaten. For instance, pizza is not typically eaten for breakfast. Baseline measurements will be made (eg, blood draw, appetite questionnaire) before participants are provided with a preload meal. This preload meal can be manipulated to determine how the manipulated variable affects satiety. After this meal, measurements are taken over a period of time ranging from 30 minutes to several hours. Satiety is generally measured by regular measurement of subjective appetite, biomarkers of appetite (often at 15, 30, 45, 60, 90, 120, 180, and 240 minutes after preload consumption), food intake at a subsequent test meal, or a combination of these measures.

METHODOLOGY FOR MEASURING APPETITE
Appetite Questionnaires

Humans have the capacity for introspection, and information can be gained by posing questions regarding their sensations or prospective eating behaviors. Because of differences in how individuals interpret appetite questionnaires, they are generally used in within-subjects studies. While many different questions are used, a standard set of questions should be asked to assess subjective appetite to facilitate comparisons across studies.[3] Following is a proposed set of questions:

- How hungry are you?
- How full are you?
- How satiated are you?
- How strong is your desire to eat?
- How much do you think you could eat right now?

The responses to these questions are typically captured using a visual analogue scale (VAS) that is 100 to 150 mm long, anchored with statements similar to "not at all" and "as hungry as I have ever felt" (see Figure 17.1).

Data from a VAS are typically presented as a graph or a table that provides the average appetite rating at each time point (eg, Zhu and Hollis[27]). However, data may also be presented as area under the curve calculated by summarizing the mean scores from adjacent time points and then calculating a weighted mean based on the duration between the two time points.[28]

Category scales may also be used. Category scales are similar to VASs except instead of a continuous line, participants are forced to choose a category (Figure 17.2). If the number of categories is very limited (eg, three to five), the scale may not allow for sufficient discrimination. However, with a large number of categories (eg, 13 or more), meaningful discrimination between adjacent categories is also questionable.

Note that both scales are not true ratio scales. That is, the difference between a rating of two and a rating of three on a VAS or category scale is not the same as a difference between an eight and nine. Moreover, a rating of eight should not be seen as a feeling twice as intensive as a rating of four.

Another approach is to use open-ended questionnaires that encourage a fuller answer regarding current appetitive sensations compared with closed-ended questions that provide limited information and may also be leading. Consequently, a strength of open-ended questionnaires is that they may provide novel insights into appetite. In appetite research, open-ended questionnaires have been used to examine the temporal pattern and intensity of appetitive sensations.[29,30]

A key limitation to the use of open-ended questionnaires is that a large number of responses is possible, and aggregating them for analysis may be

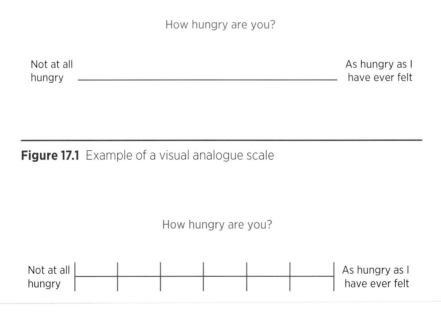

Figure 17.1 Example of a visual analogue scale

Figure 17.2 Example of a category scale

difficult. Open-ended questionnaires will commonly provide reports of sensations from different regions of the body but provide limited quantification of the intensity of these sensations. Further, open-ended questionnaires require more thought and effort than is needed to complete VASs or category scales, so motivating participants to complete the questionnaire may become an issue.[31]

While appetite questionnaires are widely used, their ability to predict food intake is modest. Studies that have correlated responses from appetite questionnaires with food intake typically report correlation coefficients less than 0.4.[32] In addition, it is not clear what magnitude of change in appetite is required to meaningfully influence food intake. Although this seems to limit the practical relevance of appetite questionnaires, it is not clear that food intake—particularly under laboratory conditions—is an objective and uncontaminated measure of appetite.

Energy/Food Intake

For registered dietitian nutritionists, food intake may seem to be the primary measure of appetite and the most practically useful measure. However, food intake is not an uncontaminated measure of appetite, and many factors may operate to uncouple this relationship.[33] As discussed in the previous section on satiation, measurement of food intake in the laboratory context should only be extrapolated to other situations with extreme caution.

Eating Behavior

Methods to measure eating parameters within a meal have been used to gain information regarding the processes that contribute to meal termination. A variety of indexes have been used, including eating rate or chewing rate. In addition, appetite ratings have also been measured during a meal.[34] However, the effect of interrupting a meal to collect data regarding the effect of subjective appetite on normal eating behavior may not be trivial. A system that has been developed to measure changes in eating parameters is the Universal Eating Monitor (UEM), which is a set of weight scales hidden under a false table top and connected to a computer.[35] During the test meal/snack, the computer can also be used to pose questions regarding motivation to eat. The UEM measures total food intake, rate of eating, and change in rate of eating during an eating episode. However, it is not clear if these measures are sufficiently sensitive to be used as a marker of appetite and thus are not commonly used.

Biomarkers of Appetite

Several physiological processes, such as the plasma concentration of gut hormones or glucose, have been linked to appetitive sensations or food intake. Consequently, researchers have proposed using them as a biomarker of appetite.[36] For a biomarker of appetite to be useful it must meet a number of criteria. The biomarker must be able to be collected without causing undue stress or requiring overly invasive procedures, must be sensitive and reliably change in response to a given appetitive sensation, must be able to be reliably measured, and should exert an effect at physiological levels. While many hormones or metabolites potentially influence appetite, a limited number are in common use and will be discussed.

Glucose

In 1953, Mayer[37] first proposed a role for plasma glucose in eating behavior, termed the *glucostatic theory of eating*. More recent studies suggest that a transient decline in plasma glucose is associated with a spontaneous request for food.[38] Another study found that meal initiation could be delayed by holding plasma glucose constant by glucose infusion.[39] These studies suggest that the concentration of plasma glucose could be a biomarker for appetite. However, there are a number of issues regarding plasma glucose as a biomarker for appetite. First, studies demonstrating that a transient glucose decline is associated with eating initiation generally infuse an insulin dose to artificially reduce plasma glucose. However, using this approach, plasma glucose declines to levels below physiological norms. Second, the link between the transient glucose decline and a food request is not robust, and individuals often request food in the absence of a change in blood glucose. Third, detecting a transient decline in blood glucose is technically difficult and is not a routine measure. Fourth, independent manipulation of glucose through euglycemic clamp (an experimental technique that maintains circulating levels of glucose at a predetermined, fixed level) studies does not alter subjective hunger or fullness.[40]

Ghrelin

The hormone ghrelin is predominantly produced by the gastric mucosa of the stomach in humans, and it is the only peripherally produced hormone that has been identified that stimulates food intake in humans.[41,42] Ghrelin circulates in two major forms: n-octanyl-ghrelin (ghrelin) and des-n-octanyl ghrelin (desacyl ghrelin). Studies indicate that plasma ghrelin concentration rises before a meal and falls after food consumption.[43] Moreover, ghrelin infusion increases subjective hunger and food intake,[44] while administration of ghrelin receptor antagonists reduces food intake in rats.[45] However, gastrectimized patients who have low ghrelin secretory capacity show normal appetite function.[46,47]

Researchers once believed only n-octanyl-ghrelin was biologically active. However, a study found that while injecting desacyl ghrelin intraperitoneally did not increase food intake, injecting it simultaneously with n-octanyl-ghrelin abolished the stimulatory effect on food intake.[48] Others have questioned whether the preprandial rise in ghrelin initiates eating or just prepares the body for ingesting food.[49] Further research is required to determine the role of ghrelin in meal initiation, how the different forms of ghrelin influence appetite, and the implications for appetite studies.

Cholecystokinin

CCK is largely secreted from I cells in the upper small intestine in response to the presence of intraluminal nutrients, in particular, fatty acids and peptides.[50] Various forms of CCK have been identified.[50] A potential role for CCK in food intake was reported by Gibbs and colleagues,[51] who demonstrated that exogenous CCK administration in rats reduced food intake and meal length. Subsequently, other researchers showed that CCK administration reduces food intake in humans.[52,53] In addition, administration of CCK receptor antagonists eliminates the appetite-suppressing effect of CCK.[54] Based on this research, CCK has potential as a biomarker of appetite, although several limitations have been identified. First, its association with appetitive sensations is not consistent because of its relative insensitivity to carbohydrate, the primary source of energy in the diet.[55] Second, it is not clear whether CCK has an effect at physiological levels and may need to be administered at supraphysiological levels to have an effect.[56] Administration of supraphysiological levels of CCK may influence food intake, in part, by increasing feelings of nausea rather than satiation.[57] Third, because of its low abundance in blood, molecular heterogeneity and homology to gastrin, which circulates at higher concentrations, measuring CCK may be technically challenging.[58]

Glucagon-Like-Peptide-1

Glucagon-like-peptide-1 (GLP-1) is produced in the L cells of the intestine and circulated in two active forms: GLP-1_{7-36} and GLP-1_{7-37}.[59] In humans, the main circulating form is GLP-1_{7-36}. GLP-1 is secreted during the postprandial period in response to stimulation by nutrients.[60] In addition, GLP-1 is stimulated by other gastrointestinal hormones, such as gastric inhibitory peptide.[61] An early peak of GLP-1 occurs approximately 15 minutes after food ingestion, whereas a second, significantly larger, peak appears later and is thought to be due to the interaction between nutrients and L cells in the ileum.[62] The infusion of GLP-1 reduces subjective hunger, increases fullness, and reduces food intake at a subsequent eating episode.[63,64] However, these responses are generally only seen at supraphysiological levels, and de Graaf[65] suggested that GLP-1 has limited utility as a marker of appetite.

Peptide YY

Two forms of human peptide YY have been identified: PYY$_{1-36}$ and PYY$_{3-36}$. PYY$_{3-36}$ is the major circulating form.[66] PYY is primarily released from the distal portion of the gastrointestinal tract and acts as an agonist on the Y2 receptor in the hypothalamus.[67] This receptor inhibits the release of neuropeptide Y, a potent stimulator of hunger and food intake.[68] Studies have shown that intravenous administration of PYY_{3-36} reduces subjective appetite and food intake over a 24-hour period.[69] While intravenous administration of PYY_{1-36} has been shown to reduce food intake in rodents, its effect is much less pronounced than that of PYY_{3-36}.[70] Moreover, PYY_{1-36} may not influence food intake in humans.[71] While PYY has promise as a marker of appetite, further research is needed to determine its relationship to subjective appetite.

Insulin

While a role for insulin in short-term appetite control has been proposed, studies that infused insulin found increased,[72] decreased,[73] or no effect on appetite.[74,75] Moreover, the relationship is further complicated by observations indicating that insulin has an appetite-suppressing effect in individuals who are lean but not individuals who are obese.[76,77] However, when glucose levels are held constant, there is no relationship between plasma insulin concentration and appetite or food intake.[74,78] Consequently, the plasma concentration of insulin concentration likely has limited use as a marker of appetite.

Leptin

Leptin is largely secreted from the adipose tissue in direct proportion to the amount of fat mass.[79] It is also secreted from the stomach, and gastric leptin may be a better predictor of eating-related changes in appetite as it is responsive to food intake.[80] However, gastric leptin is not readily measured, which limits its use as a biomarker of appetite. Studies report a strong correlation between premeal/snack leptin concentrations and energy intake.[81] Energy deficits of 24 hours result in decreases in plasma leptin concentration, whereas energy surpluses over 24 hours result in increased leptin concentrations.[82] Moreover, leptin levels are predictive of food in-

take.[83,84] Consequently, leptin may prove to be a useful biomarker to predict appetite.

Neuroimaging Techniques

Neuroimaging techniques have been used in appetite studies. In general, these studies seek to correlate neuronal activity (using markers of neuronal activity such as cerebral blood flow or oxygen consumption) with feelings of hunger or satiety (eg, Tataranni and colleagues[85] and Fuehrer and colleagues[86]). Positron emission tomography (PET) and functional magnetic resonance imaging (fMRI) have been used in studies of appetite. PET scans begin with the intravenous administration of the positron-emitting radioisotope ^{15}O, which is distributed throughout the body's tissues. As this radioisotope crosses the blood-brain barrier, it can be used to measure cerebral blood flow. At the site of brain activation, cerebral blood flow increases, which results in a greater uptake of the ^{15}O tracer and, consequently, an increase in the gamma rays detected in the activated area, which is a measure of neuronal activity. One limitation of a PET scan is that images can only be taken every 8 to 10 minutes, limiting the use of this method for studies of satiation. Another limitation is that the spatial resolution of PET is not as high as that of fMRI. As PET scans use a radioactive tracer, this method may not be used for multiple assessments in the same individual.

Magnetic resonance imaging (MRI) works on the principle that when neuronal cells are active, they consume oxygen. Therefore, active parts of the brain have a greater concentration of deoxygenated hemoglobin. Because of the magnetic resonance properties of oxygenated and deoxygenated blood, brain activity can be detected using an fMRI scanner. Typical studies involve a baseline image of the brain, followed by stimulus administration and further imaging to determine the effect on brain activity. Most of the same limitations noted for PET scanning apply to the use of fMRI to identify an appetitive biomarker. The cost of both of these techniques and the requirement for specialized instruments has limited the use of these techniques in appetite research. Another limitation of neuroimaging techniques is that the participant is required to remain still throughout the measurement. Consequently, the participant cannot eat while the measurement is being made. Participants may be able to consume food through a straw, although this would limit the generalizability of the results.

Gut Distention or Motility

Studies in which investigators inserted a balloon in the stomach and inflated it with water found that the more the balloon is inflated, the greater the reduction in food intake.[87] However, the response was less pronounced in individuals who are obese. A typical experiment may involve examining the degree and length of time the stomach is distended after a test food or meal. Several methods are available for measuring gastric distention, including ultrasound and MRI, although access to the specialized equipment required may limit the use of gut distention as a marker of appetite for the foreseeable future.

The rate of gastric emptying is associated with sensations of hunger or fullness.[88] Slower gastric emptying prolongs stomach distention and prolongs the time that nutrients are in the gut. Therefore, satiety signals arising from nutrients in the gut will be generated for a longer time, thereby promoting satiety. Methods suitable for measuring gastric emptying include ultrasound, MRI, gamma radiation cameras, measures of radioactive isotopes, breath hydrogen, or absorption of a marker such as acetaminophen (a nonmetabolized compound that can be quantified in the blood). The use of gastric emptying as a marker of appetite is limited by access to specialized equipment (ultrasound, MRI, or radioactive isotopes) or limitations in the administration of the marker (some markers, such as acetaminophen, can only be administered in liquid foods).

Evidence indicates that these markers are highly adaptive. For example, chronic distention of the stomach leads to tolerance and loss of sensitivity. The practice of ingesting a large quantity of water just before or with a food load as a means to promote satiety via gastric distention has not proven effective.[89] Moreover, evidence of normal appetitive responses

in patients who have undergone gastrectomy[47] demonstrates that the measures may, under selected conditions, be sufficient to modify appetite but are not necessary.

CONCLUSION

A large and growing number of studies have investigated the influence of a myriad of factors on appetite. While this has led to the development of new food products or strategies to promote satiety and aid weight loss, the effectiveness of these approaches is debatable. While experimental approaches to measuring satiation and satiety have been developed, they have substantial limitations, and the relevance of the results gained from these studies to eating behavior in free-living situations is debatable. New approaches will likely be required to gain new insights into human appetite.

Human appetite is expressed in an environment where an individual is exposed to a number of factors that are known to influence appetite. It is possible that several factors have yet to be identified. How all of these factors interact to influence appetite and eating behavior is poorly understood. It is not clear whether there is an additive effect (in which several factors potentiate appetite), whether there is a synergistic effect (in which the sum of the effects is greater than the individual parts), or whether various factors cancel each other out. New approaches to appetite research that determine how appetite is expressed in more naturalistic settings are required.

Clearly, the environment in which appetite is expressed is changing rapidly. Individuals have greater access to the nutritional content of a food or meal due to increased smartphone use. Moreover, access to food that is desired, rather than what is available, is becoming easier due to the emergence of meal-delivery services. Future developments, such as smart kitchens or artificial intelligence, may aid food decision making to promote healthier choices. Studies that determine how technological advances influence appetite are required so that this technology can be harnessed to promote public health. This may necessitate new approaches to appetite research and greater collaboration between researchers from different disciplines.

With their knowledge of nutrition, food science, psychology, and clinical practice, registered dietitian nutritionists are well positioned to move appetite research forward. The following areas may prove fruitful: (1) exploring new methodologies to better characterize and quantify appetitive sensations, (2) assessing the environmental and cognitive signals that modulate appetite, (3) evaluating the pattern of hormonal signals that influence appetite rather than effects of single hormones, and, (4) ultimately conducting more expansive studies that integrate these approaches and processes. With a more complete understanding, researchers and practitioners hope that appetitive sensations can be modulated for health promotion.

While efforts have been made to standardize appetite research methodology,[3] there is still no consensus regarding best approaches. The lack of consensus likely reflects the complexity of measuring appetite and the diversity of questions that can be addressed. Further discussion to standardize appetite research is required so that comparisons between studies can be made.

REFERENCES

1. Button KS, Ioannidis JP, Mokrysz C, et al. Power failure: why small sample size undermines the reliability of neuroscience. *Nat Rev Neurosci.* 2013;14(5):365-376.

2. Fabrigar LR, Wegener DT. Further considerations on conceptualizing and evaluating the replication of research results. *J Exp Soc Psychol.* 2017;69:241-243.

3. Blundell J, de Graaf C, Hulshof T, et al. Appetite control: methodological aspects of the evaluation of foods. *Obes Rev.* 2010;11(3):251-270.

4. Henrich J, Heine SJ, Norenzayan A. The weirdest people in the world? *Behav Brain Sci.* 2010;33(2-3):61-83.

5. McKieman F, Hollis JH, Mattes RD. Short-term dietary compensation in free-living adults. *Physiol Behav.* 2008; 93(4-5):975-983.

6. Speakman JR, Levitsky DA, Allison DB, et al. Set points, settling points and some alternative models: theoretical options to understand how genes and environments combine to regulate body adiposity. *Dis Model Mech.* 2011; 4(6):733-745.

7. Considine RV, Sinha MK, Heiman ML, et al. Serum immunoreactive leptin concentrations in normal-weight and obese humans. *N Engl J Med.* 1996;334(5):292-295.

8. Baver SB, Hope K, Guyot S, et al. Leptin modulates the intrinsic excitability of AgRP/NPY neurons in the arcuate nucleus of the hypothalamus. *J Neurosci.* 2014;34(16): 5486-5496.

9. West DB, Fey D, Woods SC. Cholecystokinin persistently suppresses meal size but not food intake in free-feeding rats. *Am J Physiol.* 1984;246(5): R776-R787.

10. Wansink B, Payne CR, North J. Fine as North Dakota wine: sensory expectations and the intake of companion foods. *Physiol Behav.* 2007;90(5):712-716.

11. Decastro JM, Brewer EM. The amount eaten in meals by humans is a power function of the number of people present. *Physiol Behav.* 1992;51(1):121-125.

12. McCann MT, Wallace JM, Robson PJ, et al. Influence of nutrition labelling on food portion size consumption. *Appetite.* 2013;65:153-158.

13. Wansink B, Painter JE, Lee YK. The office candy dish: proximity's influence on estimated and actual consumption. *Int J Obes.* 2006;30(5):871-875.

14. Spence C. Multisensory flavor perception. *Cell.* 2015;161(1): 24-35.

15. Archer E, Hand GA, Blair SN. Validity of U.S. nutritional surveillance: National Health and Nutrition Examination Survey caloric energy intake data, 1971–2010. *PLoS One*. 2013;8(10):e76632.

16. Hill RJ, Davies PSW. The validity of self-reported energy intake as determined using the doubly labelled water technique. *Br J Nutr*. 2001;85(4):415-430.

17. Baumrind D. Research using intentional deception—ethical issues revisited. *Am Psychol*. 1985;40(2):165-174.

18. Pocock SJ, Assmann SE, Enos LE, et al. Subgroup analysis, covariate adjustment and baseline comparisons in clinical trial reporting: current practice and problems. *Stat Med*. 2002;21(19):2917-2930.

19. Assmann SF, Pocock SJ, Enos LE, et al. Subgroup analysis and other (mis)uses of baseline data in clinical trials. *Lancet*. 2000;355(9209):1064-1069.

20. Hollis JH, Henry CJ. Dietary variety and its effect on food intake of elderly adults. *J Hum Nutr Diet*. 2007;20(4):345-351.

21. Rolls BJ, Rowe EA, Rolls ET, et al. Variety in a meal enhances food intake in man. *Physiol Behav*. 1981;26(2):215-221.

22. Rolls BJ, Morris EL, Roe LS. Portion size of food affects energy intake in normal-weight and overweight men and women. *Am J Clin Nutr*. 2002;76(6):1207-1213.

23. Levitsky DA, Youn T. The more food young adults are served, the more they overeat. *J Nutr*. 2004;134(10):2546-2549.

24. Brunstrom JM. Mind over platter: pre-meal planning and the control of meal size in humans. *Int J Obes*. 2014;38(suppl):S9-S12.

25. Wansink B, Painter JE, North J. Bottomless bowls: why visual cues of portion size may influence intake. *Obesity Res*. 2005;13(1):93-100.

26. De Graaf C, De Jong LS, Lambers AC. Palatability affects satiation but not satiety. *Physiol Behav*. 1999;66(4):681-688.

27. Zhu Y, Hollis JH. Gastric emptying rate, glycemic and appetite response to a liquid meal in lean and overweight males. *Int J Food Sci Nutr*. 2014;65(5):615-620.

28. Emilien CH, West R, Hollis JH. The effect of the macronutrient composition of breakfast on satiety and cognitive function in undergraduate students. *Eur J Nutr*. 2017;56(6):2139-2150.

29. Mattes RD, Friedman MI. Hunger. *Dig Dis*. 1993;11(2):65-77.

30. Friedman MI, Ulrich P, Mattes RD. A figurative measure of subjective hunger sensations. *Appetite*. 1999;32(3):395-404.

31. Flint A, Raben A, Blundell JE, et al. Reproducibility, power and validity of visual analogue scares in assessment of appetite sensations in single test meal studies. *Int J Obes*. 2000;24(1):38-48.

32. Parker BA, Sturm K, MacIntosh C, et al. Relation between food intake and visual analogue scale ratings of appetite and other sensations in healthy older and young subjects. *Eur J Clin Nutr*. 2004;58(2):212-218.

33. Booth DA. Lines, dashed lines and "scale" ex-tricks. Objective measurements of appetite versus subjective tests of intake. *Appetite*. 2009;53(3):434-437.

34. Yeomans MR. Rating changes over the course of meals: what do they tell us about motivation to eat? *Neurosci Biobehav Rev*. 2000;24(2):249-259.

35. Kissileff HR, Klingsberg G, Van Itallie TB. Universal eating monitor for continuous recording of solid or liquid consumption in man. *Am J Physiol*. 1980;238(1):R14-R22.

36. de Graaf C, Blom WA, Smeets PA, et al. Biomarkers of satiation and satiety. *Am J Clin Nutr*. 2004;79(6):946-961.

37. Mayer J. Glucostatic mechanism of regulation of food intake. *N Engl J Med*. 1953;249(1):13-16.

38. Campfield LA, Smith FJ, Rosenbaum M, et al. Human eating: evidence for a physiological basis using a modified paradigm. *Neurosci Biobehav Rev*. 1996;20(1):133-137.

39. Campfield LA, Brandon P, Smith FJ. On-line continuous measurement of blood glucose and meal pattern in free-feeding rats: the role of glucose in meal initiation. *Brain Res Bull*. 1985;14(6):605-616.

40. Chapman IM, Goble EA, Wittert GA, et al. Effect of intravenous glucose and euglycemic insulin infusions on short-term appetite and food intake. *Am J Physiol*. 1998;274(3 part 2):R596-R603.

41. Churm R, Davies JS, Stephens JW, Prior SL. Ghrelin function in human obesity and type 2 diabetes: a concise review. *Obes Rev*. 2017;18(2):140-146.

42. Asakawa A, Inui A, Kaga T, et al. Ghrelin is an appetite-stimulatory signal from stomach with structural resemblance to motilin. *Gastroenterology*. 2001;120(2):337-345.

43. Cummings DE, Purnell JQ, Frayo RS, et al. A preprandial rise in plasma ghrelin levels suggests a role in meal initiation in humans. *Diabetes*. 2001;50(8):1714-1719.

44. Wren AM, Seal LJ, Cohen MA, et al. Ghrelin enhances appetite and increases food intake in humans. *J Clin Endocrinol Metab*. 2001;86(12):5992-5995.

45. Asakawa A, Inui A, Kaga T, et al. Antagonism of ghrelin receptor reduces food intake and body weight gain in mice. *Gut*. 2003;52(7):947-952.

46. Cummings DE, Weigle DS, Frayo RS, et al. Plasma ghrelin levels after diet-induced weight loss or gastric bypass surgery. *N Engl J Med*. 2002;346(21): 1623-1630.

47. Bergh C, Sjostedt S, Hellers G, et al. Meal size, satiety and cholecystokinin in gastrectomized humans. *Physiol Behav*. 2003;78(1):143-147.

48. Inhoff T, Monnikes H, Noetzel S, et al. Desacyl ghrelin inhibits the orexigenic effect of peripherally injected ghrelin in rats. *Peptides*. 2008;29(12):2159-2168.

49. Frecka JM, Mattes RD. Possible entrainment of ghrelin to habitual meal patterns in humans. *Am J Physiol Gastrointest Liver* Physiol. 2008;294(3):G699-G707.

50. Liddle RA, Goldfine ID, Rosen MS, et al. Cholecystokinin bioactivity in human-plasma. Molecular forms, responses to feeding, and relationship to gallbladder contraction. *J Clin Invest*. 1985;75(4):1144-1152.

51. Gibbs J, Young RC, Smith GP. Cholecystokinin decreases food intake in rats. *J Comp Physiol Psychol*. 1973;84(3): 488-495.

52. MacIntosh CG, Morley JE, Wishart J, et al. Effect of exogenous cholecystokinin (CCK)-8 on food intake and plasma CCK, leptin, and insulin concentrations in older and young adults: evidence for increased CCK activity as a cause of the anorexia of aging. *J Clin Endocrinol Metab*. 2001;86(12):5830-5837.

53. Muurahainen N, Kissileff HR, Derogatis AJ, et al. Effects of cholecystokinin-octapeptide (Cck-8) on food intake and gastric emptying in man. *Physiol Behav*. 1988;44(4-5): 645-649.

54. Reidelberger RD, Castellanos DA, Hulce M. Effects of peripheral CCK receptor blockade on food intake in rats. *Am J Physiol Regul Integr Comp Physiol*. 2003;285(2): R429-R437.

55. Bowen J, Noakes M, Trenerry C, et al. Energy intake, ghrelin, and cholecystokinin after different carbohydrate and protein preloads in overweight men. *J Clin Endocrinol Metab*. 2006;91(4):1477-1483.

56. Lieverse RJ, Jansen JBMJ, Vandezwan A, et al. Effects of a physiological dose of cholecystokinin on food intake and postprandial satiation in man. *Regul Peptides*. 1993;43 (1-2):83-89.

57. Greenough A, Cole G, Lewis J, et al. Untangling the effects of hunger, anxiety, and nausea on energy intake during intravenous cholecystokinin octapeptide (CCK-8) infusion. *Physiol Behav*. 1998;65(2):303-310.

58. Rehfeld JF. Accurate measurement of cholecystokinin in plasma. *Clin Chem*. 1998;44(5):991-1001.

59. Holst JJ. The physiology of glucagon-like peptide 1. *Physiol Rev*. 2007;87(4):1409-1439.

60. Naslund E, Gutniak M, Skogar S, et al. Glucagon-like peptide 1 increases the period of postprandial satiety and slows gastric emptying in obese men. *Am J Clin Nutr*. 1998; 68(3):525-530.

61. Skow MA, Bergmann NC, Knop FK. Diabetes and obesity treatment based on dual incretin receptor activation: 'twincretins'. *Diabetes Obes Metab*. 2016;18(9): 847-854.

62. Wang XC, Liu H, Chen JQ, Li Y, Qu S. Multiple factors related to the secretion of glucagon-like peptide-1. *Int J Endocrinol*. 2015;2015:651757.

63. Chelikani PK, Haver AC, Reidelberger RD. Intravenous infusion of glucagon-like peptide-1 potently inhibits food intake, sham feeding, and gastric emptying in rats. *Am J Physiol Regul Integr Comp Physiol*. 2005;288(6): R1695-R706.

64. Flint A, Raben A, Astrup A, et al. Glucagon-like peptide 1 promotes satiety and suppresses energy intake in humans. *J Clin Invest*. 1998;101(3):515-520.

65. de Graaf C, Blom WAM, Smeets PAM, et al. Biomarkers of satiation and satiety. *Am J Clin Nutr*. 2004;79(6): 946-961.

66. Grandt D, Schimiczek M, Beglinger C, et al. Two molecular forms of peptide YY (PYY) are abundant in human blood: characterization of a radioimmunoassay recognizing PYY 1–36 and PYY 3–36. *Regul Pept*. 1994; 51(2):151-159.

67. Batterham RL, Cohen MA, Ellis SM, et al. Inhibition of food intake in obese subjects by peptide YY3-36. *N Engl J Med*. 2003;349(10):941-948.

68. Mercer RE, Chee MJS, Colmers WF. The role of NPY in hypothalamic mediated food intake. *Front Neuroendocrinol*. 2011;32(4):398-415.

69. Batterham RL, Cowley MA, Small CJ, et al. Gut hormone PYY3-36 physiologically inhibits food intake. *Nature*. 2002;418(6898):650-654.

70. Chelikani PK, Haver AC, Reidelberger RD. Comparison of the inhibitory effects of PYY(3-36) and PYY(1-36) on gastric emptying in rats. *Am J Physiol Regul Integr Comp Physiol*. 2004;287(5):R1064-R1070.

71. Sloth B, Holst JJ, Flint A, et al. Effects of PYY1-36 and PYY3-36 on appetite, energy intake, energy expenditure, glucose and fat metabolism in obese and lean subjects. *Am J Physiol Endocrinol Metab*. 2007;292(4): E1062-E1068.

72. Rodin J, Wack J, Ferrannini E, et al. Effect of insulin and glucose on feeding behavior. *Metabolism*. 1985;34(9): 826-831.

73. Holt SH, Miller JB. Increased insulin responses to ingested foods are associated with lessened satiety. *Appetite*. 1995; 24(1):43-54.

74. Gielkens HA, Verkijk M, Lam WF, et al. Effects of hyperglycemia and hyperinsulinemia on satiety in humans. *Metabolism*. 1998;47(3):321-324.

75. Woo R, Kissileff HR, Pisunyer FX. Elevated postprandial insulin levels do not induce satiety in normal-weight humans. *Am J Physiol*. 1984;247(4):R745-R749.

76. Speechly DP, Buffenstein R. Appetite dysfunction in obese males: evidence for role of hyperinsulinaemia in passive overconsumption with a high fat diet. *Eur J Clin Nutr*. 2000;54(3):225-233.

77. Verdich C, Toubro S, Buemann B, et al. The role of postprandial releases of insulin and incretin hormones in meal-induced satiety—effect of obesity and weight reduction. *Int J Obes*. 2001;25(8):1206-1214.

78. Lavin JH, Wittert G, Sun WM, et al. Appetite regulation by carbohydrate: role of blood glucose and gastrointestinal hormones. *Am J Physiol*. 1996;271 (2 part 1):E209-E214.

79. Friedman JM, Halaas JL. Leptin and the regulation of body weight in mammals. *Nature*. 1998;395(6704):763-770.

80. Pico C, Oliver P, Sanchez J, et al. Gastric leptin: a putative role in the short-term regulation of food intake. *Br J Nutr*. 2003;90(4):735-741.

81. Chapelot D, Aubert R, Marmonier C, et al. An endocrine and metabolic definition of the intermeal interval in humans: evidence for a role of leptin on the prandial pattern through fatty acid disposal. *Am J Clin Nutr.* 2000; 72(2):421-431.

82. Chin-Chance C, Polonsky KS, Schoeller DA. Twenty-four-hour leptin levels respond to cumulative short-term energy imbalance and predict subsequent intake. *J Clin Endocrinol Metab.* 2000;85(8):2685-2691.

83. Tomiyama AJ, Schamarek I, Lustig RH, et al. Leptin concentrations in response to acute stress predict subsequent intake of comfort foods. *Physiol Behav.* 2012; 107(1):34-39.

84. Chin-Chance C, Polonsky KS, Schoeller DA. Twenty-four-hour leptin levels respond to cumulative short-term energy imbalance and predict subsequent intake. *J Clin Endocrinol Metab.* 2000;85(8): 2685-2691.

85. Tataranni PA, Gautier JF, Chen KW, et al. Neuroanatomical correlates of hunger and satiation in humans using positron emission tomography. *Proc Natl Acad Sci U S A.* 1999;96(8):4569-4574.

86. Fuehrer D, Zysset S, Stumvoll M. Brain activity in hunger and satiety: an exploratory visually stimulated fMRI study. *Obesity.* 2008;16(5):945-950.

87. Geliebter A, Westreich S, Gage D. Gastric distention by balloon and test-meal intake in obese and lean subjects. *Am J Clin Nutr.* 1988;48(3):592-594.

88. Cecil JE, Francis J, Read NW. Comparison of the effects of a high-fat and high-carbohydrate soup delivered orally and intragastrically on gastric emptying, appetite, and eating behaviour. *Physiol Behav.* 1999;67(2):299-306.

89. Rolls BJ, Bell EA, Thorwart ML. Water incorporated into a food but not served with a food decreases energy intake in lean women. *Am J Clin Nutr.* 1999;70(4):448-455.

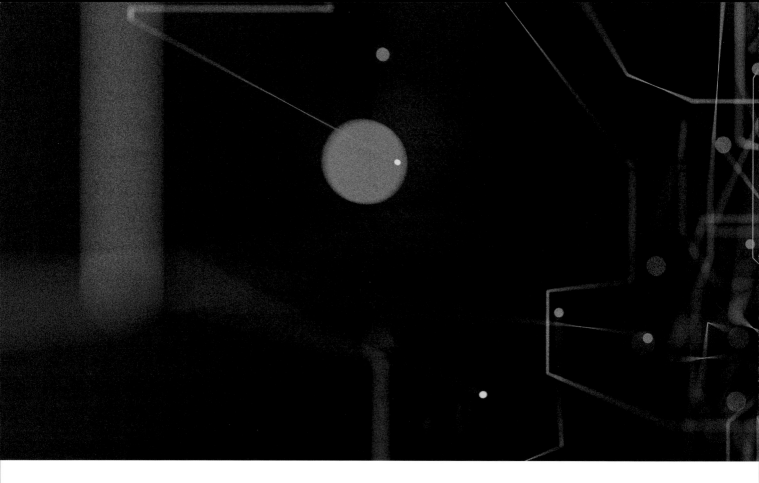

Key Aspects of Research in Food, Nutrition, and Dietetics

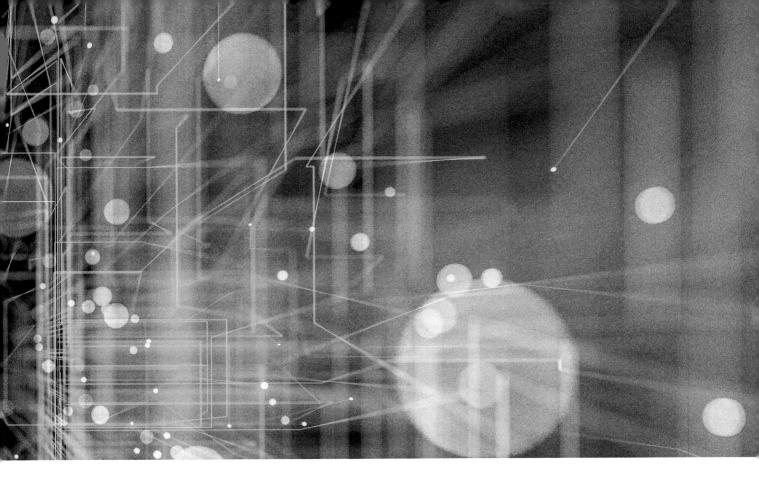

Outcomes Research and Economic Analysis

William Murphy, MS, RDN | *Rosa K. Hand,* PhD, RDN, LD, FAND

LEARNING OBJECTIVES

1. Describe the purpose and methodology of outcomes research and economic analysis.

2. Differentiate the three types of outcomes used in health care outcomes research.

3. Describe the various analytic methods used in economic analyses of nutrition research studies.

4. Evaluate practice applications of outcomes research studies and economic analyses.

In 1999, the results of a clinical trial were published that would change the landscape for congestive heart failure treatment. Results from the Randomized Aldactone Evaluation Study, commonly known as RALES, described an experiment cut short due to outstanding results and a simple change in medication regimen that could reduce complications and extend lives. After 36 months of treatment with either spironolactone or placebo, the midpoint safety review found a 35% reduction in readmissions and a 30% reduction in the death rate for the group taking the active medication.[1] Within 2 years, inclusion of spironolactone in the pharmacotherapy of patients with heart failure had risen dramatically. One analysis of data from the Ontario Drug Benefit program found a fivefold increase over the 2 years following publication of the RALES findings,[2] and the recommendation was added to evidence-based practice guidelines from the American College of Cardiology and American Heart Association in 2005.[3]

Without outcomes research, this would have been the end of a success story about disseminating and implementing research breakthroughs. However, the ultimate concern of health care providers is not the perfect implementation of research findings but the health of their patients. Juurlink and colleagues,[2] the outcomes researchers who measured the increase in spironolactone prescriptions for heart failure in Ontario, also evaluated the impact on readmissions and mortality. They found no evidence of improvements in progress on readmissions or mortality for patients with heart failure; instead, both continued to decline at rates consistent with the preceding years. They did, however, find some stark differences: increases in hospitalization for and death from hyperkalemia, one of the medication's side effects. This extraordinary example highlights the importance of outcomes research in health care and will serve as a point of reference for many concepts discussed in this chapter.

Policy makers are interested in the impact of health care, including discrete interventions as well as broader programmatic or systemic interventions, on the health outcomes of patients and populations.[4] Health care reform is changing incentives and payment models to emphasize quality and value over quantity.[5] Outcomes research serves multiple purposes: evaluating the impacts of current evidence-based practice in order to feed the findings back into the cycle of research that informs recommendations and drives practice (see Figure 18.1); contributing to the body of evidence to shape health care policy, including reimbursement; and ultimately, improving health outcomes across populations/communities. At this level, greater weight is given to the external validity and generalizability of findings so that they can be applicable across settings and population groups.

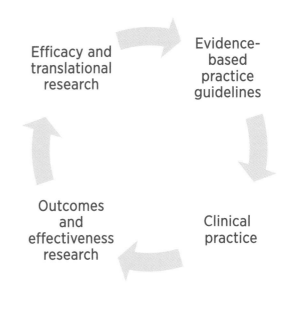

Figure 18.1 An evidence-based practice research cycle including outcomes research

OUTCOMES RESEARCH
Outcomes and Effectiveness Research

Outcomes research is "the study of the end results of health services that takes patients' experiences, preferences, and values into account."[6] This type of research, also known as *effectiveness research*, focuses on the health outcomes patients' experience as the result of health care. This is in contrast to clinical efficacy research, such as RALES from the example, which focuses on measuring the effect of interventions under ideal conditions.[7]

A range of outcomes is considered in outcomes and effectiveness research. The key outcomes of interest differ depending on who is using the information (registered dietitian nutritionists [RDNs], other health care providers, health care administrators, payers/buyers, policy makers, or patients). Carefully selected evaluation and research methods are used to determine whether the procedure or care process leads to the desired results.[8] An aim of outcomes and effectiveness research is to determine what approaches work best for most patients or clients in routine settings and at what cost. Because the goals differ from those of efficacy research, effectiveness research requires a different set of tools beyond the standard randomized controlled trial, as RALES exemplified when the findings from practice differed greatly from the clinical trial findings. Costs can also be investigated in outcomes studies— both the cost of delivering specific interventions and the costs associated with the resulting consequences, such as health care resources saved by positive health outcomes. This cost concern closely links outcomes and effectiveness research to cost-effectiveness analysis (CEA). Methods of economic analysis (discussed later in this chapter) examine effectiveness and costs to determine the cost-effectiveness of competing interventions.

The findings from outcomes research inform decisions about implementing, expanding, or changing care processes. The findings are also used, along with findings from other research approaches, to develop evidence-based protocols, clinical practice guidelines, and clinical pathway or care maps that foster the use of the most effective and cost-effective practices across the system.[9-11] Outcomes research also aids planning and decision making by providing data on which to base predictions of future clinical, cost, and patient outcomes if specific interventions, procedures, or treatments are adopted.

Types of Outcomes

Three outcome categories are traditionally assessed in health care outcomes research: health outcomes, intermediate outcomes, and cost outcomes (see Box 18.1 for examples). Health outcomes are the ultimate concern of outcomes research. However, the direct effects of nutrition care are intermediate outcomes

and help explain how nutrition care contributes to health outcomes.

Within and crossing over the types of outcomes, two notable classifications are patient-centered outcomes and surrogate outcomes, which are discussed in the sections that follow.

Patient-Centered Outcomes

Patient-centered outcomes gained notoriety when the Patient Protection and Affordable Care Act of 2010 created the Patient-Centered Outcomes Research Institute. The institute's report on standards for patient-centered outcomes research states that study designs should "identify and include outcomes the population of interest notices and cares about (eg, survival, function, symptoms, health-related quality of life) and that inform an identified health decision."[12] These outcomes of interest to patients often include health outcomes but may also include such factors as quality of life, symptom relief, adverse effects, and satisfaction with care. Notably, methodology standards require that patients or patient advocacy groups be engaged in the research design process to identify the relevant patient-centered outcomes. Research has shown that nutritional status is related to patients' functional status, including psychological and cognitive performance, psychosocial status, and activities of daily living.[13,14]

Assessment of patients' perceptions of nutrition care services and the effect of nutrition on quality of life are relatively new areas in nutrition research and outcomes assessment.[15] An early study identified a range of health and nonhealth benefits that patients gained from nutrition counseling, including reassurance, sense of control, and relief of symptoms.[16]

Type of Outcome	Examples
Health outcome	Morbidity, mortality, disease incidence, hospitalization
Intermediate outcome	Weight, low-density lipoprotein cholesterol, motivation, dietary intake
Cost outcome	Billed charges, cost of care

Box 18.1 Outcomes Examples by Type

Other studies have shown a link between nutrition-related biochemical parameters and patients' quality of life.[17]

Surrogate Outcomes

Surrogate outcomes are the near antithesis of patient-centered outcomes. When an intermediate outcome is used as the primary outcome of a study with the assumption that changes in the intermediate correspond to changes in health outcomes, the intermediate is said to be a surrogate outcome or surrogate end point. A well-known example of surrogacy is the use of low-density lipoprotein cholesterol (LDL-C) to infer the impact of medication and dietary interventions on risk for heart disease. Surrogate outcomes can be appealing to researchers because they allow for studies on chronic disease to be conducted over shorter periods of time and at less expense, but they also create a risk that the health outcomes patients experience will not follow the trend suggested by the surrogate. In 2008, the US Food and Drug Administration (FDA), faced with an influx of applications for food label health claims based on surrogate outcomes, commissioned a report from the Institute of Medicine on how to evaluate proposed surrogates. The resulting report, *Evaluation of Biomarkers and Surrogate Endpoints in Chronic Disease*,[18] describes a three-step evaluation process (see Figure 18.2) for intermediate outcomes to validate their use as surrogates, and the report authors recommended that the FDA adopt this process not just for food labels but also for all regulatory areas, including pharmaceuticals.

The analytic validation step requires that evidence be available to demonstrate that the methods used to measure the surrogate are reliable and consistent among different sites. The qualification step requires evidence that the surrogate is associated with disease states and that interventions designed to impact the surrogate also impact health outcomes. The utilization step requires an evaluation of the proposed use of the surrogate to ensure that relevant qualification evidence is available for the same intervention context. Finally, the process is represented as a cycle of cycles, indicating that each step is continually reevaluated as new evidence emerges.

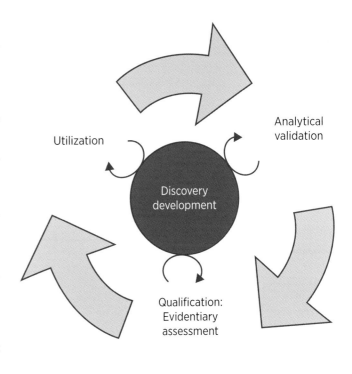

Figure 18.2 Validation process for surrogate outcome

Adapted with permission from Institute of Medicine Committee on Qualification of Biomarkers and Surrogate Endpoints in Chronic Disease, Board on Health Care Services, Board on Health Sciences Policy, Food and Nutrition Board. Michael CM, Ball JR, eds. *Evaluation of Biomarkers and Surrogate Endpoints in Chronic Disease*. Washington, DC: National Academies Press; 2010.[18]

The report also included several case study examples in which the proposed framework was applied to the body of evidence for surrogate end points being used in contemporary research, and in several cases, the report concluded that surrogates were being used in research without sufficient validation. Table 18.1 on page 354 presents selected cases relevant to nutrition. The LDL-C case highlights the importance of the utilization step, as there was ample qualification evidence to support LDL-C as a surrogate for statin medications, but the authors found inconsistent and contradictory evidence for the qualification of LDL-C in the contexts of other medications, diet, and lifestyle interventions. In one case, a pharmaceutical intervention that successfully decreased LDL-C and increased high-density lipoprotein cholesterol (HDL-C) led to poorer outcomes: increased rates of cardiovascular disease events and mortality.[19] Because of this study and others demonstrating that the relationship between

Biomarker	Analytic Validity	Qualification	Utilization: Possible Uses	Utilization: Surrogate End Point Use
C-reactive protein (CRP)	High-sensitivity tests available	Randomized controlled trials (RCTs) and observational studies available; limited data on CRP's biological role in disease progression	Risk prediction; potential expansion of statin treatment to specific populations	Current data do not support use as a surrogate end point.
Low-density lipoprotein cholesterol (LDL-C)	Validated tests are available for many uses. More accurate tests are also being developed.	Extensive data on LDL-C, both RCTs and observational studies; repeated use of LDL-C as a surrogate end point	Risk prediction	Data support use of LDL-C as a surrogate end point for some cardiovascular outcomes for statin drug interventions, but not for all cardiovascular outcomes or other cardiovascular interventions, foods, or supplements.
High-density lipoprotein cholesterol (HDL-C)	Validated tests are available for many uses. More accurate tests are also being developed.	Limited data; the biological role of HDL-C not fully understood	Risk prediction	Current data do not support use as a surrogate end point.
Beta-carotene	Validated measures of blood serum beta-carotene levels are available for many uses.	Extensive RCTs and observational trials available	Uses include a biomarker of intake of fruits and vegetables and an effective intervention to address vitamin A deficiency	Current data do not support use as a surrogate end point.

Table 18.1 Assessing Nutrition-Related Surrogate Outcomes

Adapted with permission from Institute of Medicine Committee on Qualification of Biomarkers and Surrogate Endpoints in Chronic Disease, Board on Health Care Services, Board on Health Sciences Policy, Food and Nutrition Board. Michael CM, Ball JR, eds. *Evaluation of Biomarkers and Surrogate Endpoints in Chronic Disease.* Washington, DC: National Academies Press; 2010.[18]

lipoprotein profiles and health outcomes is not absolute and the lack of qualifying evidence in other contexts, the report authors concluded that LDL-C and HDL-C were not valid as surrogate outcomes in studies involving diet and lifestyle changes. Since the publication of this report, interest in additional lipoprotein profile assays, such as LDL-C/HDL-C particle size and count, has grown,[20] yet these, too, cannot be accepted as surrogate outcomes without sufficient validation.

Figure 18.3 illustrates several scenarios in which interventions that target surrogate outcomes can fail to produce the desired health outcomes. As the chronic diseases treated by RDNs are multifactorial and dietary modifications cannot be made in isolation, it is likely that nutrition care can affect the disease process, surrogates, and outcomes independently, leading to the failure in scenarios of Figure 18.3. Figures 18.4 and 18.5 on page 356 describe a chain of consequences from nutrition care through intermediate outcomes to health outcomes. While these represent potential or ideal sequences of outcomes, the evidence for the three steps of the surrogate outcome validation process should be reviewed if the ultimate health outcomes will not be assessed in the study.

Cost Outcomes

The financial implications of a specific intervention or procedure are considered cost outcomes. Cost outcomes are derived from documented health care utilization, which can include diagnostic and treatment costs, outpatient visits, hospitalization, and medical equipment. Some outcomes studies also include the financial costs of the disease treatment (eg, cost of lost work time caused by a treatment). Cost

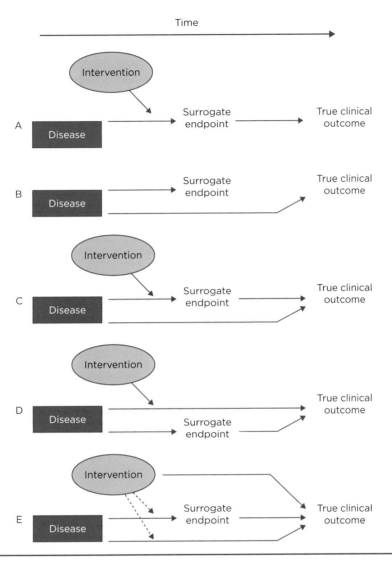

Figure 18.3 Relationships among diseases, outcomes, interventions, and valid and invalid surrogate end points

(A) A valid surrogate exists as a part of the sole causal pathway of the disease. (B) An invalid surrogate that is mediated by the disease but unrelated to health outcomes. (C) An invalid surrogate that exists on only one of multiple causal pathways of the disease. (D) An invalid surrogate that exists on a separate causal pathway from the intervention under investigation. (E) An invalid surrogate that exists on only one of the pathways of a pleiotropic intervention.[21]

Adapted with permission from Institute of Medicine Committee on Qualification of Biomarkers and Surrogate Endpoints in Chronic Disease, Board on Health Care Services, Board on Health Sciences Policy, Food and Nutrition Board. Michael CM, Ball JR, eds. *Evaluation of Biomarkers and Surrogate Endpoints in Chronic Disease.* Washington, DC: National Academies Press; 2010.[18]

outcomes can include the input cost to provide the intervention or procedure (eg, cost of enteral nutrition support) and the cost associated with the consequences of the outcomes produced—which may be positive or negative. Costs of inputs and outcomes are included in cost-effectiveness (discussed later). Cost outcomes are of major importance to health care administrators and policy makers.

METHODS USED IN OUTCOMES RESEARCH

Internal and External Validity

The concept of internal validity is a measure of how well the results of a study reflect what actually occurred in the study. Efficacy research focuses on

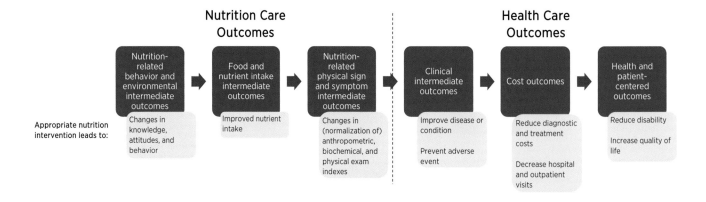

Figure 18.4 Chain of outcomes of nutrition care

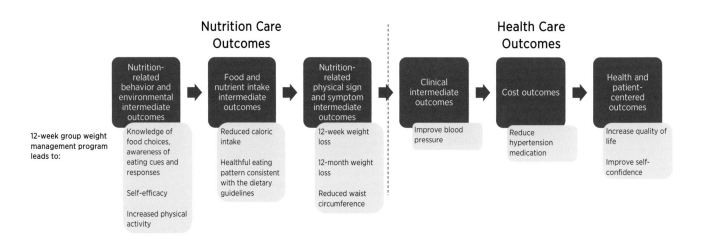

Figure 18.5 Chain of outcomes resulting from weight management program (12-month period)

maximizing internal validity by minimizing potential sources of bias. In RALES, half of the patients were given a placebo instead of an active drug to create a control group for comparison, and patients were randomly selected into these two groups to reduce the chance of underlying differences between the groups impacting the findings (selection bias). These two procedures are often considered the minimum for clinical research, the randomized controlled trial. However, there are more sources of bias and strategies to minimize them, as discussed in Chapter 10. Another common step is to limit participation in the study (inclusion and exclusion criteria) to those most likely to benefit from

the intervention and least likely to experience adverse side-effects. In RALES, one such criterion was that patients with signs of reduced renal function were excluded from participation because of the known spironolactone side effect of potassium retention.

External validity, also known as *generalizability*, is the concept of how well the results of a study can be applied to other settings and is the focus of outcomes, or effectiveness, research. The contrast between effectiveness research findings and efficacy research findings (see Box 18.2) suggests that the RALES findings lacked external validity. Indeed, additional follow-up research from Masoudi and col-

	Efficacy Study	**Effectiveness Study**
Question	Does the intervention work under ideal circumstance?	Does the intervention work in real-world practice?
Setting	Resource-intensive ideal setting	Real-world everyday clinical setting
Study population	Highly selected, homogeneous population; Several exclusion criteria	Heterogeneous population Few to no exclusion criteria
Providers	Highly experienced and trained	Representative of usual providers
Intervention	Strictly enforced and standardized	Applied with flexibility
	No concurrent interventions	Concurrent interventions and crossover permitted

Box 18.2 Comparison of Efficacy vs Effectiveness Research[7]

leagues[22] compared the inclusion and exclusion criteria from RALES to the heart failure patient population served by Medicare and found that only 25% of patients would have qualified for the study. By designing the study to maximize internal validity, the RALES investigators inadvertently reduced its external validity by studying patients that were not representative of the heart failure patient population. These nuances can be lost in the process of dissemination and implementation and can lead to undesirable patient health outcomes. While internal and external validity are not conceptually exclusive, they effectively exist at opposite ends of a spectrum for study design (see Figure 18.6), as efforts to maximize one will often minimize the other. Two common designs for outcomes research, pragmatic trials and surveillance research, are discussed in the sections that follow.

Pragmatic Trials

Pragmatic trials, the primary tool for comparative effectiveness research, are designed to maintain internal validity while making concessions to improve external validity.[23] These studies generally still use randomization to reduce selection bias, although they may randomize at the level of the provider or facility to limit performance bias. The latter is common in nutrition care research wherein providers cannot practicably be blind to the type of nutrition intervention they provide to participants. Control groups are generally provided standard of care (ie, they are cared for as they would be if they were not involved in a research study). The Pragmatic–Explanatory Continuum Indicator Summary 2 (PRECIS-2) instrument is available for rating the pragmatism of a study on nine dimensions: eligibility,

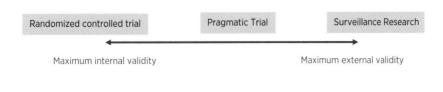

Figure 18.6 Spectrum of internal and external validity by study design

Dimension	Defining Question[a]
Eligibility	To what extent are the participants in the trial similar to those who would receive this intervention if it were part of usual care?
Recruitment	How much extra effort to engage with patients is made to recruit participants over and above what would be used in the usual care setting?
Setting	How different are the settings of the trial from the usual care setting?
Organization	How are the resources, provider expertise, and organization of care delivery in the intervention arm of the trial different from those available in usual care?
Flexibility in delivery	How is the flexibility in how the intervention is delivered different from the flexibility anticipated in usual care?
Flexibility in adherence	How is the flexibility in how participants are monitored and encouraged to adhere to the intervention different from the flexibility anticipated in usual care?
Follow-up	How is the intensity of participant measurement and follow-up in the trial different from the typical follow-up in usual care?
Primary outcome	To what extent is the trial's primary outcome directly relevant to participants?
Primary analysis	To what extent are all data included in the analysis of the primary outcome?

[a] For all questions, answers in the direction of a greater extent indicate more explanatory and less pragmatic study design.

Box 18.3 The Nine Dimensions of the Pragmatic–Explanatory Continuum Indicator Summary 2 (PRECIS-2) Instrument and the Defining Questions for Each[24]

recruitment, setting, organization, flexibility in delivery, flexibility in adherence, follow-up, primary outcome, and primary analysis (defined in Box 18.3).[24] In each of these areas, a more pragmatic trial sacrifices some control for more realistic conditions.

Surveillance Research

Surveillance research, on the other hand, is designed to maximize external validity. This research is conducted by making few alterations to the provision of care other than the collection of data. The outcomes study[2] that followed the consequences of RALES is an example of surveillance research. That design, using available population-level data, is often described as ecological research. Another well-known type of surveillance data collection is the outcomes registry, wherein health care providers submit anonymous data describing patient cases, care provided, and outcomes. Prospective registry studies can provide richer data than retrospective or ecological studies because the data collection protocols are specified in advance. When adequate protections are in place to prevent users from linking data to the identities of patients, research conducted on registry data is not considered to involve human participants and therefore does not necessitate the protections for human participants overseen by an ethical review board.[25] These factors make registry studies an appealing option for outcomes research, and the surveillance data provides the most accurate description of health care practices and patient outcomes. This design is not without caveats, however.

When attempting to compare different treatment options, surveillance data are likely to have selection bias; patient characteristics play a role in determining how the treatments are decided and eventual health outcomes. Consider an analysis of nutrition support utilization in hospitals. In a simplistic analysis, one may find that patients who receive enteral or parenteral nutrition support experience poorer health outcomes. The reality is not that the nutrition support causes poor outcomes but that the patients who receive nutrition support tend to have more significant diseases and poorer prognoses. While randomization is used to control this selection bias by balancing confounding factors in pragmatic trials, surveillance research needs to rely on alternative strategies to manage this source of bias.

Propensity Scoring

Propensity scoring and adjustment refer to the process of identifying which factors determine the likelihood that patients will receive one treatment over another, that is, their propensity to receive a treatment, and accounting for those differences via statistical methods when assessing outcomes.[26-29] When the correct covariates are used in the propensity adjustment, the resulting sample is balanced and is no longer mathematically different from a randomly selected sample as in a clinical trial. A simpler adjustment technique is propensity matching, which finds pairs of patients similar in all factors except for the treatment received; this technique has the advantage of producing a data set of control and experimental groups that is equivalent to that of an interventional study and that can be used with basic statistical analysis. However, the disadvantage of matching is that patients who do not have an adequate match are excluded from the resulting data set, so sample size is reduced. An alternative technique is propensity regression, which controls for the measure of propensity in the model that is used to assess the outcome. This method is better able to take advantage of the full set of available data, but it requires more advanced statistical techniques, such as mixed-effects linear modeling or generalized additive models to accurately partition the variance contributed by propensity.

Study Implementation

In outcomes and effectiveness research, as in any research effort, the design and methods selected must match the research question, the planned application of the findings, and the resources available to conduct the study while minimizing threats to validity. These issues are addressed throughout this book, but the steps for outcomes and effectiveness research are outlined in Box 18.4 on page 360.

Results of Outcomes Research

The key result of an outcomes study should be a quantitative estimate of (1) the magnitude of effect in outcome associated with, or attributed to, the studied intervention or interventions; and (2) the proportion of patients, clients, or population that benefits from access to, and participation in, the intervention. While statistical significance helps the researcher judge whether the study results are likely to occur by chance in the absence of a true difference between the standard intervention and comparison, it is also important to report clinical significance, or whether the magnitude of the difference is large enough to make a meaningful difference in patients' health and well-being. Other results that can be presented in quantitative or qualitative terms are variation in the provision of the intervention, costs, client characteristics associated with positive or negative outcomes (such as risk level used in case-mix analysis), other important outcomes, and intervening or confounding factors. Case mix describes the relative complexity of the health care needed by a group of patients. It is a vital factor when comparing outcomes between facilities or providers, as they may not be drawing from equivalent patient populations. Results can then be used to guide resource allocation to the most effective interventions.

The Nutrition Care Process and Outcomes Research

The Nutrition Care Process and use of standardized nutrition language support outcomes research.[30-33] Adopting the Nutrition Care Process leads to the

Phase	Steps
Question Definition	Define the research question using the PICOTS (population, intervention, comparison, outcome, time, setting) method:
	Define the patient population.
	Identify the current standard-of-care intervention, procedure, or program to be evaluated.
	Identify and describe alternative intervention(s) for comparison.
	Specify the key outcome and evaluate its validity if choosing a surrogate.
	Determine the appropriate time period for the intervention effects and outcome to manifest.
	Specify the setting of care to be studied, and evaluate evidence for surrogate validity in this setting, if applicable.
Study Design	Select the appropriate study type:
	Use pragmatic trials to establish the effectiveness of new interventions.
	Use surveillance research to evaluate the effectiveness of existing practices.
	Design the study and specify procedures for data collection:
	Determine the sample size and method of sampling.
	Establish points to measure outcomes and other indicators, considering the period of time necessary for the effect to occur.
	Define all data elements to be included, considering intervention details, patient or client characteristics, key and other outcomes, and intervening and confounding factors, and, for surveillance research, factors that determine the propensity for receiving the intervention treatments.
	Develop and pilot test forms and procedures for data collection.
	Determine data analysis methods.
Execution	Collect data according to procedures:
	Train practitioners on study procedures.
	Have practitioners record data.
	Monitor quality and completeness of data.
	Analyze the data:
	Assess the clinical importance of the data.
	Assess the statistical significance of the data.
	Interpret and report the results.
	Act on the findings.

Box 18.4 Outcomes and Effectiveness Research: Planning and Conducting a Study

documentation of pertinent information using uniform terminology. This includes relevant assessment indicators, a specific nutrition diagnosis with etiology and signs and symptoms, an explicit intervention approach, and results of the intervention measured at specific follow-up points using standard terminology for outcomes and indicators. Consistent documentation, including more relevant information about the nutrition care situation, enables study of the effectiveness of nutrition intervention alternatives used in varying circumstances and can lead to greater understanding of the results and value of dietetics services.

Using the nutrition care process and terminology in research design also has the advantage of facilitating collaboration with RDNs throughout the United States and in several other countries. The Academy of Nutrition and Dietetics Nutrition Research Network (NRN; formerly the Dietetics Practice Based Research Network)[34] helps to connect RDNs in practice with outcomes researchers, and the Academy of Nutrition and Dietetics Health Informatics Infrastructure, also known as ANDHII,[35] provides a web-based data collection and management tool that simplifies the process of multisite data aggregation.

Nutrition Informatics and Outcomes Research

In the United States, certain providers and hospitals are required to record and submit electronic clinical quality measures data. This, combined with mandated uses of coding standards and other data quality improvements in electronic health records,[36] presents growing opportunities to collect surveillance research data. Care must be taken when using quality data for research purposes, as the original intent of the data collection governs the rigor with which it is collected. Electronic clinical quality measure outcomes, for example, are not required to be substantiated as valid surrogate outcomes according to the Institute of Medicine standard, so the researcher would need to verify the status of any surrogate outcomes collected from quality measures.

ECONOMIC ANALYSIS

Economic analysis examines outcomes in relation to costs; that is, the value, or efficiency of care[37]:

$$Value = \frac{Outcomes}{Cost}$$

Methods of economic analysis are used to identify the most efficient intervention, that is, the one that achieves more of the desired outcomes for the lowest or most reasonable investment of resources. Lower costs are not inherently better; they are only better when an equivalent outcome is achieved, leading to a higher value.[37] Economic analysis requires a systematic process of defining, measuring, and valuing the costs and outcomes of two or more competing alternatives for accomplishing something.[38] The six steps of economic analysis, discussed later in the chapter, are based on a synthesis of the principles and current recommendations for economic analysis.[38-40]

Opportunity cost is a concept integral to economic analysis. As nutrition interventions or programs (or other health interventions) are implemented and produce outcomes, they consume resources. The consumed resources are then unavailable for another purpose. Opportunity cost is the value that would have been gained if the resource had been used for the next best alternative. This competition for scarce resources is the foundation of economic analysis.[41]

Economic Analysis in Nutrition

Before 1979, economic evaluation was rare in the nutrition literature. At that time, the American Dietetic Association (now the Academy of Nutrition and Dietetics) proposed a model for estimating the economic benefits of nutrition.[42]

Since that time, literature supporting the cost-effectiveness of nutrition interventions and RDN services has expanded. In 2009, the Evidence Analysis Library conducted a systematic review to answer questions related to the cost-effectiveness of medical nutrition therapy (MNT). The conclusion statements for these three questions are summa-

Question	Studies Included in Review	Conclusion	Conclusion Grade
What is the evidence to support the cost-effectiveness, cost benefit, or economic savings of inpatient medical nutrition therapy (MNT) services provided by a registered dietitian nutritionist (RDN)?	5	Five studies were reviewed to evaluate the cost-effectiveness, cost benefit, and/or economic savings of inpatient MNT services provided by an RDN, involving individualized nutrition assessment and a duration and frequency of care using the Nutrition Care Process. Three studies reported that nutrition screening, early assessment, and treatment by an RDN, leading to early discharge results in cost savings due to reduced length of hospital stay. Two studies demonstrated that appropriate parenteral nutrition use, based on recommendations from a nutrition support team including an RDN, results in cost savings. Further research is needed on the cost-effectiveness, cost benefit, and/or economic savings of inpatient MNT.	II (Fair)
What is the evidence to support the cost-effectiveness, cost benefit, or economic savings of lifestyle interventions for diabetes prevention?	6	Compared with pharmacotherapy or no intervention, lifestyle interventions for diabetes prevention were cost-effective in terms of cost per quality-adjusted life years gained based on six cost-effectiveness analyses.	I (Good)
What is the evidence to support the cost-effectiveness, cost benefit, or economic savings of outpatient MNT services provided by an RDN?	10	Ten studies were reviewed to evaluate the cost-effectiveness, cost benefit, and economic savings of outpatient MNT involving in-depth individualized nutrition assessment and a duration and frequency of care using the Nutrition Care Process to manage disease. Using a variety of cost-effectiveness analyses, the studies affirm that MNT resulted in improved clinical outcomes and reduced costs related to physician time, medication use, and/or hospital	I (Good)

Box 18.5 Academy of Nutrition and Dietetics Evidence Analysis Library Conclusion Statements Related to the Cost-Effectiveness of Medical Nutrition Therapy[43] *(continued)*

admissions for individuals with obesity, diabetes, disorders of lipid metabolism, and other chronic diseases. Further research is needed on the cost-effectiveness, cost benefit, and economic savings of outpatient MNT in other disease states.

Box 18.5 (cont.) Academy of Nutrition and Dietetics Evidence Analysis Library Conclusion Statements Related to the Cost-Effectiveness of Medical Nutrition Therapy[43]

rized in Box 18.5, but they generally indicate that MNT is cost-effective in outpatient settings and needs more research in inpatient settings.[43]

Since the Evidence Analysis Library review, other important studies that evaluate the cost-effectiveness of nutrition care include a study of North Carolina Blue Cross Blue Shield beneficiaries, which showed that MNT provided by an RDN for patients who are overweight improved health outcomes at a cost of $0.03 per insured member per month.[44] Dietitians in New Zealand also conducted a review of dietitian cost-effectiveness in primary care and identified that a savings between $NZ5.50 and $NZ99 would be achieved for every $NZ1 spent on dietitian care.[45] Philipson and colleagues[46] estimated the cost savings from oral nutrition supplements provided to malnourished adults to be $4,734 per hospitalization. And Lakdawalla and colleagues[47] used similar methodology to estimate the savings for supplements for children with malnutrition as $1,768 per hospitalization.

Economic evaluation in health care has evolved, and although the US Public Health Service convened an expert panel in the 1990s to review the theory and practice of CEA and make recommendations for standardizing CEA methodology in health and medicine,[38] variations in the use of CEA methodology and barriers to consistent use of CEA findings in decision making persist.[48]

Challenges to the consistency of CEA include the major variance in cost between facilities, even within the same region,[49] and the methodology's reliance on assumptions and hypothetical situations about which the public has inconsistent views.[50] A quick exploration of Memorial Sloan Kettering's Drug Pricing Lab website (www.drugabacus.org), which deals with costs for cancer drugs, demonstrates the many assumptions and hypotheticals required to estimate the value of a particular type of care: the discount (ie, decrease in acceptable price) based on side effects; premium (ie, increase in acceptable price) based on novelty of action and cost of development; rarity, frequency, or aggressiveness of disease; and unmet need, along with the dollar value for a year of life. Acceptable dollar values per year of life are established through hypothetical questions about how much an individual would pay to achieve a state of perfect health, which is a difficult scenario to envision and varies based on the respondent's own health status and that of their close family.[50,51] In the United States, CEA is further complicated by variance in costs and charges based on payer as well as a cultural distaste for discussing the cost of care because of the false perception that discussing costs is equivalent to discussing health care rationing.[50] Although private insurers consider cost in their coverage decisions, Congress has mandated that Medicare cannot take cost into account.[52] Other countries with single-payer health care systems have adopted CEA for decision-making to a greater extent,[50] and therefore, much of the CEA data comes from Europe and Australia. While no longer adding articles to its database, the University of York Centre for Reviews and Dissemination maintains a searchable archive of CEA articles through 2014 (www.crd.york.ac.uk/CRDWeb/AboutPage.asp).

Analytic Methods Used in Economic Analysis

Several analytic methods are used in economic analysis, including cost minimization analysis, CEA, cost-benefit analysis (CBA), cost-utility analysis,[41] and clinical decision analysis. The objectives of the investigation determine which analytic method is appropriate. Table 18.2 compares the methods and gives examples of their application in clinical dietetics.

Cost minimization analysis and CEA are used to determine the lower-cost way to achieve a specified outcome. In cost minimization analysis, the outcomes of nutrition alternatives are assumed to be equal, and only costs are measured. In CEA, the magnitude of outcome produced by each alternative is measured, along with the cost to produce the out-

Method	Focus	Application Example	Outcomes	Costs	Ways to Report
Cost minimization analysis	Identifies the lowest-cost way to do something	Should a registered dietitian nutritionist; nutrition and dietetics technician, registered; or registered nurse do nutrition assessment at hospital admission?	No data; assumes outcomes are equal	Cost analysis and comparison using cost of inputs	Costs of inputs for each alternative (dollar per activity, day, patient, or course of treatment)
Cost-effectiveness analysis	Compares the efficiency of two or more alternatives for a specified outcome	Should a special oral supplement be recommended for patients with HIV/AIDS?	Biochemical, clinical, or quality-of-life measures for each alternative	Cost of each alternative or net cost (cost of inputs + cost of consequences)	Amount of successful outcome per dollar investment, net cost per unit of outcome, dollar per unit of improvement, or per covered beneficiary
Cost-benefit analysis	Assigns dollar value to resource inputs and health outcomes; may compare alternatives with different goals	Is it cost-beneficial to initiate nutrition intervention to prevent pressure ulcers?	Dollar value assigned to outcomes	Cost of inputs over complete course of intervention	Net consumption of resources, ratio of dollar of outcomes to dollar of inputs (benefit-cost analysis), or dollar of input to dollar of outcome (cost-benefit analysis)
Cost-utility analysis	Relates cost to quality-of-life differences; other preference or satisfaction measures can also be used	Is nutrition support via enteral feeding or total parenteral nutrition worth quality-adusted life years for patients with a terminal illness?	Weeks or months of life extended and patients' perceptions of quality of life with or without intervention	Net cost for each alternative (input cost + cost of complications, cost of medical care for extended life, and any medical cost savings)	Net cost per quality-adusted life year; dollar per quality-adusted life year
Clinical decision analysis	Uses estimates from published studies or expert opinion to construct probability of events (diagnosis, treatment response, complication rate, survival)	What outcomes can be expected if elemental vs nonelemental enteral formula is used for surgical patients with hypoalbuminemia?	Intermediate and clinical outcomes	Probability estimates used to develop predictions of input costs and medical cost savings and cost of complications for each decision alternative	Decision tree with outcome probabilities and net cost estimates

Table 18.2 Analytic Methods Used in Economic Analysis

come. A ratio of cost per unit of effect (outcome) is calculated for each alternative and compared to determine which alternative is more cost-effective.[41]

CBA considers the monetary (dollar) value of both inputs and outcomes. In a cost-benefit ratio, the dollar value of input costs is related to the dollar value of outcomes (positive and negative) produced. Cost-utility analysis relates costs to the patient's years of life. However, acknowledging that a sick year is not the same as a healthy year, quality-adjusted life year (QALY) is the common unit of measure used in cost-utility analysis (see Box 18.6).[38,39] Results of cost-utility analysis are expressed as cost per QALY. Because of the standardized units, CBA and cost-utility analysis can be used to compare the efficiency of activities in different areas.[41] Thus, they can be used to inform policy and resource allocation decisions across different areas of health care or different sectors of the economy (eg, health care vs education and training) or to compare many different preventive health interventions.[53] Clinical decision analysis uses estimates of outcome probabilities and net cost to evaluate intervention alternatives.[38-40] Economic analysis is used to inform policy decision, either at a national level or at the level of a single insurance provider. It can be ex ante analysis conducted before the adoption of policy on the basis of results of pilot studies, research, or theoretical assumptions. For example, Phillips and Doley[54] report on an ex ante analysis of the anticipated cost savings from granting RDNs order-writing privileges. Economic analysis can also be conducted after policy implementation using data from actual outcomes. This ex post analysis determines the true cost-benefit of the policy in real-world conditions. The North Carolina Blue Cross Blue Shield study is an example of an ex post analysis.[44] Before and after cost-effectiveness or cost-benefit estimates can be quite different.

Various tools have been developed to assign a quality-of-life or well-being score (a number ranging from 0.0 [death] to 1.0 [optimal health]) to an individual's functioning. Numerous disease-specific quality-of-life measures have also been developed.[41]

Quality-adjusted life year (QALY) is a universal measure of health status that is expressed as the length of healthy life. It assumes that the goal is to extend the state of good health as long as possible and minimize periods of ill health or disability.

QALY takes two things into account: length of life and quality of life or state of health during various periods of time.

Length of life

- Based on actual survival data in study, or
- From a life table of the population
  - Life tables specify the proportion of the population of individuals living and dying at each age interval.

Quality of life or state of health (well-being) during various periods of time

- Measures of well-being include the following:
  - mental, physical, and social functioning (eg, social functioning includes an individual's limitations in performing usual social roles of work, school, homemaking, and the like; physical functioning can be measured in terms of being confined to a bed, chair, or home because of health reasons)
  - pain and suffering

Box 18.6 Quality-Adjusted Life Years

QALY is calculated by multiplying years times quality of life during those years.

QALYs implicitly place a higher value on the life of a healthy individual compared with an individual with a disability.[50] This does not reflect the views of the public, which believes the life of an individual with a disability is equal in value to the life of a healthy individual.[50] QALYs have been challenged as violating the Americans with Disabilities Act.[50] While QALYs are the best comparator currently available, it is important to understand the ethical drawbacks and to continue searching for a standard measure that better reflects the public's view that disability may not be a reason to adjust life years.[50]

STEPS OF ECONOMIC ANALYSIS

The process of planning, conducting, and reporting an economic analysis can be divided into six steps.

Step 1: State the Objective

First, determine the objective of the economic analysis. In general terms, the objective is to arrive at an unbiased determination of how to use scarce resources most efficiently for a specific purpose. The type of intervention or program, intended purpose (nutrition or health aims), competing alternatives, and context for application are included in the objective. How the information will be used and the primary and other expected users of the information are also stated in the purpose.

Step 2: Define the Framework for Analysis

The framework for the analysis involves decisions about three things: perspective, alternatives, and time horizon.

Perspective

The study perspective identifies whose resources are at stake. It is the basis for choosing the type of economic analysis to undertake, including the type of cost to include in the analysis. As shown in Box 18.7, different groups of people are interested in different types of information. The perspective must be spec-

ified at the planning stage because it influences which costs and outcomes are most relevant to measure for the analysis. The perspectives of the intervention provider (the program or organization) or the payer are commonly selected when comparing medical or nutrition therapies. The perspectives of the health care sector and society are frequently used in policy analysis, health care reform, and planning.[38-40]

Alternatives

To evaluate a nutrition intervention for efficiency and effectiveness, it must be compared with one or more alternatives. All reasonable alternatives should be evaluated, but at least two are necessary. The alternatives to be included are described in detail. The selected alternatives should meet the following criteria:

- address the same preventive or therapeutic aim in the same group of patients
- represent current practice and new innovations
- consider available scientific evidence
- include alternatives that have political and professional support

Sometimes the option of no intervention is included as a studied alternative.

Time Horizon

Many economic analyses track patients through a relatively short course of therapy to clinical end points. Nutrition intervention can affect longer-term outcomes, such as the patient's functional capacity at home, relapse rate, future need for health care services, or onset of disease or complications many years in the future.

When discussing the time horizon, economists use the terms cost stream and benefit stream. The *cost stream* is the period of time over which intervention resources must be invested. The *benefit stream* is the period of time over which outcomes and associated costs of consequences are accumulated. Thus, the time horizon of a study refers to the defined time periods for tracking cost and benefit streams for the economic analysis. In cardiovascular disease, for example, the study objective could be outcomes of care during the hospital stay for coronary artery bypass grafting, through a period of

Perspective	Information Interest
Clinician	Cost of preventive, diagnostic, therapeutic, and rehabilitative alternatives
	Clinical outcomes and their associated costs
Provider organization	Cost to the organization
	Resources required to deliver the intervention (eg, personnel, supplies, and equipment)
	Cost consequences associated with the clinical outcomes (eg, extended length of stay and complications)
	Impact on budget
Payer	Volume and intensity of service provided
	Claims to be paid (charges for pharmacy, ambulatory care, inpatient stays, and emergency department visits)
	Expenditures that could be avoided
Accountable care organization	Costs to provide preventive, diagnostic, therapeutic, rehabilitative, and palliative care, as well as costs associated with the outcomes (eg, illness or hospitalization prevented)
Patient	Out-of-pocket costs for diagnosis and treatment regimens
	Convenience/inconvenience, satisfaction with care
	Pain and suffering
	Functional ability and quality of life
Health care sector of economy	Resource demands across the health care system
	Hospital, community, long-term care, and outpatient services are viewed as a whole
	Considers input costs and the cost consequences of outcomes
Society	Most complex and comprehensive perspective
	Includes total economic impact of health care, disease, and disability, regardless of who bears the cost
	Can include indirect costs (eg, education potential and lost worker productivity due to disability or early death)

Box 18.7 Perspectives for Economic Analysis

cardiac rehabilitation, or several years in the future to track cardiac events.

After the framework for analysis has been specified, the next two steps are to determine costs and to determine outcomes of the compared alternatives. These procedures are undertaken for both costs and outcomes by identifying (listing and defining), measuring (quantifying the amount used or produced), and valuing (assigning units to be reported, such as natural units, dollars, or QALY). These steps are presented here as step 3 and step 4, but they can be conducted simultaneously.

Step 3: Determine Costs

The process of quantifying costs—called *cost analysis* or *cost identification*—provides a systematic and defensible estimation of resources consumed, which is necessary for all types of economic analysis. Costing often focuses on the input cost of the intervention, but it is also used to determine the monetary value of outcomes for net cost-effectiveness and for

CBA. The process is not complicated, but it must be approached in a systematic and careful manner.[38-40]

Types of Costs

Economists traditionally categorize costs into direct, indirect, and intangible costs,[41] as illustrated in Box 18.8. The researcher decides which costs to include and how to measure them based on the objectives of the analysis and the information needs of the decision makers who will use the results.

Direct costs receive attention in most economic analyses of nutrition care and programs. Direct costs include resources consumed in the prevention, diagnosis, treatment, and rehabilitation of a disease. In nutrition, direct costs are defined as the resources the provider uses in the delivery of nutrition and related care to achieve the health goals or outcome objectives of the intervention or program. They are estimated from principal resource components incurred by the provider organization. Other perspectives for analysis would require the inclusion of other kinds of costs.

Cost	Definition	Examples
Direct health care (or other sector) cost	Costs associated directly with the nutrition intervention and related health care	Nutrition education and counseling; enteral or parenteral nutrition support
	Health care or other costs resulting from the intervention	Medication use; related medical visits; hospitalization
Direct patient costs	Costs borne by patients or their families	Transportation to clinic; out-of-pocket costs for the intervention and special food products
Indirect costs	Costs of reduced productivity as a result of the condition/illness and/or the nutrition intervention	Time lost (from work, school, or normal activities) because of the condition; preparation of special feedings; time needed to participate in the intervention/program
Intangible costs	Costs difficult to quantify in monetary terms, such as the cost of pain and suffering and quality-of-life changes	Impaired mental functioning; social limitation due to dietary restriction; lost sense of control

Box 18.8 Types of Costs Used in Economic Analysis

Cost Analysis

Cost analysis can be done in two ways, using either a microcosting approach, which accounts for all costs in detail, or a macrocosting or gross-costing approach, which considers only significant economic events. Cost analysis must be carried out with equal precision for all alternatives being compared. In the microcosting/cost-accounting approach, principal resource components are identified, tracked, and assigned a dollar value based on prevailing market prices. Principal resource components commonly included are personnel, fringe benefits, food and nutrition products and supplies, office supplies, education materials, equipment, laboratory tests, other diagnostic and monitoring procedures, other ancillary services, continuing education and training of staff, facility/space, and administrative overhead.

Microcosting is a systematic process involving the following steps:

● List all activities.
● Identify principal resource components for activities (as previously described).
● Estimate resource consumption for each principal resource component by tracking/measuring actual utilization or using secondary data.
● Assign a monetary value to each component and activity using market prices.
● List all assumptions made for possible sensitivity analysis.
● Calculate total, average, incremental, marginal, and/or net cost.
● Perform discounting, if necessary.

Macrocosting may be more appropriate for making policy choices, and microcosting for making choices about an individual patient treatment.[49]

Personnel costs are a large part of the costs for nutrition interventions. Time studies may be necessary to accurately determine the quantity of personnel time required for an intervention. Time and activity records or data from productivity studies carried out nationally[55,56] or within the organization could also be used to estimate time for specific activities. This information is infrequently reported in randomized controlled trials, but collecting informa-tion about the time required for nutrition interventions that improve outcomes would be a beneficial addition to any study. A few examples of time for intervention studies have been conducted in chronic kidney disease.[57-59] Information from the Commission on Dietetic Registration Compensation and Benefits Survey for the Dietetics Profession can be used to translate time into costs.[60]

The steps of gross costing are as follows:

● Identify significant economic events relevant to the intervention (inputs) and/or outcomes. These might include outpatient care; hospitalization; nursing home placement; home health services; services of a registered RDN, physician, or other professional; medication; and durable medical equipment.
● Measure or estimate the quantity of significant events used or produced.
● Assign value to significant events using fees schedules, actual charges, or payments.
● List all assumptions made for possible sensitivity analysis.
● Calculate total, average, incremental, marginal, and/or net cost.
● Perform discounting, if necessary

Assigning Monetary Value

The value assigned to the component or significant economic event is either the actual market price the buyer pays or an assigned value. When the buyer is the provider/health care organization, the value can be based on the price paid for resources consumed, the amount billed (charges), or the amount received as payments or reimbursements. When the buyer is the third-party payer (eg, an insurance carrier, or a health plan), the value assigned is usually based on records of claims paid or estimates using organization, industry, state, or national reports of health care utilization and cost under various circumstances. Sources of such data are described by Gold and colleagues.[38]

Market price and charges often exceed the actual resource cost. To adjust for this fact, a cost-to-charge ratio is used.[38-40] Payments made by third parties are often less than charges because the amount paid includes discounts and denied claims. Thus, determining the bases for valuing health care resources must receive careful consideration when planning the cost analysis.

The value of patients' or clients' time associated with receiving the service or experiencing its consequences is an additional important cost. Time costs, including time waiting for a service to begin, travel costs, time lost from work, and child care costs are all potential indirect costs to patients and are important to the individuals receiving the service. These costs are influential in patients' decisions to keep appointments and adhere to the treatment regimen. Economists translate these indirect costs into time lost from work and lost productivity.[38-40] Wages are frequently used to value indirect costs, and in spite of the potential inequities for women, minorities, and youth, economists consider wages to be the best measure of value. Wages must be used with caution, however, and with the acknowledgment that indirect costs may be underestimated for some groups and overestimated for others. The perspective of the study determines whether indirect costs are included in the analysis.

The fear, grief, worry, and pain experienced by patients, clients, and family members are intangible costs. These costs are difficult to measure and even more difficult to value in dollar terms, but they are real to patients, clients, and families. All illnesses and treatments have intangible costs. They are less commonly addressed, although they may be influential pieces of information for decision makers. Sometimes these intangible costs are presented in narrative terms.

Each alternative included in the analysis requires a cost analysis. The same types of costs and assumptions should be used in the cost analysis for each alternative; if not, any differences must be described. The approaches to cost analysis and method of valuing costs produce different results; therefore, methods and sources used must be fully disclosed in the report. In addition, when calculating costs, assumptions are frequently used to identify relevant resource costs, estimate the amount of resources consumed, assign a value for each resource component or significant economic event, or estimate and assign a value for resources consumed. All assumptions should be documented and subjected to sensitivity analysis (described in step 4).

Summarizing and Reporting Costs

The findings of the cost analysis can be summarized and reported in a number of ways, including full (total) cost, average cost, marginal cost, and net cost. Full (or total) cost is the cost of the intervention over a period of time (usually 1 year or the usual course of treatment). Total cost estimates are made up of fixed costs (stable costs not related to the volume of service) and variable costs (resource utilization that varies with the volume [number served] or intensity [frequency and type of contact] of service). Average cost is the cost per unit of output/outcome, which is determined by dividing total costs involved by the number of units of service (eg, cost per nutrition assessment or cost per low-birth-weight infant prevented). Incremental cost is the cost difference between one alternative and another (such as the extra cost of managing obesity with an RDN visit vs standard care[44]).

When the cost of providing a little more or a little less of the intervention is calculated, it is a marginal cost calculation (eg, the added cost of a second nutrition follow-up visit for individuals completing a weight-loss program). Incremental or marginal costs are more relevant to economic analysis than are total or average costs because incremental or marginal costs relate to the extra resource requirements to produce each added effect (and the opportunity costs of removing those resources from other purposes). Total and unit costs are especially useful for budgeting, establishing fees, and negotiating reimbursement rates.

Special Considerations in Costing

In an economic analysis covering multiple years or using cost data gathered at different times in the past, dollar values for all alternatives must be expressed as a standard base year. This calculation is called *adjusting to present value*, and it uses the Bureau of Labor Statistics' Consumer Price Index (www.bls.gov /cpi/cpifact4.htm), which has a medical care component, to adjust for inflation over time. This adjustment is done before costs are related to outcomes and before discounting is done.

Discounting is a mathematical procedure used to convert future costs and future outcomes to present value. Two factors make discounting necessary in long-term analyses:

- Inflation reduces the value of money over time.
- There is a tendency to prefer both dollars and benefits now, rather than in the future.

Discounting can be done using computer accounting or statistical analysis software. The discount rate used can range between 2% and 10% per year, with 5% as the most common rate.[38] Discounting is discussed in greater detail after step 4 because it is applied to both costs and outcomes.

Applying Cost Analysis

The following example illustrates how an RDN might determine the cost of nutrition services in prenatal care from the perspective of the public health center, using data from the current program year:

- Prepare a flow chart of all activities involved in providing nutrition services to pregnant clients, including such activities as client recruitment and outreach, nutrition assessment and diagnosis, education or counseling of clients, care coordination and referral, record keeping and scheduling, client follow-up and monitoring, and program administration and evaluation.
- Identify the principal resource components necessary for each activity. This might include nutrition and clerical personnel, fringe benefits, nutrition education materials and equipment, laboratory tests to monitor anemia, office and clinic space, nutrition reference materials, office supplies, and administrative overhead.
- Specify ways costs will be measured. Use work schedules and existing reports, such as service statistics or accounting records (after verifying their completeness and accuracy), conduct time studies or productivity studies, or use other methods to accurately estimate the quantity of principal resource components necessary to carry out each activity.
- Work with the accounting staff to assign a monetary value based on the actual cost to the organization for each cost component. Keep track of all assumptions made along the way.

- Calculate the total cost for prenatal nutrition services; then divide by the number of women served to get an average or unit cost. If the cost analysis looked only at nutrition costs as a component of an existing prenatal care program, the cost could be considered incremental (the amount added to prenatal care costs for nutrition services).

Similar steps with similar assumptions should be carried out for each alternative to be compared. For example, freestanding nutrition services delivered at a different location requiring separate staffing and facilities would likely have significantly different (and probably higher) costs.

Step 4: Determine Outcomes

Once the objectives of the service are defined and the type of analysis has been determined, the effect or benefit anticipated from the dietetics services can be identified, measured, and valued. The magnitude of the outcome (effect or benefit) associated with or attributed to the nutrition intervention is determined in step 4. The researcher must have a defensible estimate of the effect of each alternative to include in the economic analysis. These estimates are made through an outcomes study, as described earlier in this chapter, or through research methods described in Chapters 8, 9, 11, and 12. In some situations effectiveness results reported by others are used to model potential outcomes. Meta-analysis is recommended as a method for critically appraising and integrating the results of past studies into an estimate of effect.[40]

Regardless of the source of outcomes data, they must be logically and scientifically linked to the interventions being studied. Furthermore, data must be appropriate, given the framework of the economic analysis (alternatives, perspective, and time horizon). The end point for the analysis can be short-term or longer-term results, with preference given to long-term patient-oriented outcomes, as discussed previously.

For CEA, a key outcome (effect) is measured and reported in natural units (eg, pounds of weight loss, percentage reduction in cholesterol, proportion of individuals with diabetes who improve their blood glucose levels, or complications avoided). For CBA, important outcomes (benefits) are measured in or converted to monetary units (dollars). For cost utility analysis, the outcomes are reported as QALYs. The magnitude of outcomes is related to cost data from step 3 for the actual economic analysis. Relating outcomes to benefits is explained in step 5.

Types of Benefits

As with costs, economists classify benefits as direct, indirect, and intangible. Direct benefits of nutrition care are in the expenditures that would otherwise have been spent on health care had the intervention not been effective. Direct benefits represent all types of health resources that are not consumed as a result of the intervention; in other words, they represent resources saved or expenditures avoided because of the nutrition intervention. Direct benefits also accrue to individuals. For example, individuals with improved nutrition status and health outcomes may save out-of-pocket expenses when medications can be reduced.

Indirect benefits of nutrition care are improvements in functional ability and capacity to carry out the daily tasks of living and resume normal social roles (eg, worker, homemaker, or student). In some studies, improvements in work attendance and performance are used as proxies for improved health status. Estimates based on measures used in the National Health Interview Survey, the National Health and Nutrition Examination Survey, and the National Medical Expenditure Survey, among others, are useful when determining the indirect benefits of health care to consumers and to society and translating those benefits into economic consequences.[38,39] The dollar savings that are due to indirect benefits are estimated as part of the burden of illness.[38]

Improvements in quality of life also represent important benefits that are difficult to measure. Intangible benefits express subjective judgments of well-being, improved independence and mobility, and avoidance of pain and suffering. These intangible benefits are real to the individuals who experience them and therefore should contribute to the decision-making process. The development of quality-of-life assessments has enabled researchers to measure how patients perceive the effect of disease and disability and the course of treatment selected on their lives and functioning.[38,39,41]

All payers are interested in direct benefits because they want to reduce their expenditures. Insurance companies pay for certain services and procedures when evidence shows that savings accrue in other areas, such as reduced hospital costs. In contrast, payers and organization administrators are less concerned about indirect benefits and intangibles because they do not produce specific dollar savings for the organization. All three categories of benefits can and do occur in the same situation; for economic analysis, however, the perspective determines which categories are measured and included in the analysis.

Study Design

After considering the aforementioned points, the researcher can determine the research design and methods to measure outcomes (effects or benefits) of the compared alternatives. As discussed, different study designs have different strengths, ranging from control of bias to real-world applicability. Including a comparison is a required aspect of these designs. Furthermore, economic efficiency is based on a comparison with the next available alternative. The stronger the design and control of confounders, either through randomization or propensity scoring, the greater the validity of results and usefulness of the economic analysis. Two examples of methods to control for confounders are demonstrated in studies on oral nutrition supplement cost savings using the Premiere data set.[46,47]

Summarizing and Reporting Outcomes

After the data are collected, they are analyzed to determine the magnitude of effect achieved by each alternative. This analysis involves aggregating the raw data into summary statistics that include a measure of variation (eg, mean with standard deviation or confidence interval), determining the statistical and clinical significance of outcomes, and comparing alternatives. Appropriate statistical tests, which are determined by the study design and type of variables measured, must be used. For each alternative the following should be reported:

- descriptive data about the sample studied and the population it represents
- magnitude of outcome associated with, or attributed to, the intervention
- assessment of the clinical importance of the outcome achieved
- comparison of results between alternatives to determine if they are significantly different or to determine the incremental effectiveness
- descriptive data about any intervening or confounding factors
- statistical adjustments of the magnitude of the outcome for preexisting group differences and intervening factors
- quantitative or qualitative summary of other outcomes
- relationship of the degree of outcome to the amount of exposure to the nutrition intervention

Application Examples

In CEA, two or more alternatives for achieving the same outcome objective are compared, and the units of measure are the same. Compared with CBA, CEA is easier to carry out because it uses natural units that are commonly measured and documented in health care. However, CEA can require considerable time and expense to access records and abstract data.

Economic analysis can use data that are actually measured for the study, as well as values that are estimated from other data sources. The clinical effect of MNT, for example, could be measured, but the value of the effect to an organization, third-party payers, or society might be estimated by using data from other sources. A frequently used application of CBA is to compare the length of stay of a group of patients receiving a new or added procedure or treatment, such as MNT, with the length of stay reported for patients with the same diagnosis in a national study or existing database. The benefit can then be calculated from the cost differences if a shorter length of stay is found in the group receiving the nutrition therapy, as was done in Philipson and colleagues[46] and Lakdawalla and colleagues.[47]

For a societal perspective in CBA, researchers often use information the government collects through state, regional, and national studies. For example, the National Center for Health Statistics conducts the National Health Survey and publishes the results on a regular basis through the *Vital and Health Statistics* series. In CBA, the benefits are expressed in dollar terms (eg, cost per day of hospital stay) so that they can be directly compared with the input costs.

As mentioned earlier, intangible benefits may be identified but not measured. These benefits are important to consumers and, depending on the perspective, may be of interest to the decision maker. A legislator considering a Medicare or Medicaid reimbursement policy, for instance, would be interested to know that the constituents' quality of life has improved through a reduction in pain or an increased ability to ambulate and care for themselves. The Medicare administrator, however, would not find this information as useful because it has no impact on the direct cost of the Medicare program. When an intervention produces significant intangible benefits, it is useful to describe them in the report because they represent added value beyond the value reflected in the cost-benefit ratio.

Discounting Costs and Benefits

Whenever the time horizon of an analysis extends beyond a year or when data for input costs or outcome estimates for compared alternatives come from different years, the issues of present value and discounting must be addressed. Discounting adjusts for the preference individuals have for immediate consumption over future consumption[38]: a bird in the hand is worth two in the bush. If money is invested in a service now, individuals prefer to have the benefits immediately rather than in 5 or 40 years in the future. Thus, immediate benefits have higher value, and future benefits are discounted or reduced in value. This puts nutrition and other preventive services at a disadvantage.[50]

The discounting procedure adjusts estimates of cost or outcomes that will be experienced in a future time period. The interest rate is commonly used for discounting. Economists recommend making and reporting a range of calculations to include conservative and more optimistic projections, including rates of 2%, 3%, 5%, and 10%.[38] If a low discount rate is used, the value of long-term costs and benefits is increased; in contrast, a higher discount rate increases the value of short-term costs and benefits. A rule of thumb is that discounting should be used in a study when the time difference between investment and benefit is greater than 1 year. When necessary, cost, outcomes, or both are discounted before step 5. Present value tables in economics and accounting reference books and in computer spreadsheet software programs simplify the process of discounting.

Step 5: Relate Costs to Outcomes

After accurate and defensible estimates of costs and outcomes have been gathered (steps 3 and 4), they are related to each other so that researchers can judge the relative economic efficiency of the compared alternatives. This economic analysis can be done and presented in several ways—ratios, net benefit or net cost-effectiveness, or an array table. The method is determined by the objectives of the study, type of economic analysis, and nature of the data, as well as by considerations about what form will be most understandable and helpful to potential users of the results.

Ratio

The ratio communicates the cost for a unit of outcome and allows direct comparison between the efficiency of one alternative and the efficiency of another. When a ratio is used, it is difficult to visualize the total costs of implementing the intervention. Another drawback is that the actual magnitude of change is not evident, so clinicians cannot determine whether the amount of change is clinically meaningful. Decision makers will need additional descriptive or graphic information to consider the budgetary ramifications and numbers of individuals who are likely to have access to and benefit from the defined nutrition intervention. Additionally, various audiences may be interested in outcomes beyond the key outcomes identified for the cost-effectiveness or cost-benefit ratio.

Array Table

Many of the drawbacks of ratio use are overcome by presenting results in an array. An array table lists the actual costs in dollars and the outcomes in their natural units of measurement and is useful for re-porting the findings across a chain of outcomes. An array table allows audiences to simultaneously consider more than one outcome measure in relation to the resource requirements to produce the outcomes. Franz and colleagues[61] used an array table to present the findings from a study of nutrition practice guidelines for type 2 diabetes mellitus.

From Ratio to Net Benefit

A ratio is traditionally used to express the results of CBA research. It may be a cost-benefit ratio, in which the numerator is the cost of inputs and the denominator is the monetary value of benefits (outcomes), or it may be a benefit-cost ratio, in which the numerator is the benefits and the denominator is the costs:

$$\text{Cost-benefit ratio} = \frac{\text{Cost of inputs in dollars}}{\text{Benefit (outcomes) in dollars}} = 1:3$$

$$\text{Benefit-cost ratio} = \frac{\text{Benefit (outcomes) in dollars}}{\text{Cost of inputs in dollars}} = 3:1$$

Net benefit (or net cost) is the dollars gained (or lost) when the monetary value of all resources consumed is subtracted from the total estimate of cost savings or averted expenditures when the alternative is implemented. It uses the same values that are used in the numerator and denominator of the cost-benefit ratio. Compared with the ratio, the net benefit calculation does a better job of communicating the magnitude of resources at stake and can be applied more directly to budgetary planning. This can also be understood as the return on investment, which is meaningful to budget creators and legislators.

Presenting only the ratio conceals the magnitude of the resources at stake. For example, benefits of $3 million gained from an expenditure of $1 million results in a 1:3 cost-benefit ratio. A benefit of $3,000 from an investment of $1,000 is also a 1:3 cost-benefit ratio. However, the net benefits would be reported as $2 million and $2,000, respectively, which certainly tells a different story.

Some experts advocate presenting the results of a CEA as net cost-effectiveness. In this method, the monetary value of cost savings generated by the improved health or averted deterioration is calculated (usually using gross costing to assign value to economically significant events). From this value, the input (intervention) costs are subtracted. The resulting value is related to a key outcome presented in natural units.[38,39]

Sensitivity Analysis and Ethical Issues in Economic Analysis

Before the final conclusions can be drawn, three more things must be considered: discounting (discussed earlier), sensitivity analysis, and ethical issues. Sensitivity analysis is used to check the robustness of the conclusions. It involves the reanalysis of data using different estimates for assumptions or uncertainties and informs the researcher and decision maker of the degree to which specific assumptions affect the results. For example, in a study of MNT in type 2 diabetes mellitus, the impact of different assumptions about RDNs' salaries, variations in the use of laboratory tests, and magnitude of glucose control outcome were assessed.[61]

In sensitivity analysis, what-if scenarios are used to determine how substitute assumptions (or other uncertainties) would affect the conclusions. Several rounds of reanalysis are done using more conservative and more liberal estimates. Reanalysis is not difficult. Using computer spreadsheets or statistical software programs, revised estimates can be substituted for a value used in the original analysis, and the program quickly recalculates the results.

Reports of CEA and CBA should describe the assumptions made and how sensitivity analysis was used to explore the impact of the assumptions on the analysis and its conclusions. If a conclusion holds up under varying assumptions, it is said to be robust. If changing some of the assumptions used to assign value to resources significantly changes the conclusion, greater efforts should be directed toward determining the true value for the cost component or the outcome estimate. When this effort is not possible, the researcher must state explicitly that the results are sensitive to the value assigned to that component. In the report of a type 2 diabetes mellitus study, the authors stated, "The results indicate that cost-effectiveness conclusions were sensitive to the outcome indicator selected." They went on to report how RDNs' salaries, laboratory tests, and outcome variations affected the conclusions.[61]

In reports of studies about the cost-effectiveness of nutrition services, questions can arise about assumptions used in estimates of costs or outcomes. RDNs and others conducting these studies must identify the potential areas for questioning. They must use sensitivity analysis to understand the strengths and limitations of the analysis and openly report them along with conclusions and recommendations.

The results of economic analysis indicate the preferred alternative based on the criterion of economic efficiency—that is, the alternative that produces the greater amount of outcomes for the lower cost. However, additional criteria come into play when setting policies, making administrative decisions, or recommending clinical practices. The findings of CBA or CEA could favor targeting MNT or a nutrition program to younger, more compliant patients with less severe disease. But is it ethical to withhold therapy from older or more acutely ill individuals? The public's opinions suggest not.[50] And although delivering a nutrition program via the internet may be efficient, is it ethical to exclude individuals who cannot afford a computer or internet access? Ethical issues like these must be considered when conducting economic analyses.

When an ethical issue, such as access to nutrition care for individuals without insurance, is incorporated into the objectives of the CEA or CBA, the study can be designed to measure and value the issue. Ethical issues can also come to light during the study and interpretation of results. Relevant ethical issues should be explored, identified, and discussed, even if it is not possible to measure or place a dollar value on them. Many individuals—especially advocates, legislators, planners, and policy analysts—who use reports about the economic implications of nutrition services and programs have no nutrition training. Ethical issues related to food and nutrition may not be evident and thus must be brought to their attention. Whenever ethical issues are identified, their implications should be explored and presented as part of the findings.

Step 6: Interpret and Use the Results

When the analysis is complete, the last step is to interpret the findings and recommend actions. The results provide information about the cost, effectiveness, and efficiency of nutrition programs and services. The study and its findings must be presented to decision makers who can use the information. Clinical nutrition managers benefit from a CEA that identifies areas in which expected outcomes are not being reached or patients' health outcomes could be achieved with fewer inputs. The results can support changes in practice necessary to make dietetics services more effective and efficient. Providing results of CBA to health plans and insurance companies can support coverage of MNT[44] and was important in advocating for order-writing privileges for RDNs.[54]

Every study has limitations that must be acknowledged. For example in the ex ante analysis of cost savings from RDN order-writing privileges, assumptions and limitations are clearly outlined so that appropriate application of the findings and the need for further study are clear.[54]

The report of an economic analysis must include enough information for users to be able to understand the conclusion, judge its accuracy, and determine the context in which it can be applied. Using a reporting checklist like Consolidated Health Economic Evaluation Reporting Standards (CHEERS)[62] helps ensure that assumptions and sensitivity to those assumptions are reported.

APPLICATIONS IN DIETETICS PRACTICE

Economic Analysis in Clinical Nutrition

Clinical nutrition involves many options for nutrition intervention: For whom? When to provide? What type? How long? By whom? Economic analysis can provide answers to these questions. Most of the recent economic analysis in clinical nutrition has focused on the identification of and intervention for malnutrition.[41,46,47]

Economic Analysis in Public Health

The Academy position paper on the role of dietetics professionals in health promotion and disease prevention includes potential cost savings associated with reducing the burden of chronic disease in the population through nutrition-related prevention strategies.[63] Under the leadership of the Centers for Disease Control and Prevention, extensive work has been done to link the principles and analytic techniques of economic analysis and epidemiology to improve the quality of CEA studies of prevention. *Prevention Effectiveness: A Guide to Decision Analysis and Economic Evaluation* provides extensive coverage of the topic.[39] In addition, the World Health Organization has identified methods to assess the costs and health effects of interventions for improving health in developing countries.[64]

CONCLUSION

Dietetics practitioners in all practice settings can contribute to knowledge about the effectiveness and efficiency of nutrition care. Using data collected for quality assurance purposes and outcomes measurement can ease the burden of conducting an economic analysis. RDNs with management responsibilities can allocate time for staff to spend on planning, conducting, and reporting outcome studies and economic analyses.

Studies may be small and carried out in one facility, or several locations may collaborate. The Academy's NRN is a way of involving RDNs from many locations in a centrally designed study.[34] In addition, the Academy of Nutrition and Dietetics Health Informatics Infrastructure was custom built with outcomes data collection for individuals and the profession in mind.[32] Ultimately, integrating nutrition in the electronic medical record will further support efforts toward documenting outcomes and costs of care. For those interested in learning more about health economics, the National Institutes of Health offers a series of self-study modules, Health Economics Information Resources: A Self-Study Course (www.nlm.nih.gov/nichsr/edu/healthecon/index.html).

Results need to be shared through professional and scientific meetings and publications. It is up to RDNs, along with other researchers and economists, to conduct the research and make the results available to the administrators, planners, regulators, legislators, and third-party payers who need this information to make informed decisions about the allocation of resources to nutrition care. By working with these policy makers, RDNs will learn about their different information needs and therefore be better able to plan, conduct, and report studies that can influence clinical administrative and policy decisions.

CEA and CBA are tools to provide more information about nutrition care and its cost and effectiveness. If used wisely, these tools will enable RDNs to continue to improve their services, increase their visibility with payers and other decision makers, and provide nutrition services that will have greater impact on the health of the public.

REFERENCES

1. Pitt B, Zannad F, Remme WJ, et al. The effect of spironolactone on morbidity and mortality in patients with severe heart failure. Randomized Aldactone Evaluation Study Investigators. *N Engl J Med.* 1999;341(10):709-717.

2. Juurlink DN, Mamdani MM, Lee DS, et al. Rates of hyperkalemia after publication of the Randomized Aldactone Evaluation Study. *N Engl J Med.* 2004;351(6):543-551.

3. Hunt SA, Abraham WT, Chin MH, et al; American College of Cardiology; American Heart Association Task Force on Practice Guidelines; American College of Chest Physicians; International Society for Heart and Lung Transplantation; Heart Rhythm Society. ACC/AHA 2005 guideline update for the diagnosis and management of chronic heart failure in the adult: a report of the American College of Cardiology/American Heart Association Task Force on Practice Guidelines (Writing Committee to Update the 2001 Guidelines for the Evaluation and Management of Heart Failure). *J Am Coll Cardiol.* 2005;46(6):e1-e82.

4. Guthrie JF, Myers EF. USDA's Economic Research Service supports nutrition and health outcomes research. *J Am Diet Assoc.* 2002;102(2):293-297.

5. Jortberg BT, Fleming MO. Registered dietitian nutritionists bring value to emerging health care delivery models. *J Acad Nutr Diet.* 2014;114(12):2017-2022.

6. Clancy CM, Eisenberg JM. Outcomes research: measuring the end results of health care. *Science.* 1998;282(5387):245-246.

7. Singal AG, Higgins PDR, Waljee AK. A primer on effectiveness and efficacy trials. *Clin Transl Gastroenterol.* 2014;5(1):e45.

8. Kane RL. *Understanding Health Care Outcomes Research.* Sudbury, MA: Jones & Bartlett Learning; 2006.

9. Research International and Strategic Business Analysis Team. *Evidence Analysis Manual: Steps in the Academy Evidence Analysis Process.* Chicago, IL: Academy of Nutrition and Dietetics; 2016. www.andeal.org/vault/2440/web/files/2016_April_EA_Manual.pdf. Accessed June 5, 2018.

10. Myers EF, Pritchett E, Johnson EQ. Evidence-based practice guides vs. protocols: what's the difference? *J Am Diet Assoc.* 2001;101(9):1085-1090.

11. Jonnalagadda SS. Effectiveness of medical nutrition therapy: importance of documenting and monitoring nutrition outcomes. *J Am Diet Assoc.* 2004;104(12):1788-1792.

12. PCORI Methodology Committee. Hickam D, Totten A, Berg A, Rader K, Goodman S, Newhouse R, eds. *The PCORI Methodology Report.* Washington, DC: Patient Centered Outcomes Research Institute; 2013.

13. Gallagher-Allred CR, Voss AC, Finn SC, McCamish MA. Malnutrition and clinical outcomes: the case for medical nutrition therapy. *J Am Diet Assoc.* 1996;96(4):361-366; quiz 367-368.

14. Gallagher-Allred CR, Voss AC, Koop KL. The effect of medical nutrition therapy on malnutrition and clinical outcomes. *Nutrition.* 1999;(156):512-514.

15. Barr JT, Schumacher GE. The need for a nutrition-related quality-of-life measure. *J Am Diet Assoc.* 2003; 103(2):177-180.

16. Hauchecorne CM, Barr SI, Sork TJ. Evaluation of nutrition counseling in clinical settings: do we make a difference? *J Am Diet Assoc.* 1994;94(4):437-440.

17. Lemon CC, Lacey K, Lohse B, Hubacher DO, Klawitter B, Palta M. Outcomes monitoring of health, behavior, and quality of life after nutrition intervention in adults with type 2 diabetes. *J Am Diet Assoc.* 2004;104(12):1805-1815.

18. Committee on Qualification of Biomarkers and Surrogate Endpoints in Chronic Disease, Board on Health Care Services, Board on Health Sciences Policy, Food and Nutrition Board. Michael CM, Ball JR, eds. *Evaluation of Biomarkers and Surrogate Endpoints in Chronic Disease.* Washington, DC: National Academies Press; 2010.

19. Barter PJ, Caulfield M, Eriksson M, et al. Effects of torcetrapib in patients at high risk for coronary events. *N Engl J Med.* 2007;357(21):2109-2122.

20. Dallmeier D, Koenig W. Strategies for vascular disease prevention: the role of lipids and related markers including apolipoproteins, low-density lipoproteins (LDL)-particle size, high sensitivity C-reactive protein (hs-CRP), lipoprotein-associated phospholipase A2 (Lp-PLA(2)) and lipoprotein(a) (Lp(a)). *Best Pract Res Clin Endocrinol Metab.* 2014;28(3):281-294.

21. Fleming TR, DeMets DL. Surrogate end points in clinical trials: are we being misled? *Ann Intern Med.* 1996;125(7): 605-613.

22. Masoudi FA, Havranek EP, Wolfe P, et al. Most hospitalized older persons do not meet the enrollment criteria for clinical trials in heart failure. *Am Heart J.* 2003;146(2): 250-257.

23. Ford I, Norrie J. Pragmatic trials. *N Engl J Med.* 2016; 375(5):454-463.

24. Loudon K, Treweek S, Sullivan F, Donnan P, Thorpe KE, Zwarenstein M. The PRECIS-2 tool: designing trials that are fit for purpose. *BMJ.* 2015;350:h2147.

25. Office for Human Research Protections, Department of Health and Human Services. Coded private information or specimens use in research, guidance (2008). www.hhs.gov /ohrp/regulations-and-policy/guidance/research -involving-coded-private-information/index.html. Accessed June 5, 2018.

26. Rosenbaum PR, Rubin DB. The central role of the propensity score in observational studies for causal effects. *Biometrika.* 1983;70 (1):41-55.

27. Rosenbaum PR, Rubin DB. Constructing a control group using nultivariate matched sampling methods that incorporate the propensity score. *Am Stat.* 1985;39 (1): 33-38.

28. Wahba S, Dehejia RH. Propensity score-matching methods for nonexperimental causal studies. *Rev Econ Stat.* 2002;84 (1):151-161.

29. Kurth T, Glynn RJ, Gaziano JM, et al. Results of multivariable logistic regression, propensity matching, propensity adjustment, and propensity-based weighting under conditions of nonuniform effect. *Am J Epidemiol.* 2006;163(3):262-270.

30. Academy of Nutrition and Dietetics. Nutrition Terminology Reference Manual (eNCPT): Dietetics Language for Nutrition Care. http://ncpt.webauthor.com. Published 2017. Accessed June 5, 2018.

31. Hakel-Smith N, Lewis NM. A standardized nutrition care process and language are essential components of a conceptual model to guide and document nutrition care and patient outcomes. *J Am Diet Assoc.* 2004;104(12): 1878-1884.

32. Hakel-Smith N, Lewis NM, Eskridge KM. Orientation to nutrition care process standards improves nutrition care documentation by nutrition practitioners. *J Am Diet Assoc.* 2005;105(10):1582-1589.

33. Thompson KL, Davidson P, Swan WI, et al. Nutrition care process chains: the "missing link" between research and evidence-based practice. *J Acad Nutr Diet.* 2015;115(9): 1491-1498.

34. Hand RK. Research in nutrition and dietetics—what can the academy do for you? *J Acad Nutr Diet.* 2014;114(1): 131-135.

35. Murphy WJ, Steiber AL. A new breed of evidence and the tools to generate it: introducing ANDHII. *J Acad Nutr Diet.* 2015;115(1):19-22.

36. Gregerson J. The great migration: opportunities and obstacles await those advancing toward electronic health record adoption. *J Acad Nutr Diet.* 2012;112(11):1710-1717.

37. Porter ME. What is value in health care? *N Engl J Med.* 2010;363(26):2477-2481.

38. Gold M, Siegel J, Russell L, Weinstein MC, eds. *Cost-Effectiveness in Health and Medicine.* New York NY: Oxford University Press; 1996.

39. Haddix A, Teutsch S, Corso P. *Prevention Effectiveness: A Guide to Decision Analysis and Economic Evaluation*. New York NY: Oxford University Press; 2003.

40. Petti D. *Meta-Analysis, Decision Analysis, and Cost-Effectiveness Analysis: Methods for Quantitative Synthesis in Medicine*. 2nd ed. New York NY: Oxford University Press; 2000.

41. Philipson T, Linthicum MT, Snider JT. Tutorial on health economics and outcomes research in nutrition. *JPEN J Parenter Enteral Nutr*. 2014;38(2 suppl):5S-16S.

42. Mason M. *Cost and Benefits of Nutrition Care: Phase 1*. Chicago IL: American Dietetic Association; 1979.

43. Academy of Nutrition and Dietetics, Evidence Analysis Library. MNT: cost effectiveness, cost-benefit, or economic savings of MNT (2009). http://andeal.org/topic.cfm?menu=5284&cat=4085. Accessed June 5, 2018.

44. Bradley DW, Murphy G, Snetselaar LG, Myers EF, Qualls LG. The incremental value of medical nutrition therapy in weight management. *Manag Care*. 2013;22(1):40-45.

45. Howatson A, Wall CR, Turner-Benny P. The contribution of dietitians to the primary health care workforce. *J Prim Health Care*. 2015;7(4):324-332.

46. Philipson TJ, Snider JT, Lakdawalla DN, Stryckman B, Goldman DP. Impact of oral nutritional supplementation on hospital outcomes. *Am J Manag Care*. 2013;19(2):121-128.

47. Lakdawalla DN, Mascarenhas M, Jena AB, et al. Impact of oral nutrition supplements on hospital outcomes in pediatric patients. *JPEN J Parenter Enteral Nutr*. 2014;38(2 suppl):42S-49S.

48. Berger ML, Teutsch S. Cost-effectiveness analysis: from science to application. *Med Care*. 2005 (7 suppl);43:49-53.

49. Drummond M, Goeree R, Moayyedi P, Levine M. Economic analysis. In: Guyatt G, Rennie D, Meade MO, Cook DJ, eds. *Users' Guides to the Medical Literature: A Manual for Evidence-Based Clinical Practice*. 2nd ed. New York, NY: McGraw Hill Medical; 2008:619-641.

50. Ubel PA. *Pricing Life: Why It's Time for Health Care Rationing*. Cambridge, MA: MIT Press; 1999.

51. King JT Jr., Tsevat J, Lave JR, Roberts MS. Willingness to pay for a quality-adjusted life year: implications for societal health care resource allocation. *Med Decis Making*. 2005;25(5):667-677.

52. Gold MR, Sofaer S, Siegelberg T. Medicare and cost-effectiveness analysis: time to ask the taxpayers. *Health Aff (Millwood)*. 2007;26(5):1399-1406.

53. Tengs TO, Wallace A. One thousand health-related quality-of-life estimates. *Med Care*. 2000;38 (6):583-637.

54. Phillips W, Doley J. Granting order-writing privileges to registered dietitian nutritionists can decrease costs in acute care hospitals. *J Acad Nutr Diet*. 2017;117(6):840-847.

55. Hand RK, Jordan B, DeHoog S, Pavlinac J, Abram JK, Parrott JS. Inpatient staffing needs for registered dietitian nutritionists in 21st century acute care facilities. *J Acad Nutr Diet*. 2015;115(6):985-1000.

56. Phillips W. Clinical nutrition staffing benchmarks for acute care hospitals. *J Acad Nutr Diet*. 2015;115(7):1054-1056.

57. Sevick MA, Piraino BM, St-Jules DE, et al. No difference in average interdialytic weight gain observed in a randomized trial with a technology-supported behavioral intervention to reduce dietary sodium intake in adults undergoing maintenance hemodialysis in the United States: primary outcomes of the BalanceWise Study. *J Ren Nutr*. 2016;26(3):149-158.

58. Ford JC, Pope JF, Hunt AE, Gerald B. The effect of diet education on the laboratory values and knowledge of hemodialysis patients with hyperphosphatemia. *J Ren Nutr*. 2004;14(1):36-44.

59. Dolecek TA, Olson MB, Caggiula AW, et al. Registered dietitian time requirements in the Modification of Diet in Renal Disease Study. *J Am Diet Assoc*. 1995;95(11):1307-1312.

60. Rogers D. Compensation and benefits survey 2017. *J Acad Nutr Diet*. 2018;118(3):499-511.

61. Franz MJ, Splett PL, Monk A, et al. Cost-effectiveness of medical nutrition therapy provided by dietitians for persons with non-insulin-dependent diabetes mellitus. *J Am Diet Assoc*. 1995;95(9):1018-1024.

62. Husereau D, Drummond M, Petrou S, et al; ISPOR Health Economic Evaluation Publication Guidelines; CHEERS Good Reporting Practices Task Force. Consolidated Health Economic Evaluation Reporting Standards (CHEERS)—explanation and elaboration: a report of the ISPOR Health Economic Evaluation Publication Guidelines Good Reporting Practices Task Force. *Value Health*. 2013;16(2):231-250.

63. Slawson DL, Fitzgerald N, Morgan KT. Position of the Academy of Nutrition and Dietetics: the role of nutrition in health promotion and chronic disease prevention. *J Acad Nutr Diet*. 2013;113(7):972-979.

64. *Making Choices in Health: WHO Guide to Cost-Effectiveness Analysis*. Geneva, Switzerland: World Health Organization; 2003.

Chapter 19

Research in Diet and Human Genetics

Marilyn C. Cornelis, PhD

LEARNING OBJECTIVES

1. Describe current methods for identifying genetic determinants of diet exposure and response and discuss key results of their application.

2. Explain gene-diet interactions, describe current methods for testing gene-diet interactions, and evaluate recent progress on these interactions.

3. Explain the concept of personalized nutrition, identify its strengths and limitations, and discuss how it may challenge existing public health nutritional guidelines

Much research has focused on identifying environmental exposures (eg, diet, tobacco smoke) that increase the risk of disease, but it is evident that not all individuals exposed to the same risk factors will develop the associated disease.[1] Dietary assessment tools, such as dietary records and food frequency questionnaires, have been instrumental in acquiring knowledge of the role diet plays in population health. However, these tools, along with other aspects of epidemiologic methods, have well-known limitations. Foods are mixtures of nutrients and non-nutrients and are often consumed with other foods, forming dietary patterns.

Separating and characterizing the causal effects of each food or food constituent is therefore a challenge. Between-person differences also add complexity. With advanced knowledge of the human genome and technology enabling affordable high-throughput measurements of individual genomes, researchers are beginning to understand the impact of differential genetic susceptibility in the etiology and pathogenesis of common diseases and in our physiological and behavioral response to the environment. This new biology offers promise of an individualized approach to preventive medicine through risk profiling and the provision of information on how to modify the potential results of genetic predisposition via dietary modification or other environmental changes.

Nutrigenetics, defined as the science of the effect of genetic variation on dietary response, is the focus of the current chapter.[2] Nutrigenomics is related but is typically defined as the science of the role of nutrients and bioactive food compounds in gene expression.[2] This chapter discusses concepts in human genetics with application to the field of nutrition. In addition, it reviews important study designs for conducting research in this area, discusses the practical and ethical concerns of implementing personalized nutrition advice, and briefly comments on the future of genetic research applied to human nutrition.

HUMAN GENETICS: A BRIEF OVERVIEW

A comprehensive review of human genetics is beyond the scope of this chapter. Interested readers may also refer to texts by Turnpenny and Ellard[3] and Alberts and colleagues,[4] from which the following overview is largely synthesized.

The genetic material within cells contains the complete set of instructions for making an organism, called its *genome*. The human genome is organized into 46 chromosomes. Of these chromosomes, 44 are in 22 pairs (autosomes), in which one chromosome is inherited from the mother and one chromosome from the father. In addition, females inherit an X chromosome from each parent, whereas males inherit an X chromosome from the mother and a Y chromosome from the father.

Each chromosome contains a unique set of many genes. A gene is a segment of a chromosome that encodes instructions that allow a cell to produce a specific protein, such as an enzyme, receptor, or carrier protein. The human genome contains approximately 19,000 predicted protein-coding genes.[5,6] The structure of a gene consists of many elements, of which the actual protein coding sequence is often only a small part (see Figure 19.1 on page 382). The open-reading frame contains *exons*, the coding regions of a gene that provide the specific instructions for making a protein. Exons are separated by noncoding stretches of DNA called *introns*. Flanking the open-reading frame are regulatory sequences that control when, and to what extent, the gene is expressed. This regulatory region can be envisioned as a series of on/off switches that respond to signals (eg, proteins and hormones) from within the cell, from neighboring cells, and from more distant parts of the organism.

Genes are composed of DNA, which exists as two paired or complementary strands forming a double helix (see Figure 19.1 on page 382). A nucleotide, which is the basic structural unit and building block of DNA, is composed of three parts: a five-sided sugar (deoxyribose), a phosphate group, and a nitrogenous base. There are four different bases in DNA: adenine (A), thymine (T), cytosine (C), and guanine (G). The two strands of DNA are held together by pairing of the bases. Base A forms hydrogen bonds with T, and C forms hydrogen bonds with G. Every three bases (called a *triplet*) along a strand of DNA specify an amino acid to be incorporated into a protein, in what is called the *genetic code*. For example, a triplet composed of the GCA sequence is the genetic triplet code for the amino acid alanine. Certain combinations of bases (eg, TAA), called *termination* or *stop codons*, will terminate the gene product. Mathematically, four bases could form up to 64 unique triplet codes; however, there are only 20 amino acids. This redundancy in the genetic code is called *degeneracy*.

Genes, through the proteins they encode, control all aspects of cell function. When a cell is switched on to make a protein, the information from a gene is copied, base by base, from DNA into a single new strand of complementary RNA. RNA differs from DNA in three ways: (1) RNA is single

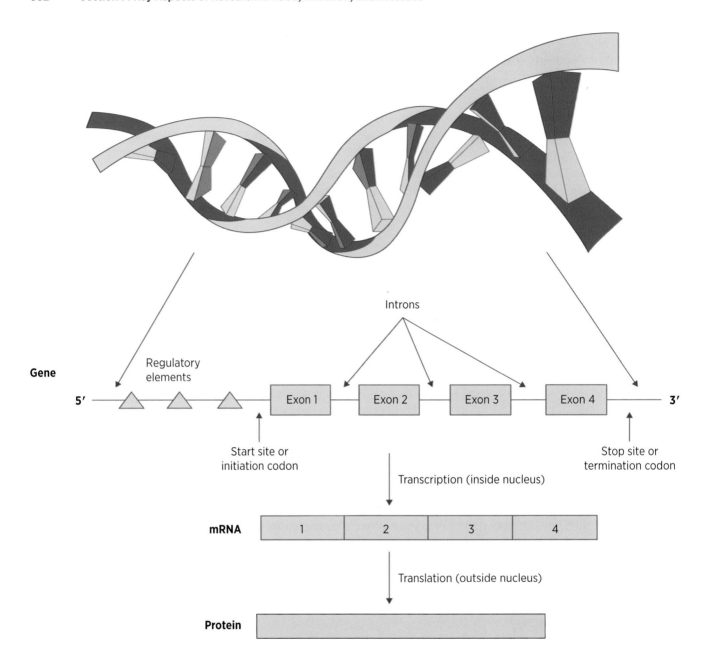

Figure 19.1 DNA and a diagram of a typical human structural gene

Adapted with permission the Academy of Nutrition and Dietetics. Patterson RE, Eaton EL, Potter JP. The genetic revolution: change and challenge for the profession of dietetics. *J Am Diet Assoc.* 1999;99:1412-1420.[7].

stranded, whereas DNA is double stranded; (2) the sugar-phosphate backbone of RNA is composed of ribose, whereas in DNA it is composed of deoxyribose; and (3) RNA contains the base uracil (U), whereas DNA contains the base thymine (T). This primary RNA molecule is spliced to remove intron sequences so that only the coding sequence from the exons are used to produce messenger RNA (mRNA).

The mRNA travels out of the nucleus into the cytoplasm, where it directs the complex set of reactions that occur on a ribosome and results in the assembly of amino acids that fold into completed protein molecules. Two other types of RNA, transfer RNA and ribosomal RNA are used in the cell to facilitate the synthesis of proteins from the mRNA template. In addition, some RNA molecules in cells function as enzyme-like catalysts rather than serving as a template for protein synthesis.

GENETIC VARIATION

Although thousands of random changes occur every day in a cell's DNA as a result of heat energy and metabolic accidents, only a few stable changes accumulate in the DNA sequence of an average cell in a year. The rest of the changes are eliminated with remarkable efficiency by a variety of DNA repair mechanisms. DNA mutations that occur in germ cells (sperm or ova) are called *germline mutations.* These inheritable DNA mutations determine the characteristics of offspring, including their susceptibility to disease. It is important to recognize that DNA mutations can occur in other body cells (that is, somatic cells). Somatic mutations are acquired from the environment (eg, from tobacco) and can transform a normal cell to a malignant cell, which can then give rise to a tumor by clonal expansion. The current chapter focuses entirely on germline mutations.

Genetic variants are typically discussed in terms of their frequency in the population (common or rare) and their nucleotide composition (single nucleotide variants or structural variants).[8] Common variants, called *polymorphisms,* are defined as genetic variants with a minor allele frequency of at least 1% in the population, whereas rare variants have a minor allele frequency of less than 1%.

Single nucleotide variants are DNA sequence variations in which a single nucleotide base (A, T, G, or C) is altered. Single nucleotide polymorphisms (SNPs) are the most common class of genetic variation among individuals and occur when corresponding sequences of DNA from different individuals differ at one base. For example, in one individual a specific sequence may be GAGCCTA and for another individual, the corresponding sequence may be GAGCTTA. This SNP involves two alleles: C and T. Because each individual has two alleles (one inherited from each parent), SNPs typically have three genotypes, denoted generically AA, Aa, and aa. In the previous example, the three possible genotypes would be CC, CT, and TT. The human genome contains at least 11 million SNPs, with approximately 7 million of these occurring

with a minor allele frequency greater than 5%.[9] The alleles of SNPs located in the same genomic interval are often correlated with one another. This correlation structure, or linkage disequilibrium (LD),[10] varies across the genome and between different populations. Comprehensive mapping efforts have nevertheless broken the genome down into groups of highly correlated SNPs that are generally inherited together (LD blocks). Such knowledge underlies, in part, the marked progress in high-throughput genotyping and, in turn, genome-wide investigations. By genotyping the DNA sample of an individual with a tagging SNP from each LD block, knowledge is gained regarding more than 80% of SNPs present at a frequency above 5% across the genome.[10-32]

Structural variants are generally all base pairs that differ between individuals and that are not single nucleotide variants.[8] Insertion–deletion variants (indels) occur when one or more base pairs are present in some genomes but absent in others. Block substitutions involve a string of adjacent nucleotides that vary between two genomes. An inversion variant occurs when the order of the base pairs is reversed in a specific section of a chromosome. Copy number variants describe cases when (nearly) identical sequences are repeated in some chromosomes but not others. The technological ability to detect structural variants is less advanced than that for single nucleotide variants; hence, the current understanding of structural variants is relatively limited.

Because the triplet genetic code is degenerate, a SNP may still code for the same amino acid (referred to as a *synonymous SNP*). Even if a DNA sequence alteration produces a change in an amino acid (nonsynonymous), it may not significantly affect the protein because the amino acid may not be at a site that is crucial to the protein's function. In contrast, other DNA alterations result in protein changes that can be disabling. For example, an indel may result in a frame-shift mutation such that all the codons downstream are now out of their usual sequence of triplets. Other alterations can convert a coding triplet into a stop codon, which tells the cell to end the protein prematurely.

In humans, hundreds of complex phenotypic traits determine how we look and behave and our propensity to develop certain diseases. Each complex phenotype is governed by a combination of inherited factors—which are largely believed to be genetic variants—and environmental influences. The vast majority of genetic variants do not contribute to phenotypic variation, achieving significant frequencies in the human population simply by chance.[14] The challenge is to determine which variants underlie or are responsible for the inherited components of phenotypes. Probably the best known genetic factors that increase risk of disease are the highly penetrant, dominant mutations associated with high disease risks. An example of this type of mutation is breast cancer gene 1 (*BRCA1*) and breast cancer gene 2 (*BRCA2*). Although this type of genetic variation can appreciably increase the individual risk of disease, the public health significance is less clear because the majority of women who develop breast cancer do not have this mutation or other highly penetrant mutations that have been identified. In contrast, genetic variants that affect susceptibility to common diseases can have a much greater effect on a population level, even though they may pose relatively low individual risk.[15]

GENETIC DETERMINANTS OF DIET EXPOSURE AND RESPONSE

Although the hunt for disease-associated genes has understandably been a priority, there is increasing interest and parallel progress in identifying genetic factors underlying physiological and behavioral responses to diet. Motivation for the latter efforts come from twin studies that report stronger correlations in diet response between monozygotic twins than between dizygotic twins, supporting an important genetic component underlying diet response.[16-18] In addition, knowledge of these genetic factors is often more actionable than equivalent knowledge concerning disease predisposition. That is, individuals may be able to modify their dietary behaviors to align with their genotype for optimal nutrition and health.

Genetic epidemiologic studies have been the most common approach to investigations of specific genetic factors and diet-related traits. Generally, linear- or logistic-type analyses are performed on nutrient biomarkers or self-reported dietary information previously collected from individuals in existing population studies and for whom DNA is also available. Early efforts to identify genetic factors associated with diet-related traits were hypothesis driven, focusing on candidate molecular pathways mediating absorption, metabolism, chemosensory detection, and physiological effects. For weight management, genes encoding the uncoupling proteins and β-adrenergic receptors were common targets for study. For bitter taste perception, the taste-receptor genes were studied, and for caffeine metabolism and response, genes encoding the xenobiotic enzymes and the adenosine receptors, respectively, were studied. This candidate approach was limited by knowledge of the relevant pathways and the variation in specific genes.

In the early 2000s, efforts to dissect the human genome into LD blocks and the technological advances in assaying SNPs enabled genome-wide association studies (GWASs).[8] A GWAS is an approach that involves rapidly scanning markers across the complete sets of DNA, or genomes, of many individuals to find genetic variations associated with a particular disease or trait. Such studies are hypothesis free, as there is no a priori list of candidate genes or SNPs that are being tested.[19] The many tests conducted, however, necessitate stringent thresholds for significance. A $P < 5 \times 10^{-8}$ is the accepted threshold, but it may be lower if multiple traits are tested. According to the latest update of the GWAS catalog, more than 7,000 SNP-trait associations have been reported, covering 17 broad categories of disease and traits. The GWAS results pertaining to diet-related traits are summarized in Table 19.1. Limitations of the early candidate gene approaches become evident in light of recent findings from GWASs, which in most cases identified genetic factors not previously thought of as a priori candidates.

Despite recent progress, SNPs associated with diet-related traits, particularly dietary behaviors, explain very little of trait variance, heritability, or trait variance combined with heritability,[20] a pattern also observed for SNP-disease associations.[21] This partly reflects the complexity of diet, which is further compounded by measurement error as-

Trait	Locus	Candidate Gene or Genes in Region	Reference
Vitamins (plasma/serum)			
Vitamin A, beta carotene	16q23.2	*BCMO1, PKD1L2 - BCO1*	24
Vitamin B-12	5q32	*PRELID2*	25
	6p12.3	*MUT*	26
	10p13	*CUBN*	26, 27
	11q12.1	*MS4A3, TCN1*	25, 27, 28
	13q32.3	*CLYBL*	25
	19p13.3	*FUT6*	25
	19q13.33	*FUT2*	25, 26, 28, 29
Vitamin B-5, pantothenate	2p23.3	*SLC5A6*	30
Vitamin B-6, pyridoxal-phosphate	1p36.12	*ALPL, NBPF3*	26, 27, 29
Vitamin D, 25-hydroxy vitamin D	4q13.3	*GC*	31-34
	11p15.2	*CYP2R1, CALCA, CALCP*	31, 33, 34
	11q13.4	*NADSYN1, DHCR7*	33, 34
	20p11.21	*SSTR4, FOXA2, CYB5AP4*	35
Vitamin E, alpha-tocopherol and response supplementation	11q23.3	*APOA5, BUD13*	24, 36, 37
Vitamin E, alpha-tocopherol	12q24.31	*SCARB1*	36
	19p13.12	*CYP4F2*	36
Minerals (plasma/serum)			
Cadmium	6q13	*CD109*	38
Calcium	2p23.3	*GCKR*	39
	2q37.1	*DGKD*	39
	3q21.1	*CASR*	39-42
	7q11.21	*VKORC1L1, GTF2IP5*	39
	10p14	*GATA3*	39
	11p15.4	*CARS*	39
	13q14.11	*KIAA0564, DGKH*	39
	20q13.2	*CYP24A1*	39
Copper	1p36.32	*CCDC27, DFFB, LRRC47, SMIM1*	43
	1q21.3	*PSMB4, POGZ, SELENBP1*	43
Iron	3q22.1	*TF*	44
	6p22.2	*HFE*	44-46
	7q22.1	*TFR2*	44
	22q12.3	*TMPRSS6*	44, 45, 47
Iron, ferritin	2q32.2	*WDR75, SLC40A1*	44, 48
	6p22.2	*HFE*	44, 45, 49
	9q34.2	*ABO - LCN1P2*	44
	17q22	*TEX14*	44
	22q12.3	*TMPRSS6*	44
Iron, soluble transferrin receptor	6p22.2	*HFE*	49
	11q23.3	*APOA, SIK3, PCSK7*	49
	22q12.3	*TMPRSS6*	49

Table 19.1 Genome-Wide Association Studies of Diet-Related Traits   *(continued)*

Trait	Locus	Candidate Gene or Genes in Region	Reference
Minerals (plasma/serum) (continued)			
Iron, total iron-binding capacity	3q22.1	*TF*	50,51
Iron, total and unsaturated iron-binding capacity	6p22.2	*HFE*	51
Iron, transferrin	2q32.2	*WDR75, SLC40A1*	44
Iron, transferrin and transferrin saturation	3q22.1	*TF*	44-46
Iron, transferrin	3q29	*TFRC*	44
Iron, transferrin and transferrin saturation	6p22.2	*HFE*	44,46
Iron, transferrin	8p22	*NAT2 - PSD3*	44
Iron, transferrin	11p15.3	*ARNTL*	44
Iron, transferrin	11q12.2	*FADS2*	44
Iron, transferrin and transferrin saturation	22q12.3	*TMPRSS6*	44
Iron, transferrin saturation	7q22.1	*TFR2*	44
Magnesium	1q22	*MUC1*	52, 53
	3q26.2	*MDS1, MECOM*	53
	4q21.1	*SHROOM3*	53
	9q21.13	*TRPM6*	53
	11p14.1	*DCDC5*	53
	12q21.33	*ATP2B1, MRPL2P1*	53
Manganese	1p34.1	*RNU5F-1*	38
	4q24	*SLC39A8*	38
Phosphorus	1p36.12	*ALPL, NBPF3*	54
	3q21.1	*CASR, CCDC58, CSTA*	54
	6p21.31	*LEMD2, MLN, ITPR3, IP6K3*	54
	6q23.3	*PDE7B*	54
	12p13.32	*FGF6, RAD51AP1, FGF23*	54
Selenium (and toenail selenium)	5q14.1	*BHMT2, BHMT, DMGDH*	43, 55
Zinc	8q21.2	*CA1, CA2, CA3, CA13*	43
	15q24.2	*SCAMP5, PPCDC*	43
	Xp11.21	*KLF8, ZXDA, ZXDB*	43
Amino acids (plasma/serum)			
Alanine	2p23.3	*GCKR*	30
Arginine	6q23.2	*MED23, ENPP3*	56
Betaine	2q34	*CPS1*	30, 57
	5q14.1	*BHMT, DMGDH, BHMT2*	30, 57, 58
	12p13.33	*SLC6A13, SLC6A12*	30, 58
	21q22.3	*CBS*	30
Glutamine	12q13.3	*GLS2*	30, 59
Glycine	2q34	*CPS1*	30, 58-60
Histidine	4p16.1	*SLC2A9*	30
Leucine	4q22.1	*PPM1K*	30
Lysine	16q22.1	*SLC7A6*	30

Table 19.1 (cont.) Genome-Wide Association Studies of Diet-Related Traits   *(continued)*

Trait	Locus	Candidate Gene or Genes in Region	Reference
Lysine (urine)	19q13.11	*SLC7A9 - CEP89*	60
Phenylalanine	5q35.3	*F12*	61
	12q23.2	*PAH*	29, 58
Proline	22q11.21	*PRODH, DGCR5*	29, 58
Serine	1p12	*PHGDH, ZNF697*	29, 57, 58
	2q34	*CPS1*	29, 58
	7p11.2	*PSPH*	29, 58
Tyrosine	6q21	*SLC22A16, SLC16A10*	29, 58
Valine	4q22.1	*PPM1K*	29
Fatty acids (plasma/serum)			
Alpha-linolenic acid	10q24.2	*SFRP5*	63
	11q12.2	*FADS1, FADS2, FADS3, MYRF*	63, 64
Arachidonic acid	3q13.33	*TMEM39A*	65
	3q23	*PCOLCE2*	64
	11q12.2	*FADS1, FADS2, FADS3, MYRF*	30, 63-65
	16p13.11	*PDXDC1, NTAN1*	65
Delta-6 desaturase activity	11q12.2	*FADS1, FADS2, FADS3, MYRF*	63
Dihomo-gamma-linolenic acid	11q12.2	*FADS1, FADS2, FADS3, MYRF*	63-65
	16p13.11	*PDXDC1, NTAN1*	65
Docosapentaenoic acid (n-3 DPA)	11q12.2	*FADS1, FADS2, FADS3, MYRF*	30, 64
	6p24.2	*SYCP2L, ELOVL2*	64
Docosapentaenoic acid (n-6 DPA)	11q12.2	*FADS1, FADS2, FADS3, MYRF*	30
Docosatetraenoic acid (red blood cells)	11q12.2	*FADS1, FADS2, FADS3, MYRF*	64, 65
Eicosapentaenoic acid (EPA)	11q12.2	*FADS1, FADS2, FADS3, MYRF*	30
Fatty acid 20:0	19p13.2	*LASS4, CERS4*	66
	20p12.1	*SPTLC3*	66
Fatty acid 22:0	19p13.2	*LASS4, CERS4*	66
Fatty acid 24:0	19p13.2	*LASS4, CERS4*	66
Gamma-linolenic acid	11q12.2	*FADS1, FADS2, FADS3, MYRF*	63-65
	11q12.3	*SCGB2A1 - SCGB1D2*	63
	16p13.11	*PDXDC1, NTAN1*	65
Linoleic acid	10q21.3	*JMJD1C, NRBF2, REEP3*	65
	12p13.31	*PHB2, MBOAT5, PTPN6, C1S*	64
	11q12.2	*FADS1, FADS2, FADS3, MYRF*	63-65
	16p13.11	*PDXDC1, NTAN1*	65
Myristoleate	10q24.31	*SCD, PKD2L1*	30
Oleic acid	1q44	*TRIM58*	64
	11q12.2	*FADS1, FADS2, FADS3, MYRF*	64, 67
	12p13.31	*PHB2, MBOAT5, PTPN6, C1S*	64
Palmitic acid	1p21.3	*TMEM56, ALG14, RWDD3, CNN3*	64

Table 19.1 (cont.) Genome-Wide Association Studies of Diet-Related Traits

(*continued*)

Trait	Locus	Candidate Gene or Genes in Region	Reference
Fatty acids (plasma/serum) (continued)			
Palmitoleic acid	2p23.3	ZNF512, XAB1, GCKR	67
	2q21.2	NAP5, NCKAP5	67
	10q24.31	SCD, PKD2L1	30, 60, 67
	11q12.2	FADS1, FADS2, FADS3, MYRF	67
Stearic acid	1p21.3	CNN3, TMEM56, ALG14	67
	1q32.3	LPGAT1	67
	10q24.31	SCD, PKD2L1	30
	11q12.2	FADS1, FADS2, FADS3, MYRF	67
Stearidonic acid	11q12.2	FADS1, FADS2, FADS3, MYRF	30
Trans fatty acid, cis/trans-18:2	11q12.2	FADS1, FADS2, FADS3, MYRF	68
Trans fatty acid, trans/trans-18:2	18q22.1	CDH19, CDH7, DSEL	68
Food-derived metabolites (plasma/serum)			
10-Undecenoate	1p33	CYP4A11	30
3-Phenylpropionate (hydrocinnamate)	16p12.3	ACSM5	30
Advanced glycation end-product levels	6p21.32	AGER, RNF5, NOTCH4	69
Arsenic metabolism (dimethylarsinate % and monomethylarsonate %, urine)	10q24.32	AS3MT, CNNM2	70
Caffeine	7p21.1	AHR	30, 71
	15q24.1	CYP1A1 - CYP1A2	71
Theophylline	15q24.1	CYP1A1 - CYP1A2	71
Campesterol	2p21	ABCG8	72
	9q34.2	ABO	72
Citrate	5p15.2	ANKH	30
	17p13.1	SLC13A5, FBXO39	30
	22q11.21	SLC25A1, GSC2	62
Erythritol	1p33	DMBX1	30
	1p34.1	NASP	30
Lead	9q32	ALAD, BSPRY	73
Lycopene	4q31.1	SETD7	74
Mannose	2p23.3	GCKR	30, 75
Taste and smell			
Odorant perception, beta-ionone	11q12.1	OR5A1 - OR4D6	76
Odorant perception, isobutyraldehyde	2q37.3	NDUFA10, OR6B2	76
Taste perception, caffeine	12p13.2	TAS2R46, PRH1-TAS2R14	77
Taste perception, 6-*n*-propylthiouracil	7q34	TAS2R38, OR9A4	77, 78
Taste perception, quinine	12p13.2	TAS2R31, TAS2R43, PRH1-TAS2R14, TAS2R19	77, 78
Dietary behaviors			
Alcohol consumption	4q23	ADH1B	79
	7q11.22	AUTS2	80
	9q22.1	LOC100129340 - RPSAP49	81
	12q24.11-.13	ALDH2	82-85

Table 19.1 (cont.) Genome-Wide Association Studies of Diet-Related Traits *(continued)*

Trait	Locus	Candidate Gene or Genes in Region	Reference
Alcohol consumption, flushing response	12q24.12	*ALDH2*	85
Alcohol dependence	1p35.2	*NKAIN1, SNRNP40, FABP3, SERINC2*	86
	2q35	*MREG - PECR*	87
	4q23	*ADH1C, ADH1B*	88, 89
	12q24.12	*ALDH2*	85
Alcohol dependence (age at onset)	3q26.1	*SLITRIK3*	90
	5q11.2	*ARL15*	90
	12q23.2	*UTP20*	90
Caffeine consumption	7p21.1	*AHR*	20
	15q24.1	*CYP1A1 - CYP1A2*	20
Coffee consumption	2p23.3	*GCKR*	91
	4	*ABCG2*	91
	7p21.1	*AHR*	91, 92
	7q11.23	*POR*	91
	7q11.23	*MLXIPL*	91
	7q31.1	*LAMB4, NRCAM*	93
	11	*BDNF*	91
	15q24.1	*CYP1A1 - CYP1A2*	91-93
	17q11.2	*EFCAB5, SSH2, CCDC55*	91
White wine liking	6p21.32	*HLA-DOA*	94

Table 19.1 (cont.) Genome-Wide Association Studies of Diet-Related Traits

cribed to assessment within and between populations.[22] In addition, most of the observed associations are in large domains of strong LD in noncoding regions of the genome and so are unlikely the causal variant. Fine mapping and functional gene assessments are necessary to pinpoint the true underlying variant.[23] With few exceptions, the results presented in Table 19.1 are derived from populations of European ancestry and have only been followed up for replication (as opposed to discovery) in other ancestries.

Knowledge of the genetic determinants of diet exposure and response may provide insight into underlying mechanisms and ways to study the potential health effects of diet more comprehensively by taking into consideration gene-diet interactions.

GENE-DIET INTERACTIONS

Most chronic diseases are thought to be a product of the interplay between genetic and environmental factors. The rapid rise in prevalence of some diseases, such as obesity and type 2 diabetes (T2D), cannot be explained by changes in the human genome alone. Susceptibility to disease is partly determined by genetic factors, but a disease-promoting environment will be necessary for its phenotypic expression. For example, Pima Indians have a high predisposition to obesity and T2D compared with other populations. However, Pima Indians living in the restrictive environment of the remote Mexican Sierra Madre Mountains have a much lower prevalence of these diseases than those living in the obesogenic environment of Arizona. Similarly, colorectal cancer rates for Japanese migrants to the United States increase rapidly and surpass the level of the host population.[94] The considerable heterogeneity observed in response to dietary interventions may also reflect a mismatch between genotype and diet rather than being the result of differences in adherence or baseline clinical factors.[96-98]

Several definitions for gene-environment interactions (or gene-diet interactions for the purpose of this chapter) have been proposed. From a biological perspective, interaction between two factors (eg, genotype and dietary intake) has been defined as their coparticipation in the same causal mechanism of disease development.[99] From a statistical perspective, an interaction exists when the joint exposure to two or more factors results in a significantly higher (or lower) number of cases of diseases than the sum of the separate factors, regardless of the biological mechanism.[1,99] This chapter uses the simplest and broadest possible definition of interaction as being two factors that act upon each other,[18] in this case in the modification of disease risk.

Regardless of the definition, the nature of an interaction need also be considered in study design and results interpretation. Interactions generally assume a fan shape or have a crossover effect.[1,100] In the fan-shaped interaction the main effect of both genotype and diet may be present, but the impact of one is far greater in one stratum or extreme of another. In a cross-over interaction, the effect of genotype on outcome in one stratum of the dietary exposure is opposite to that in a second stratum. In some cases, neither the genotype nor the environmental factor has any effect on disease risk in the absence of the other, but when both are present, the interaction increases disease risk. An example of this kind of gene-diet interaction that is well known to registered dietitian nutritionists (RDNs) is phenylketonuria, in which neither the abnormal genotype nor the environmental exposure alone is sufficient to cause mental retardation.[101]

Table 19.2 lists several gene-diet interactions reported in the literature that exemplify known or hypothesized interactions.[102-114] The literature is saturated with hypothesized gene-diet interactions: significant interactions reported but lacking adequate replication. These interactions have the potential to affect a larger number of individuals compared with the known and clinically confirmed interactions, which partly explains their persistence in the literature. Genetic epidemiologic studies have been the most common approach to investigations of gene-diet interactions on disease risk in humans. Such studies apply study designs and statistical techniques similar to those of traditional epidemiology, which were discussed in more detail in Chapters 2 and 7.

STUDY DESIGNS
Observational Studies

The cohort study and the case-control study have been the primary designs used in gene-diet interaction studies of health. Dietary exposure and outcome data are collected from unrelated individuals either prospectively (cohort) or retrospectively (case-control).[115] Genetic information, which is static, is obtained from DNA extracted from blood or buccal cells collected at any time over the course of the study. In a case-control study, individuals are identified and studied according to a single disease outcome. Individuals who have recently been diagnosed with a disease are queried about their past exposure to diet and other risk factors. A matched set of control individuals, usually drawn from the same population, are also enrolled in the study. Two major concerns with case-control studies are recall bias and selection bias.[116,117]

The classic cohort study is a design in which one or more groups of individuals who are free of disease and who vary in exposure to a potential risk factor (eg, dietary intake) are followed over time and examined with respect to the development of (any) disease. Exposure to potential risk factors is therefore assessed before the development of disease. Cohort studies address issues of temporal uncertainty and selection bias but are costly and require long follow-up.[115,117] The nested case-control or case-cohort approach balances the efficiency of a case-control study with the lower recall and selection bias of cohort studies.[117-119] A sample of cohort participants who develop a disease (cases) are matched to other individuals in the cohort who do not develop the disease (controls).

In cross-sectional studies, the outcomes of interest are quantitative traits related to the disease of interest, such as measures of insulin sensitivity (for T2D), cognitive function (for Alzheimer's disease), and body mass index (for obesity). Studying the impact of gene-diet interactions on continuously distributed traits may provide insight to some

Gene Variant Type	Gene Product Function	Dietary Exposure	Associated Disease or Condition	Study Design	References
Known					
Glucose-6-phosphate dehydrogenase (*G6PD*) Missense mutations or in-frame deletions that result in enzyme deficiency	Catalyzes rate-limiting step in the pentose phosphate pathway Helps protect red blood cells from damage and premature destruction	Fava bean consumption	Favism, acute hemolytic anemia	Clinical	102
Phenylalanine hydroxy-lase (*PAH*) Missense mutations that result in enzyme deficiency	Catalyzes rate-limiting step in phenylalanine catabolism	Dietary phenylala-nine	Phenylketonuria, an autosomal recessive inborn error of metabo-lism with a resulting accumulation of phenylalanine to neurotoxic levels	Clinical	103
Lactase (*LCT*) Missense mutations and single-nucleotide polymorphisms (SNPs) that result in deficient or reduced enzyme activity	Has phlorizin hydrolase activity and lactase activity	Dietary lactose	Lactase nonpersis-tence or adult lactose intolerance	Clinical	104
Hypothesized					
Apolipoprotein E (*APOE*)	Essential for the normal catabo-lism of triglyceride-rich lipoprotein constituents	Total fat, total saturated fat	Altered low-density lipoprotein changes in response to dietary fat	Randomized controlled trial	105
Methylenetetrahydrofo-late reductase (*MTHFR*)	Catalyzes the conversion of 5,10-methylenetetrahydrofolate to 5-methyltetrahydrofolate, a co-substrate for homocysteine remethylation to methionine	Low folate status	Occlusive vascular disease, neural tube defects, colon cancer, and acute leukemia	Observational	106
Cytochrome P450 1A2 (*CYP1A2*) SNP that alters enzyme inducibility	Enzyme involved in xenobiotic metabolism Responsible for ~95% of caffeine metabolism	Regular coffee	Myocardial infarction, blood pressure, breast cancer	Observational	107
Transcription factor 7-like 2 (TCF7L2) SNP that *may* associate with *TCF7L2* expression	A high mobility group box-containing transcription factor that plays a key role in the Wnt signaling pathway	Carbohy-drate quality	Type 2 diabetes (T2D)	Observational	108-111
T2D-genetic risk score (GRS) Multiple SNPs with known/unknown function	Multiple functions	Western dietary patterns	T2D	Observational	112
Obesity-GRS Multiple SNPs with known/unknown function	Multiple functions	Sugar-sweetened beverages	Obesity	Observational	113

Table 19.2 Examples of Known and Hypothesized Gene-Diet Interactions ● (*continued*)

Gene Variant Type	Gene Product Function	Dietary Exposure	Associated Disease or Condition	Study Design	References
Insulin receptor substrate 1 (*IRS1*) SNP that reduces basal levels of IRS1 protein and decreases insulin induction of IRS1-associated phosphatidylinositol-3-OH kinase activity	Protein phosphorylated by insulin receptor tyrosine kinase that plays a key role in transmitting signals from the immunoglobulin F-1 receptors to intracellular pathways PI3K / Akt and Erk mitogen-activated protein kinase pathways	2-year weight-loss diets of different macronutrient distribution	Insulin resistance and weight loss	Randomized controlled trial	114

Table 19.2 (cont.) Examples of Known and Hypothesized Gene-Diet Interactions

causal pathway underlying disease that is not adequately captured by studies of overt disease.[116]

Intervention Studies

Intervention studies in the genetics field aim to determine whether response to intervention is modified by participants' genotype. Randomized controlled trials (RCTs) are the gold standard and are generally crossover or parallel arm by design. In a crossover study, each participant receives all test diets in a randomized order. In a parallel-arm design, each participant is assigned at random to only one test diet and therefore different groups of participants receive different test diets. While effective in addressing several biases and potential for drawing causal inferences, RCTs tend to be small and of short duration and thus limited in power to test certain hypothesis.[120] For example, very few assess disease onset as a primary end point. This design shows greater promise for quantitative traits, such as lipid and glucose response to diet.

Most RCTs have evaluated gene-diet interactions via retrospective genotyping of participants in which phenotypic responsiveness to a specific diet or nutrient has already been undertaken. This approach is feasible in studies with large sample sizes and for polymorphisms that are highly prevalent. Another approach is to select participants a priori on the basis of genotype. This requires the investigator to identify candidate genetic polymorphisms and have some knowledge or hypothesis regarding the associated phenotypic response. In studies of this type, individuals are screened for study participation, genotyped for the polymorphism of interest, and then recruited and block randomized to treatment or treatment order by genotype. This design ensures that there is adequate, balanced representation of each genotype, which is especially valuable if the frequency of the polymorphism is low. Very few dietary intervention studies recruit individuals prospectively in order to study specific diet-genotype interactions.[121,122]

STUDY DESIGN CONSIDERATIONS AND CHALLENGES

Besides the limitations of observational and intervention studies that apply to both genetic and nongenetic research, additional considerations unique to genetic studies warrant additional discussion. Many of these concerns hold for studies of genetic main effects (see Table 19.1 on pages 385 to 389) but are especially of concern for studies of gene-diet interactions (see Table 19.2).

Study Power

A major concern in all studies of gene-diet interactions is adequate power, which is largely determined by sample size. The sample size required to study interactions is dependent upon the percentage of the sample exposed to both the main effects (eg, coffee consumption and a particular allele or genotype), the degree of increased risk conferred by each of the main effects separately, and the increased risk conferred by the interaction.[123] In general, to detect an interaction effect of the same magnitude as a postulated main effect always requires an increase in the size of a study by a factor of approximately four, and in some circumstances considerably more.[119,123] Sample-size requirements obviously increase with the number of genetic and dietary factors tested. Therefore, unless a study is specifically designed to test for gene-diet interactions, it is unlikely to have enough power to detect such an interaction.

Meta-analyses of published genetic and epidemiologic studies for main effects are increasingly common. Extending this practice to the existing gene-diet interaction literature is challenging.[124] The likelihood for publication bias and inconsistencies on how diet is assessed and modeled in analyses are especially difficult to address. A powerful alternative to literature-based meta-analyses are de novo interaction meta-analyses that allow harmonization of genetic and dietary factors and outcomes, as well as implementation of a standardized analysis protocol before combining results. The scale and distribution of the dietary exposure in each contributing study as well as the potential time-dependent nature of the gene-diet interaction may also be accounted for in this research setting.[125-127] Only recently have such ambitious studies been executed, and the results are promising.[128-131]

Diet Assessment and Selection

Reasonably uniform diagnostic criteria for disease and accurate genotyping practices have been implemented in recent studies of gene-diet interactions, but these strengths do not compensate for the use of relatively imprecise measures of diet.[132,133] Nutritional biomarkers provide more precise and comprehensive measures of diet intake but also have disadvantages, such as sensitivity, time dependency, and higher cost.[127,134] Behavioral components of dietary intake, which have genetic underpinnings (see Table 19.1, see pages 385 to 389), are also not captured by biomarkers. Most studies have used self-reported dietary intake collected via food frequency questionnaires or dietary recalls. While efficient methods for collecting dietary information

from large population studies, these tools have known biases and limits in precision.[135] Modeling dietary patterns in gene-diet interaction studies is a relatively recent practice and may have important public health relevance and attributable risk implications. However, a biological interpretation of a gene-pattern interaction is difficult if the pattern is composed of a set of heterogeneous foods.

Selecting the Genes

Early gene-diet interaction studies focused on candidate genes and dietary factors assumed to share a biological reaction or pathway and were thus entirely hypothesis driven.[120] Classic examples include genetic polymorphisms in lipoproteins, which are involved in the transport and redistribution of lipids in blood, and their interaction with dietary fat in altering low-density lipoprotein cholesterol.[105] Focusing on SNPs that are on functional pathways in terms of known nutritionally relevant metabolism and focusing on coherent metabolic pathways may allow a causal pathway approach to the interaction of nutritional factors and multiple genetic variations. In the *CYP1A2*-coffee interaction study conducted by Cornelis and colleagues,[107] an increased risk of myocardial infarction was observed only among individuals with the *CYP1A2* genotype corresponding to impaired caffeine metabolism, suggesting that caffeine is the component of coffee (and not factors correlated with the beverage or behavior) contributing to the increased risk.

Recent efforts have focused on genome-wide established disease locuses, regardless of known or unknown function, and dietary factors previously associated with the disease or that may biologically interact with the disease locus of interest. Recognizing the modest risk conferred by each locus and the impact this has on power to detect gene-diet interactions, it is also increasingly common to model susceptibility alleles together as a genetic risk score (GRS). The risk of T2D associated with a T2D-GRS may be attenuated by adopting a Western dietary pattern.[128] The risk of obesity associated with a body mass index GRS is augmented with high sugar-sweetened beverage consumption.[113] These strategies may improve power to detect an interaction and potentially lead to findings of significant relevance to public health but that are difficult to interpret biologically given potentially diverse pathways encompassed by the GRS.[115] Table 19.1 (see pages 385 to 389) presents dozens of new candidate genes worthy of study and thus potential for an optimized revival of candidate gene-diet interaction studies that offer mechanistic insights.

Replication: Protecting Against Type I Error

Most published gene-diet interactions have not been followed up for replication to rule out type I error and to assess generalizability; this has been met with much skepticism. Designing a replication study that is comparable to the original study is challenging in light of the many issues discussed earlier. Inability to replicate may not always be a function of type I error but rather real differences between populations. Publication bias may also contribute to the absence of replication reports. Significant interactions (novel or replication) are more likely to be reported and published than null reports.

PERSONALIZED NUTRITION

There is great enthusiasm to shift the current population-based one-diet-fits-all approach to personalized dietary advice potentially informed by genotype.[136] Several direct-to-consumer genetic testing services already offer consumers individualized advice based on their genetic profiles. Consumer willingness to undergo genetic testing for the purpose of personalized nutrition varies by country and age group but generally ranges between 25% and 45%.[137,138] Nevertheless, the potential ethical, legal, and social impact of individualized nutrition has attracted criticism.[139-141] The readiness of key practitioners in the field to adapt personalized nutrition in the clinic is also a concern.

Whether the scientific evidence is sufficiently strong to offer personalized nutritional advice based on genotypic information is an open question of great debate.[142] There is also limited evidence to suggest that genotype-based dietary advice will motivate appropriate behavior changes and that interventions based on such advice will be more

cost-effective than conventional population-level interventions.[143-146] Table 19.3 summarizes results of various RCTs assessing the impact of genotype-based risk estimates on risk-reducing diet behaviors.[144,147-151,156-158] In many RCTs the genotype-based risk estimate is for a particular disease (eg, diabetes, Alzheimer disease) rather than a nutritional or metabolic state (eg, low vitamin D status, rapid caffeine metabolism). Few studies support behavior modification in light of genetic information.[147,148] Food4Me is the largest (N=1,269) internet-based, personalized nutrition intervention study to date. With regards to dietary change over a period of 6 months, this study supports the effectiveness of a personalized approach (but regardless of genotype).[149] Marteau and colleagues[150] reported that genetic testing had no impact on risk-reducing behavior or perception of control, but participants in whom a mutation for familial hypercholesterolemia was found believed more strongly that their cholesterol levels were controlled by their genetic makeup and less strongly in the efficacy of diet in reducing their cholesterol level than participants in whom no mutation was found or participants with the nongenetic diagnosis. Likewise, Meisel and colleagues[151] reported that adding obesity gene (*FTO*) feedback to weight control advice enhanced readiness to control weight but had no more effect on behavior than weight control alone. Observational studies have also not generally reported significant posttesting diet or other lifestyle changes.[152-155] Recently, Nielsen and colleagues[156] assessed the impacts of genetic testing on health behaviors using customers of 23andMe and Pathway Genomics, two direct-to-consumer genetic testing companies. Web-based surveys administered before and 6 months after genetic testing revealed significant increases in vegetable intake. However, genetic results (ie, increased or decreased cardiometabolic disease risk) were not associated with any specific diet or exercise changes. It is possible that the health behavior changes were a consequence of the service experience, or the decision to pursue genetic testing was part of a broader goal to improve one's health.[155]

In an inventory of direct-to consumer genetic tests sold on the internet, Goddard and colleagues[158] identified a lack of accountability and consensus in recommendations among the service providers. The

Study	Country and Participants	Intervention	Comparison	Outcome	Results
Celis-Morales et al[156]	Germany, Greece, Ireland, Netherlands, Poland, Spain, and the United Kingdom Food4Me (web based) Adults >18 years old	Risk: obesity-related traits Personalized advice on the basis of current weight, diet, physical activity, phenotype, and *FTO* genotype	Risk: no estimate (i) or nongenetic estimated risk of obesity traits (ii, iii) (i) Standard, nonpersonalized dietary and physical activity guidelines (ii) Personalized advice on the basis of current weight, diet, and physical activity (iii) Personalized advice on the basis of current weight, diet, physical activity, phenotype, waist circumference, and blood cholesterol	Changes in obesity-related traits at 3 and 6 months	Changes in adiposity markers were greater in carriers of the *FTO* risk allele vs nonpersonalized group (i) but not vs other personalized groups (ii, iii)
Celis-Morales et al[149]	Germany, Greece, Ireland, Netherlands, Poland, Spain, and the United Kingdom Food4Me (web based) Adults >18 years old	Risk: obesity (*FTO*), n-3 fatty acid intake (*FADS1*), fat intake (*TCF7L2*), saturated fat intake (*APOE*), and folate intake (*MTHFR*) Personalized advice on the basis of current weight, diet, physical activity, phenotype, and genotypes	Risk: no estimate (i) or nongenetic estimated risk of obesity traits (ii, iii) (i) Standard, nonpersonalized dietary and physical activity guidelines (ii) Personalized advice on the basis of current weight, diet, and physical activity (iii) Personalized advice on the basis of current weight, diet, physical activity, phenotype, waist circumference, and blood cholesterol	Changes in dietary intake at 3 and 6 months	Participants randomized to any personalized group (intervention, ii, iii) consumed less red meat, salt, saturated fat, and energy; consumed more folate; and had a higher healthy eating index than those randomized to group (i) No evidence that including phenotypic (iii) or phenotypic + genotypic (intervention) information enhanced effectiveness of personalized advice
Chao et al[144]	United States Individuals with family history of Alzheimer disease	Risk: Alzheimer disease Education session, *APOE* genotype, and individualized lifetime risk estimate	Risk: Alzheimer disease Education session and individualized numeric risk estimate based on family history and sex	Change in diet, exercise, medication use, and vitamin use after 12 months	ε4+ more likely to adopt Alzheimer disease-specific health behavior changes vs ε4- (but not vs comparison group)
Godino et al[157]	United Kingdom Healthy middle-aged adults	Risk: type 2 diabetes (T2D) Genetic testing for T2D-related single-nucleotide polymorphisms	Risk: no estimate (i) or nongenetic estimated risk of T2D (ii) (i) Standard lifestyle advice (ii) Phenotypic testing for T2D risk and standard lifestyle advice	Change in physical activity and diet at 8 weeks	No difference between groups

Table 19.3 Examples of Randomized Controlled Trials Assessing the Impact of Genotype-Based Risk Estimates on Risk-Reducing Dietary Behaviors

(continued)

Study	Country and Participants	Intervention	Comparison	Outcome	Results
Hietaranta-Luoma et al[147]	Finland Healthy individuals	Risk: cardiovascular disease APOE genotype with personalized feedback and additional voluntary medical consultations	No risk estimates General health information on lifestyle and cardiovascular disease risk	Change in fruit and vegetable intake, alcohol consumption, and physical activity at 10 weeks, 6 months, and 12 months	Dietary fat quality improved in ε4+ group vs comparison group (but not vs ε4- group)
Marteau et al[150]	United Kingdom Adults with definite or possible heterozygous familial hypercholesterolemia (FH)	Risk: FH Routine clinical diagnosis of FH, cholesterol results, LDLR genotype feedback, and lifestyle advice	Risk: FH Routine clinical diagnosis of FH, cholesterol results, and lifestyle advice	Change in dietary fat intake, physical activity at 6 months	No difference between groups
Meisel et al[151]	United Kingdom University students	Risk: obesity FTO genotype and weight control advice leaflet	No risk estimates Weight control advice leaflet	Change in diet and physical activity at 1 month	No difference between groups
Nielsen et al[148]	Canada Healthy young adults	Risk: sodium-sensitive hypertension Other: caffeine metabolism, vitamin C utilization, sweet taste perception Genetic tests for caffeine metabolism, vitamin C utilization, sweet taste perception, and sodium sensitivity linked to disease risk with personalized results and dietary recommendations.	No risk estimates Dietary recommendations based on current guidelines	Change in caffeine, vitamin C, added sugars, and sodium intake at 3 and 12 months	At 12 months, participants in the intervention group who possessed a risk version of the ACE gene, and were advised to limit their sodium intake, significantly reduced their sodium intake (mg/day) compared with the control group; those who had the non-risk version of ACE did not significantly change their sodium intake compared with the control group.
Voils et al[158]	United States Veteran outpatients who are overweight/obese	Risk: T2D Genetic testing for diabetes-related genes with personalized feedback, conventional diabetes risk counseling, and brief lifestyle counseling	Risk: T2D Education on age-related macular degeneration, cataracts, and glaucoma; conventional diabetes risk counseling; and brief lifestyle counseling	Change in energy intake and physical activity at 3 and 6 months	No difference between groups

Table 19.3 (cont.) Examples of Randomized Controlled Trials Assessing the Impact of Genotype-Based Risk Estimates on Risk-Reducing Dietary Behaviors

US Government Accountability Office conducted an audit of genetic testing services and reported that the predictions made by such tests can be misleading to consumers and may lead to needless preventive actions when disease risk is believed to be low.[160] Limited understanding of genetics, particularly among those at high disease risk, is a current barrier to the communication of genotype-based risk information.[161] Health care providers might bear the responsibility of explaining such test results to consumers, but they may also lack the required resources or knowledge. RDNs are the ideal candidates to provide advice on nutrition and genetics, but the development of guidelines and research summaries for these professionals is limited. Few articles have reviewed the literature regarding nutrigenetics in an effort to collate the evidence base.[128,162-164] Colson and colleagues[164] assessed the influence of the *MTHFR* genotype on folate status followed by response to supplementation. They concluded that the *MTHFR TT* genotype was associated with increased plasma homocysteine, lowered serum folate levels, and less response to short-term supplementation at levels from 400 µg/d to the upper tolerable limit. Day and colleagues[162] systematically reviewed the literature to assess whether recommendations for zinc intake could be made according to genotype. The data extracted confirmed a connection between genetics and zinc requirements, but the direction and magnitude of the dietary modification for carriers of specific genotypes could not be defined.

Despite inconclusive findings that genotype-based nutrition recommendations are effective, RDNs need to be prepared to appropriately guide their clients, particularly in light of increasing demand and availability of genetic testing services. While nutrition practitioners acknowledge between-individuals variation in response to dietary invention and management, possibly owing to genetics, they lack knowledge and confidence regarding nutrigenetics and genotype-guided nutritional advice.[165] Earlier works discussed needs in terms of training and required knowledge for nutrition practitioners; potential ethical, legal, and social impacts on practice; and other impacts on nutrition.[166-168] Indeed, in a 2014 position paper, the Academy of Nutrition and Dietetics recognized the application of nutrigenetics in providing insight into how diet and genotype interactions affect phenotype.[169] However, the Academy also noted that the use of nutrigenetic testing to provide dietary advice was not ready for routine dietetics practice. RDNs lacked the basic knowledge and skills in genetics for understanding nutrigenetics. Motivated by this position paper, Beretich and colleagues[170] recently determined the extent to which the study of nutritional genomics is incorporated into undergraduate didactic programs in dietetics (DPDs). They concluded that the overall time devoted to genetics education was low and that DPD directors, faculty, and instructors were not adequately trained to provide this education to students enrolled in DPDs.

Issues related to potential discrimination based on genetic profiling, retrospective use of tissue samples, and protections for privacy and confidentiality have also triggered public concern.[171-173] For example, information about disease risk has the potential for discrimination with respect to insurance and employment.[174] In 2008, the Genetic Information Nondiscrimination Act was passed in the United States to protect individuals against discrimination by health insurers and employers in relation to their genetic information.[175] Such measures are important for consumer protection if personalized nutrition is to become widespread practice in public health.

CONCLUSIONS AND FUTURE PERSPECTIVES

Research on gene-diet interactions can greatly improve our understanding of how nutrition factors influence risks for common diseases. If only a subgroup of individuals is sensitive to dietary factors, the effect on disease risk may be diluted, or even undetectable, when the entire population is the focus of study. Continued research in this area will also clarify the underlying mechanisms of many nutritional factors by delineating their biological roles in relation to variations in enzyme activity. The ability to stratify individuals according to genotype has the potential to make clinical trials more cost-effective and time efficient by enrolling a much smaller number of patients with an anticipated larger treatment effect when the intervention is more precisely matched with the underlying altered biology. Eventually, increased knowledge will allow practitioners to target disease-preventing diet interventions to individuals most likely to benefit from diet modification based on their genetic susceptibility.

Despite some progress in characterizing gene-diet interactions underlying disease, there still remain many inconsistencies and significant findings in need of replication or more detailed follow-up. There are also ethical aspects of deciding how to proceed in the face of such uncertainty.[142] Large collaborative successes demonstrate a continued enthusiasm and drive that will undoubtedly fuel additional efforts in future studies of gene-diet interactions. Nutrigenetics represents an exciting and important interdisciplinary research area for RDNs in collaboration with epidemiologists and molecular scientists. However, application of research findings in clinical practice through the use of genetic testing requires that RDNs understand, interpret, and communicate complex test results in which the actual risk of developing a disease may not be known.[169] Toward this end, a standardized curriculum for genetics education in DPDs is much needed.[170] Moreover, to translate genetic information into evidence-based nutritional recommendations, clear summaries and critical analysis of the current evidence base of identified polymorphisms and their interaction with nutrition and health need to be provided.[176] These summaries can then provide the basis for the development of best-practice guidelines for nutrition practitioners to use in clinical practice.[176]

REFERENCES

1. Rothman KJ, Greenland S, Lash TL. *Modern Epidemiology*. 3rd ed. Philadelphia, PA: Lippincott, Williams, & Wilkins; 2008.

2. Fenech M, El-Sohemy A, Cahill L, et al. Nutrigenetics and nutrigenomics: viewpoints on the current status and applications in nutrition research and practice. *J Nutrigenet Nutrigenomics*. 2011;4(2):69-89.

3. Turnpenny PD, Ellard S. *Emery's Elements of Medical Genetics*. 15th ed. New York, NY: Elsevier Health Sciences; 2017.

4. Alberts B, Johnson A, Lewis J, Raff M, Roberts K, Walter P. *Molecular Biology of the Cell*. New York, NY: Garland Science Publishing; 2002.

5. Ezkurdia I, Juan D, Rodriguez JM, et al. Multiple evidence strands suggest that there may be as few as 19 000 human protein-coding genes. *Hum Mol Genet*. 2014;23(22):5866-5878.

6. Cunningham F, Amode MR, Barrell D, et al. Ensembl 2015. *Nucleic Acids Res*. 2015;43(Database issue):D662-D669.

7. Patterson RE, Eaton EL, Potter JP. The genetic revolution: change and challenge for the profession of dietetics. *J Am Diet Assoc*. 1999;99:1412-1420

8. Frazer KA, Murray SS, Schork NJ, Topol EJ. Human genetic variation and its contribution to complex traits. *Nat Rev Genet*. 2009;10(4):241-251.

9. Kruglyak L, Nickerson DA. Variation is the spice of life. *Nat Genet*. 2001;27(3):234-236.

10. Slatkin M. Linkage disequilibrium—understanding the evolutionary past and mapping the medical future. *Nat Rev Genet*. 2008;9(6):477-485.

11. Pe'er I, de Bakker PIW, Maller J, Yelensky R, Altshuler D, Daly MJ. Evaluating and improving power in whole-genome association studies using fixed marker sets. *Nat Genet*. 2006;38(6):663-667.

12. Eberle MA, Ng PC, Kuhn K, et al. Power to detect risk alleles using genome-wide tag SNP panels. *PLoS Genet*. 2007;3(10):1827-1837.

13. Clark AG, Li J. Conjuring SNPs to detect associations. *Nat Genet*. 2007;39(7):815-816.

14. Kimura M. Evolutionary rate at the molecular level. *Nature*. 1968;217(5129):624-626.

15. Malone KE, Daling JR, Thompson JD, O'Brien CA, Francisco LV, Ostrander EA. BRCA1 mutations and breast cancer in the general population: analyses in women before age 35 years and in women before age 45 years with first-degree family history. *JAMA*. 1998;279(12):922-929.

16. Pérusse L, Bouchard C. Gene-diet interactions in obesity. *Am J Clin Nutr*. 2000;72(5):1285s-1290s.

17. Yang A, Palmer AA, de Wit H. Genetics of caffeine consumption and responses to caffeine. *Psychopharmacology*. 2010;211(3):245-257.

18. Barron R, Bermingham K, Brennan L, et al. Twin metabolomics: the key to unlocking complex phenotypes in nutrition research. *Nutr Res*. 2016;36(4):291-304.

19. Altshuler D, Daly M. Guilt beyond a reasonable doubt. *Nat Genet*. 2007;39(7):813-815.

20. Cornelis MC, Monda KL, Yu K, et al. Genome-wide meta-analysis identifies regions on 7p21 (AHR) and 15q24 (CYP1A2) as determinants of habitual caffeine consumption. *PLoS Genet*. 2011;7(4):e1002033.

21. Manolio TA, Collins FS, Cox NJ, et al. Finding the missing heritability of complex diseases. *Nature*. 2009;461(7265):747-753.

22. Agrawal A, Freedman ND, Cheng YC, et al. Measuring alcohol consumption for genomic meta-analyses of alcohol intake: opportunities and challenges. *Am J Clin Nutr*. 2012;95(3):539-547.

23. Grant RW, Moore AF, Florez JC. Genetic architecture of type 2 diabetes: recent progress and clinical implications. *Diabetes Care*. 2009;32(6):1107-1114.

24. Ferrucci L, Perry JR, Matteini A, et al. Common variation in the beta-carotene 15,15'-monooxygenase 1 gene affects circulating levels of carotenoids: a genome-wide association study. *Am J Hum Genet*. 2009;84(2):123-133.

25. Lin X, Lu D, Gao Y, et al. Genome-wide association study identifies novel loci associated with serum level of vitamin B12 in Chinese men. *Hum Mol Genet*. 2012;21(11):2610-2617.

26. Hazra A, Kraft P, Lazarus R, et al. Genome-wide significant predictors of metabolites in the one-carbon metabolism pathway. *Hum Mol Genet*. 2009;18(23):4677-4687.

27. Keene KL, Chen WM, Chen F, et al. Genetic associations with plasma B12, B6, and folate levels in an ischemic stroke population from the Vitamin Intervention for Stroke Prevention (VISP) Trial. *Front Public Health*. 2014;2:112.

28. Hazra A, Kraft P, Selhub J, et al. Common variants of FUT2 are associated with plasma vitamin B12 levels. *Nat Genet*. 2008;40(10):1160-1162.

29. Tanaka T, Scheet P, Giusti B, et al. Genome-wide association study of vitamin B6, vitamin B12, folate, and homocysteine blood concentrations. *Am J Hum Genet*. 2009;84(4):477-482.

30. Shin SY, Fauman EB, Petersen AK, et al. An atlas of genetic influences on human blood metabolites. *Nat Genet*. 2014;46(6):543-550.

31. Anderson D, Holt BJ, Pennell CE, Holt PG, Hart PH, Blackwell JM. Genome-wide association study of vitamin D levels in children: replication in the Western Australian Pregnancy Cohort (Raine) study. *Genes Immun*. 2014;15(8):578-583.

32. Lasky-Su J, Lange N, Brehm JM, et al. Genome-wide association analysis of circulating vitamin D levels in children with asthma. *Hum Genet*. 2012;131(9):1495-1505.

33. Ahn J, Yu K, Stolzenberg-Solomon R, et al. Genome-wide association study of circulating vitamin D levels. *Hum Mol Genet*. 2010;19(13):2739-2745.

34. Wang TJ, Zhang F, Richards JB, et al. Common genetic determinants of vitamin D insufficiency: a genome-wide association study. *Lancet*. 2010;376(9736):180-188.

35. Sapkota BR, Hopkins R, Bjonnes A, et al. Genome-wide association study of 25(OH) vitamin D concentrations in Punjabi Sikhs: results of the Asian Indian diabetic heart study. *J Steroid Biochem Mol Biol*. 2016;158:149-156.

36. Major JM, Yu K, Wheeler W, et al. Genome-wide association study identifies common variants associated with circulating vitamin E levels. *Hum Mol Genet*. 2011;20(19):3876-3883.

37. Major JM, Yu K, Chung CC, et al. Genome-wide association study identifies three common variants associated with serologic response to vitamin E supplementation in men. *J Nutr*. 2012;142(5):866-871.

38. Ng E, Lind PM, Lindgren C, et al. Genome-wide association study of toxic metals and trace elements reveals novel associations. *Hum Mol Genet*. 2015;24(16):4739-4745.

39. O'Seaghdha CM, Wu H, Yang Q, et al. Meta-analysis of genome-wide association studies identifies six new Loci for serum calcium concentrations. *PLoS Genet*. 2013;9(9):e1003796.

40. Vinayagamoorthy N, Yim SH, Jung SH, et al. Association of common variants in the calcium-sensing receptor gene with serum calcium levels in East Asians. *J Hum Genet*. 2015;60(8):407-412.

41. Kapur K, Johnson T, Beckmann ND, et al. Genome-wide meta-analysis for serum calcium identifies significantly associated SNPs near the calcium-sensing receptor (CASR) gene. *PLoS Genet*. 2010;6(7):e1001035.

42. O'Seaghdha CM, Yang Q, Glazer NL, et al. Common variants in the calcium-sensing receptor gene are associated with total serum calcium levels. *Hum Mol Genet*. 2010;19(21):4296-4303.

43. Evans DM, Zhu G, Dy V, et al. Genome-wide association study identifies loci affecting blood copper, selenium and zinc. *Hum Mol Genet*. 2013;22(19):3998-4006.

44. Benyamin B, Esko T, Ried JS, et al. Novel loci affecting iron homeostasis and their effects in individuals at risk for hemochromatosis. *Nat Commun*. 2014;5:4926.

45. Pichler I, Minelli C, Sanna S, et al. Identification of a common variant in the TFR2 gene implicated in the physiological regulation of serum iron levels. *Hum Mol Genet*. 2011;20(6):1232-1240.

46. Benyamin B, McRae AF, Zhu G, et al. Variants in TF and HFE explain approximately 40% of genetic variation in serum-transferrin levels. *Am J Hum Genet.* 2009;84(1): 60-65.

47. Tanaka T, Roy CN, Yao W, et al. A genome-wide association analysis of serum iron concentrations. *Blood.* 2010;115(1):94-96.

48. Liao M, Shi J, Huang L, et al. Genome-wide association study identifies variants in PMS1 associated with serum ferritin in a Chinese population. *PLoS One.* 2014;9(8): e105844.

49. Oexle K, Ried JS, Hicks AA, et al. Novel association to the proprotein convertase PCSK7 gene locus revealed by analysing soluble transferrin receptor (sTfR) levels. *Hum Mol Genet.* 2011;20(5):1042-1047.

50. Li J, Lange LA, Duan Q, et al. Genome-wide admixture and association study of serum iron, ferritin, transferrin saturation and total iron binding capacity in African Americans. *Hum Mol Genet.* 2015;24(2):572-581.

51. McLaren CE, Garner CP, Constantine CC, et al. Genome-wide association study identifies genetic loci associated with iron deficiency. *PLoS One.* 2011;6(3):e17390.

52. Tin A, Kottgen A, Folsom AR, et al. Genetic loci for serum magnesium among African-Americans and gene-environment interaction at MUC1 and TRPM6 in European-Americans: the Atherosclerosis Risk in Communities (ARIC) study. *BMC Genet.* 2015;16:56.

53. Meyer TE, Verwoert GC, Hwang SJ, et al. Genome-wide association studies of serum magnesium, potassium, and sodium concentrations identify six loci influencing serum magnesium levels. *PLoS Genet.* 2010;6(8):e1001045.

54. Kestenbaum B, Glazer NL, Kottgen A, et al. Common genetic variants associate with serum phosphorus concentration. *J Am Soc Nephrol.* 2010;21(7):1223-1232.

55. Cornelis MC, Fornage M, Foy M, et al. Genome-wide association study of selenium concentrations. *Hum Mol Genet.* 2015;24(5):1469-1477.

56. Luneburg N, Lieb W, Zeller T, et al. Genome-wide association study of L-arginine and dimethylarginines reveals novel metabolic pathway for symmetric dimethylarginine. *Circ Cardiovasc Genet.* 2014;7(6):864-872.

57. Hartiala JA, Tang WH, Wang Z, et al. Genome-wide association study and targeted metabolomics identifies sex-specific association of CPS1 with coronary artery disease. *Nat Commun.* 2016;7:10558.

58. Xie W, Wood AR, Lyssenko V, et al. Genetic variants associated with glycine metabolism and their role in insulin sensitivity and type 2 diabetes. *Diabetes.* 2013; 62(6):2141-2150.

59. Draisma HHM, Pool R, Kobl M, et al. Genome-wide association study identifies novel genetic variants contributing to variation in blood metabolite levels. *Nat Commun.* 2015;6:7208.

60. Yu B, Zheng Y, Alexander D, Morrison AC, Coresh J, Boerwinkle E. Genetic determinants influencing human serum metabolome among African Americans. *PLoS Genet.* 2014;10(3):e1004212.

61. Rueedi R, Ledda M, Nicholls AW, et al. Genome-wide association study of metabolic traits reveals novel gene-metabolite-disease links. *PLoS Genet.* 2014;10(2): e1004132.

62. Kettunen J, Tukiainen T, Sarin AP, et al. Genome-wide association study identifies multiple loci influencing human serum metabolite levels. *Nat Genet.* 2012;44(3): 269-276.

63. Dorajoo R, Sun Y, Han Y, et al. A genome-wide association study of n-3 and n-6 plasma fatty acids in a Singaporean Chinese population. *Genes Nutr.* 2015;10(6):53.

64. Tintle NL, Pottala JV, Lacey S, et al. A genome-wide association study of saturated, mono- and polyunsaturated red blood cell fatty acids in the Framingham Heart Offspring Study. *Prostaglandins Leukot Essent Fatty Acids.* 2015;94:65-72.

65. Guan W, Steffen BT, Lemaitre RN, et al. Genome-wide association study of plasma N6 polyunsaturated fatty acids within the cohorts for heart and aging research in genomic epidemiology consortium. *Circ Cardiovasc Genet.* 2014; 7(3):321-331.

66. Lemaitre RN, King IB, Kabagambe EK, et al. Genetic loci associated with circulating levels of very long-chain saturated fatty acids. *J Lipid Res.* 2015;56(1):176-184.

67. Wu JH, Lemaitre RN, Manichaikul A, et al. Genome-wide association study identifies novel loci associated with concentrations of four plasma phospholipid fatty acids in the de novo lipogenesis pathway: results from the Cohorts for Heart and Aging Research in Genomic Epidemiology (CHARGE) consortium. *Circ Cardiovasc Genet.* 2013;6(2): 171-183.

68. Mozaffarian D, Kabagambe EK, Johnson CO, et al. Genetic loci associated with circulating phospholipid trans fatty acids: a meta-analysis of genome-wide association studies from the CHARGE Consortium. *Am J Clin Nutr.* 2015; 101(2):398-406.

69. Maruthur NM, Li M, Halushka MK, et al. Genetics of plasma soluble receptor for advanced glycation end-products and cardiovascular outcomes in a community-based population: results from the atherosclerosis risk in communities study. *PLoS One.* 2015;10(6):e0128452.

70. Pierce BL, Kibriya MG, Tong L, et al. Genome-wide association study identifies chromosome 10q24.32 variants associated with arsenic metabolism and toxicity phenotypes in Bangladesh. *PLoS Genet.* 2012;8(2): e1002522.

71. Cornelis MC, Kacprowski T, Menni C, et al. Genome-wide association study of caffeine metabolites provides new insights to caffeine metabolism and dietary caffeine-consumption behavior. *Hum Mol Genet*. 2016;25(24):5472-5482.

72. Teupser D, Baber R, Ceglarek U, et al. Genetic regulation of serum phytosterol levels and risk of coronary artery disease. *Circ Cardiovasc Genet*. 2010;3(4):331-339.

73. Warrington NM, Zhu G, Dy V, et al. Genome-wide association study of blood lead shows multiple associations near ALAD. *Hum Mol Genet*. 2015;24(13):3871-3879.

74. D'Adamo CR, D'Urso A, Ryan KA, et al. A common variant in the SETD7 gene predicts serum lycopene concentrations. *Nutrients*. 2016;8(2):82.

75. Korostishevsky M, Steves CJ, Malkin I, Spector T, Williams FM, Livshits G. Genomics and metabolomics of muscular mass in a community-based sample of UK females. *Eur J Hum Genet*. 2016;24(2):277-283.

76. McRae JF, Jaeger SR, Bava CM, et al. Identification of regions associated with variation in sensitivity to food-related odors in the human genome. *Curr Biol*. 2013;23(16):1596-1600.

77. Ledda M, Kutalik Z, Souza Destito MC, et al. GWAS of human bitter taste perception identifies new loci and reveals additional complexity of bitter taste genetics. *Hum Mol Genet*. 2014;23(1):259-267.

78. Reed DR, Zhu G, Breslin PA, et al. The perception of quinine taste intensity is associated with common genetic variants in a bitter receptor cluster on chromosome 12. *Hum Mol Genet*. 2010;19(21):4278-4285.

79. Kapoor M, Wang JC, Wetherill L, et al. A meta-analysis of two genome-wide association studies to identify novel loci for maximum number of alcoholic drinks. *Hum Genet*. 2013;132(10):1141-1151.

80. Schumann G, Coin LJ, Lourdusamy A, et al. Genome-wide association and genetic functional studies identify autism susceptibility candidate 2 gene (AUTS2) in the regulation of alcohol consumption. *Proc Natl Acad Sci U S A*. 2011;108(17):7119-7124.

81. Adkins DE, Clark SL, Copeland WE, et al. Genome-wide meta-analysis of longitudinal alcohol consumption across youth and early adulthood. *Twin Res Hum Genet*. 2015;18(4):335-347.

82. Baik I, Cho NH, Kim SH, Han BG, Shin C. Genome-wide association studies identify genetic loci related to alcohol consumption in Korean men. *Am J Clin Nutr*. 2011;93(4):809-816.

83. Takeuchi F, Isono M, Nabika T, et al. Confirmation of ALDH2 as a major locus of drinking behavior and of its variants regulating multiple metabolic phenotypes in a Japanese population. *Circ J*. 2011;75(4):911-918.

84. Yang X, Lu X, Wang L, et al. Common variants at 12q24 are associated with drinking behavior in Han Chinese. *Am J Clin Nutr*. 2013;97(3):545-551.

85. Quillen EE, Chen XD, Almasy L, et al. ALDH2 is associated to alcohol dependence and is the major genetic determinant of "daily maximum drinks" in a GWAS study of an isolated rural Chinese sample. *Am J Med Genet B Neuropsychiatr Genet*. 2014;165B(2):103-110.

86. Zuo L, Wang K, Zhang XY, et al. NKAIN1-SERINC2 is a functional, replicable and genome-wide significant risk gene region specific for alcohol dependence in subjects of European descent. *Drug Alcohol Depend*. 2013;129(3):254-264.

87. Treutlein J, Cichon S, Ridinger M, et al. Genome-wide association study of alcohol dependence. *Arch Gen Psychiatry*. 2009;66(7):773-784.

88. Frank J, Cichon S, Treutlein J, et al. Genome-wide significant association between alcohol dependence and a variant in the ADH gene cluster. *Addict Biol*. 2012;17(1):171-180.

89. Park BL, Kim JW, Cheong HS, et al. Extended genetic effects of ADH cluster genes on the risk of alcohol dependence: from GWAS to replication. *Hum Genet*. 2013;132(6):657-668.

90. Kapoor M, Wang JC, Wetherill L, et al. Genome-wide survival analysis of age at onset of alcohol dependence in extended high-risk COGA families. *Drug Alcohol Depend*. 2014;142:56-62.

91. Coffee and Caffeine Genetics Consortium, Cornelis MC, Byrne EM, et al. Genome-wide meta-analysis identifies six novel loci associated with habitual coffee consumption. *Mol Psychiatry*. 2015;20(5):647-656.

92. Sulem P, Gudbjartsson DF, Geller F, et al. Sequence variants at CYP1A1-CYP1A2 and AHR associate with coffee consumption. *Hum Mol Genet*. 2011;20(10):2071-2077.

93. Amin N, Byrne E, Johnson J, et al. Genome-wide association analysis of coffee drinking suggests association with CYP1A1/CYP1A2 and NRCAM. *Mol Psychiatry*. 2012;17(11):1116-1129.

94. Pirastu N, Kooyman M, Traglia M, et al. Genome-wide association analysis on five isolated populations identifies variants of the HLA-DOA gene associated with white wine liking. *Eur J Hum Genet*. 2015;23(12):1717-1722.

95. Marchand LL. Combined influence of genetic and dietary factors on colorectal cancer incidence in Japanese Americans. *J Natl Cancer Inst Monogr*. 1998;(26):101-105.

96. Bouchard C, Rankinen T. Individual differences in response to regular physical activity. *Med Sci Sports Exerc*. 2001;33(6 suppl):S446-S451; discussion S452-443.

97. Booth FW, Lees SJ. Fundamental questions about genes, inactivity, and chronic diseases. *Physiol Genomics.* 2007; 28(2):146-157.

98. Franks PW. Gene × environment interactions in type 2 diabetes. *Curr Diab Rep.* 2011;11(6):552-561.

99. Yang Q, Khoury MJ. Evolving methods in genetic epidemiology. III. Gene-environment interaction in epidemiologic research. *Epidemiol Rev.* 1997;19(1):33-43.

100. Dick DM. Gene-environment interaction in psychological traits and disorders. *Annu Rev Clin Psychol.* 2011;7:383-409.

101. Al Hafid N, Christodoulou J. Phenylketonuria: a review of current and future treatments. *Transl Pediatr.* 2015;4(4):304-317.

102. Howes RE, Battle KE, Satyagraha AW, Baird JK, Hay SI. G6PD deficiency: global distribution, genetic variants and primaquine therapy. *Adv Parasitol.* 2013;81:133-201.

103. Blau N. Genetics of phenylketonuria: then and bow. *Hum Mutat.* 2016;37(6):508-515.

104. Swallow DM. Genetics of lactase persistence and lactose intolerance. *Annu Rev Genet.* 2003;37(1):197-219.

105. Ordovas JM, Lopez-Miranda J, Mata P, Perez-Jimenez F, Lichtenstein AH, Schaefer EJ. Gene-diet interaction in determining plasma lipid response to dietary intervention. *Atherosclerosis.* 1995;118(suppl):S11-S27.

106. Sharp L, Little J. Polymorphisms in genes involved in folate metabolism and colorectal neoplasia: a HuGE review. *Am J Epidemiol.* 2004;159(5):423-443.

107. Cornelis MC, El-Sohemy A, Kabagambe EK, Campos H. Coffee, CYP1A2 genotype, and risk of myocardial infarction. *JAMA.* 2006;295(10):1135-1141.

108. Cornelis MC, Qi L, Kraft P, Hu FB. TCF7L2, dietary carbohydrate, and risk of type 2 diabetes in US women. *Am J Clin Nutr.* 2009;89(4):1256-1262.

109. Hindy G, Sonestedt E, Ericson U, et al. Role of TCF7L2 risk variant and dietary fibre intake on incident type 2 diabetes. *Diabetologia.* 2012;55(10):2646-2654.

110. Fisher E, Boeing H, Fritsche A, Doering F, Joost HG, Schulze MB. Whole-grain consumption and transcription factor-7-like 2 (TCF7L2) rs7903146: gene-diet interaction in modulating type 2 diabetes risk. *Br J Nutr.* 2009;101(4):478-481.

111. Wirstrom T, Hilding A, Gu HF, Ostenson CG, Bjorklund A. Consumption of whole grain reduces risk of deteriorating glucose tolerance, including progression to prediabetes. *Am J Clin Nutr.* 2013;97(1):179-187.

112. Qi L, Cornelis MC, Zhang C, van Dam RM, Hu FB. Genetic predisposition, Western dietary pattern, and the risk of type 2 diabetes in men. *Am J Clin Nutr.* 2009;89(5):1453-1458.

113. Qi Q, Chu AY, Kang JH, et al. Sugar-sweetened beverages and genetic risk of obesity. *N Engl J Med.* 2012;367(15):1387-1396.

114. Qi Q, Bray GA, Smith SR, Hu FB, Sacks FM, Qi L. Insulin receptor substrate 1 gene variation modifies insulin resistance response to weight-loss diets in a 2-year randomized trial: the Preventing Overweight Using Novel Dietary Strategies (POUNDS LOST) trial. *Circulation.* 2011;124(5):563-571.

115. Dempfle A, Scherag A, Hein R, Beckmann L, Chang-Claude J, Schafer H. Gene-environment interactions for complex traits: definitions, methodological requirements and challenges. *Eur J Hum Genet.* 2008;16(10):1164-1172.

116. Wareham NJ, Franks PW, Harding AH. Establishing the role of gene-environment interactions in the etiology of type 2 diabetes. *Endocrinol Metab Clin North Am.* 2002;31(3):553-566.

117. Hunter DJ. Gene-environment interactions in human diseases. *Nat Rev Genet.* 2005;6(4):287-298.

118. Clayton D, McKeigue PM. Epidemiological methods for studying genes and environmental factors in complex diseases. *Lancet.* 2001;358(9290):1356-1360.

119. Thomas D. Gene–environment-wide association studies: emerging approaches. *Nat Rev Genet.* 2010;11(4):259-272.

120. Franks PW, Mesa JL, Harding AH, Wareham NJ. Gene-lifestyle interaction on risk of type 2 diabetes. *Nutr Metab Cardiovasc Dis.* 2007;17(2):104-124.

121. Eisenach JH, Schroeder DR, Pike TL, et al. Dietary sodium restriction and β2-adrenergic receptor polymorphism modulate cardiovascular function in humans. *J Physiol.* 2006;574(3):955-965.

122. Meplan C, Crosley LK, Nicol F, et al. Genetic polymorphisms in the human selenoprotein P gene determine the response of selenoprotein markers to selenium supplementation in a gender-specific manner (the SELGEN study). *FASEB J.* 2007;21(12):3063-3074.

123. Smith PG, Day NE. The design of case-control studies: the influence of confounding and interaction effects. *Int J Epidemiol.* 1984;13(3):356-365.

124. Palla L, Higgins JP, Wareham NJ, Sharp SJ. Challenges in the use of literature-based meta-analysis to examine gene-environment interactions. *Am J Epidemiol.* 2010;171(11):1225-1232.

125. Bookman EB, McAllister K, Gillanders E, et al. Gene-environment interplay in common complex diseases: forging an integrative model-recommendations from an NIH workshop. *Genet Epidemiol.* 2011;35(4):217-225.

126. Moore SC, Gunter MJ, Daniel CR, et al. Common genetic variants and central adiposity among Asian-Indians. *Obesity (Silver Spring).* 2012;20(9):1902-1908.

127. Cornelis MC, Hu FB. Gene-environment interactions in the development of type 2 diabetes: recent progress and continuing challenges. *Annu Rev Nutr.* 2012;32:245-259.

128. Kanoni S, Nettleton JA, Hivert MF, et al. Total zinc intake may modify the glucose-raising effect of a zinc transporter (SLC30A8) variant: a 14-cohort meta-analysis. *Diabetes.* 2011;60(9):2407-2416.

129. Nettleton JA, McKeown NM, Kanoni S, et al. Interactions of dietary whole-grain intake with fasting glucose- and insulin-related genetic loci in individuals of European descent: a meta-analysis of 14 cohort studies. *Diabetes Care.* 2010;33(12):2684-2691.

130. Kilpelainen TO, Qi L, Brage S, et al. Physical activity attenuates the influence of FTO variants on obesity risk: a meta-analysis of 218,166 adults and 19,268 children. *PLoS Med.* 2011;8(11):e1001116.

131. Scott RA, Chu AY, Grarup N, et al. No interactions between previously associated 2-hour glucose gene variants and physical activity or BMI on 2-hour glucose levels. *Diabetes.* 2012;61(5):1291-1296.

132. Wild CP. The exposome: from concept to utility. *Int J Epidemiol.* 2012;41(1):24-32.

133. Moffitt TE, Caspi A, Rutter M. Strategy for investigating interactions between measured genes and measured environments. *Arch Gen Psychiatry.* 2005;62(5):473-481.

134. Martin Sanchez F, Gray K, Bellazzi R, Lopez-Campos G. Exposome informatics: considerations for the design of future biomedical research information systems. *J Am Med Inform Assoc.* 2014;21(3):386-390.

135. Willett WC. *Nutritional Epidemiology.* New York: Oxford University Press; 1998.

136. Darnton-Hill I, Margetts B, Deckelbaum R. Public health nutrition and genetics: implications for nutrition policy and promotion. *Proc Nutr Soc.* 2004;63(1):173-185.

137. Stewart-Knox BJ, Bunting BP, Gilpin S, et al. Attitudes toward genetic testing and personalised nutrition in a representative sample of European consumers. *Br J Nutr.* 2009;101(7):982-989.

138. Ronteltap A, van Trijp JC, Renes RJ. Consumer acceptance of nutrigenomics-based personalised nutrition. *Br J Nutr.* 2009;101(1):132-144.

139. Bergmann MM, Bodzioch M, Bonet ML, Defoort C, Lietz G, Mathers JC. Bioethics in human nutrigenomics research: European Nutrigenomics Organisation workshop report. *Br J Nutr.* 2006;95(5):1024-1027.

140. Gorman U. Ethical issues raised by personalized nutrition based on genetic information. *Genes Nutr.* 2006;1(1):13-22.

141. Janssens ACJW, Gwinn M, Bradley LA, Oostra BA, van Duijn CM, Khoury MJ. A critical appraisal of the scientific basis of commercial genomic profiles used to assess health risks and personalize health interventions. *Am J Hum Genet* 2008;82(3):593-599.

142. Görman U, Mathers JC, Grimaldi KA, Ahlgren J, Nordström K. Do we know enough? A scientific and ethical analysis of the basis for genetic-based personalized nutrition. *Genes Nutr.* 2013;8(4):373-381.

143. Marteau T, Senior V, Humphries SE, et al. Psychological impact of genetic testing for familial hypercholesterolemia within a previously aware population: a randomized controlled trial. *Am J Med Genet Part A.* 2004;128(3):285-293.

144. Chao S, Roberts JS, Marteau TM, Silliman R, Cupples LA, Green RC. Health behavior changes after genetic risk assessment for Alzheimer disease: the REVEAL Study. *Alzheimer Dis Assoc Disord.* 2008;22(1):94-97.

145. Hall WD, Mathews R, Morley KI. Being more realistic about the public health impact of genomic medicine. *PLoS Med.* 2010;7(10):e1000347.

146. Marteau TM, French DP, Griffin SJ, et al. Effects of communicating DNA-based disease risk estimates on risk-reducing behaviours. *Cochrane Database Syst Rev.* 2010;(10):CD007275.

147. Hietaranta-Luoma HL, Tahvonen R, Iso-Touru T, Puolijoki H, Hopia A. An intervention study of individual, apoE genotype-based dietary and physical-activity advice: impact on health behavior. *J Nutrigenet Nutrigenomics.* 2014;7(3):161-174.

148. Nielsen DE, El-Sohemy A. Disclosure of genetic information and change in dietary intake: a randomized controlled trial. *PLoS One.* 2014;9(11):e112665.

149. Celis-Morales C, Livingstone KM, Marsaux CF, et al. Effect of personalized nutrition on health-related behaviour change: evidence from the Food4me European randomized controlled trial. *Int J Epidemiol.* 2016:2017;46(2):578-588.

150. Marteau T, Senior V, Humphries SE, et al. Psychological impact of genetic testing for familial hyper-cholesterolemia within a previously aware population: a randomized controlled trial. *Am J Med Genet Part A.* 2004;128A(3):285-293.

151. Meisel SF, Beeken RJ, van Jaarsveld CH, Wardle J. Genetic susceptibility testing and readiness to control weight: results from a randomized controlled trial. *Obesity (Silver Spring).* 2015;23(2):305-312.

152. Bloss CS, Schork NJ, Topol EJ. Effect of direct-to-consumer genomewide profiling to assess disease risk. *N Engl J Med.* 2011;364(6):524-534.

153. Bloss CS, Wineinger NE, Darst BF, Schork NJ, Topol EJ. Impact of direct-to-consumer genomic testing at long term follow-up. *J Med Genet.* 2013;50(6):393-400.

154. Kaufman DJ, Bollinger JM, Dvoskin RL, Scott JA. Risky business: risk perception and the use of medical services among customers of DTC personal genetic testing. *J Genet Couns.* 2012;21(3):413-422.

155. Nielsen DE, Carere DA, Wang C, Roberts JS, Green RC, Group PGS. Diet and exercise changes following direct-to-consumer personal genomic testing. *BMC Med Genomics.* 2017;10(1):24.

156. Celis-Morales C, Marsaux CF, Livingstone KM, et al. Can genetic-based advice help you lose weight? Findings from the Food4Me European randomized controlled trial. *Am J Clin Nutr.* 2017;105(5):1204-1213.

157. Godino JG, van Sluijs EM, Marteau TM, Sutton S, Sharp SJ, Griffin SJ. Lifestyle advice combined with personalized estimates of genetic or phenotypic risk of type 2 diabetes, and objectively measured physical activity: a randomized controlled trial. *PLoS Med.* 2016;13(11):e1002185.

158. Voils CI, Coffman CJ, Grubber JM, et al. Does type 2 diabetes genetic testing and counseling reduce modifiable risk factors? A randomized controlled trial of veterans. *J Gen Intern Med.* 2015;30(11):1591-1598.

159. Goddard KA, Robitaille J, Dowling NF, et al. Health-related direct-to-consumer genetic tests: a public health assessment and analysis of practices related to Internet-based tests for risk of thrombosis. *Public Health Genomics.* 2009;12(2):92-104.

160. Nutrigenetic Testing: Tests Purchased from Four Web sites Mislead Consumers. Testimony before the Special Committee on Aging, US Senate. Statement of Gregory Kutz, Managing Director Forensic Audits and Special Investigations. GAO-06-977T. Washington, DC: US Government Accountability Office; 2006.

161. McBride CM, Koehly LM, Sanderson SC, Kaphingst KA. The behavioral response to personalized genetic information: will genetic risk profiles motivate individuals and families to choose more healthful behaviors? *Annu Rev Public Health.* 2010;31:89-103.

162. Day KJ, Adamski MM, Dordevic AL, Murgia C. Genetic variations as modifying factors to dietary zinc requirements—a systematic review. *Nutrients.* 2017;9(2). E148.

163. Shaghaghi MA, Kloss O, Eck P. Genetic variation in human vitamin C transporter genes in common complex diseases. *Adv Nutr.* 2016;7(2):287-298.

164. Colson NJ, Naug HL, Nikbakht E, Zhang P, McCormack J. The impact of MTHFR 677 C/T genotypes on folate status markers: a meta-analysis of folic acid intervention studies. *Eur J Nutr.* 2017;56(1):247-260.

165. Collins J, Bertrand B, Hayes V, et al. The application of genetics and nutritional genomics in practice: an international survey of knowledge, involvement and confidence among dietitians in the US, Australia and the UK. *Genes Nutr.* 2013;8(6):523-533.

166. DeBusk R. Diet-related disease, nutritional genomics, and food and nutrition professionals. *J Am Diet Assoc.* 2009;109(3):410-413.

167. DeBusk RM, Fogarty CP, Ordovas JM, Kornman KS. Nutritional genomics in practice: where do we begin? *J Am Diet Assoc.* 2005;105(4):589-598.

168. Rosen R, Earthman C, Marquart L, Reicks M. Continuing education needs of registered dietitians regarding nutrigenomics. *J Am Diet Assoc.* 2006;106(8):1242-1245.

169. Camp KM, Trujillo E. Position of the Academy of Nutrition and Dietetics: nutritional genomics. *J Acad Nutr Diet.* 2014;114(2):299-312.

170. Beretich K, Pope J, Erickson D, Kennedy A. Amount of genetics education is low among didactic programs in dietetics. *J Allied Health.* 2017;46(4):262-268.

171. Chadwick R. Nutrigenomics, individualism and public health. *Proc Nutr Soc.* 2004;63(1):161-166.

172. Godard B, Schmidtke J, Cassiman JJ, Ayme S. Data storage and DNA banking for biomedical research: informed consent, confidentiality, quality issues, ownership, return of benefits. A professional perspective. *Eur J Hum Genet.* 2003;11(suppl 2):S88-S122.

173. Sterling R, Henderson GE, Corbie-Smith G. Public willingness to participate in and public opinions about genetic variation research: a review of the literature. *Am J Public Health.* 2006;96(11):1971-1978.

174. Reilly PR, Debusk RM. Ethical and legal issues in nutritional genomics. *J Am Diet Assoc.* 2008;108(1):36-40.

175. National Human Genome Research Institute. Genetic Information Nondiscrimination Act of 2008: Information for Researchers and Health Care Providers. www.genome.gov/24519851/. Reviewed March 15, 2012. Accessed December 2016.

176. Murgia C, Adamski MM. Translation of nutritional genomics into nutrition practice: the next step. *Nutrients.* 2017;9(4):366.

Chapter 20

Behavior Change Theory–Based Dietary Research

Geoffrey W. Greene, PhD, RD, LDN | *Colleen A. Redding, PhD* |
Miryam Yusufov, PhD | *Jade McNamara, PhD*

LEARNING OBJECTIVES

1. Describe the importance of theory-based research.

2. Define behavior change theory constructs and how to use theories in research.

3. Distinguish among major behavior change theories used in nutrition research.

4. Describe the major constructs, strengths, and limitations of the social cognitive theory and transtheoretical model.

This chapter discusses the importance of behavior change theory–based research, provides guidelines on using theories in nutrition research, and describes the practical aspects of conducting research based on commonly used behavior change theories. The material is only an introduction to these behavioral theories and is not intended as a comprehensive review[1]; interested readers are encouraged to seek out cited sources for more details and for specific measures. The health belief model and theory of reasoned action/planned behavior are discussed only briefly here because they are extensively reviewed elsewhere in the literature[2] and are less commonly used for nutrition interventions.[3-5] The two more relevant theories focused on here, social cognitive theory and the transtheoretical model, are discussed in greater depth to provide researchers and clinicians with a better understanding of how to apply them in diet and health intervention research. Each section defines relevant theory-specific concepts or constructs in greater detail.

IMPORTANCE OF BEHAVIOR THEORY–BASED RESEARCH

According to Kerlinger, theory is "a set of interrelated constructs (concepts), definitions, and propositions that present a systematic view of phenomena by specifying relations among variables, with the purpose of explaining or predicting phenomena."[6,7] Theory describes how attitudes and beliefs related to diet and health influence behavior and behavior change. Theory guides the choice of variables/constructs and intervention strategies. Theories consist of a set of variables or constructs in clearly specified and testable relationships.[6,8] Research based on a theory involves using these specified relationships to guide choices regarding variables that are measured and, depending on the study design, using interventions designed to affect those variables.[9] Describing these mechanisms and relationships clearly is necessary for behavioral science to advance. Behavior theory–based research guides an orderly investigation of these mechanisms and relationships, which results in a better understanding of the process of behavior change, including changes in dietary and lifestyle behaviors.

It is important to distinguish between theories and planning models, such as PRECEDE-PROCEED[10] and social marketing,[11] or intervention techniques, such as motivational interviewing.[12] Planning models are like recipes: they provide step-by-step instructions about developing interventions. Techniques are similar to cooking skills: they are necessary to implement the recipes. However, theories provide the why; analogous to food science, they explain the mechanisms of behavior change.

By increasing understanding of the basic mechanisms and one's ability to influence important dietary outcomes, behavior change theory–based research has the potential to increase the efficiency and efficacy of interventions for both individuals and populations. A National Cancer Institute monograph stated, "Interventions based on health behavior theory are not guaranteed to succeed, but they are much more likely to produce the desired outcomes."[13] One meta-analysis found good evidence across many studies that theory-based research showed stronger effects.[14] This potential exists in qualitative research, where theory guides a starting place and a framework for qualitative designs (which may generate new or revised theories),[15] and in quantitative research, where theory guides the selection of validated instruments measuring key variables associated with behavior change.[6,9] Thus, researchers and clinicians can avoid reinventing the wheel. Properly conducted theory-based research produces meaningful results, both positive and negative, as well as study findings that are more easily interpretable. Theory-based research facilitates grant funding, approval of a thesis, and the publication of research results.[13,14]

Most theories used in nutrition have been applied to behavior change for health promotion. However, these theories may be applied to behavior change in clinical nutrition and nutrition management situations as well. The health belief model (HBM), for example, has defined *perceived severity* (see the HBM section for more on this construct) as a key variable predicting change. Using this example, if a patient does not believe his "touch of sugar/diabetes" is likely to affect his health, he will not be motivated to change his diet. Increasing this patient's awareness of his risk for diabetes complications and, thus, his perceived severity, may increase his motivation to change.

GUIDELINES FOR APPLYING THEORIES IN RESEARCH

Theories lay out the big picture, much like a map; they are defined in terms of constructs and relationships between constructs. For example, the HBM

Theory	Constructs		
	Self-efficacy	*Benefits*	*Barriers*
Health Belief Model	[a]	Perceived benefits	Perceived barriers
Theory of Reasoned Action/ Planned Behavior	Perceived behavior control[a]	Positive attitudes toward behavior	Negative attitudes toward behavior
Social Cognitive Theory	Self-efficacy	Positive outcome expectancies	Negative outcome expectancies
Transtheoretical Model	Confidence/temptation	Pros	Cons

Table 20.1 Similarities Across Key Constructs by Behavior Change Theory[b]

[a] Although not part of the original theory, some researchers added this construct later.
[b] This table lists the names of the comparable constructs across these four theories of behavior change.

postulates that people change those behaviors that are threatening if the perceived benefits are greater than the perceived barriers or costs of change. Perceived benefits and barriers are key constructs in this and other models (see Table 20.1).

Constructs are abstract concepts that cannot be measured directly. However, for application in research, these constructs need to be made concrete by choosing variables that reflect the construct and can be measured or operationalized. Including at least three to five items that are highly correlated provides an internally consistent and relatively stable measure of a construct, provided that expert opinion has determined that the set of items is a valid representation of the construct.[16] Constructs should be measured using reliable, validated instruments, and the instruments should be selected or developed and tested with the target population prior to the study.[17] Interested readers are encouraged to read more on selecting and measuring constructs in the health behavior area.[16] Each theory includes several similar constructs (see Table 20.1), as well as some unique and distinct constructs. The HBM includes perceived risk and perceived severity as unique constructs. The theory of reasoned action/planned behavior includes perceived norms as a unique construct. Social cognitive theory (SCT) includes reciprocal determinism as a unique construct. The transtheoretical model (TTM) includes stages of change and processes of change as unique constructs. Each of these constructs is described in more detail in its respective theory-specific section.

How to Choose a Theory

The first step in choosing a theory is to search the research literature and choose the most clearly specified research (well developed and with valid measures and interventions) in the nutrition area closest to the area for the planned intervention, with the population closest to the target population, and with the most impressive results. The next step is to define the research question in testable terms related to the theory (eg, the intervention will test the efficacy of a theory-based intervention, the survey will assess key constructs of a theory, or the study will develop/validate instruments measuring constructs). The third step is to clearly define specific and measureable primary and secondary dependent variables (eg, percentage of energy from saturated fat, number of cups of fruits and vegetables per day, body mass index or hemoglobin A1c). Key dependent variables are called *primary outcome variables*. In addition to primary outcome variables, the researcher can use theoretical constructs as intermediate or secondary outcome variables. Thus, even if the primary outcome goal of dietary change is not attained, the researcher can identify change in intermediate or secondary outcomes (eg, an increase in motivational readiness to change). A fourth step is to define the independent variables, which usually reflect the group assignment (eg, exposure or intervention group vs assessment-only control or standard care comparison group). The final step for experimental studies is to determine the expected effect size (amount of change in the primary dependent variable due to the

Effect size is a quantitative index of the strength of an observed phenomenon, in this case the difference between two groups. Other effect size estimates are also possible. Cohen used the following standardized differences between groups to reflect levels of effect size[18,19]:

0.2=small
0.5=medium
0.8=large

Box 20.1 Effect Size

independent variable; see Box 20.1) in order to conduct statistical power calculations for estimating sample size.[18] There are several ways to estimate effect size, which will not be summarized here; however, interested readers could examine other research for more detail.[18,19] In general, previous studies based on the theory can provide an estimate of the effect size.[20]

In addition to outcome analyses that examine the efficacy of a theory-based treatment group, an investigator can also conduct correlational analyses, for example, in a cross-sectional study, examining the relationships between constructs. Important research findings can emerge even when the primary dietary or health-related goal or outcome was not achieved. Thus, a study may examine mediators,[21] or intermediate variables, that influence the outcome variable; for example, self-efficacy has been shown to mediate changes in dietary behaviors.[17] Using a similar strategy, researchers could also identify moderators, that is, group differences based on demographic or other grouping variables (eg, dietary restraint), that relate to the outcome of interest. Interested readers are referred to more detailed texts for additional information on these procedures.[21] Such studies can be quite valuable, even in the absence of primary outcome findings. Investigators can also conduct process-to-outcome analyses looking at the proportion of the variance in the dependent variable that can be explained by a construct. Cohen[18] defined a large effect in the behavioral sciences as one explaining at least 14% of the variance in the out-

come. Percent variance accounted for is a different effect size estimate than the standardized effect size shown in Box 20.1; see Cohen[18] and Cohen[19] for more details about effect sizes. It is, however, difficult to detect large effects in dietary interventions because the lack of precision in assessing dietary intake usually attenuates the effect size meaning the concept may require modification of the research cycle (see Figure 20.1).[22] Nevertheless, from a public health perspective, even a relatively small change in diet can have enormous economic and public health significance when applied to a large population. Oster and Thompson,[23] for example, estimated that decreasing energy intake from saturated fat by 1% in the US population would reduce the incidence of cardiac events by 32,000 per year for a savings of $4.1 billion.

USING MAJOR BEHAVIOR CHANGE THEORIES
Health Belief Model

The first theory in health behavior was the HBM,[24] which was developed more than four decades ago, with the original intention of explaining why many people were not participating in public health programs, such as vaccination campaigns.[25] The HBM is focused on subjective perceptions, rather than objective reality and hypothesizes that individuals are more likely to change behavior if they perceive that (1) they are threatened by an adverse health condition and (2) the change will provide benefits that exceed the costs. The HBM is defined by the constructs of perceived susceptibility, perceived severity, perceived benefits, and perceived barriers. Perceived susceptibility measures a person's belief in his or her vulnerability to the adverse health condition (the likelihood of developing the condition). Perceived severity measures a person's belief in the seriousness of the adverse health condition if he or she does get it. The combination of perceived susceptibility and perceived severity leads to perceived threat. The construct of perceived benefits measures a person's belief that the behavior change will reduce threats and provide other benefits. The construct of perceived barriers measures a person's evaluation of the costs or challenges associated with behavior change.

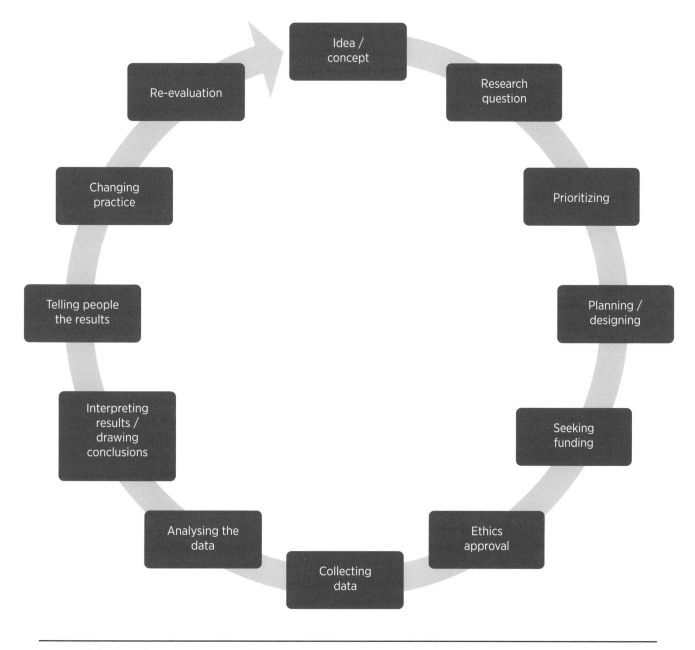

Figure 20.1 Flow diagram of interventions from concept to evaluation

Adapted with permission from Peninsula Cerebra Research Unit PenCRU, University of Exeter. www.pencru.org/research/whatdowemeanbyresearch. Accessed July 4, 2018.

One difficulty in this theory lies the necessity of developing instruments that measure the constructs for the specific health problem in the target population. Other difficulties arise when there is little variance in the constructs (eg, most people believe cancer has extremely severe health consequences). The strength of the model is in identifying and measuring perceived threats as an important mediating variable in predicting people's response to perceived benefits and barriers. This was one of the first models to define benefits and barriers and how these constructs may effect change. These constructs have been associated with behavior, as demonstrated in Table 20.1 on page 407. In the past, the HBM has not been credited with success in explaining dietary behavior change.[25] However, data suggest that the magnitude of the correlation between its constructs and dietary variables is similar to that for other theories.[26,27]

Theory of Reasoned Action/Planned Behavior

The theory of reasoned action, developed by Fishbein and Ajzen[28] and Fishbein[29] and modified later,[30] proposes that behavior change is the result of changes in beliefs defined as attitudes and subjective norms. The theory is well suited to educational interventions assuming that human beings are rational, consider the implications of their actions, and will change their beliefs.[2,28,30] A strength is that it focuses on attitudes and norms that are relevant in making decisions and forming behavioral intentions; together, attitudes and norms predict behavior, and these relationships are expressed in the following linear equation[28,30-32]:

Behavioral intention = Attitude + Subjective norm

The theory of reasoned action has been extended by adding measured behavior to the model[31,33-35] and may sometimes be expanded to include sensory factors (eg, taste and texture), making the theory particularly attractive to food scientists.[31,33-37] This leads to the following modified equation:

Behavior = Behavioral intention = Attitude + Sensor score + Subjective norm

For an illustrative example, a study by Brewer and coworkers[31] investigated the ability to predict consumption of four milk types (whole, reduced fat, low fat, and nonfat) in adult females. The researchers measured milk consumption and sensory attributes. Constructs were defined as follows: Attitude was calculated as the sum of the salient beliefs about the outcomes multiplied by the evaluations of whether these outcomes are important to the individual. Subjective norm was calculated by multiplying the normative beliefs, representing what specific people or groups of people think the individual should do, by the individual's motivation to comply, or how much the individual wishes to comply with his or her normative influences. Hedonic testing protocol produced a sensory score evaluating the taste of four milks under blinded taste testing. Behavioral intention was measured using items assessing intent

to drink milk, and behavior was defined as milk intake measured by a dairy product frequency questionnaire.

In this study, a regression model using the preceding equation with the behavior drinking "milk as a beverage" as the dependent variable explained 67% of the variability for whole or nonfat milk use, 60% for reduced-fat milk use, and 45% for low-fat milk use. Key findings in this study were that intention was a strong predictor of actual milk intake, attitudes and beliefs about health outweighed the sensory score, and subjective norms were not a significant predictor of behavior.

The theory of reasoned action/planned behavior model seems best suited to studying a specific behavior, such as drinking low-fat milk.[25,33-40] A limitation is that it is necessary to generate items measuring attitudes and norms for the behavior unless scales have previously been validated.[28,30,31]

The theory of reasoned action only applies to behaviors under volitional control. Accordingly, Madden and Ajzen[41] developed the theory of planned behavior as an extension of the theory of reasoned action by adding the concept of perceived behavior control. Perceived behavior control is measured by control belief, defined as likelihood of occurrence for each condition, and perceived power, defined as the perceived effect of each condition in making behavior performance difficult or easy. Although these additions reflect important concepts and are closely related to self-efficacy (see Table 20.1), there is conflicting evidence for their validity.[2,25,38,42-45]

Social Cognitive Theory, Reciprocal Determinism, and the Social Ecological Model

Bandura started development of SCT in 1962, defined principles of behavior modification in 1969, added the construct of self-efficacy in 1977, and broadened the scope for population-based interventions in 1978 with reciprocal determinism.[46-51] SCT postulates that behavior is not random but is a predictable result of antecedents and consequences that either increase or decrease the likelihood that the behavior will be repeated. However, the constructs of self-efficacy (a person's confidence to perform a particular behavior) and outcome expectancies (anticipated positive and negative consequences) modulate this effect. New behaviors can be learned and old ones extinguished. Thus, the overall goal of an intervention is to increase the likelihood of health-promoting behavior and to minimize the likelihood of risky health behavior. Interventions focus on skills training designed to break down complex behaviors into small steps. Practice and success will increase self-efficacy and create positive outcome expectancies, thereby enhancing the probability of successful behavior change.

Using SCT for individual change, a process referred to as *cognitive behavior modification* or, alternatively, *cognitive behavioral therapy*, involves behavior analysis and the design of a specific, individualized intervention.[47] SCT has been successfully used in a group treatment for weight control using a generalized rather than specific individualized intervention.[52] However, this generalized group approach has been less successful with minority groups and groups with literacy challenges.[52] Thus, a focus on individualization and cognitive behavior therapy has been recommended for these populations.[53]

Reciprocal determinism broadens the application from the individual to the community level.[50,51] The focus on the dynamic reciprocal relationships between person, environment, and behavior is one of the strengths of this model. A person influences the environment and in turn is influenced by the environment. Environmental interventions can increase positive outcome expectancies and positive antecedents.[27,50,51] SCT and reciprocal determinism have been adapted and used in the social ecological model (SEM), which conceptualizes the individual as the center of concentric spheres (levels) of influence ranging from the individual to the policy levels.[54] Specifically, intervening on interpersonal, organizational, and community levels increases the likelihood of change at the individual level, and there is strong evidence that changes at the policy level facilitate individual behavior change. SEM has formed the basis for a variety of community-based interventions with mixed results. The SEM-based intervention Shape Up Somerville, which was effective in reducing weight gain in children, expanded on

the environmental component of reciprocal determinism.[55,56] The reciprocal component is a key element in policy, system, and environment interventions operationalizing the SEM, which have been successful in improving dietary intake in children.[57,58] Thus, the SEM is a popular and effective adaptation of the SCT.

Modeling, another SCT construct, posits that people learn behaviors by directly observing other people performing them. Specifically, people develop ideas of how new behaviors are performed and what consequences follow, which can subsequently guide their own actions. The four conditions for modeling are attention, retention, reproduction, and motivation. Numerous factors may influence a person's attention, including prevalence, value, and characteristics (eg, seeing colleagues eating fruits and vegetables throughout the work day). Retention follows attention, as it involves remembering what one paid attention to (eg, during one's commute home from work remembering that colleagues were eating fruits and vegetables). Next, reproduction may involve self-observation of repeating a behavior (eg, bringing three servings of fruits and vegetables to work). Finally, motivation involves having sufficient reasons to imitate a behavior (eg, envisioning weight loss, lower blood pressure, lower cholesterol, fitting in with colleagues).

Although the direct translation of SCT and reciprocal determinism from the individual and group to the community has been somewhat disappointing, many SCT constructs have proven to be important predictors of behavior; for example, self-efficacy has consistently been identified as a key mediating or intermediate outcome variable.[20,27,51,59,60] In fact, self-efficacy has demonstrated so much clinical utility and predictive value that it has been widely adopted into most other behavior change theories as well (see Table 20.1). A study of 307 food shoppers across five supermarkets in Virginia underscored psychometric support for SCT. Specifically, this study found that self-efficacy and physical outcome expectancies (eg, looking thinner) were predictors of dietary behaviors.[61] A subsequent study of 201 mothers substantiated associations between SCT constructs (self-efficacy, outcome expectations) and dietary behaviors (eg, using television during dinner, fruit and vegetable consumption, consumption of fat and cholesterol).[62] One computer-based intervention revealed greater levels of nutrition-related self-efficacy ("I can bring a slice of bread with fiber to work or school for a snack" or "I can get at least four servings from every pound of ground beef I buy"), compared with the control group, as well as greater likelihood for the treatment group to attain fat, fiber, fruit and vegetable consumption goals.[63] Finally, an investigation of beliefs and barriers related to healthy eating among less educated individuals revealed differences in social cognitive construct scores between Dutch and Turkish/Moroccan adults.[64] Collectively, strong support exists for the SCT's predictive value.

Numerous successful dietary interventions for children and adults have used the SCT as a theoretical framework. For instance, recent SCT-based interventions targeting children revealed support for increased fruit and vegetable consumption.[65,66] Knol and colleagues[67] used SCT constructs to design and implement a childhood obesity prevention program that resulted in mindful eating and decreased intake of sugar-sweetened foods, desserts, and fried foods. Similarly, a teacher-taught Portuguese intervention program, based in part on social cognitive constructs, produced changes in vegetable and sodium consumption among school-age children.[68] Taken together, these studies underscore the utility of SCT in dietary interventions with populations across different ages and settings. SCT-based dietary interventions have also been successful with adult medical populations. For example, a study of 68 adults with prediabetes revealed changes in consumption of nuts/legumes, fruits/vegetables, and red/processed meats. These dietary changes were accompanied by changes in SCT constructs, including action planning (ie, generating steps to achieve a goal), action self-efficacy (ie, belief that one is able to execute a behavior), and coping self-efficacy (ie, belief that one is able to deal effectively).[69] Notably, one systematic review and meta-analysis of physical activity and nutrition behavior change programs for cancer survivors supported the efficacy of SCT-based interventions.[70] Thus, SCT constructs may be incorporated into dietary interventions for a range of populations across different ages and settings.

Box 20.2 provides an example of a SCT-based intervention.[15,26,57,58]

Despite the limited number of SCT applications in diverse populations, several studies support its cross-cultural utility. For example, a study of 148 Australian truck drivers revealed that self-efficacy and outcome expectancies predicted healthy eating.[71] Further, a study of 1,011 African Americans from 14 churches revealed that changes in self-efficacy and outcome expectations predicted changes in fruit and vegetable intake.[72] Finally, an 8-month intervention with low-income African Americans in Baltimore found that SCT constructs were effective in reducing weight.[73] As such, applying SCT interventions in diverse populations and communities has been useful when appropriately done.

Several investigations have also demonstrated some limitations of SCT. For example, a study of 172 female adolescents in Iran revealed that none of the SCT constructs predicted intake of fruits and vegetables or grams of junk food.[74] A recent study of 294 adolescent girls in low-income communities in Australia found that an SCT intervention did not have statistically significant effects on dietary outcomes.[75] In addition, a male-only weight-loss maintenance program found no effect for an SCT-based intervention; the intervention group did not do any better than the self-help control group.[76] Negative study results can be related to many things, including, but not limited to, measurement problems, inconsistent implementation or fidelity of an intervention, or other study-related problems that do not necessarily call the theory into question. Thus, continued investigation of promising SCT constructs and interventions is warranted.

Transtheoretical Model and Stages of Change

In the past three decades, the TTM has become one of the most influential models for health behavior change. The model includes four interrelated constructs: stage of change, the central organizing and clinically useful construct; decisional balance; self-efficacy (or temptation); and processes of change.[77-79] Stages of change is the most widely researched construct from this model, though decisional balance

Research Phases	Activity (Based on Shape Up Somerville)
Initial advisory meetings	Meet with advisory boards (eg, schools) in the target community to tailor intervention materials by establishing a plan for the interventions, activities, and assessments.[26]
Partnerships	Establish partnerships with schools, administrators, foodservice personnel, and restaurants to influence food and physical activity policies and systems at numerous levels.[26]
Intervention development	Develop materials that will be used in the intervention, targeting social cognitive theory (SCT) constructs, including self-efficacy, social support, modeling, and outcome expectancy for children, parents, schools, and communities.[57]
Intervention	Pilot-test intervention materials and conduct formative evaluation.[57]
Randomized controlled trial launch phase	Obtain grant funding and institutional review board approval, recruit sample in target community and comparison communities, assess consenting parents on SCT constructs (secondary outcomes), and obtain anthropometric measurements of children with parental consent.[26]
Intervention phase	Deliver intervention to experimental community for 12 months after the protocol.[58]
Follow-up phase	Sustain the intervention in the intervention community for 12 months.[15]
Outcome assessment	Assess intervention and control for outcome at conclusion of the study, for example, at 24 months. Conduct outcome analyses to evaluate results.[58]

Box 20.2 Example of a Social Cognitive Theory–Based Intervention

and self-efficacy have received considerable attention in the past decade as well. The least investigated TTM construct is processes of change.

Stage of change reflects both a temporal dimension and motivational readiness to change a behavior. Stages of change have become so popular and are so ubiquitous that they are often misconstrued as reflecting the entire TTM, which has at times been referred to as the stages of change model. The stages are: precontemplation, contemplation, preparation, action, and maintenance. Stage is both descriptive and proscriptive because different intervention strategies are important to emphasize at different stages of change. Although stage of change can be conceptualized as linear, it is better

represented as a spiral (see Figure 20.2 on page 414) because of its dynamic nature. For example, regression to an earlier stage can be as likely as progression to the next stage.[78,80] In the area of smoking cessation, for example, self-changers averaged three serious quit attempts (action stage) over 7 years before succeeding and reaching the maintenance stage.[78]

Developing a good staging algorithm is critical to all TTM applications. However, measuring stage requires defining the target behavior and the criterion for effective action.[81] The algorithm should allow for self-assessment of whether the criterion has been met for longer (maintenance) or shorter (action) than 6 months. Individuals should clearly un-

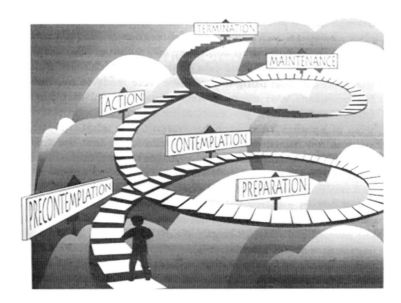

Figure 20.2 The stages of change spiral from the transtheoretical model

Reproduced with permission from Jim Prochaska. Prochaska JO, Norcross JC, DiClemente CC. *Changing For Good: The Revolutionary Program That Explains the Six Stages of Change and Teaches You How to Free Yourself From Bad Habits.* New York, NY: William Morrow and Company Publishers: 1994.[82]

derstand the amount of change necessary to meet the criterion (behavioral distance) in order to assess whether they intend to change in the next month (preparation), intend to change in 6 months (contemplation), or do not intend to change in the next 6 months (precontemplation).[83,84]

The TTM model originated from an analysis of systems of psychotherapy that identified common processes of change.[77] Processes are the covert and overt activities people use to progress through the stages (ie, how people change). Experiential processes focus on thoughts, feelings, and experiences, whereas behavioral processes focus on behaviors, social support, and reinforcement. In two studies of dietary fat reduction, use of all processes was lowest in precontemplation.[83,85] Use of experiential process increased sharply through preparation, peaked in action, and decreased in maintenance. Use of behavioral processes remained low through contemplation and rose sharply through action before decreasing in maintenance. This pattern of changes found for dietary fat reduction is consistent with patterns of process use across the stages of change that have been found in other behaviors.

Decisional balance measures the relative importance of the pros (advantages) and cons (disadvantages) of change. For 12 health behaviors, including dietary fat reduction, pros outweighed cons before action.[86] Progress from precontemplation to action required an increase of one standard deviation in pros and was associated with approximately one-half of a standard deviation decrease in cons.[87] Shifting decisional balance so that pros outweigh cons, appears to be important in explaining why people make a commitment to change behavior. A meta-analysis of decisional balance by stage confirmed these effect sizes across 48 different health behaviors, including dietary fat reduction and fruit/vegetable intake.[88]

Self-efficacy reflects situation-specific confidence to engage in behavior change and is usually operationalized as confidence.[89] This construct was adapted from Bandura's self-efficacy construct (see Table 20.1 on page 407).[47] The converse of confidence is situation-specific temptation (eg, temptations to eat high-fat foods across various challenging situations). Confidence and temptation have comparable measurement structures with three distinct factors:

positive social occasions, negative affective situations, and challenging situations (eg, when it is difficult to obtain low-fat foods).[89,90] In both smoking cessation and dietary fat studies, temptation predicted which self-changers would relapse.[89] For dietary fat reduction, temptation was lowest in precontemplation, peaked in contemplation, dipped slightly in preparation, and then declined somewhat in action and sharply in maintenance.[85] The low values in precontemplation may be typical for dietary restriction; people perceive temptation as a problem only if they are trying to avoid eating something. The sharp decline in maintenance illustrates the reduced effort needed to maintain the change after 6 months.

Several randomized intervention studies supported stage as a predictor of dietary change over 2 years.[59,80,91-102] Computerized expert systems can generate individualized materials, using stage and other key TTM constructs.[103,104] This strategy has been effective across a range of health behaviors,[14,104] including dietary fat reduction and fruit and vegetable intake.[80,106,107] Multiple risk behavior TTM interventions targeting diet have addressed conditions such as diabetes,[108] cancer prevention,[96,97] and obesity in adults,[109] as well as preventing obesity in middle school,[110] high school,[111] and college students.[112,113] TTM studies of college students also targeted fruit and vegetable consumption as part of an obesity prevention program[114,115] and sustainable or green eating.[114] Innovative research promises more applications of effective dietary behavior change programs as core components of emerging areas, such as brain and mental health. The programming and development of a TTM-tailored computerized system and required individual assessments can be expensive. However, TTM-tailored expert systems can be readily disseminated across various settings or online, which, in the long run, can make them cost-effective tools to maximize public health impact. As an alternative, tailoring interventions to the stage of a group[79] or an organization[115] has also been found to be effective. This strong program of TTM dietary research proceeded through a series of steps: applying the theory to dietary behavior, operationalizing key constructs and developing valid measures, developing tailored interventions, and conducting randomized efficacy trials in various populations. These important research steps can provide a framework for scientific progress for a range of dietary behaviors across theories. Box 20.3 on page 416 provides an example of a TTM-tailored intervention extending the model to a new population (older adults) for a new behavior (increasing fruit and vegetable intake).[116-120] If instruments have been validated for a population and behavior, measure development can be omitted.

Despite strong evidence, the TTM has critics. Some have criticized the stages-of-change concept as too developmental[121] or as failing to include the most important stages.[122] Some smoking studies found that addiction variables (eg, smoking duration, number of cigarettes smoked per day) accounted for more variance than TTM variables[123,124]; however, inconsistent and contradictory definition of variables across studies temper this criticism.[125] Further, across five smoking cessation studies, both addiction variables and stages of change were strongly related to outcomes.[99] Such debate can strengthen theories by challenging specific components or generating research that leads to reformulation producing stronger, clearer theories. This is the ideal for theoretical progress.

CONCLUSION

Although it may be difficult to operationalize all dimensions of a theory, key constructs should be measured if validated instruments exist. Constructs such as perceived benefits and barriers (originally in the HBM), self-efficacy (from SCT), and stage of change (from TTM) have consistently been found to predict behavior. Theories evolve over time in part in response to new data, and new theories will be formulated. However, it is important for nutrition researchers to strive to base their studies on specific theories because this increases the likelihood of an intervention being effective.[14] Behavior change theory–based research in nutrition has the potential to explain, predict, and influence eating behavior on both an individual and a population basis. By describing the mechanisms and interrelationships between variables, behavior change theory–based research can advance the science explaining why people eat the way they do and how to help them improve their eating habits, thereby reducing their health risks and maximizing their well-being and quality of life.

Research Phases	Activity (Based on the Study of Exercise and Nutrition in Older Rhode Islanders [SENIOR] Project)
Initial focus groups	Conduct focus groups with older adults stratified by stage of change for fruits and vegetables to identify barriers and facilitators for measurement development and natural-language phrases to tailor intervention materials.[116]
Measurement development	Develop and validate measures for transtheoretical model (TTM) constructs (decisional balance, self-efficacy, and processes of change) for older adults.[117]
Measurement cross-validation and calibration	Conduct survey of older adults assessing TTM constructs to develop stage-tailored norms and rules for each construct to inform tailoring.
Intervention development	Develop stage-tailored text files for all TTM constructs that will be used in individualized feedback reports and monthly newsletters; develop stage-based manual and telephone counselor protocol following design; and develop computerized expert system intervention tailoring delivery system and decision rules for selecting text files.[118]
Pilot and feasibility testing	Pilot-test intervention materials, including qualitative assessment of format and acceptability as well as test intervention delivery system.
Randomized controlled trial (RCT) launch phase	Obtain grant funding and institutional review board approval, recruit sample and randomize to group (experimental/control), and assess all participants on all TTM constructs as well as primary and secondary outcomes.
RCT intervention phase	Deliver baseline stage-tailored intervention to experimental group, including stage-tailored feedback using decision rules based on stage-tailored norms for each construct, and provide materials to control group according to design.
RCT follow-up phase	Reassess intervention and control groups at intervals based on research design (6 and 12 months), deliver experimental group materials that are both tailored for current stage norms for each TTM construct as well as tailored based on participant's change from previous score on that construct, and deliver follow-up control group materials.
RCT outcome assessment	Assess intervention and control groups for outcome at conclusion of study (24 months), and conduct outcome analyses to evaluate results.[119,120]

Box 20.3 Example of Transtheoretical Model–Based Intervention and Randomized Controlled Trial

REFERENCES

1. Rimer BK, Brewer NT. Intoduction to health behavior theories that focus on individuals. In: Glanz K, Rimer BK, Viswanath K, eds. *Health Behavior: Theory, Research, and Practice*. 5th ed. San Francisco, CA: Jossey-Bass Publishers; 2015:67-74.

2. Montano DE, Kasprzyk D. The theory of reasoned action, theory of planned behavior, and the integrated behavioral model In: Glanz K, Rimer BK, Viswanath K, eds. *Health Behavior: Theory, Research, and Practice*. 5th ed. San Fransisco, CA: Jossey-Bass Publishers; 2015:94-124.

3. Harrison JA, Mullen PD, Green LW. A meta-analysis of studies of the health belief model with adults. *Health Educ Res*. 1992;7(1):107-116.

4. Hagger MS, Chatzisarantis NLD, Biddle SJH. A meta-analytic review of the theories of reasoned action and planned behavior in physical activity: predictive validity and the contribution of additional variables. *J Sport Exerc Psychol*. 2002;24(1):3-32.

5. Sheppard BH, Hartwick J, Warshaw PR. The theory of reasoned action: a meta-analysis of past research with recommendations for modifications and future research. *J Consum Res*. 1988;15(3):325-343.

6. Glanz K, Rimer BK, Viswanath K. Theory, research, and practice in health behavior. In: Glanz K, Rimer B, Viswanath K, eds. *Health Behavior: Theory, Research, and Practice*. 5th ed. San Francisco, CA: Jossey-Bass Publishers; 2015:23-41.

7. Kerlinger FN. *Foundations of Behavioral Research*. 3rd ed. San Diego, CA: Harcourt Brace; 1986.

8. Spahn JM, Reeves RS, Keim KS, et al. State of the evidence regarding behavior change theories and strategies in nutrition counseling to facilitate health and food behavior change. *J Am Diet Assoc*. 2010;110(6):879-891.

9. Redding CA, Rossi JS, Rossi SR, Prochaska JO, Velicer WF. Health behavior models. In: Hyper GC, Peterson KW, Travis JW, Dewey JE, Foerster JJ, Framer EM, eds. *SPM Handbook of Health Assessment Tools*. 4th ed. Pittsburgh, PA: Society of Prospective Medicine and Institute for Health and Productivity Management; 1999:83-93.

10. Green LW, Kreuter MW. *Health Program Planning: An Educational and Ecological Approach*. New York, NY: McGraw-Hill; 2004.

11. Andereasen A. *Marketing Social Change: Changing Behavior to Promote Health, Social Development, and the Environment*. San Francisco, CA: Jossey-Bass Publishers; 1995.

12. Miller W, Rollnick S. *Motivational Interviewing: Preparing People for Change*. New York, NY: Guilford Press; 2002.

13. National Cancer Institute. *Theory at a Glance: A Guide for Health Promotion Practice*. 2nd ed. NIH Publication No. 05-3896. Bethesda, MD: US Department of Health and Human Services: 2005.

14. Noar SM, Benac CN, Harris MS. Does tailoring matter? Meta-analytic review of tailored print health behavior change interventions. *Psychol Bull*. 2007;133(4):673-693.

15. Kirby SD, Baranowski T, Reynolds KD, Taylor G, Binkley D. Children's fruit and vegetable intake: socioeconomic, adult-child, regional, and urban-rural influences. *J Nutr Educ*. 1995;27(5):261-271.

16. Redding CA, Maddock JE, Rossi JS. The sequential approach to measurement of health behavior constructs: issues in selecting and developing measures. *Calif J Health Promot*. 2006;4(1):83-101.

17. Insitute of Medicine. *Speaking of Health: Assessing Health Communication Strategies for Diverse Populations*. Washington, DC: National Academies Press; 2002.

18. Cohen J. *Statistical Power Analysis for the Behavioral Sciences*. Hillsdale, NJ: Erlbaum; 1988.

19. Cohen J. A power primer. *Psychol Bull*. 1992;112(1):155-159.

20. Sheeran P, Maki A, Montano E, et al. The impact of changing attitudes, norms, and self-efficacy on health-related intentions and behavior: a meta-analysis. *Health Psychol*. 2016;35(11):1178-1188.

21. Baron RM, Kenny DA. The moderator-mediator variable distinction in social psychological research: conceptual, strategic, and statistical considerations. *J Pers Soc Psychol*. 1986;51(6):1173-1182.

22. Thompson FE, Subar A. Dietary assessment methodology. In: Coulson AM, Rock CL, Monsen ER, eds. *Nutrition in the Prevention and Treatment of Disease*. San Diego, CA: Academic Press; 2001:5-48.

23. Oster G, Thompson D. Estimated effects of reducing dietary saturated fat intake on the incidence and costs of coronary heart disease in the United States. *J Am Diet Assoc*. 1996;96(2):127-131.

24. Becker MH. *The Health Belief Model and Personal Health Behavior*. Thorofare, NJ: CB Flack; 1974.

25. Skinner CS, Tiro J, Champion VL. The health belief model. In: Glanz K, Rimer BK, Viswanath K, eds. *Health Behavior: Theory, Research, and Practice*. 5th ed. San Francisco, CA: Jossey-Bass Publishers; 2015:75-94.

26. Abood DA, Black DR, Feral D. Nutrition education worksite intervention for university staff: application of the health belief model. *J Nutr Educ Behav*. 2003;35(5):260-267.

27. Baranowski T, Cullen KW, Baranowski J. Psychosocial correlates of dietary intake: advancing dietary intervention. *Annu Rev Nutr*. 1999;19(1):17-40.

28. Fishbein M, Ajzen I. *Belief, Attitude, Intention, and Behavior: An Introduction to Theory and Research.* Reading, MA: Addison-Wesley; 1975.

29. Fishbein ME. *Readings in Attitude Theory and Measurement.* New York, NY: Wiley; 1967.

30. Ajzen I, Fishbein M. *Understanding Attitudes and Predicting Social Behaviour.* Englewood Cliffs, NJ: Prentice-Hall; 1980.

31. Brewer JL, Blake AJ, Rankin SA, Douglass LW. Theory of reasoned action predicts milk consumption in women. *J Am Diet Assoc.* 1999;99(1):39-44.

32. McEachan R, Taylor N, Harrison R, Lawton R, Gardner P, Conner M. Meta-analysis of the reasoned action approach (RAA) to understanding health behaviors. *Ann Behav Med.* 2016;50(4):592-612.

33. Shepherd R, Sparks P, Bellier S, Raats MM. Attitudes and choice of flavoured milks: extensions of Fishbein and Ajzen's theory of reasoned action. *Food Qual Prefer.* 1991; 3(3):157-164.

34. Arvola A, Lhteenmki L, Tuorila H. Predicting the intent to purchase unfamiliar and familiar cheeses: the effects of attitudes, expected liking and food neophobia. *Appetite.* 1999;32(1):113-126.

35. Weinstein ND. Testing four competing theories of health-protective behavior. *Health Psychol.* 1993;12(4):324-333.

36. Mesters I, Oostveen T. Why do adolescents eat low nutrient snacks between meals? An analysis of behavioral determinants with the Fishbein and Ajzen model. *Nutr Health.* 1994;10(1):33-47.

37. Freeman R, Sheiham A. Understanding decision-making processes for sugar consumption in adolescence. *Community Dent Oral Epidemiol.* 1997;25(3):228-232.

38. Raats MM, Shepherd R, Sparks P. Attitudes, obligations and perceived control: predicting milk selection. *Appetite.* 1993;20(3):239-241.

39. Stafleu A, de Graaf C, van Staveren WA, de Jong MA. Attitudes towards high-fat foods and their low-fat alternatives: reliability and relationship with fat intake. *Appetite.* 1994;22(2):183-196.

40. Saunders RP, Rahilly SA. Influences on intention to reduce dietary intake of fat and sugar. *J Nutr Educ.* 1990;22(4): 169-176.

41. Madden J, Ajzen I. Prediction of goal-directed behavior: attitudes, intentions, and perceived behavioral control. *J Exp Soc Psychol.* 1986;22(5):453-474.

42. Park K, Ureda JR. Specific motivations of milk consumption among pregnant women enrolled in or eligible for WIC. *J Nutr Educ.* 1999;31(2):76-85.

43. Riebl SK, Estabrooks PA, Dunsmore JC, et al. A systematic literature review and meta-analysis: the Theory of Planned Behavior's application to understand and predict nutrition-related behaviors in youth. *Eat Behav.* 2015;18:160-178.

44. McEachan RRC, Conner M, Taylor NJ, Lawton RJ. Prospective prediction of health-related behaviours with the theory of planned behaviour: a meta-analysis. *Health Psychol Rev.* 2011;5(2):97-144.

45. Ajzen I. The theory of planned behaviour: reactions and reflections. *Psychol Health.* 2011;26(9):1113-1127.

46. Bandura A. Social learning through imitation. In: Jones MR, ed. *Nebraska Symposium on Motivation.* Lincoln: University of Nebraska Press; 1962.

47. Bandura A. *Principles of Behavior Modification.* Austin, TX: Holt, Rinehart and Winston; 1969.

48. Bandura A. *Social Learning Theory.* Englewood Cliffs, NJ: Prentice-Hall, 1977.

49. Bandura A. Self-efficacy: toward a unifying theory of behavioral change. *Psychol Rev.* 1977;84(2):191-215.

50. Bandura A. The self system in reciprocal determinism. *Am Psychol.* 1978;37(4):122-147.

51. Kelder SH, Hoelscher D, Perry CL. How individuals, environments, and health behavior interact: social cognitive theory. In: Glanz K, Rimer BK, Viswanath K, eds. *Health Behavior: Theory, Research, and Practice.* 5th ed. San Francisco, CA: Jossey-Bass; 2015:159-179.

52. Expert clinical guidelines on the identification, evaluation, and treatment of overweight and obesity in adults: executive summary. Panel on the Identification, Evaluation, and Treatment of Obesity in Adults. *Am J Clin Nutr.* 1998;68(4):899-917.

53. Fabricatore AN. Behavior therapy and cognitive-behavioral therapy of obesity: is there a difference? *J Am Diet Assoc.* 2007;107(1):92-99.

54. Stokols D. Translating social ecological theory into guidelines for community health promotion. *Am J Health Promot.* 1996;10(4):282-298.

55. Economos CD, Hyatt RR, Goldberg JP, et al. A community intervention reduces BMI *z*-score in children: Shape Up Somerville first year results. *Obesity.* 2007;15(5):1325-1336.

56. Economos CD, Hyatt RR, Must A, et al. Shape Up Somerville two-year results: a community-based environmental change intervention sustains weight reduction in children. *Prev Med.* 2013;57(4):322-327.

57. Burke NM, Chomitz VR, Rioles NA, Winslow SP, Brukilacchio LB, Baker JC. The path to active living: physical activity through community design in Somerville, Massachusetts. *Am J Prev Med.* 2009;37(6):S386-S394.

58. Folta SC, Kuder JF, Goldberg JP, et al. Changes in diet and physical activity resulting from the Shape Up Somerville community intervention. *BMC Pediatr*. 2013; 13(1):157.

59. Campbell MK, Symons M, Demark-Wahnefried W, et al. Stages of change and psychosocial correlates of fruit and vegetable consumption among rural African-American church members. *Am J Health Promot*. 1998;12(3):185-191.

60. Havas S, Treiman K, Langenberg P, et al. Factors associated with fruit and vegetable consumption among women participating in WIC. *J Am Diet Assoc*. 1998;98(10):1141-1148.

61. Anderson ES, Winett RA, Wojcik JR. Social-cognitive determinants of nutrition behavior among supermarket food shoppers: a structural equation analysis. *Health Psychol*. 2000;19(5):479-486.

62. Byrd-Bredbenner C, Abbot JM, Cussler E. Relationship of social cognitive theory concepts to mothers' dietary intake and BMI. *Matern Child Nutr*. 2011;7(3):241-252.

63. Anderson ES, Winett RA, Wojcik JR, Winett SG, Bowden T. A computerized social cognitive intervention for nutrition behavior: direct and mediated effects on fat, fiber, fruits, and vegetables, self-efficacy, and outcome expectations among food shoppers. *Ann Behav Med*. 2001;23(2):88-100.

64. Romeike K, Abidi L, Lechner L, Vries H, Oenema A. Similarities and differences in underlying beliefs of socio-cognitive factors related to diet and physical activity in lower-educated Dutch, Turkish, and Moroccan adults in the Netherlands: a focus group study. *BMC Public Health*. 2016;16(1):813.

65. Ahn SJ, Johnsen K, Moore J, Brown S, Biersmith M, Ball C. Using virtual pets to increase fruit and vegetable consumption in children: a technology-assisted social cognitive theory approach. *Cyberpsychol Behav Soc Netw*. 2016;19(2):86-92.

66. Branscum P, Housley A, Bhochhibhoya A, Hayes L. A formative evaluation of healthy heroes: a photo comic book-social cognitive theory based obesity prevention program. *J Health Educ Teach*. 2016;7(1):52-63.

67. Knol LL, Myers HH, Black S, et al. Development and feasibility of a childhood obesity prevention program for rural families: application of the social cognitive theory. *Am J Health Educ*. 2016;47(4):204-214.

68. Rosrio R, Arajo A, Padro P, et al. Health promotion intervention to improve diet quality in children: a randomized trial. *Health Promot Pract*. 2016;18(2): 253-262.

69. Miller CK, Weinhold KR, Nagaraja HN. Impact of a worksite diabetes prevention intervention on diet quality and social cognitive influences of health behavior: a randomized controlled trial. *J Nutr Educ Behav*. 2016; 48(3):169.e1.

70. Stacey FG, James EL, Chapman K, Courneya KS, Lubans DR. A systematic review and meta-analysis of social cognitive theory-based physical activity and/or nutrition behavior change interventions for cancer survivors. *J Cancer Surviv*. 2015;9(2):305-338.

71. Hamilton K, Vayro C, Schwarzer R. Social cognitive antecedents of fruit and vegetable consumption in truck drivers: a sequential mediation analysis. *J Nutr Educ Behav*. 2015;47(4):384.e1.

72. Stephens TT, Resinicow K, Latimer-Sport M, Walker L. Social cognitive predictors of dietary behavior among African Americans. *Am J Health Educ*. 2015;46(3):174-181.

73. Shin A, Surkan PJ, Coutinho AJ, et al. Impact of Baltimore Healthy Eating Zones: an environmental intervention to improve diet among African American youth. *Health Educ Behav*. 2015;42(1_suppl):105S.

74. Bagherniya M, Sharma M, Mostafavi F, Keshavarz SA. Application of social cognitive theory in predicting childhood obesity prevention behaviors in overweight and obese Iranian adolescents. *Int Q Commun Health Educ*. 2015;35(2):133-147.

75. McCabe BE, Plotnikoff RC, Dewar DL, Collins CE, Lubans DR. Social cognitive mediators of dietary behavior change in adolescent girls. *Am J Health Behav*. 2015;39(1):51-61.

76. Young MD, Plotnikoff RC, Collins CE, Callister R, Morgan PJ. Impact of a male-only weight loss maintenance programme on social-cognitive determinants of physical activity and healthy eating: a randomized controlled trial. *Br J Health Psychol*. 2015;20(4):724-744.

77. DiClemente C, Proschaska J. *The Transtheoretical Approach: Crossing the Traditional Boundaries of Therapy*. Homewood, IL: Irwin; 1984.

78. Prochaska JO, DiClemente CC, Norcross JC. In search of how people change: applications to addictive behaviors. *Am Psychol*. 1992;47(9):1102-1114.

79. Prochaska JO, Redding CA, Evers KE. The transtheoretical model and stages of change. In: Glanz K, Rimer BK, Viswanath K, eds. *Health Behavior: Theory, Research, and Practice*. 5th ed. San Fransisco, CA: Jossey-Bass Publishers; 2015:125-148.

80. Greene GW, Rossi SR, Rossi JS, Fava JL, Prochaska JO, Velicer WF. An expert system intervention for dietary fat reduction. *Ann Behav Med*. 1998;20(suppl):197.

81. Reed GR, Velicer WF, Prochaska JO, Rossi JS, Marcus BH. What makes a good staging algorithm: examples from regular exercise. *Am J Health Promot*. 1997;12(1):57-66.

82. Prochaska JO, Norcross JC, DiClemente CC. *Changing For Good: The Revolutionary Program That Explains the Six Stages of Change and Teaches You How to Free Yourself From Bad Habits*. New York, NY: William Morrow and Company Publishers: 1994.

83. Greene GW, Rossi SR, Reed GR, Willey C, Prochaska JO. Stages of change for reducing dietary fat to 30% of energy or less. *J Am Diet Assoc*. 1994;94(10):1105-1112.

84. Hargreaves MK, Schlundt DG, Buchowski MS, Hardy RE, Rossi SR, Rossi JS. Stages of change and the intake of dietary fat in African-American women: improving stage assignment using the Eating Styles Questionnaire. *J Am Diet Assoc*. 1999;99(11):1392-1399.

85. Greene GW, Rossi SR, Rossi JS, Velicer WF, Fava JL, Prochaska JO. Dietary applications of the stages of change model. *J Am Diet Assoc*. 1999;99(6):673-678.

86. Prochaska JO, Velicer WF, Rossi JS, et al. Stages of change and decisional balance for 12 problem behaviors. *Health Psychol*. 1994;13(1):39-46.

87. Prochaska JO. Strong and weak principles for progressing from precontemplation to action on the basis of twelve problem behaviors. *Health Psychol*. 1994;13(1):47-51.

88. Hall KL, Rossi JS. Meta-analytic examination of the strong and weak principles across 48 health behaviors. *Prev Med*. 2008;46(3):266-274.

89. Velicer WF, Diclemente CC, Rossi JS, Prochaska JO. Relapse situations and self-efficacy: an integrative model. *Addict Behav*. 1990;15(3):271-283.

90. Rossi SR, Greene GW, Rossi JS, et al. Validation of decisional balance and situational temptations measures for dietary fat reduction in a large school-based population of adolescents. *Eat Behav*. 2001;2(1):1-18.

91. Campbell MK, DeVellis BM, Strecher VJ, Ammerman AS, DeVellis RF, Sandler RS. The impact of message tailoring on dietary behavior change for disease prevention in primary care settings. *Am J Public Health*. 1994;84(5):783-787.

92. Brug J, Steenhuis I, van Assema P, de Vries H. The impact of a computer-tailored nutrition intervention. *Prev Med*. 1996;25(3):236-242.

93. Brug J, Glanz K, Van Assema P, Kok G, Van Breukelen GJP. The impact of computer-tailored feedback and iterative feedback on fat, fruit, and vegetable intake. *Health Educ Behav*. 1998;25(4):517-531.

94. Marcus BH, Emmons KM, Simkin-Silverman LR. Evaluation of tailored versus standard self-help physical activity interventions at the workplace. *Am J Health Promot*. 1997;12(4):246-253.

95. Steptoe A, Kerry S, Rink E, Hilton S. The impact of behavioral counseling on stage of change in fat intake, physical activity, and cigarette smoking in adults at increased risk of coronary heart disease. *Am J Public Health*. 2001;91(2):265-269.

96. Prochaska JO, Velicer WF, Rossi JS, et al. Impact of simultaneous stage-matched expert system interventions for smoking, high fat diet and sun exposure in a population of parents. *Health Psychol*. 2004;23(5):503-516.

97. Prochaska JO, Velicer WF, Redding C, et al. Stage-based expert systems to guide a population of primary care patients to quit smoking, eat healthier, prevent skin cancer, and receive regular mammograms. *Prev Med*. 2005;41(2):406-416.

98. Velicer WF, Prochaska JO, Redding CA, Rossi JS, Sun X, Rossi SR. Efficacy of expert system interventions for employees to decrease smoking, dietary fat, and sun exposure. *Int J Behav Med*. 2004;11(suppl 1):277.

99. Velicer WF, Redding CA, Sun X, Prochaska JO. Demographic variables, smoking variables, and outcome across five studies. *Health Psychol*. 2007;26(3):278-287.

100. Blissmer B, Prochaska JO, Velicer WF, et al. Common factors predicting long-term changes in multiple health behaviors. *J Health Psychol*. 2010;15(2):205-214.

101. Greene GW, Redding CA, Prochaska JO, et al. Baseline transtheoretical and dietary behavioral predictors of dietary fat moderation over 12 and 24 months. *Eat Behav*. 2013;14(3):255-262.

102. Yusufov M, Paiva AL, Redding CA, et al. Fat reduction efforts: a 24-month longitudinal comparison of a large sample of maintainers, relapsers, and non-changers. *Health Promot Pract*. 2016;17(1):116-126.

103. Redding CA, Prochaska JO, Pallonen UE, et al. Transtheoretical individualized multimedia expert systems targeting adolescents' health behaviors. *Cogn Behav Pract*. 1999;6(2):144-153.

104. Velicer WF, Prochaska JO. An expert system intervention for smoking cessation. *Patient Educ Couns*. 1999;36(2):119-129.

105. Krebs P, Prochaska JO, Rossi JS. A meta-analysis of computer-tailored interventions for health behavior change. *Prev Med*. 2010;51(3):214-221.

106. Di Noia J, Contento IR, Prochaska JO. Computer-mediated intervention tailored on transtheoretical model stages and processes of change increases fruit and vegetable consumption among urban African-American adolescents. *Am J Health Promot*. 2008;22(5):336-341.

107. Di Noia J, Prochaska JO. Mediating variables in a transtheoretical model dietary intervention program. *Health Educ Behav*. 2010;37(5):753-762.

108. Jones H, Edwards L, Vallis TM, et al. Changes in diabetes self-care behaviors make a difference in glycemic control. *Diabetes Care*. 2003;26(3):732-737.

109. Johnson SS, Paiva AL, Cummins CO, et al. Transtheoretical model-based multiple behavior intervention for weight management: effectiveness on a population basis. *Prev Med*. 2008;46(3):238-246.

110. Velicer WF, Redding CA, Paiva AL, et al. Multiple risk factor intervention to prevent substance abuse and increase energy balance behaviors in middle school students. *Transl Behav Med*. 2013;3(1):82-93.

111. Mauriello LM, Ciavatta MMH, Paiva AL, et al. Results of a multi-media multiple behavior obesity prevention program for adolescents. *Prev Med*. 2010;51(6):451-456.

112. Kattelmann KK, Bredbenner CB, White AA, et al. The effects of Young Adults Eating and Active for Health (YEAH): a theory-based web-delivered intervention. *J Nutr Educ Behav*. 2014;46(6):S27-S41.

113. Greene GW, White AA, Hoerr SL, et al. Impact of an online healthful eating and physical activity program for college students. *Am J Health Promot*. 2012;27(2):e47-e58.

114. Monroe JT, Lofgren I, Sartini BL, Greene GW. The Green Eating Project: web-based intervention to promote environmentally conscious eating behaviors in United States university students. *Public Health Nutr*. 2015;18(13): 2368-2378.

115. Prochaska JM. A transtheoretical model for assessing organizational change: a study of family service agencies' movement to time-limited therapy. *Fam Soc*. 2000;81(1): 76-84.

116. Padula C, Rossi S, Nigg CR, Fey-Yensan N, Greene GW, Clark PG. Using focus groups for instrument development: application of the transtheoretical model to fruit and vegetable behaviors of older adults. *J Nutr Elder*. 2003(22): 13-33.

117. Greene GW, Fey-Yensan N, Padula C, Rossi S, Rossi JS, Clark PG. Differences in psychosocial variables by stage of change for fruits and vegetables in older adults. *J Am Diet Assoc*. 2004;104(8):1236-1243.

118. Clark PG, Rossi JS, Greaney ML, et al. Intervening on exercise and nutrition in older adults: the Rhode Island SENIOR Project. *J Aging Health*. 2005;17(6): 753-778.

119. Greene GW, Fey-Yensan N, Padula C, Rossi SR, Rossi JS, Clark PG. Change in fruit and vegetable intake over 24 months in older adults: results of the SENIOR project intervention. *Gerontologist*. 2008;48(3):378-387.

120. Greaney ML, Lees F, Greene GW, Clark PG. What older adults find useful for maintaining healthy eating and exercise habits. *J Nutr Elder*. 2004;24(2):19-35.

121. Bandura A. The anatomy of stages of change. *Am J Health Promot*. 1997;12(1):8-10.

122. Weinstein ND, Rothman AJ, Sutton SR. Stage theories of health behavior: conceptual and methodological issues. *Health Psychol*. 1998;17(3):290-299.

123. Farkas AJ, Pierce JP, Zhu SH, et al. Addiction versus stages of change models in predicting smoking cessation. *Addiction*. 1996;91(9):1271-1280.

124. Abrams DB, Herzog TA, Emmons KM, Linnan L. Stages of change versus addiction: a replication and extension. *Nicotine Tob Res*. 2000;2(3):223-229.

125. Prochaska JO. Moving beyond the transtheoretical model. *Addiction*. 2006;101(6):768-774.

Research Methods for Dietary Supplementation Research

Cynthia Thomson, PhD, RDN | *JoAnn E. Manson, MD, DrPH*

LEARNING OBJECTIVES

1. Describe the key principles of designing and implementing dietary supplementation research studies.

2. Understand the scientific process as it applies to dietary supplement research.

3. Identify key resources for designing, implementing, and monitoring clinical research studies on the safety and efficacy of dietary supplementation.

Dietary supplements are regulated as foods under the Dietary Supplement Health and Education Act of 1994.[1] Through this act, Congress expanded the meaning of the term *dietary supplements* beyond vitamins and minerals to include other substances, such as botanical products, fish oils, amino acids, psyllium, enzymes, glandulars, bioactives, and mixtures of these.

DEFINITIONS AND CONCEPTS

Defining Dietary Supplements

The regulatory definition of a dietary supplement has not changed since 1994.[2] A dietary supplement:

- is a product (other than tobacco) that is intended to supplement the diet that bears or contains one or more of the following dietary ingredients: a vitamin, a mineral, an herb or other botanical, an amino acid, a dietary substance for use by man to supplement the diet by increasing the total daily intake, or a concentrate, metabolite, constituent, extract, or combinations of these ingredients.
- is intended for ingestion in pill, capsule, tablet, powder, or liquid form.
- is not represented for use as a conventional food or as the sole item of a meal or diet.
- is labeled as a "dietary supplement."
- includes products such as an approved new drug, certified antibiotic, or licensed biologic if marketed as a dietary supplement or food before approval as a drug, for example, psyllium.

Good Manufacturing Practices

Current Good Manufacturing Practices (CGMPs) refer to the regulations under the enforcement of the Food and Drug Administration (FDA) that guarantee proper design, monitoring, and control of dietary supplement manufacturing and processing.[3] As of 2010, the final rule for CGMPs requires manufacturing operations to control for identity, strength, quality, and purity. For more information visit the FDA's CGMPs webpage (www.fda.gov/food/guidanceregulation/cgmp). Consistency in quality also refers to composition. Each element is critical to quality research methodology in testing dietary supplement efficacy. The requirements specifically address the design and construction of manufacturing plants, cleaning, operations, quality control, tests (incoming, in process, and final materials), consumer complaint process, and records/reporting. To determine if a product is meeting standards under the CGMPs, highly trained FDA professionals inspect the manufacturing facilities using a standardized protocol for evaluating quality. While most manufacturers have successful inspection reports, the FDA can shut down manufacturing or recall orders if concerns over public safety related to a lack of CGMP compliance arise. Compliance documents for the industry are published in the *Federal Register*, and guidance documents are available at the FDA website (www.fda. gov).

Other efforts to instill consumer confidence in dietary supplement products relate to independent review and analysis of product quality. For example, the United States Pharmacopeia (USP) serves as an independent, scientific, nonprofit organization that sets standards for medications and dietary supplements. This organization maintains a dietary supplements compendium with details of the USP evaluation process, dietary supplement monographs, and industry guidance documents. The USP also offers third-party product verification services, including independent analysis of each ingredient along the supply chain. The USP logo on a dietary supplement label is assurance that the product (1) contains the ingredients listed at the listed amounts and potency, (2) does not contain contaminants, (3) is absorbable in the human body within the specified amount of time, and (4) has been manufactured using safe and sanitary practices and CGMPs.

Dietary Supplement Labeling

The FDA published guidance for dietary supplement labeling in 2005.[4] Five statements are required: (1) statement of identity, (2) net quantity of contents, (3) nutrition label, (4) ingredient list, and (5) name and place of business/manufacturer, packer, or distributer. Referred to as the Supplement Facts label, the nutrition label for dietary supplements lists any dietary ingredient whether or not it has a Dietary Reference Intake or Dietary Reference Value. The label must also include the part of the plant used as well as the source and serving size.

Dietary supplement manufacturers frequently add claims to product labels in an effort to market products. However, the government has tight regulation about the use of labeling claims. Claims vary

Type of Claim	Description	Interpretation for Nutrition and Dietetics Research
Nutrient content	Explicitly or by implication characterizes the level of nutrients	Informs about actual nutrient content relative to the Dietary Reference Intake and Dietary Reference Value
Antioxidant	Nutrient claim that characterizes the level of one or more antioxidant nutrients; must have a Reference Daily Intake and antioxidant activity	Defines what ingredients have scientifically accepted antioxidant activity and relative requirement overall, not necessarily to antioxidant activity for health
High potency	Describes individual vitamins and minerals that are present at ≥100% of the Reference Daily Intake amount commonly consumed	Refers to the amount relative to guidance on intake but does not inform about requirements relevant to health or disease
Percentage	Characterizes the percent level of an ingredient without an established Reference Daily Intake or Dietary Reference Value within the product (not Recommended Dietary Allowance)	Informs about dose for ingredients without a reference intake level
Health (authorized)	Food and Drug Administration–approved explicit or implied relationship between supplement ingredients and disease or health-related condition	Suggests significant scientific agreement for an accepted body of evidence to support the use of the supplement for disease prevention or therapeutics
Health (qualified)	Explicit or implied relationship between supplement ingredients and disease or health-related condition	Suggests some scientific evidence to support the use of the supplement for disease prevention or therapeutics; additional evidence is required to support authorized health claim
Structure/function	Describes the role of a dietary supplement ingredient to maintain the structure and/or function of the body, including mechanisms of bioactivity associated with disease	Frequently an area in need of advanced scientific study to ensure that statements have some level of evidence from well-designed studies in relation to disease risk or treatment

Table 21.1 Dietary Supplement Label Claims and Relevance to Research

depending on their focus as well as the quality and quantity of evidence. Briefly, claim areas include nutrient content, antioxidant, high potency, percentage, health (authorized and qualified), and structure/function. Table 21.1 describes these claims and their relevance to dietary supplement research.

BACKGROUND

Use of Dietary Supplements in the United States

Dietary supplement use is high across the US population. Industry estimates of dietary supplement use suggest that 76% of US adults consume at least one dietary supplement daily,[5] while data from the National Health and Nutrition Examination Survey (NHANES) suggest a more conservative estimate that 52% of US adults consume "any" supplement,

based on 2011 to 2012 data.[6] Surveys over several decades consistently report that consumers use multivitamin/multimineral supplements most commonly; however, the most recent NHANES data suggest that use within this category may be declining slightly. Supplements for which use has increased over the past 5 years include vitamin D, fish oil/n-3 fatty acids, and dietary supplements associated with weight loss and sports nutrition.[5,6] Smaller increases were reported for coenzyme Q10, cranberry, green tea, and probiotics. Use of vitamins C and E, lycopene, beta carotene, and selenium declined. These trends perhaps support the role of scientific studies in advancing consumer evaluation of dietary supplements.[6] An estimated 10% of the population sample of NHANES reported taking four or more supplements.[6]

In the 1999 to 2012 NHANES survey, the prevalence of supplement use was associated with select demographic and lifestyle characteristics.[6] Women were more likely to use dietary supplements, although the gender difference was less apparent in younger age groups.[5] Dietary supplement use also varied by age; those older than 65 years reported a higher prevalence than those age 20 to 39 years (72% vs 40%, respectively).[6] Use was also higher in consumers reporting higher levels of education and those of non-Hispanic white race/ethnicity. Dietary supplement consumers also reported eating a balanced diet, visiting their physician regularly, and having a higher prevalence of regular physical activity.[5]

Of interest to nutrition scientists and dietetics practitioners is the increasing use of dietary supplements among children. The 2007 National Health Interview Survey data suggest that 37% of US children consume dietary supplements regularly, with multivitamin/multimineral supplements accounting for an estimated 90% of use.[7] Similar to trends in adults, children using dietary supplements were more likely to be white or Asian, have parents with higher education levels, have good health, and have regular medical care. Yet, only 15% of survey respondents reported that their dietary supplement use was in response to a recommendation by a health care provider.[8] Many dietetics practitioners also work in the area of sports nutrition, where dietary supplementation is more common. A recent review suggests that supplement use is high in athletes, including supplementation with iron among female athletes and vitamin E, protein, and creatine among male athletes.[9]

Dietary Supplement Funding and Funding Priorities

Federal funding for dietary supplement research is in its infancy; federally funded research projects were initiated after 1994 when the Office of Dietary Supplements (ODS) was established at the National Institutes of Health (NIH). A portfolio analysis of the Human Nutrition Research Information Management system and the Computer Access to Research on Dietary Supplements database found that an estimated modest amount of $855 million was allocated across federal research sponsors to dietary supplement research for the 2009 through 2011 fiscal years.[10] The US Department of Agriculture's Eco-

nomic Research Service estimated that 5% of the allocated US Department of Health and Human Services human nutrition research focused on dietary supplement research in 1999, and by 2009 it had only increased to 6%.[11] Data published by the ODS suggested an extramural research portfolio in 2015 totaling $11.8 million.[12] Top research areas included cancer (61%), cardiovascular disease (47%), and women's reproductive health (38%).[10] Ingredients receiving the highest funding attention included vitamins/minerals, botanicals, phytochemicals, and fatty acids[12,13]; vitamin D alone accounted for 13% of the ODS extramural research budget in fiscal year 2015. The Computer Access to Research on Dietary Supplements database is available to individuals seeking additional information on dietary supplement research funding.[14] There is no expectation that government funding will expand, leading to recent suggestions to develop transparent and actionable public-private partnerships.[15] While the industry supports jobs and research and development efforts, no specific research funding estimates are readily available.

The need to conduct scientific study of the safety and efficacy of dietary supplements that is more robust in design and moves beyond industry-funded research has also influenced the change in funding commitment. Following are important research gaps in dietary supplement research that should be addressed:

- understanding product constituent absorption, metabolism, and bioavailability
- optimal product composition, dose, and dosing schedules
- efficacy/effectiveness for reducing disease risk, including determining when efficacy is most likely to be demonstrated in the disease process
- subgroups of the population likely to demonstrate the greatest benefit from select supplementation (eg, age, sex, race/ethnicity, nutritional status)
- interactions related to lifestyle factors, such as tobacco use, body mass index/adiposity, alcohol use, physical activity, and diet
- interactions and/or synergy with prescribed medications or over-the-counter products

This chapter provides information, resources, and suggestions for designing, implementing, and analyzing research in the area of dietary supplementation and health. Registered dietitian nutritionists (RDNs) interested in this area of research should make an effort to understand the regulatory environment (including limitations in current regulations) and their scope of practice before engaging in dietary supplement research. An analysis of the role of dietary supplementation in health is beyond the scope of this chapter, and readers are referred to a review of the topic by leaders in the field.[16] Research in this area affords RDNs an opportunity to work collaboratively within a multidisciplinary team (ideally as the principal investigator) to advance understanding and build the evidence necessary to integrate dietary supplementation into clinical and public health practice in an informed and science-based way.

RESEARCH APPROACHES

Figure 21.1 illustrates the key approaches to scientific investigation in dietary supplementation research.

Research in this area is commonly initiated when clinicians observe a phenomenon thought to be the result of dietary supplement use that requires further study. Alternatively, a patient may pose a question to the clinician related to the self-prescribed use of a dietary supplement for which evidence of efficacy and safety may be limited.

To illustrate the different approaches to scientific investigation of dietary supplements, take the example of a patient who hears (eg, from a friend or the internet) that aloe vera reduces the mucositis associated with cancer chemotherapy and decides to try the supplement. When the patient returns to the office, the RDN notes a marked improvement in the patient's clinical status and decides to gather more information and present the findings in a case report or, perhaps, a case series if additional patients have had the same or similar results. The RDN might also collect qualitative data via in-depth, structured interviews or well-designed focus group discussions. Even if the preliminary data generated by these approaches are insufficient to modify clinical practice, the data can serve as an impetus for basic mechanistic research to determine how the dietary

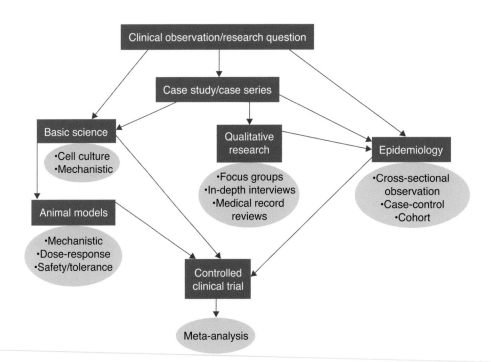

Figure 21.1 Key approaches to dietary supplementation scientific investigation

supplement may be biologically, physiologically, or biochemically altering the clinical outcome. The RDN could also look at available data on population groups that have been exposed to the dietary supplement and had the same outcome of interest. Once the basic mechanistic research is available and epidemiologic observational support exists, then the gold standard, a randomized, placebo-controlled clinical trial, is the most appropriate next step toward building the necessary evidence base to inform clinical practice. Investigators may further substantiate the evidence for or against efficacy by conducting systematic reviews and finally meta-analyses of generally homogenous, well-designed clinical trials.

Scientific Research Progression Toward Evidence

The gold standard for assessing the role of food substances in human health and disease prevention is the randomized, controlled clinical trial. In medicine, the established approach for drug development and regulatory approval is to complete a Phase I or II trial followed by a randomized, controlled clinical intervention trial. Using this approach, a Phase I study in medicine is used to determine safety, toxicity, and estimated dosage levels for new agents and, in some circumstances, the bioavailability of the agent as well (pharmacokinetics). In this case, the study investigator would enroll a small number of patients at a specific dose of medication, evaluate safety/tolerance and toxicity at this initial dose, and, if found to be sufficiently tolerated, gradually increase the dose for consecutive cohorts of patients until toxicity develops. A Phase II trial would then build on evidence from the Phase I trial to determine, in a pilot study, the potential efficacy of the agent to result in certain predefined clinical outcomes (eg, improved survival, reduced lipid levels). The Phase I/II approach to establish agent safety/tolerability, preliminary efficacy, and pharmacokinetic profile is not required for regulated dietary supplements under the definition of food.[17] The same rigor is applied to the study of many dietary ingredients used in supplements, thus enhancing the evidence base and, in turn,

clinician acceptance of dietary supplementation in clinical care.

In parallel or prior to initiating Phase I/II many of the dietary supplement ingredients or bioactive compounds may undergo experimental investigation to establish a basic understanding of product bioactivity, usually in relation to a specific mechanism of action, in a specific disease state, or in some combination of the two. These wet lab experiments may include the use of cell culture or animal studies. Once established, this basic evidence can identify products or compounds for further study in humans related to mechanisms of bioactivity, potential efficacy for specific clinical states, and early dosing estimations.

Additionally, investigators may rely on association studies to provide information on dietary supplements that may influence health and disease. Association studies, also known as observational epidemiologic studies, apply population-based (eg, NHANES) or non–population-based (eg, Nurses' Health Study, Women's Health Initiative) data to evaluate the relationship between, in this case, a dietary exposure and a health outcome. The dietary exposure would ideally be in the form of dietary supplementation, but with many nutrients, the diet-specific exposure, independent of dietary supplementation, may serve as the basis for further study. Epidemiologic studies may be case-control or prospective studies (see Chapter 5), with prospective studies usually providing greater scientific rigor than case-control studies, primarily because of the control of recall bias and the potential for selection biases inherent to case-control studies.

Overall, the availability and, ideally, consistency across experimental and association studies in conjunction with informative Phase I/II trial information on safety and early efficacy support progress toward a robust study of dietary supplementation, usually in the form of a well-designed randomized controlled trial (RCT).

A quality dietary supplement RCT requires thoughtful consideration of several design elements. A summary of the clinical trial research process specific to dietary supplement research is illustrated in Figure 21.2 on page 428. In addition, the duration of the trial is also important to consider.

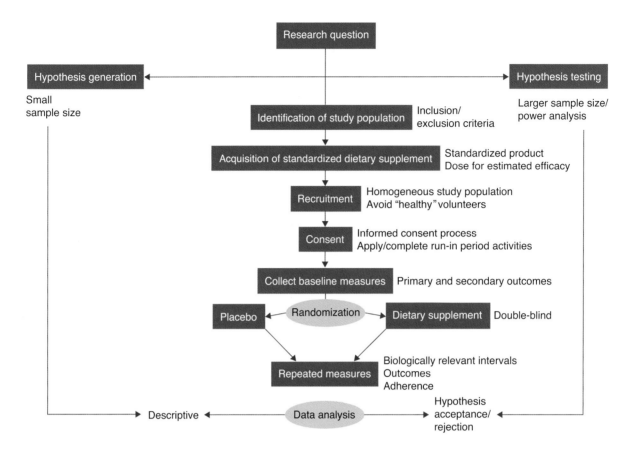

Figure 21.2 The scientific process: dietary supplement research model for a randomized controlled trial

For example, lipid-soluble vitamins or bioactives require a longer exposure period to induce a biological effect than water-soluble nutrients or compounds. Furthermore, some biological effects, such as change in body composition, require longer exposure than outcomes, such as change in oxidative stress.

Understanding the Context of Dietary Supplement Research in the Practice of Dietetics

Given that use of dietary supplements among patients has increased over time and that patients receiving dietary assessment and counseling should be evaluated in terms of dietary supplement use, it seems likely that RDNs will become increasingly involved in dietary supplementation research. Thus, it is imperative that RDNs have a working knowledge of the contexts in which they may play a role in this ever-emerging area of nutrition science. Other important roles for RDNs include assessing the use of medications or over-the-counter products that may interact with dietary supplements and educating patients and their health care providers about risks for medication–dietary supplement interactions.

All RDNs should understand two important issues regarding dietary supplement research. The first relates to intended use. When selecting study participants, note that dietary supplements are regulated as foods, and, therefore, intended for use by healthy individuals. In the prevention setting, therefore, researchers conducting a dietary supplement trial should recruit healthy, disease-free participants or high-risk participants rather than those diagnosed with the disease or health-related condition for which the product is being tested. If a participant was previously diagnosed with a disease, then the intended use could be considered as a drug and not a dietary supplement. In addition, the selection of product type will vary related to dietary function or origin,[1] such as:

- substances with an established nutritional function, such as vitamins, minerals, amino acids, and fatty acids;
- botanical products and their concentrates and extracts; and
- other substances with a wide variety of origins and physiologic roles.

The second issue relates to product quality. Sufficient product information, including product name, ingredients, justification for specific product selection, methods for standardization, and product characterization, are all essential components of any research application designed to study dietary supplementation. Detailed guidance is provided on the National Center for Complementary and Integrative Health website (https://nccih.nih.gov). Specifically, investigators are frequently required to provide prefunding information on the product, including raw and final material; in vitro study information on activity, such as the part of the plant for botanical studies; supplier and brand name; chemical profile or characterization; certificate of analysis (including batch-to-batch reproducibility); and plan for packaging and product stability testing. Manufacturing processes must also be provided, including GMPs. Dietary supplement trials frequently require an investigational new drug evaluation with the FDA, although not all products require an investigational new drug approval through FDA.[18] In addition to the product itself, randomized placebo-controlled trials require a quality placebo product. These products should be designed without bioactive substances, be presented in a similar form or package to promote blinding, and be free of contaminants. Certificates of analysis are also required for placebo products used in dietary supplement research. Importantly, meeting higher standards for scientific integrity in dietary supplement research frequently requires a multidisciplinary approach, which in this instance includes experts in botany, natural products, pharmacognosy, and analytical chemistry.

RESEARCH RESOURCES
Federal Programs

The complexity of dietary supplement research and the issues that surround the design of evidence-based research are better understood if one reviews the current governmental websites that provide extensive background information and guidance that support the development of a successful research project. Box 21.1 on page 430 lists key web-based resources along with a description of the information therein. With an annual budget of an estimated $25 million, the ODS is a leader in the funding and dissemination of dietary supplement research. More information on ODS is available on the National Insitutes of Health website (https://ods.od.nih.gov). The ODS 2017–2020 Strategic Plan states four goals: (1) expand scientific knowledge through research, (2) enhance the dietary supplement workforce through training and career development, (3) foster the development and dissemination of research tools, (4) translate research for consumer use, and (5) serve as a reliable source for dietary supplement interactions with prescription medications and over-the-counter products.

DIETARY SUPPLEMENT RESEARCH: BOTANICAL CENTERS OF EXCELLENCE

The establishment of the Centers for Advancing Research on Botanical and Other Natural Products Program, which combines the Botanical Dietary Supplements Research Centers and Centers on Advancing Natural Product Innovation and Technology across the United States (see Table 21.2 on page 430), was an important contribution to the advancement of scientific rigor and impact in dietary supplement research. With their knowledge of diet, food, nutritional biochemistry, health, and disease, RDNs are positioned to uniquely participate in and contribute to this dynamic research agenda.

Nongovernmental Research Resources

A more general resource list on the topic of dietary supplementation is provided in Box 21.2 on page 431.

Description of Site	Website
Guidelines for the National Center for Complementary and Integrative Health (NCCIH)–Supported Clinical Trials and Safety Monitoring Boards	https://nccih.nih.gov/research/policies/datasafety
Guidance on grant writing for the NCCIH	https://nccih.nih.gov/grants/resources
NCCIH Clinical Research Toolbox	https://nccih.nih.gov/grants/toolbox
NCCIH Policy: Natural Product Integrity	https://nccih.nih.gov/research/policies/naturalproduct.htm
Food and Drug Administration (FDA) Investigational New Drug Application	www.fda.gov/Drugs/DevelopmentApprovalProcess/HowDrugsareDevelopedandApproved/ApprovalApplications/InvestigationalNewDrugINDApplication
FDA guidance for dietary supplements	www.fda.gov/Food/DietarySupplements/default.htm
Dietary Supplements–How to Report a Problem	www.fda.gov/Food/DietarySupplements/ReportAdverseEvent/default.htm
Office of Dietary Supplements	http://ods.od.nih.gov
US Department of Agriculture (USDA) Food and Nutrition Information Center	www.nal.usda.gov/fnic
Computer Access on Dietary Supplements (CARDS) database	https://ods.od.nih.gov/Research/CARDS_Database.aspx
Dietary Supplement Ingredient Database (DSID)	https://dietarysupplementdatabase.usda.nih.gov
Dietary Supplement Label Database (DSLD)	www.dsld.nlm.nih.gov/dsld/index.jsp

Box 21.1 Key Web-Based Government Information for Guiding the Development of Quality Research Projects on Dietary Supplementation

Research Center	Principal Investigators and Website	Research Focus Area
Pennington Biomedical Research Center, Louisiana State University, Baton Rouge	William Cefalu, MD www.botanical.pbrc.edu	Botanicals and metabolic resiliency
University of Illinois at Chicago	Richard van Breemen, PhD https://pharmacy.uic.edu/research/botanical-dietary-supplements	Botanical dietary supplements for women's health
Icahn School of Medicine at Mount Sinai, New York	Giulio Pasinetti, MD, PhD, and Richard Dixon, PhD	Dietary botanicals in the preservation of cognitive and psychological resilience
University of Texas Southwestern Medical Center, Dallas; Simon Fraser University, Burnaby, British Columbia, Canada; University of California, Santa Cruz	John MacMillan, PhD; Roger Linington, PhD; and Michael White, PhD www.hifan.swmed.edu	High through-put functional annotation of natural products
University of Illinois at Chicago	Guido Pauli, PhD http://cenapt.pharm.uic.edu	Natural products technologies

Table 21.2 The 2015–2020 National Institutes of Health–Funded Centers for Advancing Research on Botanical and Other Natural Products (CARBON) Program Centers[19]

Resource	Website
Academy of Nutrition and Dietetics	www.eatright.org
Natural Medicine Database	http://naturaldatabase.therapeuticresearch.com
United States Pharmacopeia	www.usp.org
Herb Research Foundation	www.herbs.org
International Food Information Council	www.ific.org
Medscape Drug Interaction Checker	http://reference.medscape.com/drug-interactionchecker

Box 21.2 Additional Dietary Supplementation Informational Resources

RESEARCH METHODOLOGY

Analytical Methods and Reference Materials Program

The ODS administers a comprehensive research program, the Analytical Methods and Reference Materials (AMRM) Program, to advance scientific methods in the area of quantitative analytic chemistry and reference material development for dietary supplements. The goal is to stimulate the development of quality products using validated methodology, which ensures that standardized reference material is available for researchers testing supplement safety and efficacy. The AMRM program, established in 2002, seeks to verify dietary supplement ingredient identity, quantify individual constituents (raw and finished products), and identify any product contaminants. Having quality products and matching reference materials for verification is an essential first step in advancing the rigor and integrity of dietary supplement research. These efforts have resulted in the availability of a library of certified reference materials for dietary supplement research.[20] To date, 33 Standard Reference Materials are available through the National Institute of Standards and Technology. Partnerships to further expand the Standard Reference Materials have been developed with ODS and the National Science Foundation, USP Convention, and Association of Official Analytical Chemists International. The AMRM Program undergoes periodic external expert panel review and last received unanimous support for its research efforts in 2012. These efforts could be considered complementary to the Centers for Disease Control and Prevention's laboratory quality assurance and standardization programs, which apply standards different from but consistent with the AMRM by applying the standards of the Clinical and Laboratory Standards Institute.

Product Integrity Resources

The ODS provides a variety of resources to guide product integrity and related decision-making for dietary supplement research.[21] There is an established need for guidance on product characterization in order to advance dietary supplement research.[22] Advancements in this area have been made over the past decade, primarily as a result of National Center for Complementary and Integrative Health (NCCIH) and ODS efforts and published guidelines.[23-26] Guidelines have also been developed for laboratory quality assurance programs.[27] Led by the National Institute of Standards and Technology, the Dietary Supplement Laboratory Quality Assurance Program has performed quality testing on products from more than 75 laboratories and multiple products, including certification of elements in multivitamin/multielement products.[28,29]

Determining Appropriate Dosages

One of the earliest steps in designing randomized trials to test the efficacy of dietary supplements is determining the appropriate dosage. Early Phase I/II science that establishes feasibility, early efficacy, safety, and toxicity are also used in determining appropriate dose. Ideally, dose is based on preliminary evidence in humans. However, in the absence of human data, animal data can be applied in estimating a starting dose. Further, if dose estimation is challenged by a lack of data, a dose-escalation plan for determining the maximum tolerable dose in humans can be nested within or conducted before the RCT. Pharmacokinetics studies that are performed to evaluate bioavailability include product deposition in human tissue, urinary and hepatic clearance, peak plasma/serum levels, time course for peak, and clearance of the standardized active constituent under evaluation. All of this information supports the final dosage decisions for the research.

During the early stages of research on a specific supplement, criteria for product (in this case dietary supplement) response evaluation and safety are used to test—in a descriptive way—and determine the safest dose, the maximum tolerable dose, and the most appropriate dose to achieve the expected clinical response in most patients. Criteria for establishing a response evaluation and a safety evaluation are available for select clinical treatments and may be adapted for research using dietary supplementation. For example, the National Cancer Institute has accepted the RECIST (Response Evaluation Criteria in Solid Tumors) approach as the standard by which antitumor treatments are assessed.[30]

While guidelines specific for dietary supplement research have not been universally adopted, these standardized approaches are important for setting the most appropriate starting dose for the research, including future randomized, controlled clinical trials. Furthermore, safety related, dose-ranging, and early demonstration of effect studies allow intervention protocols to be refined, not only in terms of dose but also in terms of dose division, dose frequency, optimal administration route, patient tolerance/acceptance (including reports of adverse events), and preliminary evidence of efficacy. It is important to understand that these early studies are pilot in nature and as such are statistically underpowered to establish efficacy. The results of such preliminary research direct future study design and provide early evidence of safety/tolerance but do not inform clinical practice.

Importantly, as appropriate dose is being evaluated, selected, administered, or some combination of the three in a dietary supplement trial, some individuals will likely report adverse events that may or may not be related to the dietary supplement. In fact, with any dietary supplement trial, adverse event assessments must be routinely conducted and the results clearly documented. If the adverse event is considered serious, by law the event must be reported to the local human participants review committee, the funding sponsor, and the FDA.[31] Serious events include, but are not limited to, rashes or itching; low blood pressure; irregular heartbeat; difficulty breathing, urinating, or speaking; blood in urine or stool; severe muscle or joint pain; vomiting; marked change in mood or cognition; and visits to the emergency department or hospitalization. All events of this nature should be reported on the FDA Safety Reporting Portal.[32]

TRIAL DESIGN ELEMENTS
Qualities for Optimal Design

To have high scientific integrity, the design of a trial must be strong from inception. Generally, after product selection and dosing decisions, researchers should strive for the following three key components when designing a quality dietary supplementation trial:

● Include an appropriate intervention group and a control or placebo group.
● Randomize assignment to the treatment group.
● Use a double-blind approach to treatment and follow-up.

Including these approaches in the study design will support a quality outcome in terms of reduced bias in the assessment of efficacy. Unfortunately, these factors are often not afforded the attention required in currently published dietary supplement research.

Generally, the design of dietary supplementation trials should supplement the diets of individuals in need of supplementation. To illustrate, if a weight-loss study is initiated in normal-weight individuals to reduce cholesterol or circulating insulin, can researchers expect to see an effect if the sampled population already demonstrates a healthy body weight, low serum cholesterol level, and normal insulin response to feeding? The same will generally be true for dietary supplementation. A replete population is unlikely to demonstrate measurable clinical response to supplementation. Thus, designing studies that, at minimum, evaluate dietary or supplemental intake (and ideally measure nutrient status at baseline using biomarkers) of the proposed nutrient selected for supplementation to determine inadequacy in status affords a reasonable probability for supplementation effect. Understanding, of course, that unknowns exist in terms of inadequacies in status relative to select supplements (including bioactive compounds, botanicals, and complex combination constitutive supplements), identifying an at-risk sample for study may be more arbitrary. This healthy volunteer concern in dietary supplement research is not unique to dietary supplement studies,[33] but these studies are particularly vulnerable as individuals with higher education and a higher-quality diet and nonsmokers more commonly take dietary supplements. This bias in study participant selection can contribute to null research findings when in fact efficacy may have otherwise been demonstrated in the setting of a clinically relevant study population sample.

Capturing and evaluating placebo effects independent of the dietary supplement effect requires the inclusion of a placebo group. It is not unusual to see a significant placebo response in clinical trial research, particularly dietary supplement research.[34] The placebo should replicate the treatment as much as possible,[35] that is, it should look and taste the same and should be administered using an identical dose and dosing schedule. In terms of randomized assignment, participants should not dictate treatment arm assignment nor should the investigator. Generally, an independent body not actively involved in the research should develop the randomization plan, typically using an accepted computer-based software program. Participants should not be permitted to change treatment groups, and dropouts by treatment assignment should be closely documented, including the reason for recidivism. One caveat to the use of placebo is increasing concern regarding the ethics of denying participants treatment (ie, assigning placebo).[36,37] This may be of lesser concern in dietary supplement research where standards of practice (related to dietary supplement use) have not been established. However, circumstances exist wherein this may be an important consideration, for example, the evidence supporting the use of calcium for colorectal cancer prevention. In this case, the investigator may decide to select usual care as the placebo or a comparison group who receives usual care. In terms of blinding, it is imperative that both the investigators (and staff) and the study participant be blinded as to the treatment assignment until the end of all data collection. This is a common limitation to numerous dietary supplementation trials where an open-label approach is used.

In addition to the aforementioned factors, another key issue in designing dietary supplementation trials is an awareness of dietary intake, particularly for research using a nutrient or food-based bioactive as the dietary supplement. This requires an assessment of dietary exposure at baseline and throughout the intervention. It may also require dietary restriction throughout the study to ensure that exposure is specific to the dietary supplement under study and not largely related to intake that may be common to intervention and control participants. For example, if a group of patients is participating in an RCT assessing the efficacy of lycopene supplementation to reduce prostate-specific antigen levels in patients with elevated levels, the participants may be asked to restrict dietary lycopene sources over the course of the study to reduce confounding. In addition, participants interested in dietary supplement research may be taking a number of self-prescribed supplements at the time of study enrollment. In this case, the investigator may choose to establish an exclusion criterion for study participation that states that those taking select dietary supplements are excluded from enrollment. Another approach may be to offer a standardized multivitamin/multimineral to all study participants to replace their self-prescribed supplements or to implement a washout period during which dietary supplementation is discontinued before randomization into a trial arm. Additionally, self-prescribed dietary supplementation would ideally be restricted during the trial.

Other design decisions that need to be addressed include drop-in rates. As dietary supplements are readily available over the counter, study participants randomized to a control or placebo condition may decide to take dietary supplements independent of the study plan. This could lead to a reduced effect size between treatment arms. Generally, investigators attempt to reduce drop-in by restricting supplement use during trials, restricting, or monitoring dietary sources, acquiring detailed information on dietary supplement use (including label information) repeatedly, or some combination of these throughout the trial to control for extraneous exposures in the final data analysis.

Study Participant Homogeneity

Another problem in dietary supplement research is the lack of homogeneity in selecting patients for study participation, particularly when sample size is small, as this increases the internal validity of the study findings. For example, if a sample size of 50 patients is sufficient to determine if vitamin E supplementation reduces oxidative stress (as measured by changes in 8-epi-prostaglandin F2☒ over time) compared with the placebo, having a more homogeneous sample population is appropriate for answering the research question (not to be interpreted as reducing the diversity of study populations). In this way, there is minimization in terms of the number of potential influential confounders. Studies must also consider confounding. For example, variables that might show associations with oxidative stress include patient sex, race/ethnicity, physical activity patterns, smoking status, lean body mass, age, diet, environmental exposures, and concurrent use of other dietary supplements. Note that these factors, while easily addressed in setting the eligibility criteria for study participation, could also be addressed in the statistical analysis of study results. Furthermore, these decisions should be balanced with the need to ensure

the greatest potential for the study results to be applicable across a wider population. To ensure generalizability, the diversity and sampling approach for the study population must be carefully selected.

Sample Size

Setting a statistically appropriate sample size is critical to quality research and should involve some consultation with a biostatistician working in a similar area of research (see Chapter 24). Unfortunately, sample size may be dictated by the research budget; however, spending any amount of funding on poorly designed science is inappropriate. One way to reduce sample size is to consider a crossover study design. This approach cuts sample size in half; however, adequate washout of the supplement or placebo between treatments is essential to deriving interpretable results. Yet, cross-sectional designs are not appropriate when the intervention requires prolonged exposure to achieve the estimated effect size. Again, consultation with a biostatistician can ward off significant problems in this area.

A frequent criticism of dietary supplement research is the small sample size used in many efficacy studies. This partially relates to the relative infancy of research in this area. When establishing sample size for dietary supplement intervention trials, the investigator generally relies on previously published trials to estimate the projected effect size expected. For example, a study conducted to determine how tea polyphenol supplementation affects resting energy expenditure would evaluate all currently available peer-reviewed literature on the topic to see what effect, if any, has been previously reported. If the effect size reported in the literature ranges from a 3% to 9% increase in resting energy expenditure across studies, the investigator must then make intellectual decisions regarding how each study is relevant to the research question. Perhaps the study population differs in terms of sex, age, body mass index, or even caffeine consumption, or perhaps the supplement selected for this new research is not identical in dose or method of administration to that of the published research. Each factor would have to be considered in determining the most relevant effect size to use for estimating the sample size for the upcoming study.

The current state of dietary supplement research is such that for most dietary supplements the depth of scientific evidence (peer-reviewed papers) is generally insufficient, and thus reviewing the literature in an effort to set effect size becomes a guess by the investigator or research team. In this case, pilot or descriptive studies are warranted over hypothesis testing until more definitive effect-size estimates can be made.

In fact, a further limitation of dietary supplement research is the pilot nature of much of the published studies. As a substantive body of evidence is yet to be developed, many published studies are descriptive in nature, and no specific hypothesis is being tested; rather, varying doses of a dietary supplement are provided to small numbers of participants to determine tolerance, dose response, and optimal administration forms (eg, pill, capsule, powder). While this is important preliminary work, it does not command the level of scientific scrutiny associated with randomized, controlled clinical trials of interventions and outcomes. As this field of research progresses and additional resources are allocated, there will be a significant enhancement in trial design related to dietary supplements.

Supplement Product Selection

When selecting a product for study, the dietary supplement should be described in enough detail that other researchers would be positioned to replicate the study. As mentioned earlier, the NCCIH requires investigators to demonstrate that the biologically active test agents and placebos proposed for investigation are of sufficient quality to ensure scientific rigor. Investigators are also required to reserve the test agent and placebo samples from each batch for verification at a later date of product quality, stability over time, and comparability from batch to batch. These standards are specific requirements for NIH-funded trials and serve as excellent general guidance for a broader range of funded research in this area. An abbreviated version of these requirements is described here; a complete version can be accessed from the NCCIH website.

For single-ingredient preparations (nutrients, botanicals, animal-derived preparations, or probiot-

ics), information on the raw material and final preparation is required. For multiple-ingredient botanical preparations, identity and quality information (specifications and Certificates of Analysis for all components and for the finished product) are required for each individual ingredient and for the mixture as a whole, such as the following:

- identification of each study agent using the scientific taxonomic nomenclature (eg, genus; species; variety, if applicable; and strain) and author citation
- the name of the study-agent supplier of the final study product and, if the supplier is an intermediary, the provider of the source materials to the supplier
- description of where and how an authenticated reference specimen of the source material is reserved
- description (macroscopic) of the parts of the plant or animal from which the product is derived
- description of the extraction procedure (eg, solvent used, ratio of starting material to finished extract, time and temperature employed, type of extraction, whether fresh or dried material was used, whether any excipient materials were added, what percentage of the extract is native extract, and what percentage is composed of excipients) and definition of the entire composition of the final extract
- information regarding active and other relevant marker compounds used for standardization
- identification of the specific pharmacopoeia monograph (eg, USP) with which the material complies or a description of suitable tests performed that are specific to the proposed study material and that can be compared with results from an authenticated reference. When no pharmacopoeia monograph exists for a study ingredient, or in cases where the ingredient does not conform to the existing monograph, specifications should be provided, including all of the same tests found in the monograph
- information on the characterization (eg, chemical profile or fingerprint) of the agent as thoroughly as the state of the science allows

- any other information relevant to the standardization process to ensure reasonably consistent material suitable for scientific study (including process control, as well as chemical or biological standardization of ingredients)
- information on the analysis of the product for contaminants, such as pesticide residues, heavy metals, toxic elements, mycotoxins, microorganisms, and adulterants
- description of bioavailability, dissolution, disintegration, and release if the information is available
- information on short-term and long-term stability (including testing under extreme conditions)

Product Administration: Dietary Supplements and Placebo

Beyond the selection of the appropriate supplement in relation to composition, quality, and lack of contaminants, it is also imperative that the investigator consider other issues related to product administration. Important issues related to product packaging include the following: (1) packaging ensures that the placebo and active dietary supplement are identical, (2) packaging ensures safe shipping and transport, (3) packaging is user friendly in terms of being easy to open and containing the dosing schedule, and (4) packaging and labeling ensure optimal product storage. In relation to participant use of the dietary supplement during the trial, the investigator should develop specific labels with guidance on timing, frequency, and quantity of dose. The label should also clarify whether the product should be restricted from exposure to light or heat and whether the dietary supplement should be consumed with or without food or meals. Guidance regarding how to handle missed doses or return unused product as well as reporting of pill counts and dietary supplement or placebo diaries should also be detailed for study participants.

Additional Key Issues for Optimal Trial Design

Other concerns regarding the body of scientific evidence for dietary supplementation stem from the lack of rigor in trial design. Among the issues that must be thoughtfully addressed are the use of placebo or active supplement run-in periods and related study activities to reduce participant dropout. In addition, randomization, blinding to intervention for study participants and the investigative team, use of a placebo group, and a crossover design that includes sufficient washout between intervention periods are also important. Additional design decisions and considerations are described in detail in the sections that follow.

Dose

Selection of an appropriate dose for clinical trials develops from sound epidemiologic, animal, or basic science evidence. In the absence of such data, researchers tend to rely on common dosage from market distribution or previously published pilot studies that are commonly of insufficient sample size to test hypotheses. In addition, if the dietary supplement is a nutrient or a bioactive food constituent derived from food, evidence from studies using the whole food may provide some guidance in terms of establishing a test dose. In some circumstances, animal data may afford some guidance in dose setting. When the dose at which clinical efficacy is demonstrated is unclear, it is prudent for researchers to test more than one dose so that a more precise estimate is available for follow-up trials. Further explanation of the importance of multiple dosage testing is available at the ODS website (https://ods.od.nih.gov). Researchers should understand that dosage setting is critical in the clinical design decision-making process. Underdosing may result in null trial findings that will not hold up as they would if an appropriate dose had been selected. On the other hand, setting dosage above levels required for clinical efficacy may result in an increase in adverse events among study participants.

Duration

Determining the length of the intervention is also important in that premature termination of the dietary supplementation may result in a null trial. This may be particularly true in studies with disease-specific outcomes and for which the disease latency is prolonged. If published studies are available using the dietary supplement of interest, the duration data from trials that have shown efficacy is certainly relevant to the design of the new trial. However, null findings may indicate that a longer intervention time is needed to test efficacy. One approach to establishing duration is to understand and take into consideration the underlying biochemistry or biology that may influence the bioavailability of the nutrient or compound either systemically or at a specific tissue site of relevance to the research hypotheses. Following are relevant questions to ask:

- Is it lipid or water soluble?
- What is the chemical structure of the bioactive compound of interest?
- Does it require substantial digestion to release the biologically active compound?

Generally, it has been shown that most botanical dietary supplements (compared with prescription medications used for a similar clinical outcome) require longer duration of use before clinical efficacy is demonstrated. Again, in the absence of strong Phase I/II data, clinical trial dose estimates have a certain degree of guesswork in terms of establishing an appropriate duration of therapy.

Adherence

A major challenge in clinical research, regardless of whether the intervention is a dietary supplement, medication, or lifestyle intervention, is adherence or participant compliance. The sections that follow discuss several ways to test adherence in a clinical trial, and it is judicious to include more than one approach when designing an intervention trial.

Biomarkers of Exposure

Ideally, a valid and reliable biomarker of exposure can be used to test compliance. In this case, the biological sample (eg, blood, urine, toenail) is collected at baseline before taking the dietary supplement and repeatedly throughout the study to measure the specific nutrient, dietary constituent, or both specific nutrient and dietary constituent combined present in the supplement being studied.[38] Some of the most commonly used biomarkers of dietary compliance are plasma carotenoids as biomarkers of supplementation with specific carotenoids; plasma, serum, or red blood cell micronutrient levels (eg, retinol, vitamin D-3, folate), or fatty acid composition of cell membranes as derived from fat biopsy samples. Table 21.3 on page 438 lists common nutrient and phytochemical biomarkers that could have utility in dietary supplement trials as indicators of exposure or adherence.

Self-Report via Study Diaries

In research, investigators commonly rely on self-report to evaluate study participant compliance with regards to taking the study medication. Dietary supplementation logbooks can be used to document pill use and any adverse events the participant observes in the course of dietary supplement use. Generally, participants maintain a pill diary throughout the clinical trial, beginning during the run-in phase as an indicator of expected compliance during the treatment phases of the study. Dietary supplement logs or diaries are reviewed by study staff on a regular basis (usually weekly or bimonthly) and in conjunction with receiving each subsequent supply of dietary supplement. These diaries can also serve as a document of side effects, time of administration, missed doses, duplicate dosing, or other alterations or violations of dosage protocol.

Pill Counts

Another common approach to assessing adherence in dietary supplementation studies is the use of pill counts. Here the study participant returns to the study clinic at regular intervals with all unused dietary supplements. The investigator documents the number of dietary supplement pills provided at each clinic visit and the number returned, and then calculates the difference to determine the study participant's pill count. Pill counts are generally estimated at least monthly throughout the study period. It is important to note that regardless of whether the participant is receiving the dietary supplement or a placebo, pill counts should be kept using the same standardized approach. Some studies use calendar packs to facilitate reporting of missed pills.

Outcomes

The original hypothesis should specify the primary outcome of the research. This outcome may be clinical in nature but should *not* involve a medical diagnosis unless the RDN is collaborating with a physician.

Nutrient Exposure	Biomarkers for Exposure Assessment
Vitamins	
A	Plasma retinol, retinol-binding protein
C	Plasma vitamin C, urine deoxypyridinoline
D	Serum 25-hydroxy vitamin D-3, parathyroid hormone
E	Plasma alpha or gamma tocopherol
B-6	Plasma pyridoxal-5-phosphate
B-12	Plasma B-12
Folate	Red blood cell folate, plasma folate, plasma homocysteine
Minerals	
Calcium	Calcium retention assay, serum osteocalcin
Magnesium	Erythrocyte magnesium
Iron	Serum iron, serum ferritin, transferrin saturation
Zinc	Erythrocyte metallothionein
Selenium	Plasma or whole blood or toenail selenium
Phytochemicals	
Carotenoids	Plasma or serum carotenoids
Isothiocyanates	Urinary dithiocarbamate
Polyphenols	Urinary polyphenols (EGCG, EGC, EG, etc)

Table 21.3 Biomarkers of Nutrient or Phytochemical Exposure Available for Use in Dietary Supplement Intervention Trials

RDNs are not licensed to treat medical diagnoses, and dietary supplements, by evidence of the definition, are *not* used to treat disease (eg, vitamin C supplements are to ensure adequate intakes of an essential nutrient versus treating the common cold). Furthermore, it is imperative that the outcome selected have clinical relevance in terms of health. In other words, reducing neck circumference may be of interest, but if neck circumference has never been associated with risk for disease, then identifying neck circumference as the primary (or even secondary) outcome would waste resources. In addition, if the outcome selected has clinical relevance in terms of a disease, but not the disease of interest, then again, resources would be wasted and inappropriate conclusions might be drawn. For example, say a researcher is interested in testing the efficacy of fenugreek in reducing blood glucose levels but has no blood samples available to assess glucose; using urinary ketones (which are available) as a surrogate indicator of blood glucose levels would not be appropriate as these two biomarkers assess different biological processes.

When establishing outcomes, it can be helpful to consider what type of outcomes are of specific interest. For example, outcomes might be exposure related or related to a specific biological or pathophysiological mechanism. Exposure outcomes would involve a measurement of the level of a given nutrient or bioactive food constituent in human biological samples. These exposure outcomes may be direct or indirect. For example, measurement of folate levels may involve measuring red blood cell folate or serum folate, which are considered direct measures, or change in folate status may be indirectly assessed by measuring plasma homocysteine levels, which are known to be highly correlated with folate status. Mechanistic outcomes can also serve as relevant outcome measures in dietary supplement research, as they reflect the functional response to dietary supplementation. These outcomes are commonly used in dietary supplement research as the premise for structure-function claims on dietary supplement labels. In this case, the outcome denotes a specific (or several) biological response(s) that is(are) known to be relevant in determining the absence, presence, or severity of a disease without directly measuring a disease outcome. Examples of mechanistic outcomes include reducing biomarkers of oxidative stress; lowering fasting blood glucose, blood pressure, or serum lipid levels; increasing resting energy expenditure; or lowering body fat deposition.

When designing a clinical trial to test the efficacy of a dietary supplement, it is also imperative to establish appropriate time points for baseline and repeat measurement of the primary and secondary outcome variables. Baseline measurements must be collected before randomization and preferably before the intervention is unblinded. However, no data should be collected before informed consent. The consent process requires participants to have some understanding of the trial design and its outcome before baseline measures. Despite this limitation, baseline measurements should be taken as close to the completion of the consent process as possible and before randomization. Follow-up measures should be taken at intervals that are relevant to the biological processes under study and for which participant burden is not unduly increased. For most biological measurements, a minimum of 4 to 6 weeks of dietary supplementation is required before any biological activity can be demonstrated. For outcomes such as changes in body composition, longer intervals (6 months) are generally required to show relevant changes. In addition, trial designs are generally strengthened by having more than one outcome biomarker (generally several that are related in their biological effects). For example, a researcher who is interested in the role of vitamin E supplementation in modulating oxidative stress (outcome biomarker) could measure a biomarker of DNA damage (such as 8-hydroxydeoxyguanosine) and one of lipid peroxidation (8-epi-prostaglandin F2α). This allows the researcher to further substantiate any effect of supplementation on oxidative stress and to provide more specificity in terms of the type of oxidative stress being modulated. Other examples might include multiple biomarkers of immune function, body composition, or exercise tolerance. Examples of commonly used outcome biomarkers and appropriate time frames for assessing intervention effects are listed in Table 21.4 on page 440.

Chapter 25 provides detailed guidance regarding statistical analysis of diet- and nutrition-related research. A few important statistical approaches need to be emphasized in regards to dietary supplementation trials.

● Analysis should be driven by the a priori hypothesis(es).
● Depending on the hypothesis stated at the study onset, comparisons should be made either in terms of change in outcome measure from baseline by treatment group (best) or difference between groups at the predetermined time point(s).
● If participants are removed from the analysis, sufficient description of the statistical process leading to their exclusion should be provided.
● Associations between dietary supplement use and outcome should be evaluated in the context of confounders or effect modifiers (factors that may influence both the exposure and the outcome of interest).
● Unless prespecified, subgroup analysis should be avoided or presented only as pilot data for future prospective study.

FINAL CONSIDERATIONS
Level of Evidence

The randomized, controlled clinical trial remains the gold standard for clinical research, and adherence to this design in the development of dietary supplement trials is imperative for advancing understanding in this area. However, the randomized trial is not the only scientific approach, and the quality of trials in terms of methodology employed can vary significantly. To this end, scoring systems have been developed to rate the quality of clinical research both generally[39] and in relation to dietary supplements.[40] Also, summary reports, systematic reviews, and meta-analytic approaches have been used to evaluate the strength of the evidence, particularly in relation to dietary supplementation, by the Agency for Healthcare Research and Quality.[41] The following is a description of other research approaches that provide evidence toward our understanding of the role of dietary supplementation in health.

Outcome Biomarker	Time Frame for Repeat Assessment
Protein status	
Albumin	>6 weeks
Prealbumin	>14 days
Vitamin or phytochemical status	
Water-soluble nutrients	>3 weeks
Fat-soluble nutrients	>6 weeks
Mineral status	>12 weeks
Anthropometrics	
Weight	>1 month
% Body fat	>12 weeks
% Lean mass	>12 weeks
Circumferences	>12 weeks
Bone health	
Bone mineral density	>6 months
Osteocalcin	>8 weeks
C-telopeptide	>2 weeks
Inflammatory response[a]	
C-reactive protein	>4 weeks
Interleukin 6	>4 weeks
Tumor necrosis factor-beta	>4 weeks
Cardiac health	
Lipid response	>6 weeks
Homocysteine	>4 weeks
Oxidative stress[a]	
8-epi-prostaglandin $F_{2\alpha}$	>6 weeks
8-hydroxydeoxyguanosine	>6 weeks

Table 21.4 Possible Outcome Biomarkers for Use in Dietary Supplementation Research

[a] Given high interindividual variability, repeat measures at each time point (baseline, each follow-up) are advised, with mean of repeat measures used to estimate change score in response to dietary supplementation.

Documentation of Dietary Supplement Use in Research

Assessment of the use of dietary supplements among study participants is challenging, and that is likely the primary reason why these data were historically not routinely collected in the context of health research. The ODS at NIH has developed a centralized database of the composition of dietary supplements available on the US market. This database supports investigators in assessing nutrient, phytochemical, and botanical exposures in the context of ongoing research. However, to robustly assess exposures during a trial, researchers need to routinely collect data regarding dietary supplement usage. This ideally includes two steps: (1) participant listing of dietary supplement inventory, including what products are taken (brand name, dose), amount taken per dose, dosages per day or week, and perceived adherence frequency, and (2) onsite review of dietary supplements with study participants, including photocopying of supplement labels for entry into a study database. Other over-the-counter products and prescription medications should also be inventoried and

Supplement	Dose	When (Times/ Day/Week)	For How Long? (No. of Weeks/ Months/Years)	For Research Use (Type/Brand)	Label Collected? Yes (Y) or No (N)
Multivitamin					Y N
Multivitamin-mineral					Y N
B complex vitamin					Y N
Vitamin C					Y N
Vitamin E					Y N
Folic acid					Y N
Calcium (including antacids)					Y N
Magnesium					Y N
Iron					Y N
Selenium					Y N
Zinc					Y N
Co enzyme Q10					Y N
Echinacea					Y N
Fish oil					Y N
Garlic					Y N
Glucosamine/ chondroitin					Y N
Mixed carotenoids					Y N
Other:					Y N
Other:					Y N
Other:					Y N
Other:					Y N

Figure 21.3 Sample dietary supplement use data collection form[42]

"Other" indicates to probe participant regarding use of supplements for select conditions, such as cancer, heart disease, weight control, constipation, cognitive function, energy, and so on.

documented during the trial. A sample dietary supplement data collection form is provided in Figure 21.3

TRAINING OPPORTUNITIES

Dietetics practitioners interested in advancing dietary supplement science should consider opportunities for additional research training. One opportunity is to engage in advanced graduate studies under lead investigators in dietary supple-

ment research. These investigators are identifiable through existing NIH-funded Centers of Excellence or through a review of the website wherein all government-funded research in this area and principal investigators leading the research can be identified (www.clinicaltrials.gov). Additionally, the ODS funds administrative supplements to R01-funded research projects to support training in this area as well as in the area of analytic methods for product validation. The ODS leads a research scholars program for early career scientists to study the role of dietary supplements in health promotion and disease prevention.[43] Four to six scientists are selected annually and are assigned mentored research opportunities with investigators and research projects representing a variety of NIH institutes. Finally, several dietary supplement manufacturers hire RDNs and nutritional scientists to support their research and development efforts.

CONCLUSION

With the advent of the ODS and the NCCIH, opportunities to develop and test evidence-based research hypotheses related to dietary supplementation are unprecedented. RDNs are positioned to advance this science, both in terms of leading new projects and building collaborative multidisciplinary projects. Our understanding of dietary supplement efficacy requires a translational approach taking the best of basic science, animal science, and epidemiologic evidence to develop well-designed, randomized, double-blind, placebo-controlled trials. This chapter provides resources, guidance, and information to assist RDNs in this viable and important area of research. The following action items should be considered as dietetics practitioners explore and conduct research in dietary supplementation:

- Develop a resource library of dietary supplementation research citations and electronic and print resources.
- Develop a network of advisers and colleagues who share interest and expertise in dietary supplementation research.
- Know the regulatory issues surrounding dietary supplementation use, labeling, and marketing.
- Go beyond descriptive studies to the development and testing of research hypotheses, using robust approaches to ensure the quality of the final evidence.
- Start with strong pilot data (basic, animal, epidemiologic, or pilot trials) that support larger well-designed intervention trials.
- Ensure that adequate Phase I/II research is available to inform on safety, toxicity, and early efficacy and dosage (or develop this research).
- Publish all findings, including null and safety data (including interactions between dietary supplements and medications), to inform the broader community of scientists and consumers in regard to the role of dietary supplementation in health.

REFERENCES

1. Hathcock J. Dietary supplements: how they are used and regulated. *J Nutr*. 2001;131(3s):1114S-1117S.

2. US Food & Drug Administration (FDA). *Dietary Supplement Health and Education Act of 1994, Public Law 103-417, 103rd Congress*. https://ods.od.nih.gov/About/DSHEA_Wording.aspx#sec3. Accessed February 26, 2019.

3. US Food & Drug Administration (FDA). Guidance for Industry: Current Good Manufacturing Practice in Manufacturing, Packaging, Labeling, or Holding Operations for Dietary Supplements; Small Entity Compliance Guide. www.fda.gov/food/guidanceregulation/guidancedocumentsregulatoryinformation/ucm238182.htm. Accessed May 7, 2018.

4. US Food & Drug Administration. Dietary Supplement Labeling Guide. www.fda.gov/Food/GuidanceRegulation/GuidanceDocumentsRegulatoryInformation/DietarySupplements/ucm2006823.htm. Published April 2005. Updated March 21, 2018. Accessed April 19, 2018.

5. Council for Responsible Nutrition (CRN). *The Science Behind the Supplements*. www.fda.gov/food/guidanceregulation/guidancedocumentsregulatoryinformation/ucm238182.htm. Accessed May 7, 2018.

6. Kantor ED, Rehm CD, Du M, White E, Giovannucci EL. Trends in dietary supplement use among US adults from 1999–2012. *JAMA*. 2016;316(14):1464-1474.

7. Dwyer J, Nahin RL, Rogers GT, et al. Prevalence and predictors of children's dietary supplement use: the 2007 National Health Interview Survey. *Am J Clin Nutr*. 2013;97(6):1331-1337.

8. Bailey RL, Gahche JJ, Thomas PR, Dwyer JT. Why US children use dietary supplements. *Pediatr Res*. 2013;74(6):737-741.

9. Knapik JJ, Steelman RA, Hoedebecke SS, Austin KG, Farina EK, Lieberman HH. Prevalence of dietary supplement use by athletes: systematic review and meta-analysis. *Sports Med*. 2016;46(1):103-123.

10. Garcia-Cazarin ML, Wambogo EA, Regan KS, Davis CD. Dietary supplement research portfolio at the NIH, 2009–2011. *J Nutr*. 2014;144(4):414-418.

11. Kuchler F, Toole AA., Federal Support for Nutrition Research Trends Upward as USDA Share Declines. United States Department of Agriculture website. www.ers.usda.gov/amber-waves/2015/june/federal-support-for-nutrition-research-trends-upward-as-usda-share-declines/. Published June 1, 2015. Accessed April 19, 2018.

12. US Department of Health and Human Services, National Institutes of Health. ODS Strategic Plan 2017–2021. https://ods.od.nih.gov/About/StrategicPlan2017-2021.aspx. Accessed April 19, 2018.

13. Regan KS, Wambogo EA, Haggans CJ. NIH and USDA funding of dietary supplement research, 1999–2007. *J Nutr*. 2011;141(1):1-3.

14. Haggans CJ, Regan KS, Brown LM, et al. Computer access to research on dietary supplements: a database of federally funded dietary supplement research. *J Nutr*. 2005;135(7):1796-1799.

15. Alexander N, Rowe S, Brackett RE, et al. Achieving a transparent, actionable framework for public-private partnerships for food and nutrition research. *Am J Clin Nutr*. 2015;101(6):1359-1363.

16. Rautiainen S, Manson JE, Lichtenstein AH, Sesso HD. Dietary supplements and disease prevention–a global overview. *Nat Rev Endocrinol*. 2016;12(7):407-420.

17. Webb GP. An overview of dietary supplements and functional foods. In: *Dietary Supplements and Functional Foods*. Oxford, United Kingdom: Blackwell Publishing; 2011.

18. US Food & Drug Administration (FDA). Investigational New Drug (IND) Application. www.fda.gov/Drugs/DevelopmentApprovalProcess/HowDrugsareDevelopedandApproved/ApprovalApplications/InvestigationalNewDrugINDApplication/default.htm. Updated October 5, 2017. Accessed April 20, 2018.

19. National Institutes of Health, Office of Dietary Supplements. NIH Centers for Advancing Research on Botanical and Other Natural Products (CARBON) Program. https://ods.od.nih.gov/Research/Dietary_Supplement_Research_Centers.aspx. Accessed April 20, 2018.

20. Rimmer CA, Sharpless KE, Wise SA, Betz JM, Coates PM. Standard reference materials for dietary supplement analysis. *Anal Bioanal Chem*. 2013;405(13):4337-4344.

21. National Institutes of Health, Office of Dietary Supplements. Resources for Product Integrity for Dietary Supplement Research. https://ods.od.nih.gov/Research/ProductQualityResources.aspx. Accessed April 20, 2018.

22. Wolsko PM, Solondz DK, Phillips RS, Schachter SC, Eisenberg DM. Lack of herbal supplement characterization in published randomized controlled trials. *Am J Med*. 2005;118(10):1087-1093.

23. Swanson CA. Suggested guidelines for articles about botanical dietary supplements. *Am J Clin Nutr*. 2002;75(1):8-10.

24. Gagnier JJ, Boon H, Rochon P, Moher D, Barnes J, Bombardier C; CONSORT Group. Reporting randomized, controlled trials of herbal interventions: an elaborated CONSORT statement. *Ann Intern Med*. 2006;144(5):364-367.

25. Betz JM, Fisher KD, Saldanha LG, Coates PM. The NIH analytical methods and reference materials program for dietary supplements. *Anal Bioanal Chem.* 2007;389(1):19-25.

26. Kuszak AJ, Hopp DC, Williamson JS, Betz JM, Sorkin BC. Approaches by the US National Institutes of Health to support rigorous scientific research on dietary supplements and natural products. *Drug Test Anal.* 2016;8(3-4):413-417.

27. Phillips MM, Rimmer CA, Wood LJ, et al. Dietary supplement laboratory quality assurance program: the first five exercises. *J AOAC Int.* 2011;94(3):803-814.

28. Turk GC, Sharpless KE, Cleveland D, et al. Certification of elements in and use of standard reference material 3280 multivitamin/multielement tablets. *J AOAC Int.* 2013;96(6):1281-1287.

29. Sander LC, Bedner M, Duewer DL, et al. The development and implementation of quality assurance programs to support nutritional measurements. *Anal Bioanal Chem.* 2013;405(13):4437-4441.

30. Therasse P, Arbuck SG, Eisenhauer EA, et al. New guidelines to evaluate the response to treatment in solid tumors. European Organization for Research and Treatment of Cancer, National Cancer Institute of the United States, National Cancer Institute of Canada. *J Natl Cancer Inst.* 2000;92(3):205-216.

31. US Food & Drug Administration. Dietary Supplements - How to Report a Problem. www.fda.gov/food/dietarysupplements/reportadverseevent/default.htm. Updated November 29, 2018. Accessed April 20, 2018.

32. US Food & Drug Administration. The Safety Reporting Portal. www.safetyreporting.hhs.gov/srp2/default.aspx?sid=834d2692-ae54-460d-afe6-1cb507934e7c. Accessed April 20, 2018.

33. Austin MA, Criqui MH, Barrett-Connor E, Holdbrook MJ. The effect of response bias on the odds ratio. *Am J Epidemiol.* 1981;114(1):137-143.

34. Miller FG, Rosenstein DL. The nature and power of the placebo effect. *J Clin Epidemiol* 2006;59(4):331-335.

35. Kaptchuk TJ, Stason WB, Davis RB, et al. Sham device v inert pill: randomised controlled trial of two placebo treatments. *BMJ.* 2006;332(7538):391-397.

36. Saunders J, Wainwright P. Risk, Helsinki 2000 and the use of placebo in medical research. *Clin Med (Lond).* 2003;3(5):435-439.

37. Ellenberg SS. Scientific and ethical issues in the use of placebo and active controls in clinical trials. *J Bone Miner Res.* 2003;18(6):1121-1124.

38. Blanck HM, Bowman BA, Cooper GR, Myers GL, Miller DT. Laboratory issues: use of nutritional biomarkers. *J Nutr.* 2003;133(suppl 3):888S-894S.

39. van Tulder M, Furlan A, Bombardier C, Bouter L; Editorial Board of the Cochrane Collaboration Back Review Group. Updated method guidelines for systematic reviews in the Cochrane Collaboration Back Review Group. *Spine (Phila Pa 1976).* 2003;28(12):1290-1299.

40. Sarubin Fragakis A, Thomson C. *The Health Professional's Guide to Popular Dietary Supplements.* 3rd ed: Chicago, IL: Academy of Nutrition and Dietetics; 2006.

41. Agency for Healthcare Research and Quality. Clinical guidelines and recommendations. www.ahrq.gov/professionals/clinicians-providers/guidelines-recommendations/index.html#dietsup. Published September 2012. Updated November 2014. Accessed April 20, 2018.

42. Thomson CA, Newton T. Dietary supplements: evaluation and application in clinical practice. *Top Clin Nutr.* 2005;20(1):28-39.

43. US Department of Health and Human Services, National Institutes of Health. FY2018 referral guidelines: the Office of Dietary Supplements (ODS) Research Scholars Program. https://ods.od.nih.gov/Research/Scholars.aspx. Accessed April 20, 2018.

Chapter 22
Research in Foodservice Management

Veronica McLymont, PhD, RD, CDN | *Lianne Russo,* MS, RDN, CDN

LEARNING OBJECTIVES

1. Discuss the history of research in foodservice management.

2. Describe the areas and techniques used in foodservice management research.

3. Recognize the relevance of research in foodservice management.

4. Explore future research topics for foodservice management.

Research is critical to the integrity and evolution of the field of foodservice management, and it dates back to the early years of the profession. Through research, the field has continued to change and develop. This chapter illustrates the historical development of foodservice research, presents a matrix of foodservice management research areas, discusses current research techniques used in the field, and explores future directions for foodservice management research.

HISTORICAL DEVELOPMENT OF FOODSERVICE MANAGEMENT RESEARCH

Foodservice management has always been an important part of the dietetics profession, which formally began in 1917. Early on, contributions to research in foodservice management were significant. Soon after the launch of the *Journal of the American Dietetic Association* in 1925, Rush[1] published an article that provided some of the initial research on job analysis in foodservice management.

In the 1930s, research in foodservice management emphasized labor[2] and cost control.[3] In the 1940s, World War II had a dramatic effect on dietetics, and the literature focused on the layout and design of kitchens, food cost control and rationing, and personnel management.[4]

Work on efficiency continued through the 1960s, when researchers began to publish findings on work sampling and the use of computers in foodservice,[5] including computer simulations in cafeteria serving lines[6] and computer applications for menu planning.[7] Researchers also compared food produced using different food production systems.[8]

Research in the 1970s continued to focus on computer applications.[9,10] During this decade research related to Hazard Analysis and Critical Control Point (HACCP) and food safety[11,12] first appeared in the *Journal of the American Dietetic Association*. The HACCP research had profound significance because it directly influenced industry practices in food safety. In addition, behavioral science research, especially related to work values and job satisfaction, flourished.[13]

In the 1980s, research themes were similar to those of the 1970s. The availability of microcomputers (the personal computer or PC) in the workplace facilitated research on computer applications for training[14] and information systems.[15,16] Investigators evaluated productivity using methods from business research[17,18] and compared food production systems using new technology.[19,20]

From the 1990s to the 2000s, research covered cost-effectiveness and food waste.[21-23] Research from 2000 through 2017 will be used to illustrate the research techniques discussed in this chapter.

FOODSERVICE MANAGEMENT RESEARCH AREAS

Investigators use many ways to organize areas of foodservice management research. In the 1980s, Olsen and colleagues[24] developed a classification system for research and development in the hospitality industries, and others have identified research needs related to specific areas, such as school foodservice.[25] In 1993, Sneed[26] developed a foodservice management research area matrix, which was revised by Gerald and Cluskey in 2008.[27] This matrix was revised further and reformatted to provide a contemporary and comprehensive view of areas of research in the field (see Figure 22.1). The matrix provides an overview of areas of foodservice management research; examples of research in some of these areas are found throughout the chapter.

RESEARCH TECHNIQUES IN FOODSERVICE MANAGEMENT

Foodservice management research differs from research in other areas of nutrition and dietetics because of the complex interrelated nature of foodservice. Researchers in this field must consider the interaction of human factors, available resources, and the physical environment when designing research projects. Methods within foodservice operational units can vary, thereby limiting researchers' ability to control variables across units. For example, Wie and colleagues[28] evaluated cost-effective methods of waste disposal for four types of foodservice operations. Annual costs and net present worth for disposal methods and associated labor requirements were determined for five alternative strategies. The researchers used data collected from a previous study to determine costs for labor, supplies, transportation, utilities, and fees.[29] Foodservice management research also necessitates the use of many research techniques to answer research questions, explore research variables, and ultimately improve practice

Research Setting

Foodservice research may be conducted in a laboratory or in the field, and each setting has advantages

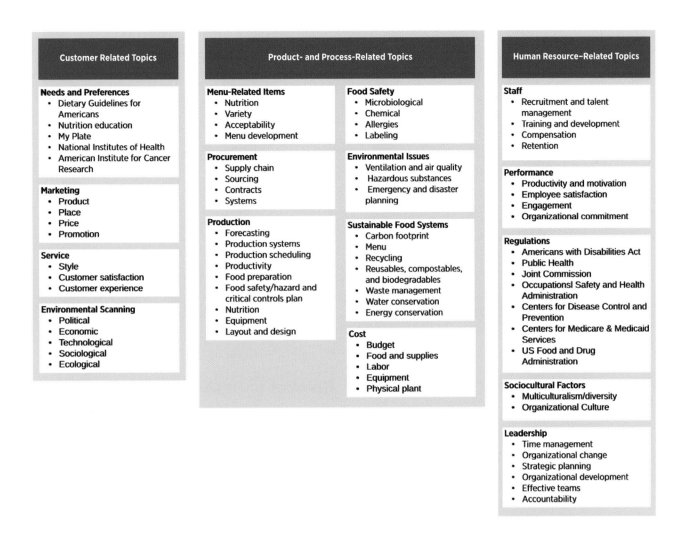

Figure 22.1 Matrix displaying research areas in foodservice management

and disadvantages. Laboratory research allows better control of research variables; however, it may not realistically reflect operational practice, which can limit the applicability of the findings. In contrast, field studies are more realistic, but researchers have less control over variables. Studies in either setting, however, produce meaningful research outcomes.

Most examples of laboratory research focus on product development, product performance, or equipment testing.[30,31] Examples of field research include studies related to food waste in schools[32]; food waste in a hospital, cafeteria, and residential home[33]; plate waste and competitive foods[34]; microbiological content of foodservice contact surfaces[35]; and pricing strategies.[36]

Data Collection

Data may be recorded using observation, self-report, or technology. Examples of each technique in the foodservice management literature are shown in Box 22.1 on page 448.

Database Review

Examinations of existing data from secondary sources can sometimes be useful in answering research questions. Greathouse and colleagues[20] obtained financial data (salaries, other direct costs, overhead, and total costs) from the Health Care Financing Administration (now known as the Centers for Medicare and Medicaid Services) to compare

Data Collection Technique	Example
Observation:	
Direction observation of participants	Researchers observed foodservice employees' compliance with food safety guidelines.[37]
Self-report:	
Participants respond to questions by themselves	After discharge from the hospital, patients were mailed a survey to determine satisfaction with foodservice.[38]
Technology:	
Use of technology to collect data	Wireless point-of-service terminals provided sales data from a farmers market.[39]

Box 22.1 Data Collection Techniques for Foodservice Research

conventional, cook-chill, and cook-freeze foodservice systems. March and Gould[40] used data from the Kansas State Department of Education, Division of Financial Services, to compare school meal programs' financial self-sufficiency and compliance with federal nutrition guidelines. Shanklin and Wie[41] determined nutrient contribution per 100 kcal and per penny for school lunches using cycle menus from two elementary schools in two school districts

Level of Analysis

For both qualitative and quantitative studies, the level of analysis is based on the research design. Qualitative analysis involves examining and coding data in an effort to identify themes, which in turn reveal answers to research questions. In quantitative studies, the level of analysis is based on how variables are measured. Data can be analyzed at the individual or the group level, depending on the research question, type of variable, and data collection method. Variables at the individual level, have been examined in research related to job characteristics, job satisfaction, and organizational commitment.[13] Analysis at the group level is the focus of much research in foodservice management, particularly in studies related to productivity and financial performance.[20]

Number of Observations

Research may be done as a one-time observation or may be replicated. Most studies using survey research techniques represent one-time data collection.[42-44] Researchers may combine observations with survey research. Sneed and colleagues[45] observed food safety practices in assisted-living facilities and interviewed staff about their food safety knowledge. The staff then completed written tests of knowledge and attitudes toward food safety. This technique compares behavior with participants' attitudes or beliefs.

Patient satisfaction, tray accuracy, and food and labor costs were measured for a 30-day period to evaluate implementation of a spoken menu.[46] To evaluate menu performance, Connors and Rozell[47] used visual estimates of lunch and dinner plate waste for four 7-day periods over the course of 1 year. Hackes and colleagues[22] conducted observations for 7 days to determine the weight and volume of service food waste in a continuing care retirement community. Replications of observations will indicate the stability of data over time, whereas one-time observations provide snapshots of the variables studied. The use of one-time observations or multiple observations depends on the research questions and variables studied. Replicated studies that reveal

Reference	Type of Research Design	Study Description
Ko and Li (2014)[48]	Delphi	Researchers administered three rounds of questionnaires to an expert panel to identify indicators of foodservice quality. The questions were based on product perspective (food character, culinary arts, hygiene, and safety) and customer perspective (environment, ambience, marketing, promotion, and service quality).
Bailey-Davis et al (2013)[49]	Focus group	Researchers examined perceptions of middle-school students and parents participating in a free school breakfast program. A moderator conducted separate focus groups for parents and students. Researchers used the analysis to identify emergent themes.
Christoph et al (2016)[50]	Survey	Researchers placed nutrition labels on sneeze guards and directly in front of food in college foodservice dining halls. They then administered surveys to determine the influence of the label placement.
Remsburg et al (2001)[51]	Preexperimental	Researchers evaluated how service style affected long-term care residents' nutritional status. After randomly assigning residents to receive regular or buffet-style service for 3 months, researchers compared data with baseline nutritional status indicators.
Freedman and Connors (2010)[52]	Quasi-experimental	To determine whether a point-of-purchase nutrition information program affected food-purchasing habits of college students at an on-campus convenience store, researchers collected baseline and postintervention sales data.
Santhi and Kalaikannan (2014)[53]	True experimental	Investigators prepared chicken nuggets with oat flour (0%, 10%, 20%) to add fiber and then examined the effects on the products.
Paquet et al (2003)[54]	Simulation	For a case study of the nutritional quality of food intake, researchers developed a service blueprint representing the patient experience from nutrition assessment to meal delivery.
Schaffner (2013)[55]	Mathematical modeling	Using predictions from the ComBase predictor and building on the 2009 US Food and Drug Administration Model Food Code and supporting scientific data in the Food Code annex, researchers developed mathematical models to manage risk of holding cold food without temperature control.

Table 22.1 Foodservice Management Research Designs

consistent results give credibility and allow for inference of results.

Research Design

A research design can be descriptive, preexperimental, quasi-experimental, or true experimental. Simulations and mathematical modeling are also used fairly extensively in foodservice management research. Table 22.1 lists examples of key research designs.

Descriptive Research

Descriptive research involves describing participants or situations without changing them. The Delphi technique, focus groups, and surveys methods of descriptive research are described in the sections that follow.

Delphi Technique The Delphi technique is a descriptive research method that brings together a group of experts in their respective fields to respond to a series of questionnaires. The first questionnaire, which typically has a few general questions, is then followed by a second, more detailed, questionnaire developed from responses gathered from the first Delphi group. The process may include several iterations, depending on the research objectives and data generated. The Delphi technique is versatile, cost effective, and time efficient for participants. When using the Delphi technique, it is important to have highly motivated participants with good written communication skills and adequate time to collect responses.[56] Table 22.1 on page 449 includes an example of the Delphi technique.

Focus Group Researchers use focus groups to collect qualitative information from carefully planned discussions designed to obtain perceptions and information from a small group of individuals (typically 7 to 10). Group members may stimulate discussion and contribute unique or divergent perspectives that are new to the researchers. Researchers prepare open-ended questions in advance, which a moderator poses to the group. Focus groups have several advantages: the method is socially oriented, offers flexibility, has high face validity, provides quick results, and is low cost. Like other qualitative research methods, it may be used to generate instruments to collect quantitative data. Some disadvantages of focus groups are that they rely on the moderator's skill and that the participants are self-selected.[57] See Table 22.1 on page 449 for an example of focus group research.

Survey Research Survey research involves the use of questionnaires or surveys. These surveys can be written and completed in person, are available online, or are conducted via interviews. Survey methods, the most frequently used research technique in foodservice management literature, can help researchers test hypotheses as well as understand, describe, or identify best practices within a population.

Survey research has many advantages as a research technique. Written surveys are relatively inexpensive and can be distributed to large, geographically dispersed participants. Thus, surveys can access nationally representative samples. Participants can respond anonymously or confidentially, which increases the likelihood that responses will be frank. The written survey format provides each participant with the same stimulus, thereby minimizing the variability in data collection.[58]

Survey research has several disadvantages, most of which are primarily related to the response rate. Ideally, the survey return rate would be 100%, which would ensure that the results were representative of the sample; in reality, return rates are rarely 100%. Researchers then need to find out whether respondents and nonrespondents are different. Furthermore, with a small response rate, results cannot be used to draw inferences about the population as a whole. Another concern is reading levels of the study sample. Pilot testing can show whether participants can read and understand the survey questions. The response format of the survey instrument may confuse respondents, making it difficult to know whether respondent interpretation is consistent with that of the researcher. In addition, respondents may not accurately or completely respond to all the survey questions; incomplete instruments may need to be eliminated, reducing the response rate.[58]

Surveys used to test hypotheses must be developed carefully to ensure the validity and reliability of the scales used to measure the research variables. For survey scales, the Cronbach α is used to determine the internal consistency (or reliability) of the measure.[58] When available, researchers should use developed scales with established validity and reliability. Some of the validated scales used in foodservice management research include the Job Descriptive Index[59] and the National Academy for State Health Policy.[60] Researchers may want to study variables with no established scale, however. In these cases, the researcher must establish the validity and reliability of the scale.[61] Table 22.1 on page 449 has an example of survey research design.

Preexperimental Designs

Field studies often use a preexperimental design,[51] which does not have the experimental control of quasi-experimental or true experimental designs. Preexperimental designs conducted in the field have the advantage of a naturalistic (or realistic) setting. This is important when the research uses applied questions. Such questions are needed to improve operations, which are often difficult or impossible to study with more controlled research designs.

A major disadvantage of preexperimental research is that the researcher has little control over extraneous variables that might confound the results. Furthermore, this design is often viewed as a case study. To be able to generalize findings, researchers would need to replicate the study in other operations or settings. Table 22.1 on page 449 shows an example of preexperimental research.

Quasi-Experimental Designs

Quasi-experimental research designs are conducted in field settings.[52] The use of intact groups in this design limits the researcher's ability to assign participants to groups but does allow the researcher to select who gets measured and to decide when the measurement takes place.

Quasi-experimental designs have the advantage of occurring in a naturalistic setting. This method addresses actual operational research questions that may apply to that operation only. The lack of control (because of the limited ability to randomly select and assign treatment to groups) means that factors unrelated to the interventions may plausibly explain the study's findings. As a result, theories cannot be proved, only explored. Quasi-experimental studies often have more external validity (results can be generalized) than internal validity (confidence in the cause and effect of a study). Table 22.1 on page 449 shows an example of quasi-experimental design.

True Experimental Designs

True experimental designs allow the researcher to manipulate the independent variable and determine the impact on the dependent variable.[53,62] These research studies are often conducted in laboratory settings, but there are examples of studies in the field as well.

True experimental designs have the advantage that all the variables are controlled and that the impact of the independent variable on the dependent variable can be determined. However, many areas in which foodservice research is needed cannot be studied in the laboratory under tightly controlled conditions. Much of what researchers need to know occurs in operations where individuals work. Thus, true experimental design is not often realistic for foodservice management research. See Table 22.1 on page 449 for an example of the true experimental research design.

Simulations and Mathematical Modeling

Simulation Researchers use computer simulations to illustrate the behavior of systems and to evaluate strategies for a system's operation. Simulations have many applications in foodservice management and provide a research model for predicting outcomes in a cost-effective manner. The use of computer simulations in foodservice dates back to the mid-1960s, when Knickrehm[63] used simulations to determine dining-room seating capacity. Guley and Stinson[64] applied computer simulation techniques to production scheduling in a ready-foods system. Nettles and Gregoire[65] used computer simulations to examine time required for tray-line flow in a school foodservice setting.

Research on the use of computers to plan menus dates back to the early 1960s. Balintfy[66] and Eckstein[67] did much of the early work related to the use of computers for menu planning. Artificial intelligence systems have been developed for computer-assisted menu planning,[68] and some hospitals use technology to offer electronic foodservice systems for patient meal ordering.[69-71]

Another type of simulation is service blueprinting, a process that looks at a service from a customer's perspective. This process, which has been used in service marketing and medical practice, has the potential to improve customer satisfaction with nutrition services. Service blueprinting may ensure that all processes are included in the patient's experience with health care services. Table 22.1 on page 449 shows an example of simulation research design.

Mathematical Modeling Several mathematical modeling techniques originally developed for use in business operations have been applied successfully in foodservice management.[40,55,72] These models use mathematical relationships to represent some aspect of reality. With mathematical models, the researcher can draw conclusions about the impact of various decisions by experimenting with the model instead of intervening in actual operations. Mathematical models have several advantages: they are a less expensive, less time consuming, and less risky way to model the impact of a decision before implementing it in an actual operation. See Table 22.1 on page 449 for an example of the mathematical modeling research design.

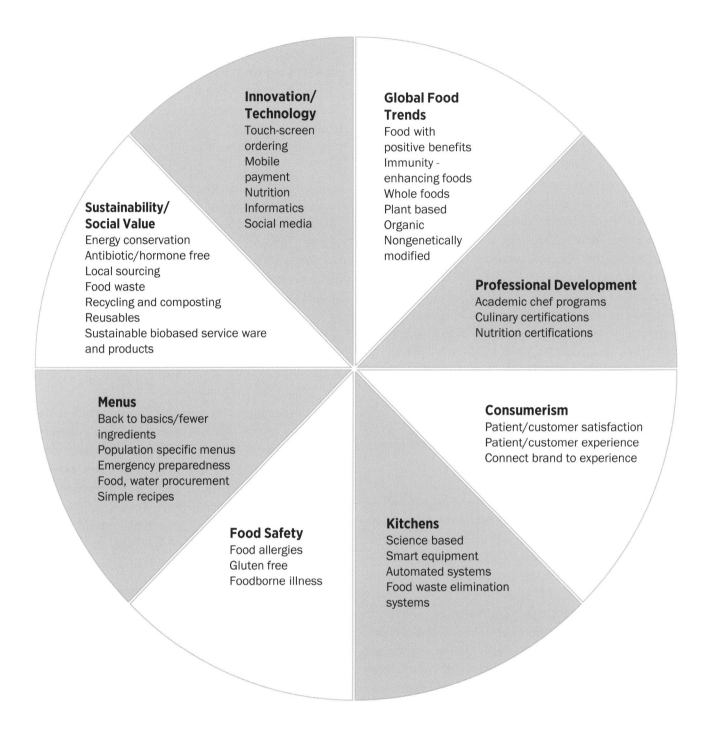

Figure 22.2 Future directions in foodservice management research

CONCLUSION

Foodservice management research has played an integral part in nutrition and dietetics practice since its early days. Investigators have used many research techniques to address foodservice management research questions. Much of the research conducted to date has used survey methodology to describe and compare foodservice operations. Future research should expand the use of qualitative techniques to build improved theories and explore relationships. Experimental research methods in foodservice management have been limited to product development and equipment testing; expanding the use of experimental methods in actual operational settings would be beneficial and would move practice forward. The foodservice management knowledge base continues to grow through the use of a variety of techniques to explore research hypotheses. Research continues to be needed to provide information on ways to most efficiently and effectively run foodservice operations in a changing environment, and research should continue to grow and develop with the industry. Interest has increased in certain foodservice topics, and there are many possibilities for research in these areas (see Figure 22.2). As nutrition and dietetics practitioners explore and learn more from future research, the possibilities are endless.

REFERENCES

1. Rush G. Job analysis of lunchroom and cafeteria management. *J Am Diet Assoc.* 1925;1:130-137.

2. Baker RT, Barlow M. Personnel study of dietary departments of hospitals. *J Am Diet Assoc.* 1931;6: 356-359.

3. Leigh MJ. Management and food control in the college dormitory. *J Am Diet Assoc.* 1939;15:179-184.

4. Bloetjes MK, Gottlieb R. Determining layout efficiency in the kitchen. *J Am Diet Assoc.* 1958;34:829-835.

5. Wise BI, Donaldson B. Work sampling in the dietary department. *J Am Diet Assoc.* 1961;39:327-332.

6. Knickrehm ME, Hoffman TR, Donaldson B. Digital computer simulations of a cafeteria service line. *J Am Diet Assoc.* 1963;43:203-208.

7. Eckstein EF. Menu planning by computer: the random approach. *J Am Diet Assoc.* 1967;51:529-533.

8. Quam ME, Fitzsimmons C, Godfrey RL. Ready-prepared vs conventionally prepared foods. *J Am Diet Assoc.* 1967;50: 196-200.

9. Orser J, Mutschler M. A computer tallied menu system. *J Am Diet Assoc.* 1975;67:570-572.

10. Wilcox MM, Moore AN, Hoover LW. Automated purchasing: forecasts to determine stock levels and print orders. *J Am Diet Assoc.* 1978;73:400-405.

11. Bobeng BJ, David BD. HACCP models for quality control of entrée production in hospital foodservice systems: I. Development of Hazard Analysis Critical Control Point models. *J Am Diet Assoc.* 1978;73:524-529.

12. Bobeng BJ, David BD. HACCP models for quality control of entrée production in hospital foodservice systems: II. Quality assessment of beef loaves utilizing HACCP models. *J Am Diet Assoc.* 1978;73:530-535.

13. Swartz RS, Vaden AG. Behavioral science research in hospital foodservice. II. Job satisfaction and work values of foodservice employees in large hospitals. *J Am Diet Assoc.* 1978;73:127-131.

14. Waddell KP, Rinke WJ. Effectiveness of a computer-assisted program for teaching sanitation. *J Am Diet Assoc.* 1985;85(1):62-67.

15. Matthews ME, Norback JP. A new approach to the design of information systems for foodservice management in health care facilities. *J Am Diet Assoc.* 1984;84(6):675-678, 681.

16. Aldrich DS, Helbig LC. A sequential procedure for implementing a computer-based information system. *J Am Diet Assoc.* 1986;86(9):1228-1231.

17. Mayo CR, Olsen MD, Frary RB. Variables that affect productivity in school foodservices. *J Am Diet Assoc.* 1984; 84(2):187-190, 193.

18. Murray IP, Upton EM. Labour productivity in hospital foodservice. *J Can Diet Assoc.* 1988;49(3):178-181.

19. Puckett RP, Boe DG, Medved CK. Management of engineering principles applied to foodservice operation. *J Am Diet Assoc.* 1987;87(6):770-774.

20. Greathouse KR, Gregoire MB, Spears MC, Richards V, Nassar RF. Comparison of conventional, cook chill, and cook-freeze foodservice systems. *J Am Diet Assoc.* 1989; 89(11):1606-1611.

21. Kim T, Shanklin CW, Su AY, Hackes BL, Ferris D. Comparison of waste composition in a continuing-care retirement community. *J Am Diet Assoc.* 1997;97(4): 396-400.

22. Hackes BL, Shanklin CW, Kim T, Su AY. Tray service generates more food waste in dining areas of a continuing-care retirement community. *J Am Diet Assoc.* 1997;97(8): 879-882.

23. Getlinger MJ, Laughlin CVT, Bell E, Akre C, Arjmandi BH. Food waste is reduced when elementary-school children have recess before lunch. *J Am Diet Assoc.* 1996;96(9): 906-908.

24. Olsen MD, Tse E, Bellas C. A proposed classification system for research and development activities within the hospitality industries. *Hospitality Educ Res J.* 1984;9(2):55-62.

25. Matthews ME, Bedford MR, Hiemstra S. Report on school food service research needs—1985. *School Food Ser Res Rev.* 1986;10:35-39.

26. Sneed J. Research needs in foodservice management. In: Sneed J, Holdt C, eds. *Issues for the 1990s: Americans with Disabilities Act, Cultural Diversity, and Research. Proceedings of the 17th Biennial Conference of the Foodservice Systems Management Education Council.* Hattiesburg: University of Southern Mississippi; 1993:73-79.

27. Gerald BL, Cluskey M. Research in foodservice management. In: Monsen ER, Van Horn L, eds. *Research: Successful Approaches.* 3rd ed. Chicago, IL: American Dietetic Association; 2008:337-351.

28. Wie S, Shanklin CW, Lee KE. A decision tree for selecting the most cost-effective waste disposal strategy in foodservice operations. *J Am Diet Assoc.* 2003;103(4):475-482.

29. Wie S, Shanklin CW. Cost effective disposal methods and assessment of waste generated in foodservice operations. *Food Serv Res Int.* 2001;13(1):17-39.

30. Daniel D, Thompson LD, Shriver BJ, Wu CK, Hoover LC. Nonhyrdrogenated cottonseed oil can be used as a deep fat frying medium to reduce trans-fatty acid content in French fries. *J Am Diet Assoc.* 2005;105(12):1927-1932.

31. Romanchik-Cerpovicz JE, Costantino AC, Gunn LH. Sensory evaluation ratings and melting characteristics show that okra gum is an acceptable milk-fat ingredient substitute in chocolate frozen dairy dessert. *J Am Diet Assoc.* 2006;106(4):594-597.

32. Cohen J, Richardson S, Austin SB, Economos CD. School lunch waste among middle school students: implications for nutrients consumed and food waste costs. *Am J Prev Med.* 2013;44(2):114-121.

33. Strotmann C, Friedrich S, Kreyenschmidt J, Teitscheid P, Ritter G. Comparing food provided and wasted before and after implementing measures against food waste in three healthcare food service facilities. *Sustainability.* 2017;9(8): 1409-1427.

34. Templeton SB, Marlette MA, Pamemangalore M. Competitive foods increase the intake of energy and decrease the intake of certain nutrients by adolescents consuming school lunch. *J Am Diet Assoc.* 2005;105(2): 215-220.

35. Sneed J, Strohbehn C, Gilmore SA, Mendonca A. Microbiological evaluation of foodservice contact surfaces in Iowa assisted-living facilities. *J Am Diet Assoc.* 2004; 104(11):1722-1724.

36. Trevino RP, Pham T, Mobley C, Hartstein J, El ghormli L, Songer T. HEALTHY study school food service revenue and expense report. *J Sch Health.* 2012;82(9):417-423.

37. York VK, Brannon LA, Roberts K, Shanklin C, Howells A, Barrett EB. Effects of observing employees for food safety compliance rates. *J Foodserv Manage Educ.* 2012;6: 17-24.

38. Barsamian AM, Gregoire MB, Sowa D, Lafferty L, Stone M. Timely resolution of patient concerns improves post-discharge satisfaction. *J Am Diet Assoc.* 2010;110(9): 1346-1350.

39. Buttenheim AM, Havassy J, Fang M, Glyn J, Karpyn A. Increasing supplemental nutrition assistance program/electronic benefits transfer sales at farmers' markets with vendor-operated wireless point-of-sale terminals. *J Acad Nutr Diet.* 2012;112(5):636-641.

40. March L, Gould R. Compliance with the School Meals Initiative: effect on meal programs' financial success. *J Am Diet Assoc.* 2001;101(10):1199-1201.

41. Shanklin CW, Wie S. Nutrient contribution per 100 kcal and per penny for the 5 meal components in school lunch: entrée, milk, vegetable/fruit, bread/grain, and miscellaneous. *J Am Diet Assoc.* 2001;101(11):1358-1361.

42. Gregoire MB, Sames K, Dowling RA, Lafferty LJ. Are registered dietitians adequately prepared to be hospital foodservice directors? *J Am Diet Assoc.* 2005;105(8): 1215-1221.

43. Brown DM. Prevalence of food production systems in school foodservice. *J Am Diet Assoc.* 2005;105(8):1261-1265.

44. Probart C, McDonnell E, Hartman T, Weirich E, Bailey-Davis L. Factors associated with the offering and sale of competitive foods and school lunch participation. *J Am Diet Assoc.* 2006;106(2):242-247.

45. Sneed J, Strohbehn C, Gilmore SA. Food safety practices and readiness to implement HACCP programs in assisted-living facilities in Iowa. *J Am Diet Assoc.* 2004;104(11):1678-1683.

46. Folio D, O'Sullivan-Maillet J, Touger-Decker R. The spoken menu concept of patient foodservice delivery systems increases overall satisfaction, therapeutic and tray accuracy, and is cost neutral for food and labor. *J Am Diet Assoc.* 2002;102(4):546-548.

47. Connors P, Rozell SB. Using a visual plate waste study to monitor menu performance. *J Am Diet Assoc.* 2004;104(1):94-96.

48. Ko WH, Li LJ. Foodservice quality: identifying perception indicators of foodservice quality for hospitality students. *Food Nutr Sci.* 2014;5:132-137.

49. Bailey-Davis L, Virus A, McCoy TA, Wojtanowski A, Vander Veur SS. Middle school student and parent perceptions of government-sponsored free school breakfast and consumption: a qualitative inquiry in an urban setting. *J Acad Nutr Diet.* 2013;113(2):251-257.

50. Christoph MJ, Ellison BD, Meador EN. The influence of nutrition label placement on awareness and use among college students in a dining hall setting. *J Acad Nutr Diet.* 2016;116(9):1395-1405.

51. Remsburg RE, Luking A, Baran P, et al. Impact of a buffet-style dining program on weight and biochemical indicators of nutritional status in nursing home residents: a pilot study. *J Am Diet Assoc.* 2001;101(12):1460-1463.

52. Freedman MR, Connors R. Point-of-purchase nutrition information influences food-purchasing behaviors of college students: a pilot study. *J Am Diet Assoc.* 2010;110(8):1222-1226.

53. Santhi D, Kalaikannan A. The effect of the addition of oat flour in low-fat chicken nuggets. *J Nutr Food Sci.* 2014;4(1):260-263.

54. Paquet C, St-Arnaud-McKenzie D, Ferland G, Dube L. A blueprint-based case study analysis of nutrition services provided in a midterm care facility for the elderly. *J Am Diet Assoc.* 2003;103(3):363-368.

55. Schaffner DW. Utilization of mathematical models to manage risk of holding cold food without temperature control. *J Food Prot.* 2013;76(6):1085-1094.

56. Delbecq AL, Van de Ven AH, Gustafson DH. *Group Techniques for Program Planning.* Glenview, IL: Scott Foresman and Company; 1975.

57. Leung FH, Savithiri R. Spotlight on focus group. *Can Fam Physician.* 2009;55(2):218-219.

58. Cronbach L. Coefficient alpha and the internal structure of tests. *Psychometrika.* 1951;16(3):297-334.

59. Smith P, Kendall L, Hulin C. *The Measurement of Satisfaction in Work and Retirement.* Chicago, IL: Rand McNally; 1969.

60. Chao S, Hagisavas V, Mollica R, Dwyer J. Time for assessment of nutrition services in assisted living facilities. *J Nutr Elder.* 2003;23(1):41-55.

61. Dienhart JR, Gregoire MB, Downey R. Service orientation of restaurant employees. *Hosp Res J.* 1990;14(2):421-430.

62. Hautenne-Dekay D, Mullins E, Sewell D, Hagan DW. Wet-nesting of foodservice dishware: investigation and analysis of potential bacterial contamination. *J Am Diet Assoc.* 2001;101(8):933-934.

63. Knickrehm ME. Digital computer simulation in determining dining room seating capacity. *J Am Diet Assoc.* 1966;48:199-203.

64. Guley HM, Stinson JP. Computer simulation for production scheduling in a ready foods system. *J Am Diet Assoc.* 1980;76:482-487.

65. Nettles MF, Gregoire MB. Use of computer simulation in school foodservice. *J Foodserv Syst.* 1996;9:143-156.

66. Balintfy JL. Menu planning by computer. *Commun ACM.* 1964;7:255-259.

67. Eckstein EF. Menu planning by computer: the random approach. *J Am Diet Assoc.* 1967;51:529-533.

68. Petot GJ, Marling C, Sterling L. An artificial intelligence system for computer-assisted menu planning. *J Am Diet Assoc.* 1998;98(9):1009-1014.

69. Roberts S, Marshall A, Chaboyer W. Hospital staffs' perceptions of an electronic program to engage patients in nutrition care at the bedside: a qualitative study. *BMC Med Inform Dec Mak.* 2017;17:105-116.

70. Hartwell H, Johns N, Edwards J. E-menus–managing choice options in hospital foodservice. *Int J Hosp Manag.* 2016;53:12-16.

71. Maunder K, Lazarus C, Walton K, Williams P, Ferguson M, Beck E. Energy and protein intake increases with an electronic bedside spoken meal ordering system compared to a paper menu in hospital patients. *Clin Nutr ESPEN.* 2015;10(4):e134-e139.

72. Blecher L. Using forecasting techniques to predict meal demand in Title IIIc congregate lunch programs. *J Am Diet Assoc.* 2004;104(8):1281-1283.

Chapter 23

Dietetics Education Research

Mary B. Gregoire, PhD, RD, FADA, FAND |
Kevin Sauer, PhD, RDN, LD, FAND

LEARNING OBJECTIVES

1. Categorize nutrition and dietetics education research studies.

2. Describe the various methodologies used to collect data in nutrition and dietetics education research.

3. Understand the importance of nutrition and dietetics education research.

Nutrition and dietetics education prepares students with the needed competence to effectively compete for entry-level positions and positively contribute to the nutrition and dietetics profession. The formal education of registered dietitian nutritionists (RDNs) began in the 1920s.[1] At nearly the same time, research on nutrition and dietetics education began as a way to discover the best ways of educating future RDNs and establish principles for nutrition and dietetics education. The first issue of the *Journal of the American Dietetic Association*, published in 1925, contained a questionnaire from the education section of the American Dietetic Association designed to solicit information on the courses given to student dietitians in the hospital.[2]

This chapter categorizes research in nutrition and dietetics education, discusses techniques and tools used when conducting nutrition and dietetics education research, and suggests future directions for nutrition and dietetics education research. This chapter is not intended to be an exhaustive review of the research that has been conducted on nutrition and dietetics education but rather cites selected studies as examples within each section.

CATEGORIES OF NUTRITION AND DIETETICS EDUCATION RESEARCH

Several categories of research are described in other chapters in this text. Much of the research done in nutrition and dietetics education could be categorized as descriptive, observational, or experimental.

Descriptive Research

Types of descriptive studies include survey research, case reports, and qualitative research. Surveys, a commonly used descriptive research design in nutrition and dietetics education, have been used to describe attitudes, beliefs, or practices. These descriptive studies have focused on issues of concern to nutrition and dietetics educators at particular points in time.

Often, descriptive studies include a focus on program content and teaching techniques.[3-10] Researchers have also examined such topics as simulation,[11-14] interprofessional education,[13-16] cultural competence,[17,18] and diversity[19,20] in nutrition and dietetics education using descriptive methods.

Case studies in nutrition and dietetics education are twofold, as they can serve as a form of research methodology or can be used to describe the scope of the research being undertaken. These case studies usually describe teaching techniques and innovative course content implemented at an individual nutrition and dietetics education program.[12,21-26]

Qualitative research has only begun to be used as a methodology for nutrition and dietetics education research. Kruzich and colleagues,[27] for example, used qualitative techniques with practicum preceptors to evaluate a dietetics internship. Others have used interviews or reflection exercises to capture student perceptions of different modes of education or content delivery.[12,13,17,28]

Observational and Experimental Research

Very little nutrition and dietetics education research could be categorized as observational or experimental. Studies that have been structured as more experimental, that is, with the goal of hypothesis testing, have focused primarily on testing methods for teaching information to students. Most commonly a pre- and postsurvey design is used to assess student attributes, such as satisfaction with or knowledge of education methods.[11-14,29] See Box 23.1 on page 458 for more information about types of descriptive research in nutrition and dietetics education.

DATA COLLECTION TECHNIQUES

Researchers in the field of nutrition and dietetics education use a variety of data collection techniques. Questionnaires are the most common data collection technique used, but tests, interviews, and observation have also been used. This section gives examples of nutrition and dietetics education research studies using each technique and discusses potential concerns.

Questionnaires

A questionnaire is a group of printed questions, either on paper or in an electronic format, used to elicit information from respondents by self-report. The questions may be open ended, that is, requiring respondents to answer in their own words; closed ended, that is, requiring respondents to select one or more answers from among the answers provided; or a combination of the two. Recent research studies have used questionnaires to collect data primarily from students[7,9,28,30,31] although some studies have also collected data from preceptors,[9] program directors,[3,6] and practitioners[19,22] to address issues related to nutrition and dietetics education. Researchers have surveyed current

Research Aim

Observational and experimental studies are characterized by broad statements of desired research outcomes.

Example: Researchers set out to understand how varied classroom lecture styles influence student learning outcomes.

Observational Study

Investigators measure variables by observing participants (students) without assigning specific treatments or interventions.

Example: Researchers observe 100 students in different classrooms, take note of the lecture styles, and record learning outcomes.

Experimental Study

Investigators apply and control treatments to the environments where participants have been randomly assigned and observe the effects of the treatments.

Example: Two distinct lecture styles are used to cover the same topic. Researchers observe the effects of 50 students randomly assigned to each lecture style and draw conclusions from the data.

Box 23.1 Definitions and Examples of Observational and Experimental Studies in Nutrition and Dietetics Education

RDNs to assess their perceived educational needs and intent or barriers on completing graduate education in clinical nutrition.[32]

Questionnaires are an affordable and standardized data collection tool, and they allow researchers to gather a large amount of data in a reasonable time frame. However, these instruments are prone to error, such as response bias and researcher subjectivity as to what is important to include or interpret from the findings. The accuracy of data collected using a questionnaire can be jeopardized when a question's meaning is misinterpreted. The timing of survey distribution and online vs physical mailing can also influence the accuracy of results and response rates. Guides for effective questionnaire development are discussed elsewhere in this text. Dillman and colleagues[33] also provide valuable information for investigators using this technique for data collection. Pretesting the questionnaire can help reduce the chance that respondents will misinterpret questions.[33]

Tests

According to Ary and colleagues,[34] a test is a set of stimuli or questions to be answered by the study sample members and to which a numeric score can be assigned. Tests are categorized as being either norm referenced or criterion referenced. A norm-referenced test allows investigators to compare a particular respondent's performance against a reference, or normative, group. A criterion-referenced test describes what a respondent can or cannot do compared with the criterion, but these results cannot be compared against others. Researchers can develop tests for particular studies or may obtain or purchase standardized tests from other researchers.

Standardized tests have consistent and uniform procedures for administration and for scoring and interpreting behavior and have been demonstrated to have strong validity and reliability.[35] Moore[36] suggested that tests that are not standardized usually do not have an established procedure for administration and have likely not been constructed using procedures to minimize error.

Numerous standardized tests have been developed for measuring such things as personality, reading, intelligence, behavior, and achievement. Researchers often access commercially available measuring instruments through the *Mental Measurement Yearbooks*[37] and the companion volume, *Tests in Print*.[38] These resources provide a variety of research tools and standardized psychological tests. The *Mental Measurement Yearbooks*[37] include descriptions and professional reviews of standardized test instruments. *Tests in Print*[38] provides detailed information about standardized tests, such as author, publisher, price, purpose, intended test population, scoring information, and administration time.

Purchased standardized tests are not commonly used in nutrition and dietetics education research. Two examples, however, are the work by Mitchell and Nyland[7] and Arendt and Gregoire.[9] Mitchell and Nyland[7] used the Learning Styles Inventory to compare learning styles of nutrition and dietetics students and faculty; Arendt and Gregoire[9] used the Student Leadership Practices Inventory to identify leadership behaviors in nutrition and dietetics students. More recently, Holthaus and colleagues[13] used the Readiness for Interprofessional Scale to assess an education simulation exercise among dietetics and multidisciplinary health care professionals.

Researcher-developed standardized tests are used less frequently in nutrition and dietetics education research, though researchers who have developed their own tests have documented the steps taken to ensure the reliability and validity of the tests. Buckley,[39] for example, developed culinary knowledge and skills assessments to measure the culinary prowess of students and reported the methods used to assess validity and reliability in the development of the instruments.

Nutrition and dietetics education researchers collecting data using tests must be concerned about the effect of retesting and test anxiety.[34,40] The retesting effect is of primary concern in designs that use a pretest and a posttest as part of the methodology. The retesting effect is the improvement in test scores that occurs on subsequent tests because a previous test was taken on the same material. The amount of this effect varies depending on the type of test, the sophistication of the test taker, and the amount of time between the two tests. Anderson and colleagues[40] suggested that although reducing the retesting effect may be difficult, having a control group that takes both the pretest and the posttest provides researchers with a way to statistically control for the effect of retesting.

Test anxiety is a concern because it may affect the meaning of test scores and thus influence inferences based on those scores. Test anxiety is believed to have both cognitive and emotional components. The cognitive (worry) component has been shown to affect performance on tests—the greater the level of worry, the poorer the test performance.[41] Nutrition and dietetics education researchers can try to reduce the likelihood of test anxiety before data are collected by having students use such techniques as relaxation or positive self talk, or they can try to assess the level of test anxiety and then take its influence into account when analyzing and interpreting results.

Interviews

Gay and Airasian[42] define an interview as "the oral, in-person administration of a questionnaire." Interviews vary in the amount of structure imposed and thus are categorized as structured or unstructured. Lennie and Juwah,[43] for example, interviewed preceptors to obtain information on assessment methods used to evaluate student performance in supervised practice.

Interviews allow for greater response accuracy, additional probing, and access to hard to reach audiences. However, nutrition and dietetics educators using interviews must consider the possible increased cost involved with this technique and the bias the interviewer can create. Training and using skilled interviewers is expensive, and the time involved is often long. Interviewer training is critical to help reduce bias. Furthermore, when several individuals serve as interviewers, interrater reliability must be assessed to reduce potential rater bias in the results.[36]

Observation

As a data collection technique, observation allows researchers to document visual perceptions of behavior as it occurs rather than rely on self-reports of behavior and knowledge in tests, questionnaires, and interviews. Researchers may observe situations as they exist or contrived, simulated conditions.[34] Research by Vickery and associates,[44] for example, videotaped students conducting mock–diet counseling interviews in a classroom setting after they had completed a unit on interviewing. Trained observers documented 61 skills using a scale ranging from 0 (absent) to 3 (excellent).

According to Ary and colleagues[34] and Anderson and colleagues,[45] observation data can be collected using ratings, systematic observation, coding scales, or sequential narratives. Ratings are subjective assessments made on an established scale.[45] For example, an observer in a classroom might rate the quality of the answers the instructor provides to student questions on a scale ranging from poor to excellent. Ary and colleagues[34] explain that systematic observation instruments include two types of recording systems: sign and category. Sign systems list a large number of variables, and each variable that occurs during a given period of observation is marked. For example, a list of classroom behaviors might include "student asks question," "teacher gives directions," and so forth. An observer using a sign system observation instrument would check each of the behaviors observed. Behaviors occurring more than once during the observation period are checked only once. Category systems generally include a more restricted number of variables. These variables are recorded continuously and as often as they occur to produce an ongoing, moving record of behaviors. In the classroom example, the observer would record continuous behavior, documenting each time the student asks a question, each time the teacher provides direction, and so on. Data collected using the category system of observation would include a sequence of events in the classroom and the frequency at which each particular behavior occurs. Coding scales are descriptive scales used to help describe behaviors observed. Each observation of a behavior, such as the instructor interacting with a student, would be coded from a list of possible descriptors of the behavior. Classic work by Flander,[46] for example, provided the following options for coding teacher talk:

- accepts feelings
- praises/encourages
- accepts students' ideas
- asks questions
- lectures
- gives direction
- criticizes or justifies authority

Sequential narratives are a written description of all behaviors that occur during an observation session.[36]

The type of scale used depends on the objectives of the research project. If the goal is to determine whether certain behaviors occur in the classroom, a systematic observation instrument with a sign system for recording might be most appropriate. If the goal is to determine the frequency or sequence of specified behaviors, a systematic observation instrument with a category system of recording would be used. When more detail about the actual behaviors and interactions are desired, coding scales or sequential narratives are most commonly used.

Researchers in nutrition and dietetics education who use observation techniques for data collection must consider the potential for several sources of error, including the Hawthorne effect, halo effect, generosity error, and error of severity.[42] The Hawthorne effect refers to changes in behavior that occur when participants in an experiment or evaluation are aware that they are being observed. Students may work more eagerly or teachers teach more enthusiastically if they know they are being observed or think they have been specially chosen to be part of a research project. To help reduce the Hawthorne effect, researchers often need to minimize the newness of the program to students or find ways to make both the treatment and the control groups believe they are receiving equal treatment; alternatively, students may need to be unaware they are being observed. The halo effect occurs when raters allow their general impressions to influence their judgment when documenting observations. Generosity error occurs when raters give the participant the benefit of the doubt and give a more positive rating on the behavior being observed. The other extreme, the error of severity, occurs when a rater has a tendency to give less positive ratings on all characteristics. Thorough training of observers is usually needed to help reduce the impact of the halo effect and generosity or severity errors.

LEVELS OF RESEARCH

Anderson[45] proposes four levels of educational research: descriptive, explanatory, generalization, and basic. According to Anderson,[45] descriptive research is used to describe what has happened in the past or what is happening currently. Research methods such as case studies, needs assessment, program evaluation, and survey research are often used to describe past or current practice. Statistics are often used to quantify and simplify description by grouping observations.

Explanatory research focuses on what is happening in a specific setting rather than on the implications for the world at large.[45] Explanatory research addresses two major questions:

- What is causing this to happen?
- Why did it happen?

Research methods used to address these questions include case studies, comparative or correlational studies, observation, or time-series analysis (see Box 23.2 for definitions of these methods).

Determining whether the same thing will happen in different circumstances is the goal of generalization research. For example, can a new teaching technique that has demonstrated effectiveness at one university be implemented at another university and produce the same outcome? Experimental, quasi-experimental, meta-analysis, and predictive approaches are often used in this type of research.[13,45]

Basic or theoretical research attempts to determine whether there is an underlying principle to explain an observed phenomenon. Such research often involves experiments, meta-analysis, or time-series analysis.[45] Very limited basic or theoretical research has been published in nutrition and dietetics education.

FUTURE RESEARCH NEEDS

Research in nutrition and dietetics education is important to the growth and development of the profession of nutrition and dietetics and is essential for educating future RDNs to be effective. The 1994 Future Search Conference[47] set forth recommendations for the nutrition and dietetics profession that prioritized immediate action to enhance the research skills of practitioners. The 1998 American Dietetic Association environmental scan[48,49] encouraged nutrition and dietetics education researchers to look to the future and develop projects that would help provide the information needed to better guide nutrition and dietetics education. Research priorities

Case study	Study in which a real-life example is described and examined
Comparative study	Study that explores similarities and differences in two or more cases, events, or specimens
Correlational study	Study that examines the relationship between two variables
Observation	Study in which researchers observe outcomes without implementing a treatment or intervention
Time-series analysis	Study in which researchers analyze data collected at predefined points during a period of time

Box 23.2 Types of Methods Used in Explanatory Research

identified by the Academy of Nutrition and Dietetics research committee in 2004 and 2014, included nutrition and dietetics education as a key research priority.[50,51] The 2014 report[51] specifically encouraged research to determine knowledge, skills, and competencies that are critical for effective entry-level and advanced practice, effective teaching methods and strategies, career paths and employment trends in nutrition and dietetics, and strategies for attracting diverse practitioners.

The multiyear project by the Accreditation Council for Education in Nutrition and Dietetics (ACEND) exploring the future education needed to prepare entry-level nutrition and dietetics practitioners provides an example of the use of multiple research methodologies to collect data and validate research findings. ACEND's *Rationale Document*[52] summarizes interviews, focus groups, online data collection, and qualitative input that have been collected and used to help shape the future of nutrition and dietetics education.

Researchers in nutrition and dietetics education might explore and replicate research and research topics and methods used in the field of education, such those reported in education research journals (eg. *American Educational Research Journal, Educational Research*). Moving nutrition and dietetics education research from its reliance on descriptive-level research using surveys, case studies, and observation toward the generalization and basic levels of research that use experimental, meta-analysis, and predictive approaches would improve its quality.

Nearly all the nutrition and dietetics education research conducted to date has been quantitative in nature. Future research of a more qualitative nature might provide new insights into the underlying intentions and feelings of students that affect the nutrition and dietetics education process. Interprofessional research projects conducted with education researchers could produce information on why students learn and on factors that help motivate students in the learning process. In addition, with the proliferation of online education programs, several forms of online delivery of education have surfaced. This brings opportunities to examine ideal learning styles for different forms of content delivery, such as face to face, online, or simulated.

Nutrition and dietetics education research has provided valuable information for nutrition and dietetics educators. Research has focused on strategies and program outcomes. Systematic research also seeks to determine future competencies to ensure a competent and competitive nutrition and dietetics workforce. Many studies have focused on a single program, which limits generalization beyond that program.

Publication of nutrition and dietetics education research findings is limited. Although such research projects are being conducted, as evidenced by the number of abstracts for poster presentations at the annual Academy of Nutrition and Dietetics Food and Nutrition Convention and Expo, few of these projects are published as more complete research papers. The Academy's research publication, *Journal of the Academy of Nutrition and Dietetics*, includes reports of dietetics education research projects in "Topics of Professional Interest," a section designed to highlight practice-related topics rather than research summaries. The Nutrition and Dietetics Educators and Preceptors quarterly newsletter, *NDEP Line*, includes manuscripts detailing research being done to enhance nutrition and dietetics education.

CONCLUSION

To date, researchers in nutrition and dietetics education have focused primarily on descriptive and quantitative methods for collecting and analyzing data and most often present their research findings through poster sessions at national conferences rather than publication in peer-reviewed journals. Exploring why this is occurring could help researchers develop strategies for expanding publication of research results. In the future, nutrition and dietetics education research must expand from the descriptive level to more analytic approaches. Researchers should select the best measurement techniques for their studies while being aware of the strengths and limitations of the various techniques that could be used

Research in nutrition and dietetics education is paramount to ensure that students and future practitioners acquire the evidence-based knowledge and competencies expected by employers and the recipients of nutrition and dietetics care and services. Research opportunities and methods in nutrition and dietetics are diverse and will mirror new frontiers in education that address various modes of teaching, learning styles and assessment, simulation, and online education initiatives.

REFERENCES

1. Chambers MJ. Professional dietetic education in the US. *J Am Diet Assoc.* 1978;72:569-599.

2. Questionnaire for the education section. *J Am Diet Assoc.* 1925;1:31.

3. Scheule B. Food-safety educational goals for dietetics and hospitality students. *J Am Diet Assoc.* 2000;100(8): 919-927.

4. Lorenz RA, Gregory RP, Davis DL, Schlundt DG, Wermager J. Diabetes training for dietitians: needs assessment, program description, and effects on knowledge and problem solving. *J Am Diet Assoc.* 2000; 100(2):225-228.

5. Rhee LQ, Wellman NS, Castellanos VH, Himburg SP. Continued need for increased emphasis on aging in dietetics education. *J Am Diet Assoc.* 2004;104(4): 645-649.

6. Short JE, Chittooran MM. Nutrition education: a survey of practices and perceptions in undergraduate dietetics education. *J Am Diet Assoc.* 2004;104(10):1601-1604.

7. Mitchell AW, Nyland NK. Learning styles differ between senior dietetics students and dietetics faculty members. *J Am Diet Assoc.* 2005;105(10):1605-1608.

8. Vickery CE, Cotugna N. Incorporating human genetics into dietetics curricula remains a challenge. *J Am Diet Assoc.* 2005;105(4):583-588.

9. Arendt SW, Gregoire MB. Dietetics students perceive themselves as leaders and report they demonstrate leadership in a variety of contexts. *J Am Diet Assoc.* 2005; 105(8):1289-1294.

10. Gould S. Potential use of classroom response systems (CRS, clickers) in foods, nutrition, and dietetics higher education. *J Nutr Educ Behav.* 2016;48(9):669-674.

11. Todd J, McCarroll C, Nucci A. High-fidelity patient simulation increases dietetic students' self-efficacy prior to clinical supervised practice: a preliminary study. *J Nutr Educ Behav.* 2016;48(8):563-567.

12. McKay T, Jimenez EY, Svihla V, Castillo T, Cantarero A. Teaching professional practice using interactive learning assessments to simulate the Nutrition Care Process. *Top Clin Nutr.* 2016;31(3):257-266.

13. Holthaus V, Sergakis G, Rohrig L, et al. The impact of interprofessional simulation on dietetic student perception of communication, decision making, roles, and self-efficacy. *Top Clin Nutr.* 2015;30(2):127-142.

14. Gibbs H, George K, Barkley R, Meyer M. Using multiple-patient simulations to facilitate interprofessional communication between dietetic and nursing students and improve Nutrition Care Process skills. *Top Clin Nutr.* 2015; 30(3):230-238.

15. Gilchrist M, McFarland L, Harrison K. Dietetics students' perceptions and experiences of interprofessional education. *J Hum Nutr Diet.* 2011; 24(2):135-143.

16. Turner P, Eliot K, Kent S, Rusnak S, Landers P. Level of implementation of the Institute of Medicine recommended core competencies among dietetics education programs. *J Acad Nutr Diet.* 2017;117(11):1709-1716.

17. Wright L, Lundy M. Perspectives of cultural competency from an international service learning project. *J Acad Nutr Diet.* 2014;114(7):996-997.

18. McArthur L, Greathouse K, Smith E, Holbert D. A quantitative assessment of the cultural knowledge, attitudes, and experiences of junior and senior dietetics students. *J Nutr Educ Behav.* 2011;43(6):464-472.

19. Wynn C, Raj S, Tyus F, et al. Barriers to and facilitators of dietetics education among students of diverse backgrounds: Results of a survey. *J Acad Nutr Diet.* 2017; 117(3):449-468.

20. Olivares L, Burns-Whitmore B, Kessler L. Retaining Hispanic dietetic undergraduate students through mentoring and professional development. *J Acad Nutr Diet.* 2014;114(2):189-195.

21. Brehn BJ, Rourke KM, Cassell C. Enhancing didactic education through participation in a clinical research project. *J Am Diet Assoc.* 1999;99(9):1090-1093.

22. Hampl JS, Herbold NH, Schneider MA, Sheeley AE. Using standardized patients to train and evaluate dietetics students. *J Am Diet Assoc.* 1999;99(9):1094-1097.

23. Litchfield RE, Oakland MH, Anderson JA. Improving dietetics education with interactive communication technology. *J Am Diet Assoc.* 2000;100(10):1191-1194.

24. Harman T, Bertrand B, Greer A, et al. Case-based learning facilitates critical thinking in undergraduate nutrition education: students describe the big picture. *J Acad Nutr Diet.* 2015;115(3):378-388.

25. Plaine EK, Hamady CM, Ludy MJ. Use of web-based timelines to enhance patient care skills of dietetics students. *J Acad Nutr Diet.* 2017;117(3):347-352.

26. Smith AR, Christie C. Facilitating transdisciplinary teamwork in dietetics education: a case study approach. *J Am Diet Assoc.* 2004;104(6):959-962.

27. Kruzich LA, Anderson J, Litchfield RE, Wohlsdorf-Arendt S, Oakland MJ. A preceptor focus group approach to evaluation of a dietetic internship. *J Am Diet Assoc.* 2003; 103(7):884-886.

28. Novotny D, Novik M. Complementary and integrative health attitudes and education of dietetics students about complementary and alternative medicine therapies. *Top Clin Nutr.* 2015;30(3):209-221.

29. Turner RE, Evers WD, Wood OB, Lehman JD, Peck LW. Computer-based simulations enhance clinical experience of dietetic interns. *J Am Diet Assoc.* 2000;100(2):183-190.

30. Lakshman R, Strohbehn CH. Student attitudes toward podcasting for food safety education: an example-based approach. *J Foodserv Manage Educ.* 2011;5(1):28-31.

31. Lambert L, Kim YH, Molaison EF, Tidwell DK. Dietetics students' cultural food knowledge and experiences with various cultures, *J Foodserv Manage Educ.* 2012;6(2):6-9.

32. Tatum C, Touger-Decker R, Brody R, Byham-Gray L, O'Sullivan-Maillet J. Perceived needs for graduate level clinical nutrition education for registered dietitians. *Top Clin Nutr.* 2008;23(4):320-330.

33. Dillman DA, Smyth JD, Christian LM. *Internet, Phone, Mail and Mixed-Mode Surveys.* 4th ed. New York City, NY: John Wiley & Sons; 2014.

34. Ary D, Jacobs LC, Razavieh A. *Introduction to Research in Education.* 6th ed. Belmont, CA: Wadsworth/Thomson Learning; 2002.

35. McMillan JH. *Educational Research.* 2nd ed. New York, NY: HarperCollins; 1996.

36. Moore GW. *Developing and Evaluating Educational Research.* Boston, MA: Little Brown and Co; 1983.

37. Carlson J, Geisinger KF, Jonson JL, eds. *The Twentieth Mental Measurements Yearbook.* Lincoln: University of Nebraska Press; 2017.

38. Anderson N, Schlueter JE, Carlson JF, Geisinger KF, eds. *Tests in Print IX.* Lincoln: University of Nebraska Press; 2016.

39. Buckley NH. Culinary Competence: Skills and Knowledge Assessment for Dietetic Students. Master's thesis. 2016. http://scholarworks.uark.edu/etd/1701. Accessed March 2, 2018.

40. Anderson SB, Ball S, Murphy RT. *Encyclopedia of Educational Evaluation.* San Francisco, CA: Jossey-Bass Publishers; 1975.

41. Cassady J. The stability of undergraduate students' cognitive test anxiety levels. *Pract Assess Res Eval.* 2001; 7(20):1-5.

42. Gay LR, Airasian P. *Educational Research.* 7th ed. Upper Saddle River, NJ: Prentice Education; 2003.

43. Lennie SC, Juwah C. Exploring assessment for learning during dietetic practice. *J Human Nutr Diet.* 2010; 23(3): 217-223.

44. Vickery CE, Cotugna N, Hodges PA. Comparing counseling skills of dietetics students: a model for skill enhancement. *J Am Diet Assoc.* 1995;95(8):912-914.

45. Anderson G. *Fundamentals of Educational Research.* 2nd ed. Bristol, PA: Falmer Press, Taylor & Francis; 1998.

46. Flander NA. *Analyzing Teacher Behavior.* Boston, MA: Addison-Wesley; 1970.

47. Parks SC, Fitz PA, Maillet JO, Babjak P, Mitchell B. Challenging the future of dietetics education and credentialing—dialogue, discovery, and direction: a summary of the 1994 Future Search Conference. *J Am Diet Assoc.* 1995;95(5):598-606.

48. Maillet JO, Rops MS, Small J. Facing the future: ADA's 1998 environmental scan. *J Am Diet Assoc.* 1999;99(3):347-350.

49. Bezold C, Kang J. Looking to the future—the role of the ADA environmental scan. *J Am Diet Assoc.* 1999;99(8): 989-993.

50. Castellanos VH, Myers EF, Shanklin CW. The ADA's research priorities contribute to a bright future for dietetics professionals. *J Am Diet Assoc.* 2004;104(4): 678-681.

51. Academy of Nutrition and Dietetics. *Priorities for Research: Agenda to Support the Future of Dietetics.* Chicago, IL: Academy of Nutrition and Dietetics; 2014.

52. Accreditation Council for Education in Nutrition and Dietetics. *Rationale for Future Education Preparation of Nutrition and Dietetics Practitioners.* Chicago, IL: Accreditation Council for Education in Nutrition and Dietetics; 2017.

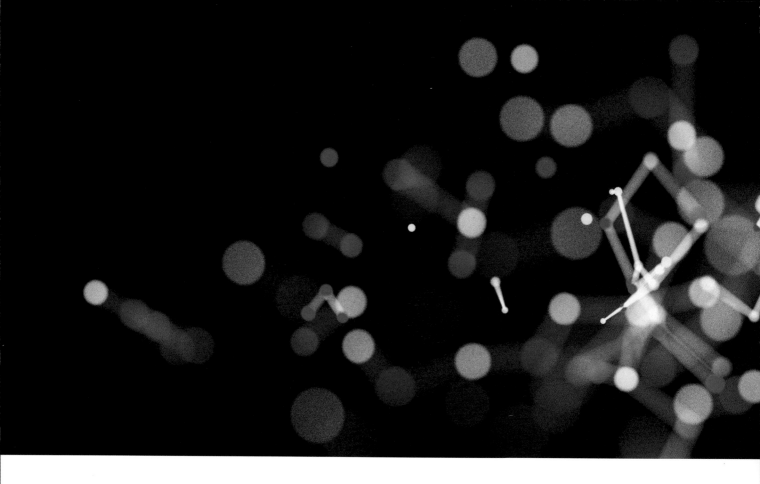

SECTION 8

Application of Statistical Analysis in Nutrition and Dietetics Research

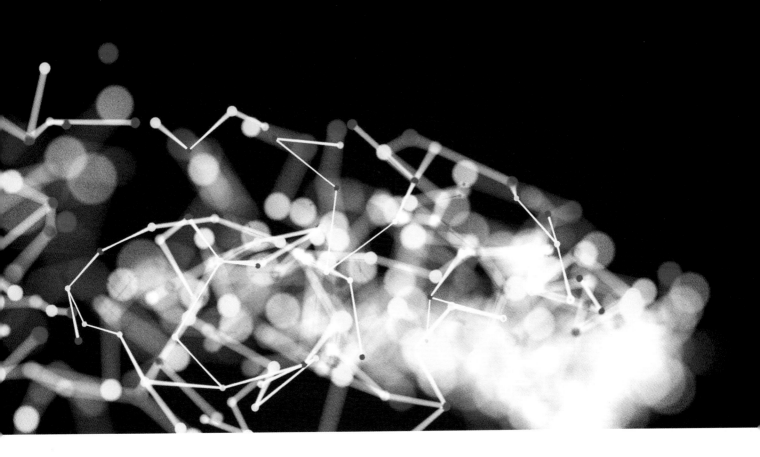

Chapter 24

Estimating Sample Size

Jeffrey Harris, DrPH, MPH, RDN, LDN, FAND |
Carol J. Boushey, PhD, MPH, RDN

LEARNING OBJECTIVES

1. Describe the steps in sample size determination.
2. Calculate sample sizes for various research and data situations.
3. Use software and websites for calculating sample size.
4. Explain the difference between clinical and statistical significance.

Almost all studies rely on the selection of samples from populations and not data from an entire population. Estimating sample size is a vital initial step in designing a successful study so the right size sample can be chosen from a population. Insufficient sample sizes can result in failure to detect meaningful effects and low confidence in the validity and reliability of results. Studies with excessive sample sizes may result in the inefficient and ineffective use of resources, financial and otherwise. This chapter focuses on the determination of sample sizes for a variety of study designs and data types. More specifically, this chapter highlights the issues underlying the logic of sample size calculations, outlines the general procedure that is common to all situations, describes the procedures specific to common research situations, recommends useful statistical software and calculation websites, and provides references for further information.[1] Finally, the distinction between clinical and statistical significance will be addressed in relation to determining appropriate sample size. This chapter will not address conditions in which a set sample size is known or assumed to determine the standard deviation, α, and β to estimate a minimum relevant effect size.

THE LOGIC OF SAMPLE SIZE CALCULATIONS

The process of estimating the required sample size involves several steps and can be technically complex. A knowledgeable statistician as well as statistical software and calculation websites can be very valuable.

The use of statistics allows the investigator to estimate the unknown. By using statistics, the investigator can estimate characteristics of a population based on observations of a sample drawn from it. The size of the sample largely determines how accurate or precise the estimates from the sample are; the larger the sample, the more information about the population and the more precise the estimate. Uncertainty always exists. The investigator, however, can specify in advance the amount of uncertainty that is acceptable for the study and perform appropriate sample size calculations.

Two hypotheses, the null hypothesis and the alternative hypothesis, provide the framework for the logic of sample size calculations. Before an investigation is undertaken, the investigator formulates an alternative hypothesis that serves as the basis of the investigation.[2] The null hypothesis—that there is no

difference or effect—typically serves as a standard of comparison. Statistical analysis is conducted to determine whether the results of a study are consistent with the underlying null hypothesis. If the results do not demonstrate the presence of a difference or an effect, the investigator concludes that the data fail to refute the null hypothesis.

When drawing conclusions from statistical results, there are four possible outcomes—two correct and two incorrect (Table 24.1). First, one can correctly conclude that there is no difference or effect when there is none (probability=$1-\alpha$; for convenience in sample size calculations, it is often incorrectly assumed that failure to reject the null hypothesis is the same as concluding that the null hypothesis is true; however, this assumption is not appropriate when interpreting results). Second, one can conclude that there is a difference or effect when there is none (probability=α; false-positive, type I error). Third, one can conclude that there is no difference or effect when there is one (probability=β; false-negative, type II error). Finally, one can conclude that there is a difference or effect, which is truly present (probability=$1-\beta$; power). All four possible outcomes are expressed statistically as probabilities of reaching the appropriate conclusions.

The type I error, or α error, is also known as the significance level of the study; its complement, $1-\alpha$, is the correct conclusion if the null hypothesis is true. By convention, α is usually set at 5%, or 0.05. This means that the maximum acceptable risk of drawing a false-positive conclusion when the null hypothesis is true is 5%. Obviously, the smaller the α, the lower the risk of drawing a false-positive conclusion. The investigator specifies the α level when planning the study and compares the resulting P value with α at the end of the study. If the observed

		Truth About Study Hypothesis	
		True alternative, H_1 (real difference)	False (null, H_0) (no real difference)
Statistical test result	True: Reject H_0 (difference)	Correct ($1-\beta$, power)	False positive (type I error, α)
	False: Do not Reject H_0 (no difference)	False negative (type II error, β)	Correct ($1-\alpha$)

Table 24.1 Possible Outcomes When Drawing Conclusions from Statistical Results

P value is less than α, the result is considered to be statistically significant.

The type II error, or β error, expresses the probability of missing a difference; its complement is power, or $1-β$. If the null hypothesis is not true and a difference or effect exists, the β probability quantifies the risk of missing that difference, and power quantifies the chance of finding it. As β decreases, power increases. The investigator specifies β when planning the study, which then determines power. For example, if the risk of missing a difference were set at 20% (0.20), the chance that the study would find a real difference would be 80% (0.80).

The probability that if a true effect exists, a study will detect power largely depends on the sample size. Increasing the sample size increases the power. At the same time, increasing the sample size decreases the risk of a false-positive conclusion (ie, α or type I error) because the ability to detect a true difference increases.

The power of a study also depends to some degree on the true magnitude of difference or effect under study (often termed *effect size*). For any given power, a large difference can be detected with a smaller sample size more easily than a small difference can be detected. Accordingly, for any given sample size, the study will be more likely to detect a large difference than a small difference. The investigator determines in advance the magnitude of difference or effect that is important for the study to be able to detect, sometimes referred to as the target effect size or target minimum detectable effect size, and this becomes the research hypothesis for the purposes of power and sample size calculations.

There is a general relationship among sample size, type I error, power, and the magnitude of the difference or minimum effect sought. The required sample size is inversely related to the magnitude of the difference and the type I error rate (α), and it is positively related to the standard deviation and desired power $(1-β)$.[3]

If the sample size is not restricted, the investigator will want to determine the sample size required to ensure a high probability of detecting a meaningful difference or effect. If, in contrast, the sample size is limited (ie, predetermined), the investigator can use sample size calculations to determine the prob-ability (power=$1-β$) that the study will be able to detect a meaningful difference. In practice, the final determination of the size of the research project will be a judicious balance of power and resources (financial and otherwise).

GENERAL PROCEDURE FOR SAMPLE SIZE CALCULATIONS

Sample size estimates are based on a number of assumptions about the conditions of the study. It is not possible for an investigator to know in advance what the conditions of the study and unanticipated changes in design will be; thus, the calculations provide only an estimate. The general procedure for calculating the required sample size involves seven steps, which are discussed in the sections that follow.

Step 1

Choose the main outcome of interest in the study and the method by which it is to be measured (eg, bone density of the radius as measured by dual photon absorptiometry). A series of sample size calculations may be performed if the study has more than one important outcome. In such cases, the largest estimated sample size is generally used. Note that α may need to be adjusted for the increased number of simultaneous significance tests (see step 5).

Step 2

Choose the statistical test that is appropriate for the data and the research question (eg, the independent *t* test). It is best to consult with a statistician at this point.

Step 3

Specify the magnitude of the difference or effect that is meaningful to detect. Often this information is gleaned from previous similar studies. The magnitude of the difference or effect selected should be practical—that is, an important difference in practice. As noted later in this chapter, the meaningful difference or effect (clinical significance) is not always the same as a statistically significant difference. If too large a sample size is chosen, small differences that are statistically significant may not be clinically significant. Additionally, the sample should be sufficiently small that a negative study outcome (ie, no significant difference) would be assurance that if a true difference existed, it would be too small to be of practical importance.

Step 4

Estimate the expected variability of the difference in outcome between two groups—that is, the estimated standard deviation (SD). Preferably, this value comes from a pilot study conducted earlier or previously published research results. Lacking either of these, investigators must make a best guess.

Step 5

Specify the maximum acceptable risk of a false-positive conclusion (α, or type I, error). For a given sample size, alterations in α concomitantly alter both power and β. As α is lowered, power decreases and β increases; as α is increased, power increases and β decreases. By convention, the α probability is set at 0.05, although some situations may warrant setting a lower or higher risk. The seriousness of a false-positive conclusion determines whether the maximum acceptable risk should be set lower. Only under rare circumstances is α set greater than 0.05, as doing so can make the results less convincing. An increased α would be warranted, however, in circumstances in which there are serious consequences of a false-negative conclusion (β error) and investigators want to decrease β without increasing the sample size beyond what is feasible.

Another consideration in choosing α is whether the statistical test is to be one tailed or two tailed. A one-tailed test attempts to detect a difference in only one direction. The more conservative approach of applying a two-tailed significance test enables the investigator to test for a difference in either direction from the null and is generally preferred.

When a study has more than one primary outcome, it is important to test each with the same level of rigor, that is, $\alpha=0.05$ or lower. Some (but not all) statisticians believe the appropriate way to ensure that the α level remains at less than or equal to 0.05 (or the desired level) for all significance tests is to account for more than one test. Accounting for more than one primary outcome is usually achieved by dividing the desired α by the number of significance tests being conducted. For example, if investigators plan to test the difference between treated and control groups on three primary outcomes and choose $\alpha=0.05$ as acceptable, they should compute the sample size based on $0.05 \div 3 = 0.017$ to preserve the type I error probability of 0.05. This is one of a number of approaches to adjust for multiple comparisons.

Step 6

Specify the probability of successfully detecting the difference or effect, if it exists (power $=1-\beta$). Alternatively, the probability of a false-negative conclusion can be specified (β, or type II, error). By convention, power is usually set at 0.80 to 0.90, and β is set at 0.20 to 0.10. Again, the seriousness of a false-negative conclusion guides the decision.

Step 7

Apply the appropriate calculations. Note that there are different formula variations based on the specific data situation and research designs (see the examples and calculations in the next section).

SAMPLE SIZE DETERMINATION FOR SPECIFIC RESEARCH SITUATIONS
Paired Continuous Data

A paired *t* test is usually used in an investigation in which a continuous response measure that is normally distributed is observed before and after the participant receives a treatment or in an investigation in which observations in two groups with similar characteristics are linked by pairing, such as determining statistical differences between identical twins. In this instance, the sample size formula accounts for the correlation between the measurements within the pairs.[4,5]

Take the example of a study assessing whether a particular intervention will decrease dietary cholesterol intake as measured by 3-day food records (step 1). For a one-sample, before-and-after study design, an experimental effect can be tested with a paired t test (step 2). Using the data of Cohen and associates,[6] it can be determined that a change of -75 mg would be meaningful and practical (step 3). Furthermore, the SD of the difference (SD_{diff}) can be estimated (step 4) as 158.9 mg, according to the study of Van Horn and colleagues,[7] which used 3-day food records.

The α is specified in advance with a two-tailed test (step 5) as 0.05. The investigators set power, or $1-\beta$, at 0.80, making $\beta=0.20$ (step 6). The appropriate calculations (step 7) can now be applied. The calculation of the sample size needed to conduct a test with a significance level of α and a power of $1-\beta$, follows. See Table 24.2 for the Z values.

$$n=\left[\frac{(Z_{1-\beta}+Z_{1-\alpha})\times SD_{diff}}{(Mean_1-Mean_2)}\right]^2$$

(formula for sample size for paired t situation)

$Z_{1-\beta}=0.84$ (from Table 24.2)

$Z_{1-\frac{\alpha}{2}}=1.96$ (from Table 24.2)

$SD_{diff}=158.9$

$Mean_1-Mean_2=75$ mg

$$n=\left[\frac{(0.84+1.96)\times158.9}{75}\right]^2$$

$$=\left[\frac{444.92}{75}\right]^2$$

$$=35.2, \text{ or 35 partcipants}$$

If the investigators also planned to measure the difference in other nutrients (eg, saturated fat intake), these calculations would be repeated for each nutrient of interest using $\alpha=0.05\div k$, where $k=$ the number of nutrients of interest. The appropriate Z value would be chosen based on a lower α. The final sample size would correspond to the calculation with the highest n. Finally, the investigators would enroll extra participants to allow for attrition during the intervention without compromising the study's power (dropout rates and noncompliance are discussed later).

Two-Sided Test[a]		
α *or* β	$Z_{\left(1-\frac{\alpha}{2}\right)}$	$Z_{(1-\beta)}$
0.01	2.58	2.33
0.025	2.24	1.96
0.05	1.96	1.64
0.10	1.64	1.20
0.20	1.28	0.84
0.30	1.04	0.52

Table 24.2 Standard Normal Distribution Multipliers (Z Values) for Values of α and β

[a]If using a one-sided test, the $Z_{1-\alpha}$ values would be the same as those in the $Z_{1-\beta}$ column

Tables are available to help investigators estimate sample size and power for a variety of differences and levels of α and β errors.[4,8] These tables are useful because they eliminate the need to use a formula to calculate the sample size.

Group Comparison with Continuous Data

Two Independent Groups

Study designs addressing nutrition questions usually involve a comparison of two samples, such as in the case of randomized trials. Investigations are often planned to observe the response measures on participants who receive either of two treatments, typically an experimental treatment and a control treatment. The response variable (eg, serum high-density lipoprotein cholesterol level) is measured on a continuous scale with the assumption that it conforms to a normal distribution. A specified magnitude of difference is set at a level thought to be important with a particular power. The comparison is usually made using an independent t test.

For example, suppose members of the dietetics department of a health maintenance organization (HMO) are concerned that the current screening criteria for anemia using the hemoglobin value may need to be revised. Nordenberg and colleagues[9] suggest that hemoglobin cutoff values should be adjusted upward for smokers. The HMO collects detailed smoking information on each new enrollee and determines hemoglobin value, so an investigation is planned to determine whether women smokers and nonsmokers between the ages of 18 and 44 years have significantly different hemoglobin values. One of the study components involves comparing the mean hemoglobin values of a random sample of smokers with those of a random sample of nonsmokers.

In this case, the main end point of interest is hemoglobin, a continuous variable (step 1). To compare the means of the two randomly selected groups, an independent t test can be used (step 2). The results reported by Nordenberg and colleagues[9] indicate that the mean hemoglobin value is 137 g/L among female smokers and 133 g/L among female nonsmokers. The calculated difference of interest is 4 g/L (step 3). A standard error of 0.4 g/L for smokers and 0.5 g/L for nonsmokers was reported.[9] By converting these values (step 4) to their corresponding SDs (standard error = SD/square root of n), setting α at the conventional 0.05 (step 5) and power at 90% (step 6), and applying the appropriate formula, the sample size for the two groups can be determined. Following is the formula for calculating the sample size for each group for a two-sided test (assuming unequal variances).[3,10]

$$n = \frac{\left(Z_{1-\beta} + Z_{1-\frac{\alpha}{2}}\right)^2 (SD_1^2 + SD_2^2)}{(Mean_2 - Mean_1)^2}$$

SD_1 (nonsmokers) = 17.37
SD_2 (smokers) = 12.37
$Z_{1-\beta}$ = 1.28 (from Table 24.2)
$Z_{1-\frac{\alpha}{2}}$ = 1.96 (from Table 24.2)
$Mean_2 - Mean_1$ = 4 g/dL

$$n = \frac{(17.37^2 + 12.37^2)(1.28 + 1.96)^2}{(-4)^2}$$
$$= \frac{(454.7338)(10.4976)}{16}$$
$$= 298 \text{ in each group (596 total)}$$

Three or More Independent Groups

Studies that compare a continuous response measure in more than two groups usually use an analysis of variance model for data analysis rather than

several t tests. Based on analysis of variance, Zar[11] provides a nomogram to estimate the required sample size when comparing three or more treatment groups. In addition, later in this chapter software and websites will be listed where investigators may calculate sample size for different situations. Note that if the sample sizes were being calculated using formulas and so on, the previously described seven-step procedure would be used.

Cross-Sectional Studies/Surveys, Proportions, and Continuous Variables

Often the goal of cross-sectional studies and surveys is to estimate population parameters from a sample drawn from the population. It is important to be able to estimate the sample size needed for an effective estimate. Charan and Biswas[12] present great examples of calculating sample sizes for the estimation of population proportions and continuous variables. The formulas and calculations presented here illustrate a sample size calculation to estimate the proportion of children who have hypertension in a city population. The seven steps for calculating sample sizes are presumed. This calculation differs from previous sample size calculation situations because a large enough sample size must be chosen to achieve a sufficiently low sampling error.

$$n = \frac{\left(Z_{1-\frac{\alpha}{2}}\right)^2 (p)(1-p)}{d^2}$$

$Z_{1-\frac{\alpha}{2}}$ = 1.96 (based on two-tailed α of 0.05; see Table 24.2)
p = 0.15 (expected proportion of children with hypertension in the population from previous or pilot studies, 15%)
d = 0.05 (the amount of error in the estimate investigators are willing to tolerate, 5% error)

$$n = \frac{(1.96)^2 (0.15)(1 - 0.15)}{(0.05)^2}$$
$$= \frac{(3.84)(0.15)(0.85)}{0.0025}$$
$$= \frac{0.49}{0.0025}$$
$$= 196$$

To estimate the proportion of children with hypertension with a type I error of 5% and 5% error, 196 children must be selected randomly from the city population. Charan and Biswas[12] also present an example of calculating the sample size for estimating a continuous variable for a population. They use the example of estimating the mean systolic blood pressure of children in a city population. Again, presume that the seven steps for sample size calculations are followed.

$$n = \frac{\left(Z_{1-\frac{\alpha}{2}}\right)^2 (SD)^2}{d^2}$$

$Z_{1-\frac{\alpha}{2}} = 1.96$ (based on two-tailed α of 0.05; see Table 24.2)

SD = 25 mmHg

(SD from previous or pilot studies)

d = 5 mm Hg (amount of error acceptable on either side of the mean)

$$n = \frac{(1.96)^2 (25)^2}{(5)^2}$$
$$= \frac{(3.84)(625)}{25}$$
$$= 96$$

In this case, the investigator must choose a random sample of 96 children from the city pediatric population to estimate the mean systolic blood pressure with a 5% chance of type I error and an error ±5 mm Hg.

Independent Groups and Proportions

Das and colleagues[13] present an excellent illustration for calculating the appropriate sample size when comparing proportions related to two independent groups. In this case investigators would use an independent t test to compare proportions. Suppose an investigator was studying the ability of phenylephrine to reduce the proportion of patients who develop hypotension after spinal anesthesia. One group would get the phenylephrine and the other a placebo. The calculation that follows presents the sample determination. Presume that all seven steps are followed.

$$n = \frac{\left(Z_{1-\frac{\alpha}{2}} + Z_{1-\beta}\right)^2 (p_1 q_1 + p_2 q_2)}{x^2}$$

$Z_{1-\frac{\alpha}{2}} = 1.96$ (based on two-tailed α of 0.05; see Table 24.2)

$Z_{1-\beta} = 0.84$ (based on a β of 0.20 and a power of 0.80; see Table 24.2)

$p_1 = 0.20$ (proportion of subjects with hypotension in the treated group based on previous or pilot studies)

$q_1 = 0.80$ proportion of participants without hypotension in the treated group; $1 - p1$)

$p_2 = 30$ (proportion of participants with hypotension in the control group based on previous or pilot studies)

$q_2 = 0.70$ proportion of participants without hypotension in the control group; $1 - p2$)

$x = 0.10$ (the difference in proportions between the groups that is clinically relevant as determined from previous or pilot studies)

$$n = \frac{\left[(1.96+0.84)^2\right]\left[(0.20)(0.80)+(0.30)(0.70)\right]}{(0.10)^2}$$
$$= \frac{(2.80)^2 (0.16 + 0.21)}{0.01}$$
$$= \frac{(7.84)(0.37)}{0.01}$$
$$= \frac{2.90}{0.01}$$
$$= 290 \text{ per group}$$

In this case, 290 participants must be recruited for each group. Once investigators collect the data for each group they can conduct an independent t test for proportions with a power of 80%, risk of type I error at 5% and sensitivity to a minimum proportion difference between groups of 10%.

Paired Observations and Proportions

Rosner[3] presents a formula for determining the sample size for a situation in which investigators want to compare proportions before and after a treatment or among matched pairs of participants. In this case a paired *t* test would be used for proportions to analyze the data. For example, suppose a sample of children in which 50% are malnourished and investigators want to apply an intervention to attempt to reduce the proportion of malnourished children in the sample. The following calculation shows how to estimate the sample size in this situation. Again, presume the seven steps.

$$ n = \frac{p_0 q_0 \left(Z_{1-\frac{\alpha}{2}} + Z_{1-\beta}\sqrt{\frac{p_1 q_1}{p_0 q_0}} \right)^2}{(p_1 - p_0)^2} $$

n = number of pairs or participants if they have before and after measurements

$Z_{1-\frac{\alpha}{2}} = 1.96$ (based on two-tailed α of 0.05; see Table 24.2)

$Z_{1-\beta} = 0.84$ (based on a β of 0.20 and a power of 0.80; see Table 24.2)

$p_0 = 0.50$ (estimated proportion of children who are malnourished before the intervention)

$q_0 = 0.50$ (estimated proportion of children who are not malnourished before the intervention; $1-p_0$)

$p_1 = 0.40$ (estimated proportion of children who will be malnourished after the intervention based on previous or pilot studies)

$q_1 = 0.60$ (estimated proportion of children who will not be malnourished after the intervention; $1-p_1$)

$$ n = \frac{(0.50)(0.50)\left[(196) + (0.84)\sqrt{\frac{(0.40)(06.0)}{(0.50)(.50)}} \right]^2}{(0.40 - 0.50)^2} $$

$$ = \frac{(0.25)\left[1.96 + 0.57 \right]^2}{0.01} $$

$$ = \frac{(0.25)(6.40)}{0.01} $$

$$ = 160 $$

In this case 160 participants with before and after measurements of malnutrition will be needed to have a power of 80%, a risk of type I error of 5%, and a minimum sensitivity to detect a change in proportion by 10%.

Case-Control Studies

Case-control studies involve choosing participants with and without a disease. These groups of participants are compared retrospectively to determine if there are statistically significant differences between the groups. Often these groups are matched demographically. Appropriate sample sizes must be calculated to minimize type I and type II errors as well as to be able to detect differences between groups. Groups can be compared for both categorical and continuous variables. The two types of variables use separate sample size formulas.[12,14] Separate formulas and calculations are provided for categorical and continuous variables. Presume the seven procedural steps.

In the case of a categorical variable, suppose investigators want to examine women with and without bulimia nervosa. The women are asked about childhood sexual abuse retrospectively to examine a potential association between bulimia and sexual abuse. The investigators need a sample size that allows them to effectively explore this association. The formula and data are as follows:

$$ n = \frac{r+1}{r} \frac{(p^*)(1-p^*)(Z_{1-\frac{\alpha}{2}} + Z_{1-\beta})^2}{(p_1 - p_2)^2} $$

n = number of participants in each group (cases and controls)

r = 1 (ratio of cases to controls; in most cases this will be 1 to keep equal numbers in the groups)

$p^* = 0.25$ average proportion exposed [(estimated proportion of exposed cases + estimated proportion of exposed controls) ÷ 2]

$Z_{1-\frac{\alpha}{2}} = 1.96$ (based on two-tailed α of 0.05; see Table 24.2)

$Z_{1-\beta} = 0.84$ (based on a β of 0.20 and a power of 0.80; see Table 24.2)

$p_1 = 0.30$ estimated proportion of cases exposed to sexual abuse determined from previous or pilot studies

$p_2 = 0.20$ estimated proportion of controls exposed to sexual abuse determined from previous or pilot studies

$$n = \frac{1+1}{1} \frac{(0.25)(1-0.25)(1.96+0.84)^2}{(0.30-0.20)^2}$$

$$= \frac{2}{1} \frac{(0.25)(0.75)(2.80)^2}{(0.10)^2}$$

$$= \frac{2.94}{0.01}$$

$$= 294$$

In this situation 294 cases and 294 controls must be recruited. This will ensure only a 5% chance of type I error, 80% power, and minimum estimation of difference in proportions of 10%.

For a case-control study examining the difference between cases and controls for a continuous variable the formula is different. Suppose an investigator wants to examine the potential association between birth weight and diabetes in adulthood.[12] The cases in this situation are adults with diabetes and the controls are those without. The groups will be compared for their birth weights. The formula and calculations follow.

$$n = \frac{r+1}{r} \frac{(SD)^2 \left(Z_{1-\frac{\alpha}{2}} + Z_{1-\beta}\right)^2}{d^2}$$

n = number of participants in each group (cases and controls)

r = 1 (ratio of cases to controls; in most cases it is 1 to keep equal numbers in the groups)

SD = 1 kg (this is the SD that might be expected in birth weight derived from past and pilot studies)

$Z_{1-\frac{\alpha}{2}} = 1.96$ (based on two-tailed α of 0.05; see Table 24.2)

$Z_{1-\beta} = 0.84$ (based on a β of 0.20 and a power of 0.80; see Table 24.2)

d = 250 g (0.25 kg) (estimated mean difference in birth weight between cases and controls from past and pilot studies)

$$n = \frac{1+1}{1} \frac{(1)^2(1.96+.084)^2}{(0.25)^2}$$

$$= \frac{2}{1} \frac{(1)(7.84)}{0.06}$$

$$= \frac{15.68}{0.06}$$

$$= 261$$

For this example, 261 cases and 261 controls would need to be recruited. Investigators can be assured that there is only a 5% risk of type I error, 80% power, and minimum detectable difference of 0.25 kg in birth weight.

Cohort Studies

In cohort studies, researchers select participants with and without exposure to a risk factor. They then monitor participants for a substantial time period and document an outcome of interest.

Suppose researchers want to conduct a cohort study examining a possible association between tree nut consumption and myocardial infarctions. They propose recruiting participants who eat tree nuts as a normal part of their diets. In addition, they want to select a comparison group of participants who do not eat tree nuts. The researchers will track these participants and document the number of myocardial infarctions (MIs) in each group after 30 years. The proportion of the participants with MIs in each group will be compared for statistically significant differences. Following are the steps for calculating the sample size needed for this study[12,15]:

$$n = \frac{\left[Z_{1-\frac{\alpha}{2}}\sqrt{\left(1+\frac{1}{m}\right)p^*(1-p^*)} + Z_{1-\beta}\sqrt{\frac{p_0(1-p_0)}{m} + p_1(1-p_1)}\right]^2}{(p_0-p_1)^2}$$

$Z_{1-\frac{\alpha}{2}} = 1.96$ (based on two-tailed α of 0.05; see Table 24.2)

$Z_{1-\beta} = 0.84$ (based on a β of 0.20 and a power of 0.80; see Table 24.2)

m = 1 (number of control participants per study participants; 1 should be selected if the groups should be the same size)

p_1 = 0.10 (estimate that 10% of study participants will develop MIs)

p_0 = 0.20 (estimate that 20% of controls will develop MIs)

p^* = 0.15 (average proportion between study participants and controls)

$$n = \left[(1.96)\sqrt{\left(1+\frac{1}{1}\right)(0.15)(1-0.15)} \right.$$

$$\left. + (0.84)\sqrt{\frac{.020(1-0.20)}{1}+0.10(1-0.10)} \right]^2$$

$$\overline{(0.20-0.10)^2}$$

$$= \frac{\left[(1.96)\sqrt{2(0.15)(0.85)} + (0.84)\sqrt{0.20(0.80)+0.10(0.90)} \right]^2}{0.10^2}$$

$$= \frac{\left[(1.96)(0.50)+(0.84)(0.50) \right]^2}{0.01}$$

$$= \frac{(0.98+0.42)^2}{0.01}$$

$$= \frac{1.40^2}{0.01}$$

$$= 196$$

This calculation indicates that 196 participants must be recruited for each group. This will ensure that the risk of type I error is 5%, the power is 80%, and the proportion difference is 0.20. However, it would be prudent to oversample to compensate for the possibility that some participants will drop out or die during the prospective period.

Complex Situations

This chapter has explored the most basic situations for calculating sample size. The calculations for nutrition studies that involve factorial designs, crossover designs, repeated measures, complex analysis of variance, regression, reliability estimates, and multivariate statistical techniques are best done using specialized software or websites. The same is true for more complex epidemiologic studies and nonparametric statistical testing situations. A variety of references are available for reading about these more complex situations.[16-20] When determining sample sizes using software or websites, investigators must make similar decisions about α and other values.

SOFTWARE AND WEBSITES

Though estimating sample size is much easier through the use of calculation software or websites,

it is important for registered dietitian nutritionists to know how sample sizes are calculated. Box 24.1 on page 478 presents a variety of free and fee-based software and websites for calculating sample size and where to access them.[12,18]

The most comprehensive applications are G*Power, GLIMMPSE, PASS, and the UCSF Sample Size Calculators. Most nutrition investigators use these applications to determine sample sizes rather than calculating by hand.

CLINICAL AND STATISTICAL SIGNIFICANCE

Sample size and power calculations incorporate the concepts of clinical and statistical significance. Of these two concepts, clinical significance is more important. The finding that the effect of two treatments is statistically significantly different is of little value if the size of the difference is of no practical importance. For example, a study might find that a weight loss medication produces a statistically significant 5% reduction of original body weight; however, a 15% reduction is required to produce a significant improvement in metabolic syndrome (clinical significance). When planning a study, clinical or practical significance should be the driving force.[21]

Investigators have the option of several methods to determine the degree of difference or strength of association needed to obtain clinical significance. Commonly, they use information from peer-reviewed published experimental studies, case reports, systematic reviews, or data from pilot studies recently conducted. Clinical experience in practical situations can also inform as to the clinical significance. A registered dietitian nutritionist may develop an intuition about determining when interventions are leading to practical improvement in patients. Thus, investigators can look to their own experience or that of colleagues as a basis for a meaningful outcome. Lindgren and colleagues[22] describe a procedure for choosing a size of treatment effect that is based on the underlying distribution of the measurement of interest in the target population. This procedure has the benefit of minimizing any subjectivity in selecting clinical significance and is useful in generating a range of values to use for the size of the effect.

Software or Website	Description and Access Information
G*Power	Free software for calculating statistical power
	Download from the G*Power home page at the University of Dusseldorf (www.gpower.hhu.de/en.html)
GLIMMPSE	Free software for calculating accurate sample size and power
	Download from the Sample Size Shop website (http://samplesizeshop.org/software-downloads/glimmpse)
SPSS Sample Power 3	Software for calculating sample size; a free 14-day trial period is offered, after which the software must be purchased
	Download from the IBM website (www-01.ibm.com/marketing/iwm/iwmdocs/tnd/data/web/en_US/trialprograms/U741655I36057W80.html)
Open Epi	Free open-source software for epidemiologic statistics
	Download from the Open Epi website (www.openepi.com/Menu/OE_Menu.htm)
EpiTools	The Ausvet website offers a number of free epidemiologic calculators (http://epitools.ausvet.com.au/content.php?page=home)
UCSF Sample Size Calculator	The University of California, San Francisco, Clinical and Translational Science Institute offers free sample size calculators (www.sample-size.net)
PowerandSampleSize.Com	The PowerandSampleSize.com website has more than 30 free calculators (http://powerandsamplesize.com/Calculators)
Power Analysis for ANOVA	This website, maintained by Michael Friendly, runs an SAS program that calculates power or sample size needed to attain a given power for one effect in a factorial analysis of variance design (www.math.yorku.ca/SCS/Online/power)
ClinCalc	The ClinCalc website offers a free sample size calculator (http://clincalc.com/stats/samplesize.aspx)
PASS Sample Size Calculator	A free trial of the NCSS Statistical Software sample size program is available before purchase (www.ncss.com/software/pass)

Box 24.1 Sample Size Calculation Software and Websites

CONCLUSION

Researchers want to avoid performing a study that may fail to find a statistically significant difference when a true difference does exist. This is an example of a type II error, and such a result can be avoided through the use of sample size calculations during the design of the study. The calculation provides the researcher with the number of individuals needed in each group of study participants to produce statistically significant results. The specific calculation needed will depend on the type of study and the outcome measure. Many resources are available to aid the researcher, including sample size calculators and consultations with a statistician. Before using any resource, the researcher needs to estimate the level of outcome that would be meaningful and the variation surrounding the outcome measure. This can be achieved through a review of the literature or by performing pilot studies.

REFERENCES

1. Browner WS, Newman TB, Cummings SR, Hulley SB. Estimating sample size and power: the nitty-gritty. In: Hulley SB, Cummings SR, Browner WS, Grady D, Hearst N, Newman TB, eds. *Designing Clinical Research: An Epidemiological Approach.* 2nd ed. Philadelphia, PA: Lippincott Williams & Wilkins; 2001:65-91.

2. Field A. *An Adventure in Statistics.* Thousand Oaks, CA: Sage; 2016:337-339.

3. Rosner B. *Fundamentals of Biostatistics.* 7th ed. Boston, MA: Brooks/Cole; 2011:231, 302, 383.

4. Dixon WJ, Massey FJ Jr. *Introduction to Statistical Analysis.* 4th ed. New York, NY: McGraw-Hill; 1983.

5. Lachin JM. Introduction to sample size determination and power analysis for clinical trials. *Control Clin Trials.* 1981; 2(2):93-113.

6. Cohen NL, Laus MJ, Stutzman NC, Swicker RC. Dietary change in participants of the Better Eating for Better Health course. *J Am Diet Assoc.* 1991;91(3):345-346.

7. Van Horn L, Moag-Stahlberg A, Liu K, et al. Effects on serum lipids of adding instants oats to usual American diets. *Am J Public Health.* 1991;81(2):183-188.

8. Noordzij M, Tripepi G, Dekker FW, Zoccali C, Tanck MW, Jager KJ. Sample size calculations: basic principles and common pitfalls. *Nephrol Dial Transplant.* 2010;25(5): 1388-1393.

9. Nordenberg D, Yip R, Binkin NJ. The effect of cigarette smoking on hemoglobin levels and anemia screening. *JAMA.* 1990;264(12):1556-1559.

10. Turner RM, Walter SD, Macaskill P, McCaffery KJ, Irwig L. Sample size and power when designing a randomized trial for the estimation of treatment, selection, and preference effects. *Med Decis Making.* 2014;34(6):711-719.

11. Zar J. *Biostatistical Analysis.* Upper Saddle River, NJ: Pearson; 2010: 861.

12. Charan J, Biswas T. How to calculate sample size for different study designs in medical research? *Indian J Psychol Med.* 2013;35(2):121-126.

13. Das S, Mitra K, Mandal M. Sample size calculation: basic principles. *Indian J Anaesth.* 2016;60(9):652-656.

14. Cai J, Zeng D. Sample size/power calculation for case-cohort studies. *Biometrics.* 2004;60(4):1015-1024.

15. Kasiulevičius V, Šapoka V, Filipavičiūtė R. Sample size calculation in epidemiological studies. *Gerontologjia.* 2006; 7(4):225-231.

16. Ryan T. *Sample Size Determination and Power.* Hoboken, NJ: John Wiley and Sons; 2013.

17. Candel MJ, Van Breukelen GJ. Sample size calculation for treatment effects in randomized trials with fixed cluster sizes and heterogeneous intraclass correlations and variances. *Stat Methods Med Res.* 2015;24(5):557-573.

18. Guo Y, Logan HL, Glueck DH, Muller KE. Selecting a sample size for studies with repeated measures. *BMC Med Res Methodol.* 2013;13:100.

19. Konikoff J, Brookmeyer R. Sample size methods for estimating HIV incidence from cross-sectional surveys. *Biometrics.* 2015;71(4):1121-1129.

20. Viechtbauer W, Smits L, Kotz D, et al. A simple formula for the calculation of sample size in pilot studies. *J Clin Epidemiol.* 2015;68(11):1375-1379.

21. Page P. Beyond statistical significance: clinical interpretation of rehabilitation research literature. *Int J Sports Phys Ther.* 2014;9(5):726-736.

22. Lindgren BR, Wielinski CL, Finkelstein SM, Warwick WJ. Contrasting clinical and statistical significance within the research setting. *Pediatr Pulmonol.* 1993;16(6):336-340.

Philip Gleason, PhD | *Mary C. Naglak, PhD, RD* |
Carol Koprowski, PhD, RDN

LEARNING OBJECTIVES

1. Recognize the key elements of a study design and analysis that affect the selection of statistical methods.

2. Describe the basic process of selecting statistical methods to use for a specific research question.

3. Develop working knowledge of basic statistical procedures used to estimate relationships and assess significance in different study design situations.

Selecting the statistical method to apply for best analyzing research data can be a challenge to a researcher or investigator who is not a statistician. Guidance from a statistician throughout a research project can help address this challenge, but to facilitate this communication, the investigator should be familiar with the fundamentals of statistical analysis. Having a working knowledge of statistics is also important for understanding the research literature and assessing the quality of research articles. This chapter reviews these fundamentals in the first section, describes basic statistical concepts and outlines the general process of conducting statistical analysis in the second section, and provides a tool kit of statistical procedures to address a variety of research questions along with extended examples of the application of some of these procedures in the third section.

FUNDAMENTAL ELEMENTS OF STUDY DESIGN AND STATISTICAL ANALYSIS

Elements that guide the selection of a statistical method in a research study include the research question, type of data collected (scale of measurement), and number and type of samples being analyzed along with their relationship. Another central aspect of most statistical analysis is the testing of research hypotheses, which allows researchers to draw conclusions based on the data being analyzed. The process of testing hypotheses raises a number of additional considerations, including assumptions about the distribution of the data, whether the hypothesis is directional (one-sided) or nondirectional (two-sided) and whether the investigator is interested in a single research question or more than one question (multiple comparisons).

The Research Question

The starting point in any research study is the research question. It is critically important for the investigator conducting a dietetics study to carefully define the question being addressed because this determines the type of analysis to be conducted. The research question lays out what the researcher is interested in knowing and what the consumer of research should expect to learn.

There are different kinds of research questions. One important distinction is between causal and descriptive questions. Causal questions seek to identify causal relationships, those of cause and effect between variables in a population. For example, a causal question might determine if a long-chain n-3 enriched diet improves cognition in the elderly.[1] Descriptive questions seek to describe the attributes of a population or relationships or associations among variables in that population, without necessarily attributing causality. An example of a descriptive question is, "What was the mean intake of sodium (mg/d) by US adults from 1999 to 2016?"[2]

Other types of distinctions between research questions are also possible. For example, some distinguish between comparative and relational research questions. Each of these questions has a different, though closely related, aim. Comparative research questions seek to examine differences between two (or more) groups on one (or more) dependent variable(s). A simple example of a comparative question is, "What is the difference in energy intake of male and female high school students?" On the other hand, relational research questions seek to estimate the relationship between two variables, an independent variable such as sex or family income, and a dependent variable, such as an individual's health status, nutritional intake, or preferred type of exercise. Researchers should be careful when interpreting relational questions as many are not causal relationships but rather associations, trends, or interactions. Establishing a causal relationship most convincingly requires an experimental study design, whereby study participants are randomly assigned to either an experimental condition—such as a prespecified long-chain n-3 enriched diet—or a control condition—such as participants' usual diet.

Ultimately, research questions should define the variables of interest in an analysis and lead directly to research hypotheses about the way these variables might be related. In other words, the research questions determine what hypothesis testing the investigator will be conducting in a study. The process of hypothesis testing is described later in the chapter.

Scale of Measurement (Type of Data Collected)

Characteristics that can be measured or counted are referred to as variables. Variables can be classified as categoric or numeric. Categoric variables can be further classified as nominal or ordinal, and numeric categories can be further classified as continuous or discrete (see Figure 25.1 on page 482). The statisti-

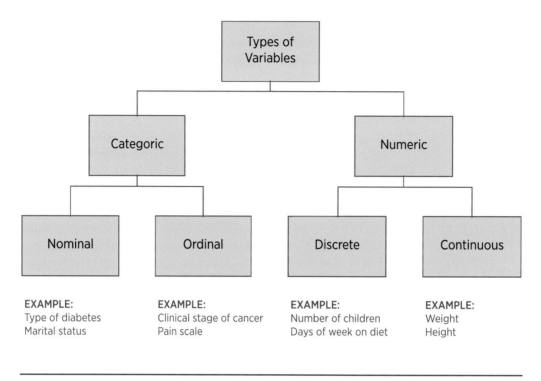

Figure 25.1 Classification of types of variables

cal methods used for categoric variables differ from the methods used for numeric variables.

Categoric: Nominal vs Ordinal Variables

Categoric variables have values that do not have meaning as numbers but instead group participants into categories; in other words, these kinds of variables are not cardinal measures (number that specifies a quantity, something that can be counted). Categoric variables represent names or categories, and they may have values that are nonordered (nominal) or ordered (ordinal). Nominal variables have values that represent categories that have no ordered meaning. An example of a nominal variable might be the following categories regarding marital status: never married, married, widowed, and divorced. Nominal variables that fit into two categories are termed *binary*. For example, a researcher may create a binary variable where a value of 1 indicates the presence of a particular condition in an individual—such as having type 2 diabetes, and a value of 0 indicates the absence of the condition.

Ordinal variables take on values that represent ordered categories, such that higher values indicate more of a particular attribute than lower values.

Clinical stage of cancer (1 through 4) is an example of an ordinal variable. With ordinal variables, the space between values is undefined. In other words, if an ordinal variable has a value of 3 for an individual, then that individual has more of the attribute than those with a value of 1, but that does not mean the individual has three times as much of the attribute. An ordinal variable might be created from another, more detailed variable. For example, a continuous total energy intake measure could be divided into quartiles (1 through 4), but the highest quartile (4) would not necessarily have four times the energy intake of the lowest quartile (1).

Numeric: Discrete vs Continuous Variables

Discrete variables take on only a limited number of values and are typically whole numbers rather than decimals or fractions. The number of days per week someone consumed sugar-sweetened beverages is an example of a discrete variable. In this example, it is discrete in the sense that there are only eight possible values (zero times per week to seven times per week). In this case, the discrete variable is a cardinal measure because its values have meaning as numbers and the space between the values is defined (eg,

2 days is twice as many as 1 day). Thus, it makes sense to perform arithmetic operations on these values (such as adding, subtracting, or averaging them). Discrete variables can be counted, as in how many apples are in the bowl.

Continuous variables also have a defined space between numeric values, but they can have any value within a measurement scale, and the differences between values also have meaning. They can take on any value, at least within a range of values (eg, any value between 0 and 100 or even 0 and 1) and are not limited to whole numbers but can include decimals or portions. There are several types of continuous variables. Variables with interval data have numeric values with no natural zero point, such as temperature scales measured in degrees Celsius or degrees Fahrenheit. Ratio data are numeric but have a natural zero point. An example of a ratio variable is weight, since a weight of zero means the absence of weight. Continuous variables with interval or ratio data are treated the same way statistically and may also be referred to as *quantitative variables*. Other examples of continuous variables include height, energy intake, and body mass index.

Relationships Among Samples

A common type of analysis in dietetics and other fields is to compare the value of one or more variables between individuals in different samples. For example, a researcher might want to compare the incidence of a particular disease between samples of men vs women or between individuals who have received a particular treatment and those who have not. In conducting analyses such as these, an important distinction is whether the samples being compared are independent or dependent.

Independent Samples

The assumption underlying many statistical tests is that the sample data are independent. Samples are independent if members from one group are not related or linked to members of another group. For example, an investigator may be interested in the relationship between smoking and hemoglobin levels in women between the ages of 18 and 44 years. If an investigator randomly selects a group of smok-

ers and a group of nonsmokers from a given health plan and measures their hemoglobin levels, the two samples would be independent because the data were obtained from unrelated groups of women.

Dependent Samples

Samples used in statistical tests are dependent when the data points in one sample are related to (or not independent of) the data points in the second sample. For example, an investigator may be interested in the change in hemoglobin levels in women between the ages of 18 and 44 years before and after their participation in a 6-month smoking cessation program. If the investigator measures their hemoglobin levels before the program and again 6 months later, the data would be dependent because the data would have been obtained from the same women at different points in time. Several different circumstances might result in dependent samples.

Pairing and Matching Study designs sometimes pair or match samples before analysis to get the best possible estimate of the effect of a treatment. Investigators often match samples on the basis of characteristics like age and sex, particularly if these characteristics are likely to be related to the primary outcome of interest. In a study of the influence of exercise on cholesterol levels, for example, an investigator may first match adults of the same sex and similar age, and then randomly assign members of each age/sex to either a high or low exercise group. Age and sex are associated with cholesterol levels. Matching on these variables helps to control the effect they have on cholesterol when examining the relationship between exercise and cholesterol. The fact that the groups were matched to have similar characteristics implies that the high and low exercise groups are dependent.

In a paired or matched study, specially designed tests that account for the pairing or matching and the resulting dependence among measurements must be used. Examples of such tests are the paired *t* test and the Wilcoxon signed rank test, which are described in standard statistics textbooks.[3,4]

Serial/Repeat Measurements Besides matching and pairing, another situation giving rise to dependent measures is the practice of obtaining repeated or se-rial measures of the same characteristic or attribute (eg, blood pressure) on the same sample of individuals. It is common to repeat measurements of a variable at several points in time according to a predetermined schedule and then examine changes in its value over time, perhaps to evaluate the influence of an intervention implemented during that period. If the study includes more than one sample or group, this change over time may be compared between groups. For example, Rider and colleagues[5] sought to determine if television (TV) viewing while exercising increased participants' enjoyment in the exercise experience. Study participants exercised by walking on a treadmill for 30 minutes, three separate times, with a minimum of 48 hours between sessions. The researchers captured a variety of data, including heart rate and rating of physical activity enjoyment at several points in time—10, 20, and 30 minutes after starting their walk. In other words, these were repeated measures of heart rate and reported enjoyment of exercise.

Investigators must take care when analyzing data from serial measurements. For example, the dependence between measures implies that it is not appropriate to simply apply paired t tests at each time point. Instead, a two-stage method described by Matthews and colleagues[6] should be used. This approach first summarizes the observations of the individuals' responses over time and then analyzes the summary measure using standard univariate techniques that would be appropriate when using a single measurement per participant (eg, mean). Another method would be to use repeated measures analysis of variance to determine whether groups differ in their responses over time. Investigators who are not familiar with this procedure should consult a statistician.

Replicate Measurements Another situation leading to dependent samples occurs when replicate measurements are used. Replicate measurements are several measurements taken for the same individuals as part of repeated implementation of a given treatment or intervention. Using the TV viewing while exercising study as an example, replicate measurements (eg, heart rate) would occur if each study participant completed all three viewing conditions more than one time (see Figure 25.2). Analysis of variance can be used for replicate measurements of a continuous variable, provided the number of observations is the same for each participant. If this is not the case, the analysis is more complex, and statistical advice should be obtained.

Testing Hypotheses

The process of specifying hypotheses designed to address an investigator's key research question or objective is central to conducting research studies. The hypotheses determine what type of analysis should be used. They should be specified in advance of other parts of the study. Once a hypothesis is specified, then the investigator collects the data and actually tests the hypothesis. In their study of TV viewing during exercise, for example, Rider and colleagues[5] specified and tested hypotheses stating that participants who watched TV during exercise had greater (or less) enjoyment of the activity than those who did not watch TV.

Defining Null and Alternative Hypotheses

Hypothesis testing requires the investigator to specify both a null hypothesis and an alternative hypothesis. For analyses that involve examining the relationship between two variables, the null hypothesis is typically that there is no relationship between these variables (or no relationship in the anticipated direction). In the previous example, one of the null hypotheses is that there is no relationship between TV viewing during exercise and the enjoyment of that exercise. In other words, the null hypothesis states that the average level of enjoyment is the same for participants who do and who do not watch TV during exercise.

The alternative hypothesis is the opposite of the null hypothesis. It states that there is a relationship between the two variables of interest, possibly in a particular direction. Following the previous example, an alternative hypothesis from Rider and colleagues[5] is that TV viewing during exercise is related to enjoyment of that activity—those who watch TV during exercise have a different level of enjoyment than those who do not.

In defining the null and alternative hypotheses, investigators are usually more interested in the latter than the former. In other words, the theory

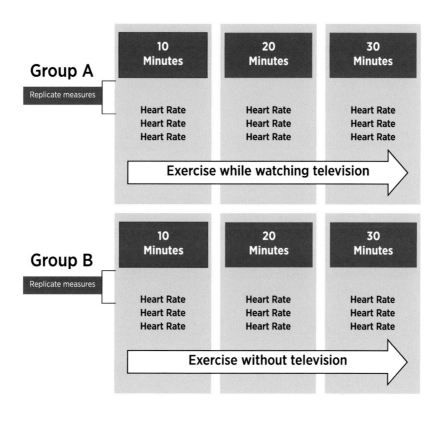

Figure 25.2 Example of serial and replicate measures

that motivated the research is usually consistent with the alternative hypothesis. For example, Rider and colleagues[5] were most interested in determining whether there is a relationship between TV viewing and enjoyment during exercise because they had reason to believe there is such a relationship. This determined how they defined the alternative hypothesis. The null is just the opposite of the alternative hypothesis.

One-Sided and Two-Sided Hypothesis Tests

Alternative hypotheses state that there is a relationship between two variables, and this departure from the null hypothesis can occur in two possible directions. If there is a relationship, the two variables can either be positively or negatively correlated. A one-sided (or directional) hypothesis test uses an alternative hypothesis that states a specific direction of the relationship. No direction is specified in a two-sided test, only that there is a nonzero relationship.

For example, an alternative hypothesis stating that participants who watch TV during exercise ex-

perience greater enjoyment of the exercise than participants who do not watch TV would be used in a one-sided test. The corresponding null hypothesis would be that participants who watch TV during exercise do not experience greater enjoyment (without distinguishing between whether they experience less enjoyment or the same enjoyment). A two-sided version of this test would use an alternative hypothesis that there is a relationship between TV watching during exercise and enjoyment without specifying whether the relationship is positive or negative—that is, whether those who watch TV experience more or less enjoyment of exercise.

Investigators sometimes use two-sided hypothesis testing, not committing in advance to a particular direction of the relationship and preserving the ability of the test to detect a relationship in either direction. This is because there is usually uncertainty about the nature of the relationship and interest in a finding that goes in either direction. A one-sided hypothesis test would be appropriate only if the investigator had strong prior beliefs that the relationship went in a particular direction and little interest in distinguishing between finding a relationship in the opposite direction vs no relationship at all.

The Logic of Hypothesis Tests

After specifying the null and alternative hypotheses, the investigator collects and examines the data to see whether observed data are consistent with the null hypothesis. Note that the focus here is on the null hypothesis, even though the investigator may be more interested in the alternative hypothesis. A hypothesis may be considered a thought experiment. After specifying the null hypothesis, the investigator initially presumes that it is true, then examines the sample data to see whether there is a relationship between the variables being studied, and finally asks the question: How likely would it be for us to observe the sample data that we see if it were really the case that the null hypothesis were true?

In reaching conclusions about the null hypothesis, investigators need to consider the possibility of making either of two types of errors. A type I error occurs if the investigator rejects the null hypothesis when it is true—in other words, the investigator incorrectly concludes there is a relationship. A type II error occurs if the investigator does not reject the null hypothesis when it is false or incorrectly concludes there is no relationship. In hypothesis testing, the idea is to select a criteria for determining whether or not to reject the null hypothesis that minimizes the chances of either error, given the trade-off involved. The more the investigator minimizes the chances of a type I error, the more likely they are to have a type II error.

The P value indicates the probability of observing the sample data conditional on the null hypothesis being true. If the data are not consistent with the null hypothesis, then the P value will be lower. If it is less than a prespecified "critical value" (often 5%, or $P<.05$), then the investigator concludes that this likelihood is so low that the null hypothesis must be false. In this case, the investigator rejects the null hypothesis and concludes that the data support the alternative hypothesis. When the null hypothesis is rejected, the relationship between the variables being examined is said to be statistically significant. Another way to interpret the P value is that it gives the probability that the

test will result in a type I error if the null hypothesis is rejected.

If the P value is higher than the critical value ($P>.05$) then the investigator concludes that there is not enough evidence to determine that the null hypothesis is false. In this case, the investigator does not reject the null hypothesis and cannot say that the data support the alternative hypothesis; the estimated relationship between the variables is not statistically significant. This does not necessarily mean the null hypothesis is true, just that there is not enough evidence to conclude that it is false.

In conducting hypothesis tests, two types of error are possible. If the null hypothesis is true and the researcher rejects the null hypothesis and reports that there is an association, this is a type I error or a false positive. If the alternative hypothesis is true but the researcher fails to reject the null hypothesis, this is a type II error or false negative.

In the analysis of the relationship between TV viewing and enjoyment during exercise, Rider and colleagues[5] rejected the null hypothesis of no relationship between these variables. They found a statistically significant relationship between watching TV during exercise and reported enjoyment of the exercise, and the relationship was positive. If no association existed between watching TV during exercise and reported enjoyment of the exercise, Rider and colleagues would have made a type I error (reported a false positive). By contrast, the results of another hypothesis test they conducted were different. They failed to reject the null hypothesis of no relationship between TV viewing during exercise and participants' heart rate during the activity. The heart rate of those who watched TV was not significantly different from the heart rate of those who did not. If the difference between heart rates of those who did and those who did not watch TV during exercise was in fact significantly different, then a type II error would have occurred.

Another way of illustrating hypothesis testing is a courtroom analogy (see Box 25.1).

Other Considerations

Beyond the basics of defining research questions, understanding different kinds of variables and

The logic behind hypothesis testing in statistical analysis is analogous to that of jury decisions in criminal trials.

Hypothesis Test	Criminal Trial

Hypothesis Test

Investigator

Null hypothesis: No relationship

Alternative hypothesis: Relationship

Initial presumption: Null is true

Data

P value: How likely is the sample data if the null hypothesis is true?

If $P < .05$:

- Reject the null hypothesis
- Data support alternative hypothesis
- Statistically significant relationship

If $P > .05$:

- Fail to reject null hypothesis
- Data do not support alternative hypothesis
- Not a statistically significant relationship

Rejecting null hypothesis does not mean null is true, just that there is not enough evidence from the data to rule it out.

Criminal Trial

Jury

Null: Defendant is not guilty

Alternative: Defendant is guilty

Initial presumption: Presumed innocent

Evidence from witnesses and exhibits

Reasonable doubt: How consistent is the evidence with the presumption of innocence?

If no reasonable doubt:

- Reject the presumption of innocence
- Jury finds defendant guilty
- Beyond reasonable doubt

If reasonable doubt:

- Do not reject the presumption of innocence
- Jury finds defendant not guilty
- Reasonable doubt remains

Reaching a verdict of not guilty does not mean defendant is innocent, just that there is not enough evidence to prove guilt.

Box 25.1 Hypothesis Testing and Criminal Trials

samples, and testing hypotheses, researchers will likely encounter many other issues in the process of conducting statistical analysis. This section highlights two of these additional considerations—assumptions about the variables' distributions and the consequences of conducting studies that involve testing large numbers of hypotheses.

Assumption of Normality

The validity of many statistical tests depends on the assumption that the data are drawn from a normal distribution and that the variability of the data within different groups is similar. For many variables and populations, this is a reasonable assumption, but for some variables and populations the data may be skewed or otherwise not follow a normal distribution. For example, the variable height among individuals from the same sex, age group, and background generally follows an approximately normal distribution, but variables capturing an individual's daily intake of many nutrients is highly skewed. In other words, many individuals in a population have low intakes of the nutrient on a given day, but a few have very high intakes, well above the overall average value. A distribution like this is said to be skewed to the right, with the right-hand tail of the distribution extending far from the rest of the distribution.

Statistical tests that rely on the assumption that the distribution of variables is normal (or has some other specific shape) are examples of parametric

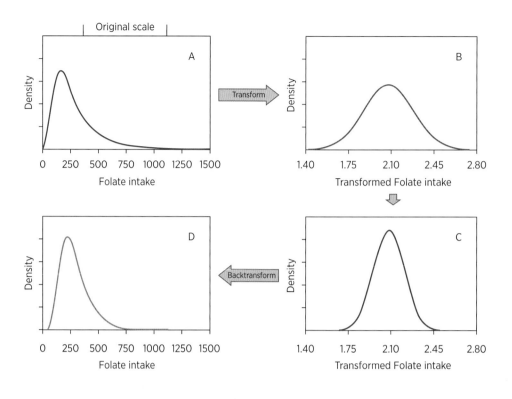

Figure 25.3 Example of transforming data (folate intake) used in statistical modeling of usual dietary intake

Adapted from Centers for Disease Control and Prevention. NHANES Dietary Web Tutorial. Task 2: Key concepts about statistical methods that have been used to estimate the distribution of usual intake with a few days of 24-hour recalls. www.cdc.gov/nchs/tutorials/dietary/Advanced/ModelUsualIntake/Info2.htm. Accessed July 19, 2018.[7]

tests. The results of such tests may be sensitive to violations of the assumption of normality. Two options for addressing the situation are described in the following sections.

Transformations When faced with a distribution that is not normal, such as a skewed distribution, a researcher may transform the skewed data using a mathematical function so that the transformed version of the data becomes approximately normal and parametric tests can be performed on the transformed data. The researcher can transform the data back to the original scale once the statistical test has been performed. An example of such a scale transformation is the log transformation, where the researcher uses the natural log or log base 10 of a variable that is skewed. After the transformation, the researcher can plot the transformed data using a histogram to determine whether the transformation resulted in an approximately normal distribution.

The drawback of this option is that interpretation of the results may not be straightforward.

The graph in the upper left of Figure 25.3 shows an example of the distribution of usual intake of folate, which is skewed to the right. The transformation of this measure results in a distribution that is approximately normal, as shown in the graph in the upper right. The bottom two graphs show the back-transformation of the distribution to its original scale.

Nonparametric Methods The second option in accounting for violations of parametric assumptions is to use a distribution-free or nonparametric statistical method. These methods do not depend on the assumption of normality and thus are valid with skewed data or with data that are collected in categoric form. These tests are easy to apply and most require minimal calculations. The disadvantage is that they are usually less powerful than their

Analysis Type	Parametric	Nonparametric
Compare two quantitative measurements taken from the same individual	Paired *t* test	Wilcoxon signed rank test
Compare means from two distinct independent groups	Independent *t* test	Mann-Whitney U test
Compare means from two or more distinct independent groups	One-way analysis of variance (ANOVA)	Kruskal-Wallis test
Estimate the degree of association between two quantitative variables	Pearson correlation	Spearman rank correlation

Table 25.1 Parametric Statistical Tests and Their Nonparametric Counterparts

parametric counterparts, especially if the assumptions are met and the parametric method can be applied.[8] In other words, the nonparametric tests may be less sensitive in finding effects and produce wider confidence intervals (confidence intervals are discussed later in this chapter). However, nonparametric statistical methods are useful and should be considered when sample sizes are small, the distribution is skewed, or categoric data are used. For more information on nonparametric statistical methods, several resources are available.[9,10] Table 25.1 provides examples of common parametric and nonparametric tests.

Multiple Comparisons

Researchers may use statistical procedures or tests to summarize the data from a single sample, compare two samples (or two subgroups from the same sample), or compare more than two samples or subgroups. For two groups, only one comparison is possible. But when more than two groups are being compared, more than one comparison is possible. In comparing groups A, B, and C, for example, the researcher can compare A to B, A to C, or B to C. When researchers make more comparisons in a single study—that is, conduct more hypothesis tests—the chances of finding a spurious significant result increase. This is the statistical problem of multiple comparisons, sometimes referred to as *multiplicity* or *multiple hypothesis testing.*[11]

More Than Two Groups With any statistical test, there is a possibility that even if there is no relationship between variables in reality, the data will—by chance—falsely lead to a finding of statistical significance. The likelihood of a false positive or type I

error like this is referred to as the *level of statistical significance,* or α, and is set by the investigator to be low, often at 5% (which corresponds to a *P* value of .05).

With more than two groups and more than one comparison, the likelihood that standard statistical tests will falsely find at least one significant result increases to more than 5%. For example, there is a 14% chance of a false positive when there are three groups and three comparisons. This likelihood of a false positive increases to 40% when there are five groups (10 comparisons).

The common practice of conducting separate and independent *t* tests to examine each pair in such situations is not appropriate because the *t* tests do not account for the multiplicity present in the data. Multiple comparison techniques are described by Schochet[11] and standard statistics texts. The standard approach involves first examining the data across all groups to determine whether there is an overall significant relationship or difference among the groups. If a significant difference does exist, the investigator then applies the appropriate multiple comparison technique to determine whether individual pairs of samples differ. Examples of these techniques include the Bonferroni, Scheffé, Tukey, Benjamini-Hochberg, Newman-Keuls, and Duncan tests.

Unrestrained Statistical Testing Multiplicity is also present when researchers look for significant differences between just two samples but for a large number of variables. Inappropriate methods, such as the unrestrained repeated use of *t* tests, are frequently used in nutrition research since many analyses involve a large number of potential outcome measures (such as intakes of a large number of different nutrients or dietary components). This may result in too many findings of statistically significant results.[8,11,12]

One approach to addressing this issue is to define in advance the primary research questions and hypothesis tests that are the focus of the research and to use the standard approach to testing and defining the level of significance for these tests only. If other tests are to be performed, they should be regarded as exploratory and a more conservative (lower) significance level should be used. For example, the Bonferroni adjustment involves dividing α by the number of comparisons. If differences between program participants and nonparticipants are compared for 20 different dietary outcomes, the standard α of 0.05 would be divided by 20 so that a significant finding would result only if the *P* value were below .0025.

THE GENERAL PROCESS OF CONDUCTING STATISTICAL ANALYSIS

The process of conducting statistical analysis for a research study consists of three general steps. First, the investigator describes the basic characteristics of the sample. Second, the investigator estimates statistics of particular interest using sample data to make inferences about the characteristics of a broader population. Third, the investigator conducts hypothesis tests and assesses statistical significance based on the sample data. The first step is sometimes referred to as *descriptive statistics*, while the second and third steps are referred to as *inferential statistics*.

Using Statistical Analysis to Summarize Data

Plotting the Data

As a first step, it is often helpful to present and describe or summarize the sample data visually. This can provide a sense of the central location of the data and its distribution. An investigator can also use visual presentations of the data to quickly identify outliers—cases with values of a variable far outside the range of typical values for other cases (Figure 25.4). Outliers may arise for various reasons. In some cases, outliers indicate a problem such as a data entry error. In this case, the researcher should either correct the error in the original data (if possible) or exclude the outlying data point from the analysis. In other cases, an outlier may simply reflect an unusual case or a highly skewed distribution. Here, the researcher may decide to exclude this data point so that the analysis reflects patterns among more typical cases, or the researcher may use statistical procedures that minimize the influence of outliers (eg, measuring central location using the median rather than the mean value).[13]

The investigator may focus on summarizing just one variable (or one variable at a time) using a histogram, which shows the frequency distribution of the variable. The frequency distribution shows the number or percentage of observations in which the variable has a particular value or falls within a particular range of values. Figure 25.5 on page 492 shows an example of a histogram from a study of remission of type 2 diabetes among patients undergoing bariatric surgery (see Box 25.2 for a description of this study). This figure shows the type of treatment for diabetes among 86 study participants. The taller center bar indicates that more than 50 of these participants were treated with oral medication, much more than were treated with insulin or diet.

To visually summarize the relationship between two variables, a scatterplot may be used. In a scatterplot, each single point on the graph shows the values of the two variables for one sample observation. The value of one variable is shown on the graph's x-axis and the value of the other variable is shown on the y-axis. The investigator then assesses the shape of the data by examining all of the data points collectively. If, for example, the data appear to take on an upward sloping shape, this would suggest a positive relationship between the variables, as shown in Figure 25.4. In this example (ignoring the outlier), observations that have more positive values of the variable shown on the x-axis also tend to have more positive values of the variable shown on the y-axis. By contrast, if the data points form a mass without any apparent upward or downward slope, this would suggest that there is no strong relationship between the variables.

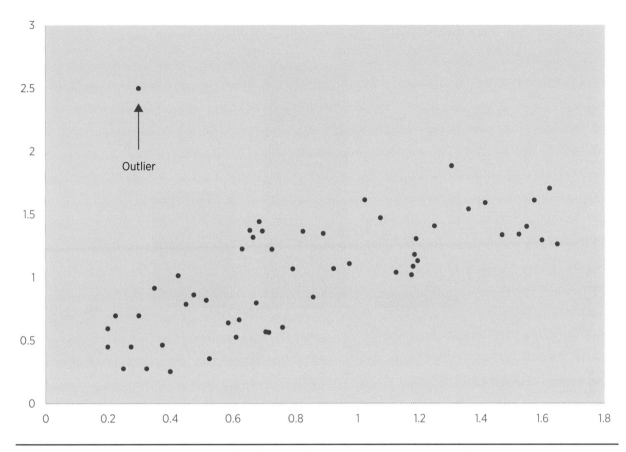

Figure 25.4 Example of a statistical outlier illustrated via scatterplot

Background: Adults who are obese and undergoing bariatric surgery frequently suffer from type 2 diabetes mellitus. Bariatric surgery may help improve this condition, and researchers are interested in whether the surgery and resulting weight loss may be associated with remission of type 2 diabetes or other health benefits.

Null hypothesis: All proportions are equal. In other words, diabetes underwent remission for an equal proportion of each of the four groups of patients.

Study design: Retrospective observational cohort study of patients undergoing one of four types of bariatric surgery (gastric banding, sleeve gastrectomy, laparoscopic gastric bypass, and biliopancreatic diversion with duodenal switch).

Methods: Patients with type 2 diabetes undergoing bariatric surgery are routinely monitored closely before and after surgery. Data from a group of 86 patients with type 2 diabetes were reviewed to determine the rate of remission of their diabetes after surgery. Data were collected before surgery, 1 month after surgery, and then at 3-month intervals for 1 year. Variables collected included race, sex, age, weight, height, body mass index, hemoglobin A1c, and fasting blood glucose. Remission of diabetes was defined as discontinuation of all medications and return of blood glucose to normal (fasting blood glucose <100 mg/dL, hemoglobin A1c<6.5%).

Box 25.2 Clinical Study Example Used to Illustrate Statistical Methods: Remission of Type 2 Diabetes in Patients Undergoing Bariatric Surgery

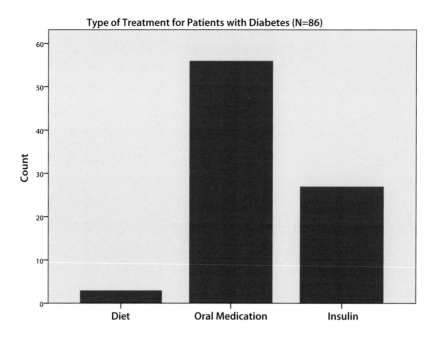

Figure 25.5 Example of how a histogram can be used to summarize a single variable such as type of diabetes treatment (diet, oral medication, insulin)

Using Summary Statistics to Describe Discrete Data

A frequency distribution is a useful way to describe the distribution of discrete data. In the diabetes study described earlier, for example, the researchers created a discrete (nominal) variable indicating the type of surgery that each participant underwent. A frequency distribution of this variable indicates that 18 participants (20.9%) had gastric banding, 13 (15.1%) had sleeve gastrectomy, 31 (36.0%) had laparoscopic gastric bypass, and 24 (27.9%) had biliopancreatic diversion with duodenal switch.

It may also be useful to compare the frequency distribution of a discrete variable for different groups within a sample. In the diabetes study example, the distribution of surgery type can be prepared for the participants with diabetes who went into remission after surgery and those who did not go into remission. Figure 25.6 uses a histogram to show the distribution of remission of diabetes and surgery type. Each bar represents the sample that underwent a particular type of surgery and the height of the bars show the percentage in each group whose diabetes did and did

not go into remission. The figure shows that the majority of the participants with diabetes who had the laparoscopic gastric bypass or biliopancreatic diversion with duodenal switch went into remission after surgery. For those who had gastric banding, the majority did not go into remission after surgery.

Using Summary Statistics to Describe Continuous Data

Statistical summaries of continuous variables are more complex than those of discrete variables. Since continuous variables can take on a wide range of potential values, a complete frequency distribution is often not useful as it would result in many categories of values containing only one observation, but it may be useful to present a modified frequency distribution showing the likelihood that the continuous variable falls into ranges of possible values. In a study of weight status and obesity among adults in the United States, for example, Flegal and colleagues[14] started with a continuous variable—body mass index (BMI) in adults—that could take on any value over a

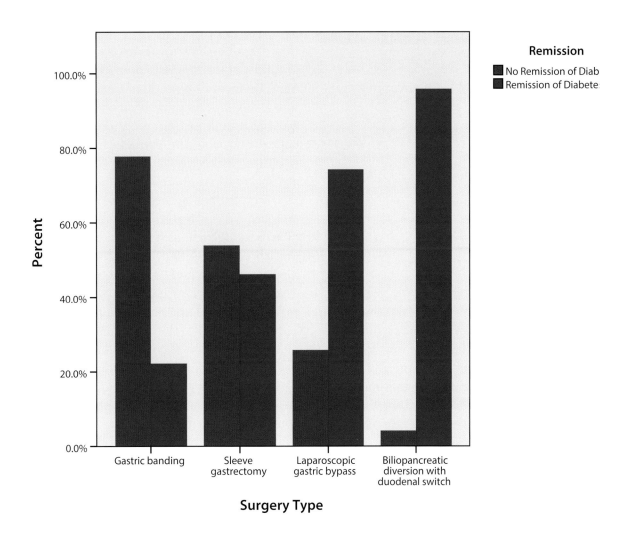

Figure 25.6 Histogram showing the distribution of diabetes remission among four different types of bariatric surgery

See Box 25.3 for additional statistical analyses based on this example.

range from less than 20 to well above 40, but instead, they included a frequency distribution of BMI by showing the percentage of participants with values at or above 30 (obese) or less than 30 (not obese) (see Table 25.2). In other analyses, they created additional categories based on the original BMI value, including class C obesity (BMI ≥ 40).

Aside from describing continuous data using a frequency distribution, an investigator can do so using a measure of central location along with a measure of the width or variation of the variable (see Table 25.3) on page 494.

Obesity status	Adults (Age 20+ Years)
Not obese (body mass index [BMI] < 30)	62.1%
Obese (BMI ≥ 30)	37.9%
Status including class C obesity	
Not obese (BMI < 30)	62.1%
Obese, not class C (30 ≥ BMI < 40)	30.2%
Class C obesity (BMI ≥ 40)	7.7%

Table 25.2 Prevalence of Obesity Among Adults in the United States[14]

Body Mass Index (N = 86)	Value
Mean	45.47
Median	44.18
Mode	36.95[a]
Standard deviation	5.97
Standard error of the mean	0.644
Variance	35.62
Range	24.82

Table 25.3 Measures of Central Tendency and Dispersion for Prestudy Body Mass Index[b]

[a] Multiple modes exist. The smallest value is shown
[b] See Box 25.2 for the related study description.

Measure of Central Location

A statistic that measures the central location of a variable's values captures the average or typical value of that variable. Examples include the mean, median, and mode. The mean value of a variable is the mathematical average value. The median is the middle value, or the value for which half of the observations have a higher value and half have a lower value. The mode is the most common or frequent value. For numeric variables, the mean value is probably the most commonly used measure of central tendency. However, for highly skewed variables or if an investigator is concerned about outliers the median may be used—unlike the mean, the median value of a variable is not influenced by outliers. For categoric variables, the mode is often used.

Measure of Variation

A statistic that measures variation captures the extent to which different observations of a variable have different values. The most common such statistic is the standard deviation, which measures the amount by which the value of a variable's typical observation differs from the mean value. The square of the standard deviation is the variable's variance.

Another common measure of variance is the range of a variable, which is the amount by which the highest and lowest values of the variable differ. The range of a variable is highly sensitive to the presence of outlier or extreme values. The more extreme a single value of a variable, the greater the range. Outlier values also have an influence on the standard deviation, although not as great.

Shape of the Distribution

The shape of a distribution describes how a variable's values are grouped around the mean, median, or both mean and median. Do most observations have values fairly close to the mean or median, with equal numbers above and below and just a few values far above and far below? This would be characteristic of a normal distribution, which would have a bell-shaped curve. Or are observations grouped in some other way?

A key distinction between distributions is whether or not they are symmetric or skewed. In a symmetric distribution—such as a normal distribution—there are an equal number of observations at various distances above and below the mean. In a skewed distribution, there are not an equal number of observations above and below the mean. If the distribution is skewed to the right, for example, there are more values below the mean than above it, but the low values are mostly clustered close to the mean while the values above the mean are more likely to be far from it. Distributions skewed to the right are common in nutrition, as described previously. For example, individuals' daily intakes of many nutrients follow this distribution. On most days, an individual will have very little or none of the nutrient, which leads to a fairly low mean value overall. On days in which the individual happens to consume a food rich in that nutrient, however, their daily intake of the nutrient will be very high. In other words, the distribution looks compressed to the left and stretched out to the right.

The shape of a distribution determines the appropriate summary statistics for a variable. A normal distribution has a convenient property—95% of the sample observations lie within two standard deviations of the mean. Thus, the mean and standard deviation are sufficient to fully describe a normal distribution. For skewed distributions, more than two summary statistics may be necessary. The median and range are helpful additional statistics in this case, as are statistics such as the 5th and 95th percentiles or statistics capturing a distribution's degree of skewness.

Describing the Relationship Between Two Continuous Variables

The statistics discussed previously all focus on approaches to describing data from a single continuous variable. In addition, there are many different ways of describing the relationships between two or more such variables. A simple example is a correlation coefficient, which can vary between −1 and +1 and indicates whether the variables have a positive relationship (correlation coefficient>0), no relationship (correlation coefficient=0), or negative relationship (correlation coefficient<0). Another example of a statistical approach to measuring the relationship between variables is regression, which provides an estimate of how the value of one variable (the independent variable) can predict the value of another variable (the dependent variable). These statistical procedures are described in greater detail in the "Developing a Tool Kit of Statistical Procedures" section.

Estimating Population Values Based on Sample Statistics

Using Samples to Estimate Population Values

Researchers often want to describe some characteristic of an entire population, such as adult women in the United States, school-aged children in a single city, or men with diabetes in Canada. It is usually not feasible to measure the characteristic among all members of the population, so a sample (preferably a random sample) is selected to represent the population. Summary statistics from that sample—for example, the mean, standard deviation, a correlation coefficient—are single value or point estimates of the analogous measure in the full population. For example, Flegal and colleagues[14] wished to estimate the prevalence of obesity among all adults in the United States, but measuring each adult's BMI would have been too costly. Thus, they relied on data from the National Health and Nutrition Examination Survey, which measured BMI among a randomly selected sample of about 5,500 adults. The estimated prevalence of obesity among this sample of adults served as the authors' point estimate of the overall prevalence of obesity among all adults in the United States.

Measuring the Degree of Uncertainty in Estimates of Population Values

If a point estimate of a population mean value is based on a sample, this implies that there is uncertainty surrounding its accuracy as an estimate of the true population mean. For example, if additional samples were drawn from the same population one might get somewhat different sample mean estimates. To measure the degree of certainty—or precision—of an estimate, researchers calculate the standard error and confidence interval for the estimate.

Standard Error Imagine if an investigator were to select a large number of random samples from the same population and then calculate a given summary statistic, such as a variable's mean value from the data in each sample. The estimated mean values resulting from these samples would themselves differ from sample to sample, and this set of estimates would form what is known as the sampling distribution of the mean. Statistical theory says that if the samples are sufficiently large (usually n>30), this sampling distribution will be normal. In addition, the mean value of all of these sample means will be at or very close to the true mean value in the population. And as with any normal distribution, 95% of the values in the sampling distribution will be within two standard deviations of the overall mean.

The standard deviation of the sampling distribution described previously is equivalent to the standard error of an estimated mean value from a single sample. The standard error reflects how certain the researcher is that the estimated mean from this one sample is actually close to the true population mean. In the case of mean values, the standard error can be calculated by dividing the standard deviation of the original variable being studied by the square root of the sample size (n). Because the sample size appears in the denominator of this calculation, the resulting standard error will be smaller when researchers calculate a sample mean using a larger sample. This lower standard error means that the researcher should have more confidence that the sample mean is close to the true population mean—there is greater precision and less uncertainty.

Although the names are similar, there are important differences between a standard error and a standard deviation. The standard deviation describes variation in a characteristic among individual participants in a sample. The standard error describes uncertainty in a sample estimate of the characteristic based on that sample. The standard error can be used to make probability statements

Standard Deviation (SD) vs Standard Error of the Mean (SE)

Statistic	Type	Description	
SD	Descriptive	Measure of the variability of the scores (data points) around the mean; average distance between the data points and the mean	$SD = \sqrt{\dfrac{\Sigma(x - M)^2}{n - 1}}$ Where x = score (data point) M = mean n = number of observations
SE	Inferential	Measure of the precision (accuracy) of the mean; standard deviation of the mean SE is always smaller than SD	$SE = \dfrac{SD}{\sqrt{n}}$ Where SD = standard deviation n = number of observations

Figure 25.7 Comparison of standard error and standard deviation

about statistics like the mean value of the characteristic, such as how likely it is that the mean value of the characteristic in the population falls within a particular range of values, known as the *confidence interval*. Figure 25.7 describes the differences between the standard error and standard deviation, along with the range and confidence interval.

Confidence Interval The confidence interval is the range of values within which it is likely (eg, with 95% probability) that the true population value falls. The calculation of the confidence interval is based on the standard error from the study sample, so it depends on both the true amount of variation in the characteristic of interest (the standard deviation of this variable) and the size of the sample used to estimate the relevant sample statistic. It also depends on the degree of confidence the investigator wishes to place in the results, conventionally set at the 95% level. This implies an $\alpha = 0.05$ level of significance, or that there is a 5% chance of incorrectly concluding that the true population value lies within the confidence interval when in fact it does not.

The confidence interval is mathematically expressed as shown in the following equation, in which

CI indicates confidence interval and SE indicates standard error:

$$CI = \text{Point estimate} \pm \text{Confidence } (1-\alpha) \text{ factor} \times SE$$

Typically, the investigator will present the confidence interval along with the point estimate of the population value. The point estimate represents the investigator's best guess as to the true population value, while the confidence interval shows the level of uncertainty surrounding this estimate. A wide confidence interval means the point estimate lacks precision and that the true population value of the statistic could actually fall elsewhere within a wide range of values. A narrow confidence interval indicates a more precise estimate and that the true population value is likely to fall somewhere close to the point estimate.

Like the standard error, the confidence interval is related to sample size. All else being equal, point estimates based on larger samples will have narrower confidence intervals. The confidence interval is useful in understanding the practical or clinical importance of estimates. For example, the confidence interval surrounding the point estimate of a correlation coefficient would help investigators understand the strength of the relationship between two variables. If the confidence interval only includes positive values that are close to one, this would suggest that we can be confident that the two variables have a strong positive relationship. However, if the confidence interval includes a wide range of both positive and negative values—that is, the confidence interval includes zero, investigators would not be able to say much about the relationship between the variables— it could be positive, it could be negative, or there could be no relationship.

Flegal and colleagues,[14] in their study of obesity among adults in the United States, present confidence intervals for their estimates of obesity. For example, they estimate that the overall rate of obesity in this population is 37.9%, and the 95% confidence interval is 36.1% to 39.8%. This implies that it is 95% likely that the true rate of obesity among adults in the United States in 2013 to 2014 was between 36.1% and 39.8%.

Assessing Statistical Significance

Statistical procedures are concerned with uncertainties, and a challenge to nutrition researchers is determining when a sample estimate provides enough certainty about a population value to allow a researcher to state a specific conclusion about that population value with confidence. Statistical significance is a tool that helps researchers make that determination. Statistical significance comes out of hypothesis testing. As described previously, researchers test null vs alternative hypotheses as a way of addressing their research questions.

Testing Hypotheses

As described previously, the focus of hypothesis testing is on the null hypothesis. If an investigator is examining the relationship between two variables (eg, using a correlation coefficient), the typical null hypothesis in a two-sided test is that there is no relationship or that the correlation coefficient is zero. The corresponding alternative hypothesis is that there is a relationship between the variables or that the correlation coefficient is not equal to zero. For example, in an investigation of a parenteral amino acid

solution rich in branched-chain amino acids and its effect on nitrogen retention, the null hypothesis (H_0) would be that the branched-chain solution has the same effect on nitrogen retention as a standard amino acid solution. The alternative hypothesis (H_1) would be that the branched-chain solution does not have the same effect as the standard amino acid solution.

After defining the null and alternative hypotheses, the investigator would select a sample and calculate the sample statistic, such as a correlation coefficient. The investigator would then conduct the hypothesis test based on the correlation coefficient estimated from the sample data, the standard error of that estimate, and some additional information about the test, such as the level of statistical significance, or α. The exact nature of the test would depend on the specifics of the hypotheses and variables involved, but two common types of hypothesis tests are t tests and χ^2 tests. For example, a t test could be used to estimate whether men and women within a given population have different mean BMI values— that is, whether there is a relationship between sex and BMI. A χ^2 test might be used to assess whether there is a relationship between an individual's race/ethnicity (as measured by three or more categories) and their BMI. Additional information about these and other tests is provided in the "Developing a Tool Kit of Statistical Procedures" section.

One result of the hypothesis test is a P value, which indicates the likelihood of obtaining the correlation coefficient estimated from the sample data if, in fact, the null hypothesis of no relationship is true. If the P value is less than the level of statistical significance being used as a threshold (that is, if $P < .05$), then the investigator would reject the null hypothesis. The conclusion in this situation would be that there is a statistically significant correlation between the variables being tested (consistent with the alternative hypothesis). The direction and strength of that relationship would depend on the exact value of the point estimate.

If there is a large P value, greater than the level of statistical significance, this indicates that it would not be unusual to get the correlation coefficient estimated from the sample data if the null hypothesis were true. In other words, the estimated correlation coefficient is not inconsistent with the null hypothesis of no relationship between the variables. This could occur if the point estimate of the correlation coefficient were close to zero or if it were not close to zero but the standard error of that estimate was very large, indicating substantial uncertainty. In this case, the investigator would not reject the null hypothesis and would conclude that there is not a significant correlation between the two variables.

Interpreting Statistical Probability Values

Caution and common sense must guide the use and interpretation of statistical probability values. Statistical significance is important, but it is not the only important result of the analysis worth the attention of the investigator. As noted by Rothman[15] and Guyatt and colleagues,[16] statistical significance classifies results into dichotomous outcomes of significant or not significant using a somewhat arbitrary threshold to distinguish the two cases. It ignores the size of any effect that was observed and the study's level of statistical power, or the probability that a statistical test will correctly reject the null hypothesis in situations when the alternative hypothesis is true (and the null hypothesis is false).

It is also important to consider the practical or clinical significance—or meaningfulness—of the results. A study that uses very large samples may find statistically significant relationships that are small in magnitude and of little practical significance. For example, in many contexts a change in an individual's systolic blood pressure of less than 5 mm Hg would not be considered clinically meaningful. So if a costly and time consuming dietary intervention had the true effect of reducing this measure by 5 mm Hg (or less), the intervention would not be considered worth the cost. However, a study of the effectiveness of this intervention based on a very large sample could find that the estimated effect of an intervention that reduced systolic blood pressure by this amount was statistically significant. If the researcher failed to consider the clinical significance of the effect, the study could have misleading conclusions.

Conversely, a less well-powered study may fail to find a significant relationship, even though the point estimate of the correlation coefficient is

substantial enough in magnitude to have clinical significance or policy relevance. So researchers should always consider the magnitude of the estimates from their studies along with the estimates' statistical significance. The point estimate and confidence interval provide useful information about the size of an effect and its clinical or practical importance.

DEVELOPING A TOOL KIT OF STATISTICAL PROCEDURES

Most nutrition research studies are ultimately concerned with how two characteristics or variables relate to each other. For example, a study might examine how receiving a particular treatment relates to some outcome, such as a measure of dietary intake, the presence or absence of a health condition, or an individual's BMI. While the first two sections of this chapter provided information on the fundamentals of statistical analysis, this section describes how the statistical analysis should be carried out in specific research situations.

Comparing Differences Between Groups

A common situation is when an investigator wants to examine whether there is a relationship between an independent variable that is categoric (such as a binary variable) and a dependent or outcome variable representing some individual characteristic or outcome measure. To examine this relationship, the investigator can first use the categoric variable to define separate groups within the sample, and then—if the outcome is continuous—compare the mean value of the outcome variable between groups to see whether there are meaningful or statistically significant differences.

To test the null hypothesis of no difference between the groups in the outcome vs the alternative hypothesis of a difference, the investigator should assess the situation along several dimensions. One key issue is whether just two groups are being compared or more than two groups. In other words, is the categoric variable binary or does it have more than two values? Second, are the samples represented by the groups being compared independent or dependent, such as serial or repeated measures? Third, what type of variable is the outcome measure—is it continuous, nominal, ordinal, or binary?

The answers to these questions determine how the investigator should specify the null hypothesis and carry out the analysis. Different situations call for different approaches to summarize and present descriptive statistics on the outcome, different kinds of estimates of the relationship between the variables and the standard error and confidence interval of this estimate, and different formal statistical tests of the null hypothesis. Table 25.4 on page 500 provides a guide that shows a number of different situations and the appropriate approach for the statistical analysis. [3,4,6,17-24]

Estimating Relationships or Associations

A common situation is when an investigator wants to examine whether there is a relationship between categoric variables (such as a binary variable) and another variable representing some individual characteristic or outcome measure. To examine this relationship, the investigator can first use the categoric variable to define separate groups within the sample, and then compare the value of the outcome variable between groups to see whether there are meaningful or statistically significant differences.

Knowing whether there is a statistically significant difference between two groups or a significant relationship between two variables is useful but incomplete. This does not indicate the nature or strength of the association being examined or its practical or clinical importance. For this reason, it is important to estimate a measure of the strength of the association.

Discrete Data

The strength of the association between binary variables can be measured by various methods. The most straightforward approach is to simply calculate the difference in proportions between samples or groups and then interpret the magnitude of the difference in light of the context of the study being conducted. It will often be clear whether the difference in proportions that has been calculated has practical importance given the nature of the research question being studied. However, a statistical test of the null hypothesis of no differences between groups in these proportions will allow the investigator to determine the significance of any differences observed. An example of such a situation is described in Box 25.3 on pages 501 through 502.

Another measure of the strength of associations between binary variables is the ϕ coefficient, which is interpretable as a correlation coefficient with values ranging from –1 to +1. Values of ϕ at or near 0 indicate little or no association between the two variables. However, Fleiss and colleagues[18] caution that the ϕ coefficient has serious limitations and should be avoided in areas of research requiring a comparison of findings among investigations.

Fortunately, better measures of associations exist. Two of the most useful measures are the relative risk and odds ratio. Relative risk is used when the investigation is a cohort or prospective design, and the odds ratio is appropriate for investigations that are a case-control or cross-sectional design. Both measures describe the degree of association between an antecedent factor and an outcome event, such as morbidity,[25] so both are important in observational analytic studies that evaluate potentially causal relationships. Methods for calculating and interpreting the relative risk and the odds ratio are discussed in Chapter 7. Readers are also referred to Fleiss and colleagues[18] for details on deriving the confidence intervals for both measures and for assessing statistical significance.

Logistic regression methods are another way to measure the relationship between variables when at least one of them is a binary variable. Like other regression methods, logistic regression allows the researcher to examine how well one or more independent variables predict the value of a dependent variable (a binary variable in the case of logistic regression). More specifically, logistic regression can be used to estimate the relationship between an independent variable and the log odds of a particular outcome. Logistic regression is similar in many ways to linear regression (discussed later), and is described in greater detail by Sheean and colleagues.[26]

Sampling Situation	Outcome Variable Type	Null Hypothesis	Summary Statistic	Estimate	Statistical Test
Two independent samples	Binary	Proportions are equal	Frequency table (2×2 table)	Difference in proportions, with confidence interval (CI)	χ^2 test[3,4,17,18]
	Ordinal	Median values are equal	Median value, interquartile range	Difference in medians, with CI	Mann-Whitney test, Wilcoxon rank sum test[3,4,17,19]
	Continuous	Mean values are equal	Mean value, standard deviation	Difference in means, with CI	Independent samples t test[3,4,17,20]
More than two independent samples	Binary	All proportions are equal	Group frequencies (contingency table)	Difference in proportions; pairwise CI from multiple comparisons of groups	Global χ^2 test followed by multiple comparisons analysis[18]
	Binary, but groups are ordered	All proportions are equal	Group frequencies (contingency table)	Difference in proportions	Bartholomew test[18]
	Ordinal	All medians are equal	Medians, interquartile range	Difference in medians	Kruskal-Wallis (Jonckheere), nonparametric test[19]
	Continuous	All mean values are equal	Group means, standard deviations	Difference in means; pairwise CI after multiple comparison analysis	One-way analysis of variance followed by multiple comparison analysis[20,21]
Crossover, single sample but measures taken at two times for that single group	Nominal or ordinal	Median values for the group equal in each time period	Median values, interquartile range	Change over time in median value, with CI	Wilcoxon sign rank test[9,19,20]
	Continuous	Mean values for the group equal in each time period	Mean values, standard deviation	Change over time in mean value, with CI	Paired t test[3,4,20]
Two independent samples, but measures taken at two time for each group	Binary	Change in proportion over time equal for each group	Group frequencies (2×2 table)	Difference between groups in the change in proportions, with CI	Normal approximation to binomial or χ^2 test; matched study— McNemar test[17,18]
	Continuous	Change in mean values over time equal for each group	Mean values and change in mean values, standard deviations	Difference between groups in the change in mean values, with CI	A t test of mean changes, or analysis of covariance[22-24]
Two independent samples, but serial measures at multiple time points	Continuous	Changes over time in mean values equal for each group	Plot response over time to determine how mean values change (peaked or growth curves); select appropriate summary	Difference between groups in appropriate measure of change over time, with CI	A t test of mean difference (from summary), or repeated measures analysis of variance, or multivariate analysis of variance[3,4,6]

Table 25.4 Suggested Statistical Methods for Evaluating Differences Between Samples or Groups

Using data from the study described in Box 25.2, an investigator might wish to examine the relationship between type of bariatric surgery and remission of diabetes mellitus. Since patients in the sample had one of four different types of bariatric surgery, this is a situation with more than two independent samples—the four groups of patients having different forms of surgery. The outcome measure is binary—whether or not patients' diabetes had gone into remission at 12 months. The statistical analysis then follows the approach suggested in Table 25.4.

Null hypothesis: All proportions are equal. In other words, diabetes went into remission for an equal proportion of each of the four groups of patients.

Summary statistics: Group frequencies

Count	Surgery Type				Total
	Gastric Banding	**Sleeve Gastrectomy**	**Laparoscopic Gastric Bypass**	**Biliopancreatic Diversion with Duodenal Switch**	
No remission of diabetes	14	7	8	1	30
Remission of diabetes	4	6	23	23	56
Total	18	13	31	24	86

Remission × Surgery Type Cross-Tabulation

Estimates: Differences in proportions, with confidence intervals. With four different groups, there are six possible differences that could be compared. The following equations show the difference in the proportion whose diabetes went into remission between the first two groups—those who had gastric banding (GB) versus those who had a sleeve gastrectomy (SG) procedure.

$$\text{Difference in proportions} = \frac{4}{18} - \frac{6}{13} = 0.222 - 0.462 = -0.242$$

$$\text{Confidence interval (CI)} = \text{Point estimate} \pm Z_{1-\frac{\alpha}{2}} \times \text{Standard error (SE)}$$

$$SE = \sqrt{(P1Q1)/n1 + (P2Q2)/n2} = \sqrt{\frac{22.2 \times 77.8}{18} + \frac{46.2 \times 53.88}{13}} = 16.94$$

$$95\% \text{ CI} = 24.2 \pm (1.96 \times 16.94) = 9.00, 57.40$$

$$95\% \text{ CI} = 24.2 \pm (1.96 \times 16.94) = 9.00, 57.40$$

For this study population, patients who had a SG had a 24.2 percentage point higher remission rate than those who had GB. The researchers are 95% confident that the true difference in these remission rates in the population lies between 9.0 and 57.4. In other words, the researchers are confident that the SG remission rate is greater than the GB remission rate by somewhere between 9.0 and 57.4 percentage points.

Statistical test: Global χ^2 following by multiple comparisons analysis. The global χ^2 test examines the null hypothesis that all four proportions are equal. If this test is rejected, the investigator knows there are some differences, but the test result does not indicate which differences are important so the investigator should then examine the pairwise differences in proportions to understand the nature of the relationship.

Box 25.3 Examining the Relationship Between Bariatric Surgery and Diabetes Remission   *(continued)*

Results:

Count	Gastric Banding	Sleeve Gastrectomy	Laparoscopic Gastric Bypass	Biliopancreatic Diversion with Duodenal Switch	Total
No Remission of Diabetes	14 (0.78)$_x$	7 (0.54)$_{x,y}$	8 (0.26)$_{y,z}$	1 (0.04)$_z$	30
Remission of Diabetes	4 (0.22)$_x$	6 (0.46)$_{x,y}$	23 (0.74)$_{y,z}$	23 (0.96)$_z$	56
Total	18	13	31	24	86

Remission × Surgery Type Cross-Tabulation

[a]Each subscript letter denotes a subset of surgery type categories whose column proportions do not differ significantly from each other at the .05 level. Column proportions with different subscripts do differ significantly from each other at the .05 level. Column proportions are in parentheses.

The results of the Pearson χ^2 test revealed a two-sided $P=.0001$ which indicates a statistically significant difference in the remission rate for the four types of surgery since the P value is <.05. The multiple comparisons analysis, which is reported as subscript letters in the table, indicates that there is a significant difference, at the .05 level, in the rate of remission for both GB and biliopancreatic diversion with duodenal switch (BPD/DS). The rate of remission for GB (22%) is significantly different than laparoscopic gastric bypass (LGB) (74%) and BPD/DS (96%). SG (46%) is also significantly different than BPD/DS (96%). Interestingly, while the majority of patients who had GB (14/18 or 78%) did not experience remission, nearly all (23/24 or 96%) of the BPD/DS patients did have remission of diabetes. For those patients who had LGB, there was no statistically significant difference compared with BPD/DS; however, 74% (23/31) of these patients did experience remission, which is a clinically significant result.

Box 25.3 (cont.) Examining the Relationship Between Bariatric Surgery and Diabetes Remission

Continuous Data

The relationships among continuous variables are commonly explored by scatterplot and summarized by linear regression or correlation coefficient. Other methods are possible for examining the relationship between continuous variables—such as the independent samples test or analysis of variance (ANOVA) (see Box 25.4)—but the remainder of this section focuses on correlation and linear regression (see Box 25.5 on page 506). Although these two measures are related, they are used for different purposes and have different interpretations. Linear regression expresses the relationship between two variables using a mathematical model that fits a straight line that best describes the relationship—how the value of the outcome or dependent variable changes when there is a change in the value of the independent or predictor variable. Investigators can use linear regression to predict the value of the outcome given the value of the other variable. The correlation coefficient is a standardized measure that is used to simply show the strength of the relationship between two continuous variables. It cannot be used to make predictions about the value of one of the variables based on the value of the other.

Correlation The linear correlation coefficient (r) is a measure of the strength of the linear association between two variables (typically continuous). It is related to the slope coefficient in the regression equation but does not depend on the units of measurement of the original observations. The value of the correlation coefficient ranges from –1 to +1. When it is 0, the slope of the regression line is also 0. A value of either –1 or +1 indicates that the data fall on a straight line with either a negative or positive slope. A positive correlation coefficient indicates a positive relationship between the two variables—that as the value of one of the variables increases the value of the other also tends to increase. A negative correlation coefficient indicates the opposite—that as one variable increases the other tends to decrease.

While the correlation coefficient indicates the direction and strength of the association between two variables, it provides no other quantitative information to describe the linear relationship. For example, it does not describe how much the outcome variable changes for each one-unit change in the predictor variable, as does a regression coefficient. Furthermore, the correlation coefficient can be influenced by both the steepness of a regression line and the degree to which the data points cluster about the line. Thus, it can sometimes be misleading. A large value can arise because the variables are scaled in such a way that the slope is steep, and a change in the scaling of the variables can result in a change in the correlation coefficient. It is useful to interpret the correlation coefficient when it is paired with a plot of the data or the regression coefficients.

A scatterplot can also be used for ordinal, or ordered, categoric data. Unlike continuous data, however, ordinal data should not be analyzed with a linear correlation coefficient. Categoric data are better summarized with a distribution-free correlation procedure, such as the Spearman or Kendall correlation coefficient (see Table 25.4 on page 500).

The first step in regression or correlation analysis is to plot the values of the two variables, assess the linearity of the data, and look for outliers (see Figure 25.8 on page 505). Because both of these

---

Using data from the study described in Box 25.2, an investigator wants to determine if there is a significant difference in the hemoglobin A1c (HbA1c) level before surgery (prestudy) and 12 months after surgery for four types of bariatric surgery. Analysis of variance (ANOVA) is the appropriate statistical test to use because it determines whether any differences exist among two or more groups of participants on one or more continuous variables. Since the dependent grouping variable (type of surgery) has four groups and HbA1c is a continuous variable, one-way ANOVA is the most appropriate statistical test (recall that the independent *t* test only compares two groups) (see the first table shown on page 504). Of course, this assumes that the data meet the assumptions for this test. Assumptions for an ANOVA are (1) the dependent variable is continuous, (2) observations (or measurements) are independent of each other, (3) the population from which the sample was drawn is normally distributed, and (4) samples are taken from populations with equal variances.

Null hypothesis: The means of all four types of surgery are equal before surgery and 12 months after surgery.

Statistical test: One-way ANOVA compares the four types of surgery in terms of participants' mean HbA1c levels before surgery and 12 months after surgery. If this test is rejected, the investigator knows there are some differences but does not necessarily know which differences are important. Thus, the investigator performs a multiple comparisons test to determine which types of surgery have significantly different mean HbA1c levels.

Results: The second table shown on page 504 provides the means, standard deviations, and 95% confidence intervals for the prestudy HbA1c and 12-month HbA1c levels for each of the four types of surgery. Table 25.6 on page 504 provides the results of the ANOVA, which indicates that while the HbA1c levels before surgery were not significantly different ($P=.717$) among the four types of surgery, they were significantly different after 12 months ($P<.0005$). The results of the multiple comparisons test revealed a statistically significant difference between gastric banding and laparoscopic gastric bypass (mean difference of 0.9462 [$P=.023$]), gastric banding and biliopancreatic diversion with duodenal switch (BPD/DS) (mean difference of −2.1109 [$P<.005$]], BPD/DS and sleeve gastrectomy (mean difference of −1.5947 [$P<.005$]), and BPD/DS and laparoscopic gastric bypass (mean difference of −1.1647 [$P=.001$]).

Box 25.4 Comparing Mean Hemoglobin A1c Levels at Different Time Periods by Type of Surgery   *(continued)*

	Type of Surgery	N	Mean	Standard Deviation	95% Confidence Interval for Mean	
					Lower Bound	Upper Bound
Presurgery hemoglobin A1c level	Gastric banding	18	7.37	1.19	6.78	7.97
	Sleeve gastrectomy	13	7.57	1.36	6.75	8.39
	Laparoscopic gastric bypass	31	7.20	1.37	6.69	7.70
	Biliopancreatic diversion with duodenal switch	24	7.57	1.29	7.03	8.11
	Total	86	7.39	1.29	7.12	7.67
12-month hemoglobin A1c level	Gastric banding	13	6.85	0.81	6.36	7.34
	Sleeve gastrectomy	10	6.33	0.81	5.75	6.91
	Laparoscopic gastric bypass	17	5.90	0.92	5.43	6.39
	Biliopancreatic diversion with duodenal switch	17	4.74	0.82	4.31	5.16
	Total	57	5.84	1.15	5.54	6.15

Descriptive Statistics for Analysis of Variance Comparison of Mean Hemoglobin A1c Levels Before and After Four Types of Bariatric Surgery

		Sum of Squares	Degrees of freedom	Mean Square	F Value	P Value
Presurgery hemoglobin A1c level	Between groups	2.325	3	0.775	.452	.717
	Within groups	140.653	82	1.715		
	Total	142.978	85			
12- month hemoglobin A1c level	Between groups	36.368	3	12.123	16.770	<.0005[a]
	Within groups	38.312	53	0.723		
	Total	74.680	56			

Analysis of Variance Comparison of Mean Hemoglobin A1c Levels Before and After Four Types of Bariatric Surgery

[a]Statistically significant difference in the hemoglobin A1c levels 12 months after surgery among four types of bariatric surgery (see Table 25.5 for types of surgery).

Box 25.4 Comparing Mean Hemoglobin A1c at Different Time Periods by Type of Surgery

measures assume a linear relationship between the variables, if the scatterplot suggests important non-linearities, alternative methods should be used.

Regression Analysis If the scatterplot suggests a linear relationship, the investigator uses the data to estimate the straight-line association between the variables using the following equation: $y = a + b \times x$, expressed conceptually as

$$\text{Outcome variable} = \text{Intercept} + (\text{Slope} \times \text{Predictor variable})$$

In other words, y is the outcome (dependent) variable that is regressed on x, the predictor (independent) variable. The data allow the investigator to estimate values for two model coefficients, the intercept (a) and slope (b). The intercept represents the estimated value of y when $x = 0$. The slope describes the relationship between x and y—how the value of y changes when there is a one-unit change in x. The estimates of both the intercept and slope have some error or uncertainty (ie, variance), which can be used to calculate confidence intervals and conduct significance tests for these coefficient estimates. For example, it

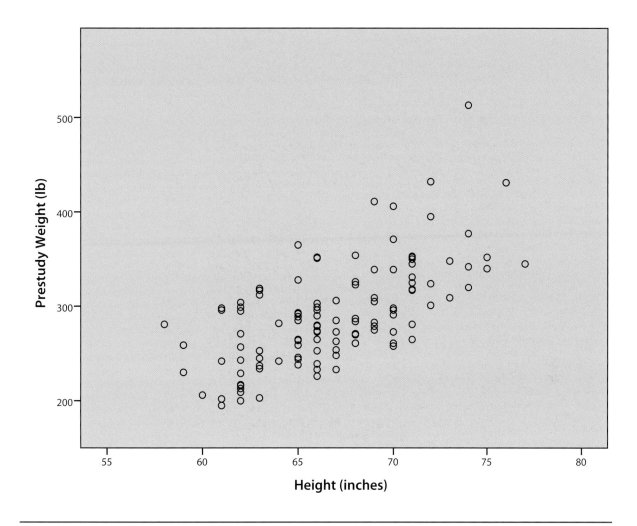

Figure 25.8 Scatterplot of prestudy weight and height

is common for investigators to test whether the slope coefficient is significantly different from zero. This test tells the researcher whether the estimated relationship between *x* and *y* is statistically significant.

An important summary statistic that comes out of regression analysis is the R^2 value, or the square of the correlation coefficient. The R^2 expresses the proportion or percentage of the variation in *y* that is explained by the linear relationship with *x*. The R^2 value varies between 0 and 1, with lower values indicating a weak relationship in which the values of *x* do not predict *y* very well, and higher values indicate a strong relationship where knowing the value of *x* tells the investigator a great deal about the value of *y*.

In addition to the coefficients, the degree to which data points cluster around the regression line

is also important to quantify.[27] The difference between the observed value of *y* and the value predicted by the regression is known as the residual. The residual variance measures the amount by which the actual values of *y* differ from their predicted values. A good regression minimizes the residual variance, which will—in turn—maximize the R^2 value.

It is important to verify, at least roughly, that the regression equation accurately summarizes the data.[28] This procedure involves examining the residuals by plotting them on the *x*-axis to show how they are related to the values of *x*. A relatively accurate regression equation should show no distinctive pattern, whereas a less accurate equation shows a systematic trend, such as progressively higher values or a V-shaped spread. The regression equation requires

Using data from the study described in Box 25.2, an investigator wants to construct a linear regression equation to predict hemoglobin A1c (HbA1c) levels 12 months after bariatric surgery. A linear regression is a way to model the relationship between two variables. Based on clinical experience, the investigator suspects that the 12-month HbA1c level (dependent variable) is correlated with the patients' weight loss during the same time period (independent variable). A correlation analysis and a simple linear regression are the appropriate statistical tests to use. But first there are a few assumptions to check: (1) all variables in the model must be continuous; (2) independent and dependent variables are correlated and have a linear relationship; (3) independent variables (assuming there is more than one) are not strongly correlated with each other (referred to as multicollinearity); and (4) outliers, normality, linearity, and independence of residuals must be checked.

Results: The correlation analysis indicates that there is a statistically significant ($P<.0005$) correlation between the 12-month HbA1c level and weight loss between baseline and 12 months with a Pearson correlation coefficient of −0.587. This indicates that the greater a participant's weight loss, the lower their 12-month HbA1c level. Since there is only one independent variable, there is no need to test for multicollinearity Checks for outliers, normality, linearity, and independence of residuals all met required assumptions.

The next page shows the results for the linear regression analysis. The model summary section provides the R^2 value, which says how much of the dependent variable (12-month HbA1c) is explained by the model (which includes weight loss between baseline and 12 months). The adjusted R^2 value corrects for the number of variables in the model and suggests that the model explains 33.1% of the variance in participants' 12-month HbA1c level.

The coefficients section provides the information necessary to construct the regression equation, which can be used to predict the 12-month HbA1c level. It is also used to determine whether the weight loss variable is significantly related to 12-month HbA1c in the sample. In this case, the weight loss variable is negatively and significantly related to 12-month HbA1c ($P<.005$). The negative value of the coefficient indicates that the greater the weight loss, the lower the HbA1c level. In the unstandardized coefficients, the values in the B column show the regression equation.

A simple **linear regression equation** is denoted as $y=a+b\times x$, where y is the outcome or dependent variable, x is the independent variable, b is the slope, and a is the y-intercept. For this study, the regression equation is:

12-month HbA1c$=7.275+(-0.015)\times$(Weight loss between baseline and 12 months)

Box 25.5 Constructing a Linear Regression Equation to Predict Hemoglobin A1c Levels 12 Months After Bariatric Surgery

continued

further refinements if a trend is detected. Details on residual analysis are provided by Kleinbaum and colleagues[29] and Godfrey.[28]

CONCLUSION

This chapter focused on the area of statistics that deals with analyzing and drawing conclusions from the data. The field of nutrition and dietetics offers many opportunities to carry out research. This introduction to statistical methods is intended to enhance the investigator's skills in this area as well as facilitate communications with statisticians in planning and completing research projects and interpreting study results. Numerous references were cited to encourage further reading on this topic and to provide guidance for developing a resource library. The basic steps discussed in this chapter will help with the many decisions that need to be made in approaching and executing successful research.

Model Summary[a]

Model	R	R^2	Adjusted R^2	SE of the Estimate
1	0.587[b]	0.344	0.331	0.9444

ANOVA[a]

Model	Sum of Squares	df	Mean Square	F	P Value
Regression	23.420	1	23.420	26.260	<.0005[b]
Residual	44.593	50	0.892		
Total	68.012	51			

Coefficients[a]

Model	Unstandardized Coefficients B	Unstandardized Coefficients SE	Standardized Coefficients Beta	t	P Value
(Constant)	7.275	9.308		23.589	<.0005
Weight loss between baseline and 12 mo	-0.015	9.003	-9.587	-5.124	<.0005

Model summary for linear regression analysis with weight loss as the independent variable and 12-month hemoglobin A1c level as the dependent variable

Abbreviations: ANOVA = analysis of variance; df = degrees of freedom; SE = standard error

[a] Dependent variable: 12-month hemoglobin A1c level

[b] Predictors: (Constant), weight loss between baseline and 12 months

Box 25.5 (cont.) Constructing a Linear Regression Equation to Predict Hemoglobin A1c Levels 12 Months After Bariatric Surgery

REFERENCES

1. Causal relationships between LC-omega-3-enriched diet and cognition (MOP201109). US National Library of Medicine. https://clinicaltrials.gov/ct2/show /NCT01625195. Accessed February 9, 2017.

2. Rehm CD, Peñalvo JL, Afshin A, Mozaffarian D. Dietary intake among us adults, 1999-2012. *JAMA*. 2016;315(23): 2542-2553.

3. Moore DS, McCabe GP, Carig BA. *Introduction to the Practice of Statistics*. 8th ed. New York, NY: W.H. Freeman; 2015.

4. Rosner B. *Fundamentals of Biostatistics*. 8th ed. Boston, MA: Cenage Learning; 2016.

5. Rider BC, Bassett DR, Strohacker K, Overstreet BS, Fitzhugh EC, Raynor HA. Psycho-physiological effects of television viewing during exercise. *J Sports Sci Med*. 2016; 15(3):524-531.

6. Matthews INS, Altman DG, Campbel MJ, Royston P. Analysis of serial measurements in medical research. *BMJ*. 1990; 300(6719):230-235.

7. Centers for Disease Control and Prevention. NHANES Dietary Web Tutorial. Task 2: Key concepts about statistical methods that have been used to estimate the distribution of usual intake with a few days of 24-hour recalls. www.cdc.gov/nchs/tutorials/dietary/Advanced /ModelUsualIntake/Info2.htm Accessed July 19, 2018.

8. Ried M, Hall IC. Multiple statistical comparisons in nutritional research. *Am J Clin Nutr*. 1984;40(1): 183-184.

9. Higgins JJ. *Introduction to Nonparametric Statistics*. Belmont, CA: Duxbury Press; 2003.

10. Corder GW, Foreman DI. *Nonparametric Statistics for Non-Statisticians: A Step by Step Approach*. Hoboken, NJ: John Wiley and Sons; 2009.

11. Schochet PZ. An approach for addressing the multiple testing problem in social policy impact evaluations. *Eval Rev*. 2009;33(6):539-567.

12. Horgan GW. Statistical analysis of nutritional studies. *Br J Nutr*. 2001;86(2):141-144.

13. Grace-Martin K. Outliers: To drop or not to drop. The Analysis Factor website. www.theanalysisfactor.com /outliers-to-drop-or-not-to-drop. Accessed February 16, 2017.

14. Flegal KM, Kruszon-Moran D, Carroll MD, Fryar CD, Ogden CL. Trends in obesity among adults in the united states, 2005 to 2014. *JAMA*. 2016;315(21):2284-2291.

15. Rothman KJ. A show of confidence. *N Engl J Med*. 1978; 299(24):1362-1363.

16. Guyatt G, Jaeschke R, Heddle N, Cook D, Shannon H, Walter S. Basic statistics for clinicians: 2. Interpreting study results: confidence intervals. *CMAJ*. 1995;152(2): 169-173.

17. Gardner MJ, Altman DG. Confidence intervals rather than P values: estimation rather than hypothesis testing. *BMJ*. 1986;292(6522):746-750.

18. Fleiss JL, Levin B, Paik MC. *Statistical Methods for Rates and Proportions*. New York, NY: Wiley; 2003.

19. Forrest M, Andersen B. Ordinal scale and statistics in medical research. *BMJ*. 1986;292(6519):537-538.

20. Rimm AA, Hartz AJ, Kalbfleisch JH. *Basic Biostatistics in Medicine and Epidemiology*. New York, NY: Appleton-Century-Crofts; 1980.

21. Godfrey K. Comparing means of several groups. *N Engl J Med*. 1985;313(23):1450-1456.

22. Kaiser L. Adjusting for baseline: change or percentage change? *Stat Med*. 1989;8(10):1183-1190.

23. Samuels ML. Use of analysis of covariance in clinical trials: a clarification. *Control Clin Trials*. 1986;7(4):325-329.

24. Egger MJ, Coleman ML, Ward JR, Reading JC, Williams HJ. Uses and abuses of analysis of covariance in clinical trials. *Control Clin Trials*. 1985;6(1):12-24.

25. Jaeschke R, Guyatt G, Shannon H, Walter S, Cook D, Heddle N. Basic statistics for clinicians: 3. Assessing the effects of treatment: measures of association. *CMAJ*. 1995; 152(3):351-357.

26. Sheean PM, Bruemmer B, Gleason P, Harris J, Boushey C, Van Horn L. Publishing nutrition research: a review of multivariate techniques—part 1. *J Acad Nutr Diet*. 2011; 111(1):103-110.

27. Motulsky HJ. Common misconceptions about data analysis and statistics. *J Pharmacol Exp Ther*. 2014;351(1): 200-205.

28. Godfrey K. Simple linear regression in medical research. *N Engl J Med*. 1985;313(26):1629-1636.

29. Kleinbaum DG, Kupper LL, Nizam A, Rosenberg ES. *Applied Regression Analysis and Other Multivariable Methods*. 5th ed. Boston, MA: Cenage Learning; 2014.

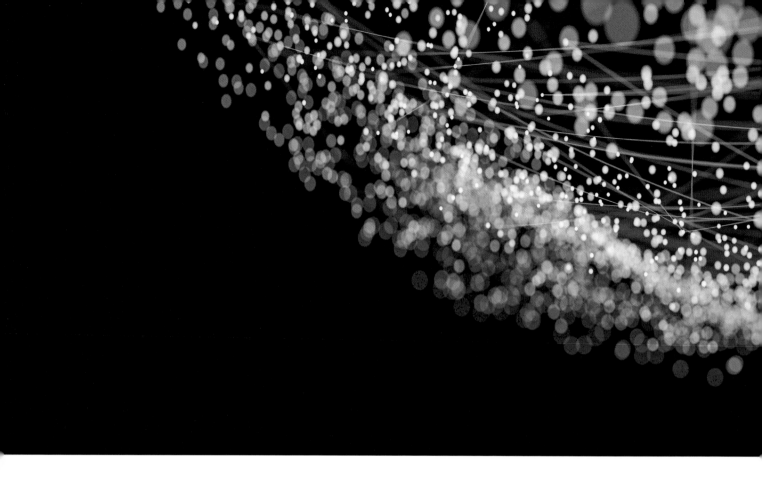

Presentation of Research Data

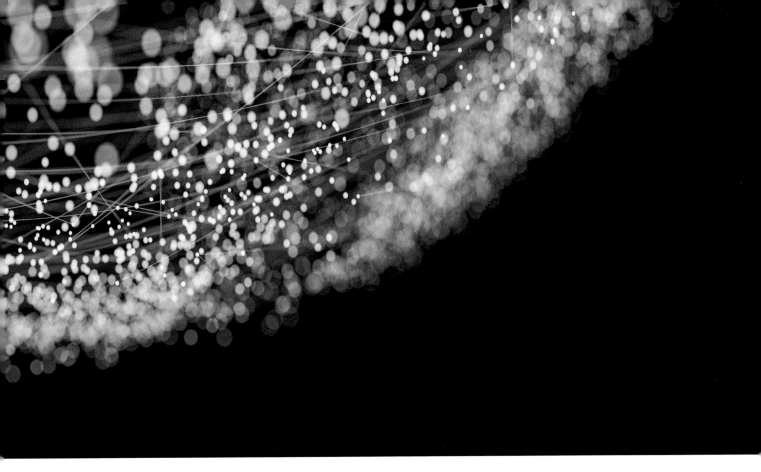

Techniques and Approaches for Presenting Research Findings

Joanne Kouba, PhD, RDN

LEARNING OBJECTIVES

1. Describe the importance of disseminating research results to professional and consumer audiences.

2. Explore diverse ways to disseminate research using multiple media methods.

3. Develop a plan for effective written and oral research dissemination methods.

4. Formulate effective poster presentations.

Researchers have an ethical obligation to share their research findings with communities that may benefit from the knowledge gained from their work. This knowledge transfer should be active and collaborative to ensure that the research findings are relevant and useful. Typically, disseminating new knowledge through peer-reviewed journal articles or professional conference presentations is one of the concluding activities of a research project. Often these outputs are used as evidence of the research team's capacity to seek future grant funding to extend research activities in the same general field of study. However, a more integrated knowledge translation approach is also recommended. The knowledge translation approach is more innovative, dynamic, and interactive; has an enhanced awareness of multiple stakeholders, professions, and platforms; and allows shared authority of evidence, all of which leads to a more relevant and responsive dissemination of knowledge. Those involved in the knowledge translation approach include practitioners, health care or public health program managers, policy makers, and study participants. Outputs of this approach include evidence-based position papers, practice protocols, training programs, and policy briefs.[1] Examples are presented in this chapter.

AUDIENCES FOR RESEARCH DISSEMINATION

In determining where to disseminate research findings, both broad and specific communities of interest should be considered. From a broad perspective, the information gained from a research project should be shared with other professionals, research participants, and the communities representing the research participants. Those who gain knowledge from research findings range from bench scientists (eg, microbiologists or immunologists) to various health care providers, patients, and the general public depending on the topic of the research. Because of the diverse nature of food, nutrition, and health, even policy makers and food manufacturers may be important recipients of the research findings of registered dietitian nutritionists (RDNs).

For example, the findings of a study evaluating food-handling practices of senior citizens living at home using microbiological assays of food samples from their homes would likely be of interest to microbiologists, RDNs, home health nurses, primary care physicians, food manufacturers, those who manage community programs for seniors, social workers, and older adults and their family members. A research project assessing how a Grab'N'Go salad project in a high school cafeteria affects fruit and vegetable intake of adolescents may be of interest to anyone who works with adolescents or schools, including RDNs, foodservice managers, school administrators, parents, and students. Results of a study that evalu-

ates the role of vitamin D in the fatigue experienced by patients with breast cancer may be of interest to oncologists, RDNs, and physical therapists in addition to those diagnosed with breast cancer and their families and caregivers.

Research findings are also reported to very specific audiences, although this probably applies to the professional arena more than consumer groups. Even within the nutrition and dietetics profession, research reports may be targeted to specialty areas based on life cycle (eg, breastfeeding or infant nutrition), disease or disorder (eg, cardiovascular disease or cancer), type of practice setting (eg, acute care or telehealth), or dietary constituents or interventions (eg, vitamin D, Mediterranean eating pattern, or total parenteral nutrition). Narrower topics and audiences may be defined. Researchers should also think about reporting findings to other professionals who work in these specialized fields. For example, a study that evaluates how vitamin D levels affect mood in people who are obese may be of interest to mental health professionals, primary care physicians, and obesity researchers.

The Academy of Nutrition and Dietetics has identified interprofessional collaboration as a theme for future dietetics practice. This involves sharing research findings and may result in future collaborations with other professionals.

PURPOSES OF RESEARCH DISSEMINATION

Disseminating information gained from research to a broad spectrum of audiences can achieve multiple goals. For this reason, research should be disseminated in a timely fashion to anyone who could benefit. In the example of food safety among older adults living at home, some basic concepts about common lapses in food safety should be widely shared with older adults and their families right away and accompanied by strategies or resources to correct problems. Practitioners who provide care, services or programs for older adults would be interested in this research, as would those who develop policies, systems, or environmental structures for older adults. For example, RDNs involved in community nutrition programs could use this as a topic for nutrition education in congregate feeding programs or for home health nurses who make home visits. A related policy change might involve advising the food manufacturing and packaging industries to enlarge the font size of expiration dates to reduce the prevalence of expired foods in the homes of older adults. Finally, research findings should be shared with a broad range of professional communities to inform future research and contribute to knowledge gains in that specific field without unnecessary redundancy or error. This allows others to learn which research methods or protocols were effective and which were not to maximize efficiency of labor, time, and cost with optimal study protocols for future research projects.

When organizing knowledge dissemination, researchers should think about the various ways this information could be transferred. For example, a well-written abstract could be easily modified to a one-page press release, or a comprehensive, final technical report to the funding agency could be edited to a peer-reviewed paper. Adjustments may be necessary considering audience and formatting guidelines. Early on, the research team should discuss the knowledge translation process so they identify integrated, multiple outputs at the start.

PLAN FOR RESEARCH DISSEMINATION

Researchers and authors should develop an organized knowledge dissemination plan with input from the research team and stakeholders. Reviewing the success of and audience response to past dissemination efforts is always a good place to start. Efforts that were not fruitful should still be considered to learn from past unsuccessful attempts. Establishing several objectives for the dissemination project is important, including purposes (eg, raise awareness of problem or promote community engagement in new programs), key messages, and stakeholder groups. Establishing objectives helps researchers develop a dissemination plan that identifies specific audiences, messages, approaches, or methods as well as a time frame for each. For example, if a project evaluated how a telehealth session with an RDN affected weight loss in adults with hypertension at a particular clinic, then an objective might be to increase awareness of the use of telehealth approaches to reach adults who are trying to improve lifestyle for hypertension management. The likelihood of gathering the clinic patients together for a presentation about the research findings is very small. Best approaches may be a 2-minute video clip that could be viewed by patients in the clinic reception areas, a summary in an electronic newsletter, or even a bulletin board. The messages should be patient focused, highlighting the benefits of telehealth in saving time and cost, reducing transportation barriers, and increasing health outcomes of patients. A policy brief to the clinic administrators and health care providers would reach important stakeholder groups who make decisions about models of care and equipment purchases.

The key messages are the core of dissemination. The level of detail, method of delivery, or future implications should be tailored to the specific audience. These messages should be limited to three to five main ideas, findings, concepts, or recommendations that are direct, clear, and concise and that take into account the needs and ability of the audience. The key messages are then transferred via a selected method to the target audience. Available resources, including personnel, skill sets, and finances, should be reviewed to select the best methods. Pilot testing a draft version of the product with at least one member of the particular stakeholder audience is always a good idea. Feedback is also important. In the earlier telehealth example, feedback from one or two patients would be helpful to ensure that the intended audience will understand the message. For example, a message containing acronyms or medical jargon could confuse the target audience. Minor yet critical revisions could be made, such as defining a technical term or adding several words of detail.

The dissemination plan should consider both product and channel. For example, a 2-minute video for patients in a clinic may be a good product, but if the video cannot be shown in the waiting room or patients are not there long enough to see it, then the channel will not effectively meet the objective. The dissemination plan should also include a realistic projected time line and assignment of responsibilities. Members of interprofessional research teams have a variety of talents and strengths. Whereas some team members excel at statistical writing, others are effective at presenting to policy makers or consumer groups.

WRITTEN DISSEMINATION OF RESEARCH

Research Reports

At the conclusion of a research project, researchers are typically required to submit a report to the funding agency. The principal investigator or coinvestigators usually complete this responsibility. Most funding agencies provide detailed instructions about reporting requirements and procedures, and it is important for investigators to understand these at the start of a project. For example, some funders require updates throughout the project, not just at the end. Researchers funded by the US Food and Drug Administration, for one, are required by law to register their projects and provide regular progress reports through the ClinicalTrials.gov electronic portal (https://clinicaltrials.gov).[2] Registering current research projects provides benefits for various constituents: it meets investigators' ethical obligation to share research activity with the public, provides information on trends in research and potential future treatments to practitioners, and minimizes duplication of resources for funders. This is also an excellent resource for investigators to review when formulating research proposals, so they can learn what is currently funded. Report format, length, and time expectations are usually specified when funding is awarded. Many organizations provide electronic report templates. Researchers should be aware that large organizations, such as universities or health care systems, often require reports to be vetted by additional internal offices (eg, research services) or a university administrator (eg, dean or provost). Some funders require additional documents, such as a financial report of expenditures or a cover letter. All of these steps take additional time.

Journal Articles

Reporting research project findings in a professional journal is the most common way to disseminate study results, is considered a measure of scholarly activity in many professions, and provides evidence that a research team merits continued funding. Reporting accurate and honest results in articles submitted to professional journals is important to ensuring safety and integrity as research findings are applied in such areas as patient care, program delivery, policy development, and future research, and many professionals use information from journal articles to guide practice. The task of publishing a journal article may seem daunting, largely because of the potential impact of the work. However, the potential benefit may also be great. And by not reporting findings, researchers may do a disservice to professional and consumer groups. Keeping these considerations in mind, the following sections offer some practical ideas about publishing research findings in a professional journal.

Selecting a Journal

Publishing research findings in a scholarly, professional journal is a common goal. The International Association of Scientific, Technical and Medical Publishers[3] estimates that 2.5 million articles were published in 28,100 active scholarly, peer-reviewed, English-language journals in 2014; US researchers contributed about 23% of these, the largest portion from any country. The number of research articles published increases by about 3.0% to 3.5% annually, and about 30% of articles are categorized as biomedical. The growth in the number of articles published yearly is partly because more researchers are submitting articles for review. The International Association of Scientific, Technical and Medical Publishers estimates that 7 to 9 million researchers submitted articles in 2014, and only 20% were repeat authors. Most researchers read about 270 articles annually and spend about 30 minutes per journal article, down from 45 to 50 minutes in the 1990s. This suggests that authors should be thorough yet succinct and design their article to flow quickly to the important results.

Most RDNs can name several key journals in their field of work without hesitation. However, with so many competing publication options, it is worth spending some time reviewing journals to identify a good fit for your submission.[1] Key points to consider include the journal's mission, types of articles accepted for review and possible publication, topics of interest to readers, and characteristics that would disqualify a study or manuscript from publication. Highly regarded journals conduct double-blinded peer review of articles (meaning the authors and reviewers are not known to each other) before publication. Reviewers are expected to evaluate the article according to the journal's publication criteria. Typical criteria include timely nature of the topic, relevance to the readership, accuracy and strength of the study design and methods, originality or novel contributions of the work, accuracy, implications for future work, and whether the research is practice related or continues previous work. Researchers may also want to consider the approximate time frame from review to publication and any publication fees. Implications of open access publication, such as costs, will be discussed in more detail later in the chapter. Researchers should carefully review the author guidelines to determine how these factors are handled and explore other features of the journal.

The *Journal of the Academy of Nutrition and Dietetics* describes itself as the "official research publication of the Academy of Nutrition and Dietetics." The introductory material for authors clearly identifies the value placed on evidence-based, original research articles, including preferred study designs, as well as on topics that advance nutrition dietetics practice. The *Journal of the Academy of Nutrition and Dietetics* covers a broad array of topics ranging from nutrigenomics to public policy, dietetics education, and leadership. Potential authors are also cautioned on characteristics that may disqualify a manuscript or study from publication, such as an untestable hypothesis, lack of definition in measuring study aims, or unvalidated research methods; portions of dissertations and market research studies are not accepted.[4]

Many other journals publish nutrition and dietetics research, including *The American Journal of Clinical Nutrition, Journal of Parenteral and Enteral Nutrition, Journal of Nutrition Education and Behavior, The Journal of Nutrition, Topics in Clinical Nutrition*, and *Public Health Nutrition*. In addition, RDNs should consider submitting manuscripts to journals that specialize in the topic of their research. Many excellent peer-reviewed journals publish research in cardiovascular disease, diabetes, food science, obesity, public health, renal disease, geriatrics, and other areas of dietetics-related research.

Information scientists use bibliometric measures to evaluate scholarly journals, and researchers should consider these during the journal selection process.[5] Clarivate Analytics Web of Science maintains a database of metrics on professional literature, including the *Journal Citation Reports,* which offer data on citation and article counts, cited and citing half-life, citing journals, publisher information, and impact factors for journals in the areas of science, social science, and technology. The impact factor is a commonly used quantitative tool to evaluate and compare the prestige or importance of a journal. These indexes were established in the 1960s with the advent of computer-generated data. One criterion authors may consider when selecting a journal for manuscript submission is impact factor, which estimates the number of times the average article from a particular journal is cited in a specific year or period. The impact factors in the *Journal Citation Reports* are based on the ratio between the number of citations in the current year and citable items published in that journal for the 2 previous years. The calculation adjusts for variations in the frequency of issues, number of articles, and other factors for each publication. This reduces bias and levels the playing field between larger vs smaller journals and between quarterly vs monthly publications. The ISI, a leader in indexing journals and other scientific publications representing major publishers, reports impact factors for many fields of research. In the medicine category, ISI lists impact factors for 6,186 medical journals, 255 food journals, and 151 nutrition journals.[6] A higher impact factor indicates a more important journal. Because impact factors consider citations in a recent period, usually 2 to 5 years, they change on an annual basis. The 2017 impact factor for the *Journal of the Academy of Nutrition and Di-*

Journal	Impact Factor	Guidelines for Authors
New England Journal of Medicine	72.4	www.nejm.org/author-center/new-manuscripts
Diabetes Care	11.9	http://care.diabetesjournals.org/content/instructions-for-authors
American Journal of Clinical Nutrition	6.9	https://academic.oup.com/ajcn/pages/General_Instructions
Pediatrics	5.7	www.aappublications.org/content/pediatrics-author-guidelines
Nutrition Reviews	5.3	https://academix.oup.com/nutritionreviews/pages/General Instructions
Journal of Parenteral and Enteral Nutrition	4.2	www.nutritioncare.org/Publications/JPEN_Author_Instructions
American Journal of Public Health	3.9	https://ajph.aphapublications.org/page/authors.html
Journal of the Academy of Nutrition and Dietetics	4.0	http://jandonline.org/content/authorinfo
Public Health Nutrition	2.3	www.cambridge.org/core/journals/public-health-nutrition/information/instructions-contributors

Table 26.1 International Scientific Institute Impact Factors 2016–2017 for Selected Journals[6,7] and Guideline Websites

etetics was 4.021. The most recent 5-year impact factor is 4.534.[7] Impact factors for some key journals are listed in Table 26.1

While authors should be aware of impact factors or other similar metrics, they should also use them wisely. The impact factor is just one of several criteria to consider, just like deciding about hiring a new employee or assessing a patient's nutritional status involves numerous criteria. One number does not tell the whole story. Impact factors may be more meaningful within a subset of journals in a specialized field. For example, it may be useful for an author to review three to five dietetics or nutrition journals to help decide where to submit a manuscript rather than comparing the impact factors of journals in dietetics, major medical, and specialized practice areas.

Journal selection should also be realistic. For example, journals with a high impact factor are likely to have the highest number of submissions, partly due to their prestigious ranking, and therefore can be very selective. It may be more realistic for a beginning researcher to select a journal with a more modest ranking to maximize the likelihood that the manuscript will be accepted. Similarly, results of a pilot study with a small sample size are not likely to be published in a top-tier journal with a high impact factor but may be of interest to a journal with a lower

impact factor. Factors that increase citation of articles from a particular journal are inclusion of review articles and timeliness of article topics. These factors ultimately influence the impact factor.

Table 26.1 also includes URLs for author guidelines for a sampling of journals appropriate to dietetics practice. Author guidelines vary considerably among journals from the fine points, such as style details (eg, font type and size) to major features, such as cost of publication and required checklists.

Publication Access

Many journals offer authors several options related to access of their manuscript once accepted for publication. Open access, as a publication option, began between 2001 and 2003 with the work of several organizations, including the Budapest Open Access initiative and the Bethesda Statement on Open Access Publishing.[8] The goal of open access publication is to make information freely available without the costs of journal subscription or library privileges. This trend may also maximize the impact of research findings by extending the reach and distribution of the work. Technological advances of online resources in contemporary society allow for easy access to journal articles without physically going to a library or being affiliated with a university or health system. Several open access categories are available. Authors are advised to read the journal policies to understand the details and implications of the open access categories. Many open access articles are peer reviewed; however, authors should confirm this.

Gold open access with Elsevier, for example, generally implies that consumers have immediate, no-cost access to a published article. The cost of publication is usually transferred from the reader to the author. In this case, a publication fee is required for the article to be published; this may be paid by the author, an affiliated institution (eg, university, medical center, or other agency), or funder. For example, Elsevier, which publishes the *Journal of the Academy of Nutrition and Dietetics*, charges $2,750 (excluding taxes) for an article to be published as open access. Additional user rights or restrictions are defined by the journal's user license agreements and agreed upon by the author. The user license outlines the ways readers can use an article, including permission to access, read, print, download, distribute, translate, extract, or even sell portions of the article. User license details may specify, for example, if distribution or sharing is limited to classroom use, grant applications, social media, or other platforms.[8] Green open access with Elsevier provides no-cost public access to the article, although an embargo period may be applied. In this case, the article may not be available without cost for a specific time period. The benefit of this option is that the author generally does not pay a fee as the cost is subsidized by library subscriptions. Various options are available for green open access.

Types of Research Articles

Most journals accept several types of research articles, including original research reports, research briefs, case studies, reviews, and research commentaries or editorials. Once a researcher selects the journal for submission, it is worth spending time reviewing its specific guidelines for authors so the manuscript can be written with the appropriate focus and formatting. This includes such details as font style and size, heading format, reference style, and page numbering. For example the *Journal of the Academy of Nutrition and Dietetics* specifies using 12-point Times New Roman font and double-spaced pages.[4]

The author guidelines typically also provide information on the use of abbreviations, such as online sources for standard abbreviations. Generally, an abbreviation should be defined parenthetically the first time the word or phrase is used. Standard abbreviations may also apply to statistical terms such as n for the number of observations or SD for standard deviation.[4] Journals may also provide a list of abbreviations that do not require definition. For example the *American Journal of Clinical Nutrition* does not require BMI (body mass index) or DNA to be defined.[9]

Units of measure and their abbreviations must also be reported according to the journal's specified standards. When preparing a manuscript, take care to determine whether the journal uses the metric or International System of Units (SI units) classification. Importantly, for reporting dietetics research, authors should note the journal's preferred term and abbreviation for energy (ie, kilocalories or kilojoules). Conversion factors are often included in author guidelines.

Author guidelines for the *American Journal of Clinical Nutrition* note that key criteria are "originality, validity of data, clarity of writing, strength of the conclusions and potential importance of the work to the field of clinical nutrition."[9] This tells a researcher that a report of increased customer satisfaction in a worksite cafeteria, unrelated to nutrition, might not be a good fit for this journal.

Since the original research report is the primary mechanism for reporting original data-based research findings, the following section highlights guidelines for that format.

Original Research Reports

Original research manuscripts describe a research project, preferably generated from original data-based work; sections typically include introduction, hypothesis, study aims, methods, results, discussion, strengths and limitations, and conclusion. A secondary data analysis project generated from an original project may also be accepted. The narrative report, that is, the body of the manuscript, is typically about 3,500 to 5,000 words and, if accepted for publication after peer review, results in a full-length journal article. Besides the narrative report, additional required components usually include a title page, an author page, abstract, references, and, if applicable, tables, figures, and acknowledgments (see the sections that follow for descriptions). A cover letter, which provides a brief introduction to the topic and type of article being submitted, often accompanies the manuscript upon submission; this may be required or optional. A variety of research designs are acceptable, though key characteristics to include are clear study aims, a robust sample size that represents the population of interest, valid methods, high response and retention rates, and appropriate statistical analysis. Many journals provide a checklist specific to the study design and require authors to demonstrate that each item on that checklist has been met.

Title Titles are often the first thing to catch the reader's attention, so they need to be clear, concise, and appealing. The old adage "easier said than done" applies here. Avoid the passive voice, as it can be confusing to the reader. Jargon should be avoided also. If readers cannot determine the main topics of an article, they are less likely to read it through. A catchy title may be enticing, but not if it diminishes the importance of the work. Since many readers will use online searching to find the article, authors should think about key terms that would result in a match through this technique. Some journals do not allow authors to use words from the title as key words, so authors should think about creating titles that would allow unique key terms to be used for searching while still maintaining similar meaning. For example, unique key words for an article titled "Teenagers meet selected Dietary Guidelines for Americans" could be adolescents, health promotion, and nutrition.

Abstract An abstract is a concise summary of a research report that provides the reader with a preview of the full article. A 300- to 500-word limit is common for abstracts, so authors must learn to distill the most important information about their study. Putting the abstract through several rounds of revisions or having colleagues read the abstract and provide feedback on clarity is helpful. Abstracts are categorized as structured or unstructured. Unstructured abstracts are typically a one-paragraph

description of the study. Structured abstracts follow a specified outline using subheads specified by the journal (see Figure 26.1 on page 520 for an example). The *Journal of the Academy of Nutrition and Dietetics*, for example, uses the following subheads in structured abstracts: background, objectives, design, participants, intervention, main outcome measures, statistical analysis, results, and conclusions.[4] The background section should clearly identify the problem concisely, describe its importance, and link it to the research project and journal readers. The objective section states the primary study aims and hypothesis. The study design section includes the type of study, duration, comparison group, and methods. The participants section describes characteristics, setting, and number of study participants, briefly relating this to the general population of interest. The intervention section describes key features (if this was part of the study design). For example, this may describe manipulation of eating patterns, such as the Mediterranean diet; use of a nutrient supplement, such as calcium; a novel type of care delivery, such as telehealth for diabetes management; or a method of self-management, such as coping skills training to address adolescent obesity. An intervention section is not appropriate for observational studies, systematic reviews, or meta-analyses. The main outcome measures section summarizes the primary outcomes based on the original hypothesis. If subsequent outcomes were evaluated after the original research outcomes were completed, this should be noted.[4] In addition to measures used, the statistical analysis section should include confounding factors.[4,9] The results section should provide a quantitative summary of the primary outcomes based on the original hypothesis and any additional post hoc hypothesis and outcomes. The conclusion section summarizes the evidence generated by this study. A well-written abstract is not easy. The word limit is challenging, and the first version is usually longer than it should be. But after a few thoughtful revisions, authors can condense each sentence to the essential information. Some authors find it helpful to draft the abstract before writing the full manuscript, but it is critical to ensure that there are no inconsistencies between the final drafts of the abstract and manuscript.

Abstract

PURPOSE Osteoporosis increases the risk of fracture and is often considered a late effect of breast cancer treatment. We examined the prevalence of compromised bone health in a sample of exclusively African-American (AA) breast cancer survivors since bone mineral density (BMD) varies by race/ethnicity in healthy populations.

METHODS Using a case–control design, AA women in a weight loss intervention previously diagnosed and treated for stages I–IIIa breast cancer were matched 1:1 on age, race, sex, and BMI with non-cancer population controls (n=101 pairs) from National Health and Nutrition Examination Survey (NHANES). Questionnaires and dual-energy x-ray absorptiometry (DXA) scanning were completed, and participants were categorized as having normal bone density, low bone mass, or osteoporosis using the World Health Organization (WHO) definition for femoral neck *T*-scores.

RESULTS The majority of these overweight/obese survivors were 6.6 (±4.7) years post-diagnosis, had stage II (n=46) or stage III (n = 16) disease, and treated with chemotherapy (76%), radiation (72%), and/or adjuvant hormone therapies (45%). Mean femoral neck BMD was significantly lower in cases vs. matched non-cancer population controls (0.85±0.15 vs. 0.91±0.14 g/cm^2, respectively; p=0.007). However, the prevalence of low bone mass and osteoporosis was low and did not significantly differ between groups (n = 101 pairs; p = 0.26), even when restricted to those on adjuvant hormone therapies (n =45 pairs; p = 0.75). Using conditional logistic regression, controlling for dietary factors and education, the odds of developing compromised bone health in AA breast cancer survivors was insignificant (OR 1.5, 95 % CI 0.52, 5.56).

CONCLUSIONS These null case–control findings challenge the clinical assumption that osteoporosis is highly prevalent among *all* breast cancer survivors, providing foundational evidence to support differences by race/ethnicity and body weight.

IMPLICATIONS FOR CANCER SURVIVORS Routine bone density testing and regular patient–provider dialogue is critical in overweight/obese AA breast cancer survivors to ensure that healthy lifestyle factors (e.g., ideal weight, regular weight-bearing exercises, dietary adequacy of calcium and vitamin D) support optimal skeletal health.

Figure 26.1 Example of a structured abstract in a journal

Adapted with permission from *Journal of Cancer Survival.* Sheean P, Huifang L, Schiffer L, Arroyo C, Troy K, Solley M. Assessing the prevalence of compromised bone health among overweight and obese African-American breast cancer survivors: a case–control study. *J Cancer Surviv.* 2016;10(1):21–30.[10]

Manuscript Body The manuscript body, the main narrative section of the article, allows for a thorough yet clear and succinct description of the study. The journal's author guidelines usually outline manuscript sections, which typically include introduction, methods, results, discussion, and conclusion, though there may be variations.

The introduction or background section should summarize the problem that led the researchers to conduct the study. This usually includes some basic data on the prevalence and nature of the problem, its negative impact on individuals and society, and gaps in scientific knowledge related to prevention or solutions.[4,9] The section often concludes by positioning the research as filling some of those gaps, creating a compelling rationale for the importance of the report. The primary aims, objectives, or study hypothesis are often stated in the final paragraph of the background section and should be clearly identified. It is easy to devote too much space to this section because so much information about epidemiology or health consequences is available, but, similar to the abstract, it is important to keep this section focused and concise so that adequate space is available for the details of the work being presented.

The methods sections should describe the study design, including time frame, variables, methods to measure the variables, study participants, and setting.[4,9] A brief description, with references, of the validity and reliability of study instruments used to measure outcome variables is expected and adds credibility to the work. This might include a summary of anthropometric measurement protocols, type of equipment or methods for lab analyses, or software used for nutrient analysis with version and release date. Inclusion criteria should summarize characteristics that made persons eligible for the study, such as age, health conditions (eg, diabetes, cancer, or malabsorption problems), sex, and physiologic measures (eg, BMI or glycated hemoglobin level). Exclusion criteria that disqualify a candidate as a study participant should also be outlined. Institutional review board approval for research with human subjects should be noted with a description of the consent process. If the study was exempt from institutional review board review, this should be noted. Additional information can be obtained from

the US Department of Health and Human Services Office for Human Research Protections (www.hhs.gov/ohrp). A brief description of recruitment strategies should be outlined highlighting any novel methods, such as social media, and their effectiveness. Statistical approaches are included in the methods section; researchers should list types of analysis and software and version used. Consulting a statistician may be helpful when writing this section.

Once the foundation of the research project has been established with the introduction and methods sections, the results section should follow. A description of study participants is a logical starting point and is often summarized in the first table, including subgroup demographic and baseline characteristics. A diagram that visually and quantitatively outlines recruitment, screening, eligibility or exclusion, enrollment, assignment to intervention groups, attrition, and completion is helpful. The results of the study aims or hypotheses should be presented in an objective and sequential fashion using tables and figures to provide detail, including statistical measures and significance levels.[4,9]

The discussion section reviews the results of this study in comparison to other similar research projects, noting differences in participant characteristics, measures, study design, or duration that may account for inconsistencies or similarities in findings.[4,9] This section should also include an honest appraisal of the study's strengths and limitations as well as suggestions for continued research in the area to extend the research and narrow the knowledge gaps.

Depending on the focus of the journal selected, additional sections may be optional or required. For example, many journals whose readers are predominantly practitioners include a section that discusses implications for practice and applies the research findings to patient care, nutrition services, or programs. A conclusions paragraph summarizing findings and suggestions for future directions of this work is customary.

Tables and Figures Tables allow authors to present aggregate data in a way that provides a wealth of information in a concise format. Tables should be clearly organized and include a complete title and column headings with properly abbreviated units of measure. Superscript letters or symbols are typically used to refer to footnotes explaining statistical significance, abbreviations, confounding variables, or other important information to make interpretation easy for the reader. Author guidelines will provide details about font size, type, spacing, numeric or mathematical style (eg, number of decimal places), number of columns or rows allowed, and more. Typically, tables are labeled with Arabic numbers in the order in which they appear in the article. See Figure 26.2 for an example of how to improve a poorly constructed table. Figures, such as bar graphs and line charts, provide visual data to illustrate important findings. Figures are also typically labeled with Arabic numbers in the order in which they appear, and each has a descriptive caption.[4] Each table and figure is submitted as a separate document and should not be embedded in the manuscript body. Any tables or figures reproduced from another source should be accompanied by copyright permission. This might apply, for example, to a drawing of the gastrointestinal tract.

Supplementary Materials Some important items in a journal article fall into the supplementary materials category. These are fairly quick to complete but should not be overlooked. The conflict of interest statement discloses financial or personal relationships of all authors with a company or organization that sponsored the research or provided materials during the project duration. Funding sources (similar to but not always the same as financial relationships) should also be acknowledged, including government, foundation, or corporate resources. Governmental support can be federal, state, or local. If federal grants are involved, the granting agency (such as the National Cancer Institute) and grant number are included. At times funding comes from within the organization, such as a university or health care system; such funding should likewise be noted. The acknowledgments section is a way to recognize people who are not coauthors or investigators but who contributed to the project in a meaningful manner. This might include research assistants who helped with recruitment, collected or entered data, or edited manuscripts. Their per-

mission should be obtained and care should be taken to correctly list names, credentials, and affiliations. Many journals require authors to complete an online checklist for these situations.

Author Checklists Checklists are useful tools for authors to ensure that their research reports meet expectations and include required components for a specific study design. The Strengthening the Reporting of Observational Studies in Epidemiology (STROBE) checklist applies to cross-sectional, case-control, and cohort observational study designs.[11] The Consolidated Standards of Reporting Trials (CONSORT) 2010 guidelines were developed by a consensus of experts for reporting randomized, controlled clinical trials. Resources from this exceptional collaborative include a 25-item checklist and a template for summarizing recruitment, screening, enrollment and participation of study participants.[12] Even for those not reporting a randomized clinical trial, the examples are valuable and worth reviewing at the CONSORT website (www.consort-statement.org).

Research Briefs Many journals publish brief reports, approximately 2,500 to 3,000 words, of original research. These generally report on pilot studies with smaller sample sizes, secondary analysis of another study, a series of case studies with a common theme, or studies that validate a research method.[3] The format is a condensed version of the original research report format described earlier.

Organizational Publications

Organizational publications are another place to share research results. Many organizations produce a number of print and electronic publications that are distributed to various internal and external target audiences.[1] These publications allow for a wide distribution of research findings to those who may not subscribe to professional journals or have access to library resources. One example would be the annual report of the researcher's employer. Other sources for sharing research are professional organizations, educational institutions, community service, and not-for-profit service organizations that

EXAMPLE: POORLY CONSTRUCTED TABLE

Table 1. Diabetes Self-Management Questionnaire Scores

DSMQ Score	Baseline	6 months	Change	P for change
Glucose Management	7.09	8.34	+1.25	.12
Nutrition Management	5.73	7.71	+1.98	.004
Physical Activity	7.49	6.52	–1.97	.17
Health Care Use	9.17	8.9	–.027	.24
Sum Score	7.32	8.08	+.76	.085

Can you identify ways that this table should be improved?
1. The title should reflect the sample population.
2. The sample size is not provided.
3. The abbreviation DSMQ is not defined. It could easily be in the table title.
4. An explanation of the scores is not provided, such as the unit of measure, maximum score and if the values are the mean or median.

EXAMPLE: REVISED AND IMPROVED TABLE

Table 1. Diabetes Self-Management Questionnaire (DSMQ) Scores from participants with diabetes in the Care Connect Program, 2014 (n = 28)

DSMQ Subscale and Sum Scores	Baseline	6 months	Change	P for change
Glucose Management[1]	7.09	8.34	+1.25	.12
Nutrition Management[1]	5.73	7.71	+1.98	.004
Physical Activity[1]	7.49	6.52	–1.97	.17
Health Care Use[1]	9.17	8.9	–.027	.24
Sum Score[1]	7.32	8.08	+.76	.085

[1] DSMQ scores are based on an ideal score of 10.0 for each subscale and sum. Values provided are the mean for each row.

Figure 26.2 Techniques for improving the presentation of research data in table format

are connected in some way with the researchers, represent stakeholders, or highlight the topic of research. Most of these articles are typically briefer and less structured than a full research article for a professional journal. Photos are often included, along with a citation or link to the full research article. These informal publications often provide networks that might lead to future research ideas, collaborators, recruitment of study participants or sites, or funding sources. Figure 26.3 on page 524 presents an example from a university magazine.

Newsletters

Newsletters are a popular type of publication that may be a vehicle for sharing research results. The Academy of Nutrition and Dietetics has more than 20 dietetic practice groups (DPGs), most of which produce electronic or print newsletters on a bimonthly or quarterly basis.[13] Issues are distributed to the DPG membership, and current issues may be accessed via the DPG website. In addition, other professional and consumer groups produce newsletters targeted toward specific audiences or topics. For example, the

MAINTAINING A BALANCED DIET POSES A UNIQUE CHALLENGE IN COMMUNITIES WITH LIMITED FOOD ACCESS

by Zoë Fisher ('17)

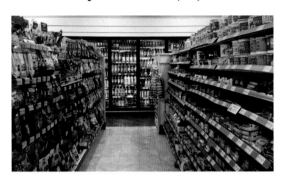

Eating healthy starts with picking the right foods from grocery store shelves, but what happens when the options in the aisles are much more limited? Joanne Kouba, PhD, RDN, LDN, associate professor and director of Niehoff's dietetics education programs; and Annemarie Cahill (BSN '98, MSN '06), FNP, MSN, RN, clinical nursing instructor; sent a group of 20 dietetic, nursing, and medical students from Loyola to find out.

As part of a research project on food availability in Maywood, presented at this year's Palmer Research Symposium, students were sent into the neighborhood with a shopping list. They quickly discovered there are no grocery stores in Maywood and instead found that most residents do their shopping at mom-and-pop shops, gas station mini-marts, or dollar stores. The research project is similar to one Kouba managed in 2007, where she compared food availability in Chicago's Austin neighborhood to that of Oak Park.

The 2007 study paired Loyola students with community residents and a geographer. In the new study, students were separated into collaborative teams with at least one representative of each discipline and sent out to collect data. Early on, the students found it difficult to confirm the location of food sources. Some places they found listed on the internet had closed, and when students drove through the neighborhoods, they also discovered stores that weren't listed online.

Once in the stores, students shopped for 60 items from the USDA Thrifty Food Plan and checked the availability, price, and quality of each item. They found that the most common food source, gas station mini-marts, don't sell fresh fruits or vegetables. The only two items from the list that they found in all surveyed stores were juice and salt.

An unexpected finding was that many items in stores weren't priced. While students were surveying one convenience store, they found a carton of expired eggs. When they asked the store manager the price, he shrugged and said, "'I don't know, $8?'" Another team of students had a similar story, but this time the eggs were $1.

Students were surprised to learn that neighborhood residents encounter these types of barriers on a regular basis when shopping for food. "It makes getting what you need more difficult and intimidating sometimes," says Kouba.

Currently, Kouba is working with the Proviso Partners for Health (PP4H) community group to address chronic disease in Maywood. When it comes to managing and preventing diseases, she says, there's nothing more crucial than a healthy diet. A recent PP4H project provided 100 salads a day for students at Proviso East High School, providing a faster, healthier lunch alternative.

For Maywood residents with limited food access, Kouba suggests they seek out food at community gardens or farmer's markets. She also says residents could connect with community organizations or shop owners to explain their needs.

One goal of the project was to bring students of different disciplines together to understand their different professions. Cahill adds that the experience left many students awestruck. She says it was important for the students to learn about the obstacles patients face in order to advise them more effectively. "Practitioners of the future should understand the community," she says.

Figure 26.3 Example of an organizational publication

Adapted with permission from *Loyola Magazine*. www.luc.edu/loyolamagazine/stories/features/archive/fooddeserts.shtml.[14]

National Cancer Institute's Division of Cancer Prevention publishes a quarterly enewsletter, *Nutrition Frontiers*, which highlights discoveries and new developments in our understanding of the relationships among food, nutrition, and cancer prevention. Information and past issues are available at the National Cancer Institute website (https://prevention.cancer .gov/research-groups/nutritional-science/nutrition -frontiers).

The length and formatting of research reported in newsletters varies. Some feature a 150- to 300-word synopsis of the research, without tables or figures, and direct interested readers to the full article by a citation or electronic link. Others publish comprehensive articles of about 3,000 words with tables, figures, and references. Many professional newsletters are peer reviewed, some provide continuing education credit for longer articles, and others are indexed in medical journal databases. For example, the newsletter of the Dietitians in Nutrition Support Dietetic Practice Group, *Support Line*, is indexed in the *Cumulative Index to Nursing and Allied Health Literature*.[13] For many sources, author guidelines are available online or can be obtained by contacting the newsletter editor. Some DPG newsletters welcome student submissions and literature reviews. Newsletters provide a mechanism to increase exposure to research and researchers, which may increase future collaboration between like-minded investigators and direct readers to full journal articles.

Press Releases

Knowledge gains through research can be quite effective when disseminated through print, broadcast, and web-based media platforms. Media outlets reach a large, diverse audience, beyond that of many professional publications.[1] Keep in mind, however, that because media outlets focus on newsworthiness, media pieces may be overly dramatic or exaggerate findings, while missing such important details as study design, measurement methods, or sample size. A press release is a format by which researchers can convey important highlights of a research project to media organizations. Press releases should start with an interesting, concise, and attention-grabbing head-line that compels media representatives to continue reading. The newsworthy essence of the research findings should be captured in the headline in a way that avoids excessive technical jargon and is understandable to consumers. The body of the press release should be about two paragraphs and should tell who, what, where, why, and how of the study. Press releases are generally one double-spaced page and may include a photo or institutional or project logo.

Policy Briefs

Policy briefs are another method of disseminating research knowledge to a targeted professional audience that may be involved in legislation or policy development. Policy briefs focus on a single topic, highlighting a study's evidence-based results and implications for solving societal problems. Considering the demanding schedule of policy professionals, lengthy details about statistical methods or validity of measures are not necessary. Authors of policy briefs should make a convincing argument that the research findings provide evidence and insights into proposed solutions about an important problem in today's society. A common format includes a title, executive summary, problem statement with some background facts, critique of policy options, policy recommendations, references, and resources for further reading in about four to six pages with a clear, logical flow of information.[1] These need to be readable and may include logos, photos, or quotes.

VERBAL DISSEMINATION OF RESEARCH
Professional Conferences

In addition to the aforementioned written strategies, research is widely communicated to professional and consumer audiences verbally via conferences and other settings. With advances in technology, verbal presentations may also be distributed via synchronous or asynchronous electronic formats. The following sections summarize key considerations for presenting research verbally.

Poster Presentations

A poster presentation combines visual and verbal methods, as illustrated in Figure 26.4.[15] The poster reports research in a condensed, high-impact, visual format that blends creativity and scholarship.[16] Posters provide a snapshot of a project and a way for researchers to interact in a more personal manner than can be done with large podium presentations. Conference planners often arrange sessions so that a large number of posters are exhibited in a common space over several hours. Posters are often categorized by a theme, such as a life cycle stage, diagnosis, or type of dietetics practice (eg, sports nutrition). This format allows hundreds of research projects with a similar focus to be displayed simultaneously. Posters are exhibited on rows of boards in exhibit spaces. Ordinarily, a representative of the research project stands near the poster and is available to interact with conference attendees by sharing insights and chatting informally.[17] The advantage of this format is the opportunity for small-group dialogue, as conference attendees can ask specific questions about a project and review many posters in a limited time.[17,20] Disadvantages are that conference at-

---

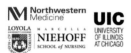

MEDICAL NUTRITION THERAPY FOR PATIENTS WITH ADVANCED SYSTEMIC SCLEROSIS (MNT PASS)

Bethany Doerfler MS, RD;[1] Tara Allen, MS, RD;[2] Courtney Southwood, MS, RD;[3] Darren Brenner, MD;[1] Ikuo Hirano, MD;[1] Patricia Sheean PhD,RD;[4]

Northwestern Medicine[1]; Advocate South Suburban Hospital[2]; Advocate Children's Hospital[3]; Loyola University Chicago[4]

Introduction

- Systemic Sclerosis (SSc) is incurable and 90% of cases involve the GI tract.
- Pain, dysmotility, malabsorption, GI reflux, SBBO and weight loss often occur.
- Limited pharmacological therapies are available to manage symptoms.
- This study: 1) assessed the prevalence of malnutrition and sarcopenia, and 2) tested the impact of a 6-week dietary intervention on symptom burden in patients with SSc.

Methods

- Non-randomized intervention
- 40 patients referred to gastro-enterology with GI symptoms & weight loss were screened (18 mos.)
- 22 were ineligible due to illness acuity (e.g., PN needed within 3-6 months; n=12), transportation issues (n=4) or lack of interest (n=6).
- Nutritional status, quality of life, body composition, diet and physical activity were assessed.

MNT intervention techniques:
- ✓ ↑ calories (500-100 kcals/d) → snacks & regular eating
- ✓ Modify textures, volume or CHO → use fats for oral lubrication, puree foods, consume liquid meals
- ✓ Lifestyle changes → small, frequent meals, elevate HOB

Results

Of the 18 participants enrolled:
- Predominantly white (n=14), females (n=16), 51 (± 11) years of age
- 100% endorsed GERD & 50% reported symptoms R/T gastroparesis
- 83% (n=15) were malnourished
- Using DXA and sex-specific cut-points, 50% (n=9) were sarcopenic.

Pre vs. post-intervention:
- 1400 ± 624 vs. 1577 ± 647 kcals; p=0.12
- No differences in % CHO, PRO or FAT.

Table 1. Anthropometrics, nutrition scores, quality of life and symptom scores pre- and post-intervention for MNT PASS participants

Characteristic	Mean (± SD)		P value
	Baseline (n=14)	Follow-up (n=14)	
Weight (kg)	63.5 ± 9.2	63.6 ± 9.0	0.35
Waist Circumference (cm)	76.2 ± 9.9	75.2 ± 9.8	0.84
BMI (kg/m2)	21.7 ± 3.3	21.8 ± 3.6	0.17
Physical Activity (days)	2.4 ± 2.1	2.5 ± 2.6	0.56
abPG3GA (points)	13.1 ± 7.2	7.6 ± 5.2	0.01
CDC HRQOL Score* (days)	7.7 ± 6.6	6.6 ± 6.5	0.34
Overall Health	2.6 ± 1.0	2.6 ± 1.0	1.00
UCLA SCGI Total Score	0.87 ± 0.44	0.66 ± 0.49	0.20
Reflux	1.80 ± 0.80	0.79 ± 0.61	0.13
Distention	1.80 ± 0.76	1.39 ± 0.93	0.14
Soilage	0.16 ± 0.38	0.07 ± 0.27	1.00
Diarrhea	0.85 ± 0.75	0.54 ± 0.74	0.73
Social Function	0.63 ± 0.47	0.52 ± 0.68	0.26
Emotional Well Being	0.56 ± 0.47	0.52 ± 0.49	0.54
Constipation	0.63 ± 0.63	0.73 ± 0.68	0.89

* Trends toward improved % body fat (p=0.14) and sarcopenia (p=0.02)

Conclusions

- This study provided an MNT PASS allowing malnourished patients with SSc free access to Registered Dietitian specialized in GI disorders.
- Our pilot findings establish the feasibility and positive association of providing MNT to patients with SSc involving the GI tract.
- Adequately powered studies are warranted to better assess the impact of MNT on a broader array of outcomes in this patient population.

Funded by: ADAF Dietitians in Nutrition Support; Northwestern Medicine; NCI (R25CA057699)

Figure 26.4 Example of a poster presentation

This poster was presented at Clinical Nutrition Week, Austin, TX, 2016 and at the Ruth K. Palmer Research Symposium, Maywood, IL 2016.

Reproduced with permission from Doerfler B, Allen T, Southwood C, Brenner D, Hirano I, and Sheean P.[15]

tendees may be overwhelmed by the volume of exhibits, congestion, noise levels; and difficulty in locating specific posters or researchers.[18,19] Evidence for the last point is illustrated in evaluations of four conferences on medical education in the United Kingdom in which attendees reported that the times a presenter accompanied a poster varied from 21% to 86%.[18] The implication is that the poster needs to visually entice the attendee to review it yet provide enough content to be meaningful and scholarly.[17] Some conferences arrange a limited number of poster presentations in a room, perhaps 10, and each researcher is given several minutes to provide an oral synopsis of the project, followed by unstructured time for interaction with everyone in attendance.

Few studies have reported on the extent to which posters are a good strategy to disseminate research findings.[18] The data from these studies, though sparse, can still be useful in planning poster presentations. A small study (n = 34) by Rowe and Ilic[16] surveyed conference participants after they attended poster presentations. The majority (62% [21 participants]) agreed that poster presentations are a good method of knowledge transfer, but fewer (41% [14 participants]) believed this method allows for academic debate, and still fewer (32% [11 participants]) agreed that a poster provides sufficient depth of information. The majority of participants (94% [32 participants]) in this study reported that the visual aspects of posters, such as images, tables, and figures, captured more attention than the text and subject matter. Participants also thought it was important for the poster to be enhanced by verbal communication with the researcher. These findings highlight the importance of first impressions. Saperstein and colleagues[17] reported low retention rates (14.9% and 11.3% at 3 and 90 days, respectively, after the conference) in another small study (n = 26) of physicians who viewed posters at a medical conference. The study noted one limitation: Participants were assigned to review posters that may not have reflected their areas of interest and later knowledge retention. The authors suggest using more interactive measures to enhance retention.

Traditionally, posters have been printed on paper and mounted with pushpins on bulletin boards. This is still common, though it requires care so that the poster is not damaged. Digital poster displays were introduced in 2001 and offer several advantages, including ease of transport (on a portable disk or stored in a digital box), accuracy of color, ability to embed video clips, capability to highlight or magnify sections, opportunity to include sound, and ease of archiving.[17,19] However, digital posters are less common due to the increased cost of the electronic display boards, which is assumed by the organization sponsoring the conference.

Preliminary Review: Submit the Abstract

Before a poster presentation is accepted for display at a conference, an abstract of the work typically undergoes peer review by a panel of content experts. It is important for the researcher to read and adhere to the specific guidelines for the conference, which will dictate word or character limits, format (structured vs unstructured), font size, type, and spacing margins. Most often the abstract is submitted blinded, that is, with all identifying information removed (eg, author names, employers, affiliations or field sites, and geographic location) to minimize reviewer bias. This information may be included in a separate unblinded abstract or on a separate cover page. The abstract generally should include sections similar to a manuscript abstract, including study aims, hypothesis, methods, design, participant characteristics, results, conclusion, and implications for practice. Most abstracts are limited to 150 to 350 words. Conveying key points that make a compelling case for the importance of the research within this word-count limitation is tricky but important. Conference abstracts are usually published in supplemental issues of the journal affiliated with the professional association, and this acknowledges their scholarly worth. Figure 26.5 on page 528 presents an example of an abstract.

After Acceptance: Prepare the Poster Presentation

Similar to preparing a manuscript for publication, the first step in preparing a poster presentation is to thoroughly read the instructions for the specific conference.[18]

Poster Development A variety of software programs are available to create a poster. Popular options include PowerPoint or Publisher (Microsoft

WHAT'S FOR DINNER IN MAYWOOD?
An Environmental Scan of Local Food Availability

Purpose: The purpose of this study is to characterize retail food availability in Maywood, Illinois. This information may provide insights for current and future health care providers and be useful for community initiatives related to health and commerce.

Significance: Healthy People 2020 includes four objectives aimed at increasing healthier food access including retail sources that provide a variety of items consistent with the Dietary Guidelines for Americans (NWS-4).

Methods: Interprofessional teams of students from the Loyola University Chicago Health Sciences Division surveyed retail food availability in Maywood using a modified-version of the USDA Market Basket tool. A list of retail food outlets was developed by an online search. Student teams included a mix of medical, nursing, and dietetic students.

Results: The list of 27 stores included groceries, gas stations, convenience stores, and a pharmacy. Nine store surveys were completed. The remainder were no longer in business, or unable to be surveyed. Availability of food items varied by category. The three categories of highest availability were staples, sweets, and spices with an average of 65%, 56%, and 42%, respectively, of items in these categories available. The three with lowest availability were frozen vegetables, fresh fruits, and fresh vegetables at 11%, 17%, and 20%, respectively. Only two items, salt and juice, were available in 100% of the stores surveyed. On average, stores carried 22% of items on the list. This ranged from 5 to 98%. Details will be provided in the poster. Surveys of remaining stores are in progress and will be added to this preliminary data.

Conclusions: The foods that are most available in Maywood are characterized as high in caloric density, low in nutrient density, and shelf stable. This creates challenges for community members and health care providers in promoting eating patterns consistent with health.

Implications: Health care providers and health science students should be aware of these challenges experienced by patients who reside locally. Strategies for individuals and families will be provided, in addition to initiatives for community partners.

Figure 26.5 Example of an abstract in which the authors have been blinded for a poster presentation at a professional conference

Corporation, Redmond, WA); Illustrator, Photoshop, and InDesign (Adobe Systems, San Jose, CA); and PosterGenius (SciGen Technologies, Chicago, IL).[19] Presenters should pay attention to the dimensions and orientation of the poster as it is designed. A poster that stands out because it hangs over the edges of the poster board or has a different orientation from others is not a good thing. Many universities and employers provide poster templates with the institutional logo. This makes it easier for the researcher and also creates a branded style in terms of color scheme, fonts, and other features. Because of the bustling atmosphere of many poster presentation spaces, a poster format that makes review easy is recommended. As with manuscripts, key points should be organized in sections that describe the title, authors, background, study aims, methods, results, discussion, and conclusion. Some organizations require disclosure of funding or conflicts of interest. All of this should be done in an abbreviated manner. Succinct writing is a skill. Several revisions are often required. Complete sentences are typically used for background and discussion sections,[20] but the other sections may use bullet points, phrases, flow charts, and graphs.[18] Researchers often include too much information because they are proud of their project, but in a high-volume exhibition, lengthy posters discourage attendees from taking the time to review. Box 26.1 on page 530 lists more suggestions for effective posters. Giving the poster a critical review for accuracy and completeness is wise, including the list of authors and their credentials. All authors should have the chance to review the poster before printing.

After the poster has been developed, proofread, and revised, it is ready for printing. Options for printing are to (1) print locally and carry the poster to the destination, (2) print locally and ship, or (3) print at the conference location. Local printing can often be ordered through an in-house printing service available through many universities or employers or through a private printing company. The print order is usually submitted electronically by uploading the computer file. Ideally, the researcher will have the option to review a draft before the final production. This is a critical step, and it is important to allow time for a thorough review. Mistakes are not uncommon, and it would be disappointing to ap-

prove without review and to find errors in the poster at the conference. If the poster is printed locally, ensure delivery several days before travel and secure transport. Usually, researchers will carry the poster with them in a rigid poster tube. Posters can be shipped to the conference, but ensure adequate time and confirm the exact location of delivery, as delivery is not risk free. Finally, printing services may be available near the conference location; arrangements can be made in advance to print and pick up the poster so it does not need to be transported, though this may be more costly.

The Poster Session Presenting a poster exhibit can be a rewarding experience and can prompt a lively exchange of ideas and experiences with attendees who view the poster. The goal of the presentation is to share information about the research with interested attendees. Thought and preparation to accomplish this goal is important. Pay attention to simple but important details like reviewing the time frame and location of the session and bringing a supply of pushpins, copies ($8 \frac{1}{2} \times 11$ in) of the poster to share, and business cards. The presenter should prepare for the exhibit session by summarizing the key points of the research in several sentences and practicing those orally. Anticipating attendees' questions and formulating responses is advised.[20] A practice session with colleagues is recommended, and be sure to have them ask questions.

Presenters should arrive at the exhibit as soon as allowed and place the poster on the designated board. McCleod and Stover[19] identified three types of people who view poster exhibits and offered suggestions on ways the presenter should interact. The first type—the browser—scans all posters to determine which are of interest. The presenter should be cordial and say hello but allow the person time to review the poster. Presenters should not interrogate the reviewer or infringe on his or her time. The second type reads the abstracts or program information before the session and seeks out specific posters for careful review. This person will often start a conversation to gain a comprehensive understanding of the research project, so the presenter can engage in a longer discussion. The third type is a coworker or peer who comes to acknowledge the re-

Suggestion	Reason
Print the poster number on the top corner of poster	Number allows participants to easily locate a specific poster. The poster might cover the poster numbers on the board.
Keep it simple and highlight main points	Readability is key in large venues with many people. The presenter can expand on main points or bring more detailed information to share.
Make it easy to read	*Section headings:* Use boldfacing and a large font (36 point). *Text:* Use a font no smaller than 24 point. *Font styles:* Times New Roman and Palatino are easy to read. *Tables, graphs, flow charts:* Summarize information well. *Organization:* Use the software's grid and ruler functions to align and organize content for a professional look.
Proofread carefully	Accuracy, completeness, and aesthetics are important. Ask for help. Double-check dimensions. Make sure all authors are properly listed.
Limit references	A lengthy reference list takes up space, makes your poster look cluttered, and distracts from the key points.

Box 26.1 Practical Suggestions for Conference Poster Presentations[17,18-21]

searcher's presentation.[20] This is primarily a social interaction. McCleod and Stover[19] suggest that presenters be collegial but keep it brief to allow adequate time for interactions with others.

Podium Presentations

Similar to the process of preparing a journal article, the process of presenting research at a professional conference requires careful thought and planning. The call for speaker session proposals is generally announced 6 to 12 months before the conference. This announcement includes conference themes, types of presentations, important dates for speakers and sessions, levels of content (from 1 [basic] to 3 [advanced]) for continuing education purposes, and instructions for submitting a proposal to be a speaker.

Selecting a Professional Conference

Research presentations should be a good match with the conference themes. For example, the 2017 Food and Nutrition Conference and Exhibition (FNCE) sought speakers to present "original ideas that challenge us to embrace change."[21] The theme of the 2017 American Public Health Association Annual Meeting was "creating the healthiest nation: climate changes health," although the 33 specialty sections listed for proposal submission ranged from food and nutrition to aging to vision care.[22] Each section had a distinct review panel and sought to present a robust program of research, so researchers considered the best fit for their topic. The research example given earlier about the habits of elderly persons and food safety would fit the aging section or the food and nutrition section. The theme of the 2017 Society for

Nutrition Education and Behavior annual conference was to "honor the past, embrace the present and define the future" but stated that behavior change and food choice were important presentation topics.[23] Other identified themes in 2017 ranged from electronic devices to help people sustain healthy lifestyle patterns to policy, systems, and environmental initiatives to promote health. Finding a good fit for the research project is important. Many professional associations sponsor a large annual conference, and regional affiliates offer smaller meetings; some even provide opportunities for student presentations. Reviewing the mission, vision, and strategic plan of the particular professional association is another way to ensure a good match.

After identifying the appropriate meeting, the research team should review the types of conference presentation options. For example, FNCE accepts abstracts for presentations in three categories: (1) research, (2) projects or programs, and (3) innovations in dietetics practice or education.[21] Research podium presentation formats vary and are specified by the hosting association in preconference announcements. Keynote research presentations may feature an established research team or research on a hot topic that highlights key conference themes. These are generally in an auditorium seating hundreds and have a generous time allotment of an hour or more. More common is a format in which four to six brief research presentations with a common theme are presented. Each person is allowed about 10 to 15 minutes to present. This is often followed by a 20- to 30-minute moderated panel discussion with the researchers. Typically, the audience is invited to ask questions, which provides the opportunity for dialogue. This format is sometimes termed *concurrent research presentations.* The conference planning team may ask potential speakers to identify preferred presentation formats in their submission materials. Options may include a podium, poster, or roundtable presentation. The designated format will be included in the decision notification.

Preliminary Review: Submitting the Proposal and Abstract

After deciding on a conference and presentation type, the next step is to prepare the presentation proposal materials for review. The principal submission is the abstract (often both blinded and unblinded versions are required). The abstract should precisely match the specifications, so read the conference guidelines carefully. For example, FNCE research abstracts are required to be no more than 250 words and in a structured format with sections on research outcome, methods, analysis, results, conclusions, and overall scientific merit. Note that research findings presented are usually expected to be original, to be completed, and not to be presented or published elsewhere. Statements suggesting that "data collection is ongoing," "results will be discussed," or "analysis is pending" are not highly regarded by reviewers. Abstract reviewers are looking for results. If space is still available for a presentation or poster after the first round of abstract review and acceptance, then a second round, often termed "late breaking" abstract submission is opened. FNCE abstracts are judged by a panel of three content experts.[21] Keep in mind that the review is a competitive process, and any deviations from directions are cause for disqualification. Reviewers may cull abstracts that exceed word or character limits, do not follow the structured format (if required), lack supplemental materials, or are late.

The abstract should have a good title: one that is brief, accurately describes the project, and is clever enough to catch the reader's attention. This is followed by the abstract body. Most organizations have an online submission form that requires applicants to provide basic information about researcher and presenter demographics; affiliations; contact information; and disclosures related to funding, conflict of interest and ethical conduct of human subjects in addition to the abstract. Approximately two-thirds of abstracts submitted to FNCE are accepted. Conference rules differ as to the number of abstracts one researcher can submit or have accepted, so pay attention to these details. Conference planners want to spread the opportunity widely and provide a program with a variety of diverse research projects and presenters. Researchers are informed about the acceptance decision 2 to 3 months after submission.

Preparing for the Presentation

After the abstract is accepted, researchers should prepare the presentation using details specified in the conference resources. Time allocation and number of research team members who will be presenting are primary considerations. Generally, the presentation format follows that of a written research manuscript submitted for publication. Of course, the important difference is the delivery. Podium presentations generally combine oral and visual modes.

Visual Component for Podium Presentation

An outline provides a framework and can help allocate time and speaker assignments for a session. If the presentation is in the concurrent session format, that is, with multiple presenters in one session, it is critical that everyone adheres to the time limit so that each person is able to present as expected. Exceeding the time allocation is disrespectful to the other speakers and moderator. The sponsoring association will provide information about software and hardware, due dates for supporting materials, room assignment and size, date and time assignment, moderator, and other presenters in the session. Some organizations provide standard templates for visual presentations; Box 26.2 has a sample outline for a 10- to 30-minute research presentation focusing on one study.

In terms of graphics, simplicity is generally best. Images should summarize data to support spoken content. Graphs and diagrams are very useful to display results. Tables and charts are also useful, but make sure they are readable and not overly busy or packed with information. Copyright permissions must be obtained and submitted to the conference staff for any diagrams or graphics used from other sources. Use of colors, complicated designs, cartoons, transitions, fancy fonts, and similar features should be limited to increase readability and keep audience members focused on content.[24] The appearance of color schemes can vary with different computers and projection systems, so doing a trial run in the room being used for the presentation is recommended, if possible, to make any necessary adjustments.

In terms of text, as with poster presentations, complete sentences are not necessary.[24] Information can be presented in a bullet-point format using a large font, at least 24 points, and high-contrast colors between background and text. Use no more than four to five bullet points per slide. Avoid blocks of text as audience members will not have time to read the text and absorb the oral details simultaneously. It is

always wise to ask a colleague to proofread the final presentation.

Once the visual part of the presentation is finalized, it is often sent electronically to the conference planners so that it can be archived for easy retrieval before the presentation. Additionally, the presenter should ensure that the presentation is available by bringing it on a personal laptop or flash drive, uploading it to a web-based archival site (eg, Dropbox, OneDrive), or emailing it to one's self in case there is a problem with the file sent to the conference planners.

Oral Component for Podium Presentation

The audience and professional association should be considered when structuring the oral component of the presentation. If the audience is a specialized group, then certain abbreviations or acronyms may be used without definition. For example, if presenting to a group of RDNs, it is safe to use the term BMI without defining it as body mass index in the presentation. However, if speaking to a variety of health care providers, it would be wise to define BMI at first use.

Time frame is also important to consider when preparing the oral presentation. The presenter should supplement the visual content with additional detail and explanation lasting approximately 45 to 60 seconds per slide, and not more than one slide per 30 seconds.[24] If the time frame is 30 minutes or more, then the presenter may describe background, methods, and results in greater detail, spending several minutes per slide. Established researchers may present a body of work with several studies in one presentation if the time allotment is generous.

As a starting point, many presenters prepare notes or a brief script with key points for each slide so that important details are not overlooked and information is given in logical order. It is also a good idea to practice the presentation multiple times with the slides to coordinate flow of the visual and oral information, ensure that smooth transitions occur as slides are advanced, and guarantee appropriate timing and good pronunciation. A respectful and professional tone is an important part of delivery. This is not the venue for casual comments like "we all know . . ." or "you guys," which may sneak into a presentation if one is nervous but can be perceived as un-

Slide	Main Idea	Key Information to Include
1	Title	Project title identical to abstract
		Authors with credentials and titles
		Author affiliations, institutions
2–3	Background	Significance of the problem (brief)
		Graph or diagram to summarize key points
		Gaps in knowledge leading to the research being presented
		Note: Be careful to limit this section so as not to exceed time allocation
4	Purpose	Research question, purpose or study aims (primary, secondary, exploratory) in several clear and concise statements
5	Study design	Design: observational, clinical trial, other
		Time frame: cross-sectional, retrospective, prospective
		Time period: days, weeks, months, other
		Recruitment strategies
		Data sources
		Institutional review board: consenting process
6	Criteria for participation	Inclusion and exclusion criteria
		Screening process
7	Variables	Outcome measures
		Independent and confounding variables
		Methods and time frame of measurements
8	Statistical measures	Sample size, power analysis, statistical methods
		Significance level
9–12	Results	Key results to answer the purpose stated in slide 4
		Use tables, charts, and graphs to summarize and display data and findings (may need to limit the number)
		Supplementary data can be available if questions arise
13	Strengths and limitations	Generalizability
		Challenges
14	Conclusions	Summary of findings
		Implications for practice, if applicable
		Next steps for future research
15	Final slide	Acknowledgments
		Disclosures
		Question prompt

Box 26.2 Sample Slide Organization for Research Presentation[24]

prepared or unprofessional. A practice run will also help the presenter minimize reliance on notes. Room arrangements and lighting may be such that the presenter cannot see notes during the presentation, so it is best to be ready to deliver the narrative without notes but to have them available just in case. After completing several solo practice rounds, deliver the presentation to a small group of colleagues to get their feedback and solicit questions. This will be valuable in clarifying information, fine-tuning the visual or oral components, and preparing for possible questions from the audience. Feedback from colleagues may also help identify distracting, nervous behaviors such as relying on verbal fillers like "um" or fiddling with hair.

Delivering the Podium Presentation

Additional arrangements warrant attention to prepare for a smooth and professional presentation, including travel arrangements, conference registration, and logistics. Information provided to speakers upon acceptance may include details about registration requirements and compensation for travel. Though it is customary for presenters to pay the conference registration fee, in some cases the fee may be waived. Planning travel well in advance of the conference is advised. Upon arrival at the conference center, speakers should register, identify themselves as a speaker, and ask about resources for speakers. This often includes a speaker room with equipment to check media, a secure space to leave luggage (if needed), refreshments, and other assistance. Many conference venues are large, spanning several city blocks, and have wings and pavilions sprawling in different directions. Thus, it is important to locate and view the exact room where one will be presenting well in advance. Doing this increases the likelihood that the speaker will arrive at the room without getting lost or arriving late. If possible, attend another session in the room to observe the lighting, sound system, seating arrangements, podium, hardware, and projection placement. Situational awareness beforehand allows time to consider ways to manage the presentation delivery and minimizes last-minute surprises. For example, if the podium is in the middle of the room and the projections are on either side of the speaker, the speaker

will want to think about the need to make eye contact with those on both sides of the podium.

Speakers should arrive 30 to 60 minutes before the start of the presentation so they can introduce themselves to the moderator and other speakers and clarify any questions, such as name pronunciation. Flow of the session can also be discussed, such as whether the moderator will introduce all speakers at the start or if each will be introduced immediately before his or her presentation. Another logistical detail is the manner in which questions will be answered. This is also a good time to ensure that visuals (slides) are loaded and cued up for the presentation. A quick run-through to ensure that everything is in working order is a good idea.

When cued by the moderator, speakers should smile, start with a quick note of thanks to the moderator and conference planners, and deliver their presentation in a clear and paced manner. Important messages are lost when the presentation is rushed and overwhelmed with details. Depending on the format and timing, with coordination from the moderator, questions may be answered at the conclusion of the presentation or held until all speakers have completed their presentations. If questions arise, the speaker should repeat them so that the audience can hear it. If a question is unclear, the speaker should ask for clarification. If the answer is not available, the speaker should note this and perhaps offer to communicate information later to the person who asked. Any criticism of the work should be graciously accepted. Speakers should stay in the room, often at the speaker table, until the moderator concludes the session. Whatever the format, speakers should remain in the room until all speakers in that session have completed their presentations as a professional courtesy, even if they were the first speaker.

After the session, speakers and audience members may continue to discuss questions or collaborations, exchange business cards, or distribute handouts. If the room is needed for the next session, this can be done in the hallway. To establish positive professional relationships with potential future collaborators, speakers should promptly follow up on any requests as agreed upon, such as emailing slides or providing references.

Presenters should dress neatly and be prepared for technological mishaps, such as a projector light bulb burning out without a nearby replacement. The prepared speaker should be able to stand alone and deliver an elevator speech that conveys key research findings in an unflustered and enthusiastic manner.

Roundtable Presentations

Roundtable presentations offer another option for researchers to present their projects. The preliminary work of identifying an appropriate conference and submitting a proposal with abstract and supplementary materials is generally the same as for podium and poster presentations. The difference is the format of the session. Roundtable presentations are generally categorized by broad theme (eg, stage of the life cycle), a specific disease (eg, diabetes), an area of practice (eg, community or school food service), or an innovative technique (eg, telehealth or social media). A dozen or more presenters whose work can be classified under the common broad category are assigned to a shared space containing round tables. Generally, but not always, each round table is assigned a number that corresponds to an abstract in the conference program. Presenters are available at their table to provide a brief overview of their work and guide a discussion with those who join them. This format is more flexible in time frame and movement than a podium presentation. Participants are allowed to move from one table to another, at preset intervals, based on their interest. A roundtable session may be planned to allow two or three rotations during the entire session. The presenter should be prepared to repeat the presentation and discussion several times. The casual format allows for more individualized exchange between the presenter and participants. This venue is excellent for meeting colleagues with similar interests and sharing experiences and deeper discussions than some of the other formats. Because of the smaller group environment, people often participate in discussions though they might be hesitant to ask a question in a large auditorium.

Preparing for the Presentation

Research should be summarized in a brief, approximately 15-minute, talk that has a conversational tone. Presenters should have key points written for reference and supplementary materials available if additional detail is needed. The talk is generally followed by a 20- to 30-minute discussion that ideally engages all those present. The presenter should prepare three to five open-ended discussion questions and encourage audience interaction. Examples of questions are listed in Box 26.3. Additional questions specific to the project should be included. Visual aids are minimal as there is typically no technology in roundtable sessions. A few diagrams or graphs can be printed on standard-sized paper and displayed on the table or as a tabletop flip chart. A one-page handout should be prepared that includes additional references and contact information. The presenter should bring approximately 50 to 100 copies of the handout along with business cards and other printed visuals to the session.

Delivery of the Presentation

As with other formats, presenters should locate the assigned room ahead of time, arrive early, identify themselves to the session moderator, and be at their table about 15 minutes before the session is scheduled to start. As participants arrive, the presenter should greet them in a welcoming fashion. At the beginning of the session, the moderator will provide an overview of and perhaps some introductions. The presenters should then give a summary of their research project. Key concepts of respect and professionalism still apply, though the delivery can be more casual than a podium presentation. After the project

Now that you have heard a summary of this project, what else can I tell you about it?

What questions do you have for me?

What is your interest or experience in this topic?

If you have done work in this area, how does it relate to this project?

What are your suggestions for continued work in this area?

Box 26.3 Sample Roundtable Discussion Questions

summary, the table presenter leads the discussion. If only a few participants are at the table, the discussion may start with brief introductions. However, it is important that this not take most of the discussion time. The presenter should manage group dynamics so that everyone has an opportunity to contribute and ask questions. When the moderator announces that it is time for the next round to begin, the researcher should thank participants for their attention and contributions and begin the next round.

Community Presentations

The importance of sharing research findings with communities of interest was noted earlier in this chapter. This is also pertinent when considering oral communication of research findings. The effectiveness of traditional modes of research dissemination—writing papers and didactic presentations—has been challenged, especially for community groups.[25] Vaughn and colleagues[26] advises researchers to take this seriously, particularly in light of the variety of stakeholders with which RDNs work. Stakeholders range from physicians to pot washers, newborns to grandparents, pharmaceutical firm empolyees to farm workers. Some may be considered vulnerable because of limited literacy, language, health status, or disability. Many do not have access to professional, peer-reviewed journals through subscriptions, libraries, or even open access mechanisms. Understanding the perspectives of the audience, including community stakeholders, is important in planning community sessions.[27] Planning a community presentation may take more time than planning a professional presentation because the rules may not be spelled out as clearly. Experts in community relationships emphasize the importance of connecting with community partners to obtain their ideas about planning presentations. Feedback from community members should be valued and incorporated into the session. The researcher still has the obligation to share research findings with these groups so that everyone can benefit from knowledge discovery, especially those who may experience the problems studied. The goal of research is also to ultimately translate this new knowledge into improved

environments, practice, and policy at the organizational or systems level for improved health outcomes. Yet a gap exists between knowing and doing.[27] Including members of the communities of interest has been suggested as necessary to narrow the "know-do" gap, particularly considering health disparities.[26,28] A systematic literature review of knowledge transfer specific to scaling up public health interventions recently identified some ways to deal with the know-do gap. Success factors included active engagement of implementers and the target community, training, political will, and advocacy.[28] One barrier, poor engagement between thought leaders and stakeholders, may be addressed by giving research presentations to health care providers and patient or consumer groups where they work and live, and not just at professional venues.

Often a researcher can arrange for 10 to 15 minutes on the agenda of a regularly scheduled staff meeting to share research findings that might be particularly relevant to that group. For example, if study participants were recruited from an endocrinology clinic for a study on diabetes outcomes with a telehealth project involving an RDN, then the clinic staff might be very interested to learn about the process and outcomes. This might lead to a revised model of health care in the clinic and improved patient outcomes, thereby narrowing the know-do gap. Usually, piggybacking on an existing meeting is more successful in reaching people than asking people to come to a meeting before or after work.

Partnerships are key to accessing community groups for research presentations. Researchers should attempt to incorporate their presentations into existing community meetings. Health care systems, schools, faith-based groups, park districts, and others often host gatherings that would be perfect for sharing research findings. Key concepts in planning and delivering presentations to community groups include designing a concise, clear story of the research project encompassing the background or rationale, a brief description of methods and participants (including ethical conduct compliance), results, discussion, and implications for the community of interest. This is similar to the professional presentation framework but must be revised to make the language and terms appropriate to the audience. Researchers should avoid using highly technical terms or abbreviations that may intimidate listeners. Two to three clear results should be highlighted. Visuals are helpful but again should be appropriate to the audience. Any tables and graphs should be explained. Questions and dialogue should be encouraged.

Fullilove and colleagues[25] suggest a community research group model as a novel method to engage stakeholders for research dissemination that includes a "lived experience" aspect. This model includes not only the community members but also those external to the community so that advocacy and political will are built. They accomplished this with neighborhood tours. RDNs might do this with community gardens, school cafeterias, and grocery stores. Communication of research findings need not be limited to didactic monologues. Thinking outside the box is encouraged by the model of research dissemination proposed by Fullilove and colleagues.

Electronic Means of Disseminating Research

Web Seminars and Electronic Presentations

Web seminars, also known as *webinars* or *web conferences*, are online meetings that provide a means to share information and deliver a presentation without everyone being physically present in the same space. Documents such as slides or video clips can be included.

A webinar is usually a live format (though most are recorded for later use, too), allowing participants an opportunity to discuss content or interact around questions and answers. A number of different technologies and services are available to deliver web-based programs. Producing a webinar requires extra consideration and planning.

Planning the Webinar Most professionals face plenty of competition for their valuable time. This means that a clever and appealing title is important for announcing a webinar. If the goal is to have real-time interaction, then timing is critical; thus, a lunchtime or early evening event may be ideal.

A team is useful in preparing the webinar. Having more than one voice or presenter adds interest. For example, one person may be a moderator, introducing each presenter who speaks for a 10- to 15-minute block. A webinar format also means that not all presenters need to be in the same space and may connect remotely to do their part. A backstage buddy, who plays a supportive role in dealing with technical problems or assisting with audience queries, is recommended. This person can answer easy or common questions during the webinar via chat features or texting, screen and organize questions during live sessions, monitor time, and resolve technical problems for participants.[28]

A hosting service provides technical mechanisms to set the framework and control the webinar. For example, a hosting service is able to restrict the audience, register participants, create announcements with photos or graphics, and distribute announcements through multiple channels (eg, email, social media, and newsletters). After the webinar, the hosting service may also be able to conduct evaluations and ask participants to rate relevance and satisfaction and suggest ideas for improvement or future topics.

Sending announcements at least three times using various mechanisms is recommended as each reaches and may generate a different subset of participants.[27] A last chance announcement the day before the webinar is advised. Take care to collect only relevant information during registration, such as name and email address. A generic job title or work environment may also be helpful so speakers know their audience and can personalize presentation. Asking the audience for questions during the registration process may also be helpful in designing the presentation. For example, when preparing a webinar about diabetes management, it would be helpful to know if the audience is 100% outpatient RDNs; a mix of inpatient and outpatient RDNs; or if some nurses, pharmacists, social workers, physicians, or dietetics students are attending. Avoid asking too many questions at registration, however, as it may ultimately deter registration.

The presenters should write an introductory script that includes the items shown in Box 26.4 on page 538. The moderator should rehearse the script

Name of webinar

Name of moderator

Names of presenters

Acknowledgment of sponsors, funding sources, partners, disclaimers, and conflicts of interest

Location of webinar slides and recording, if applicable

How to get technical help during webinar, if needed

Contact information for questions after webinar

Box 26.4 Information to Include in a Webinar Introductory Script

out loud, and the backstage buddy should also have a copy in case of technical problems.[28]

In general, the body of the webinar follows the pattern of podium presentations described earlier. However, the webinar format allows for additional features. For example, polling the audience during the webinar is a means to interact with them and evaluate their understanding of the content or relevance to their work. Polling allows presenters to adjust the content during the session. Before the webinar, presenters may want to think about ways to personalize their presentation depending on how participants respond to polling. Though this would take more advance preparation, the webinar will be smoother and more informative if the presenter is not constructing responses during the session.

Similar to a podium presentation at a face-to-face conference, practice sessions are essential, especially if more than one presenter will be involved. This includes learning how to use all features of the hosting service, such as transitioning screen control from one presenter to another or from webcam to screen, starting and ending recording, polling, and tallying polling results quickly. Rehearsals with the moderator, presenters, backstage buddy, and any other team members all together ensures smooth transitions, accurate timing, and appropriate coverage of content without redundancy. Also be sure to rehearse use of

polls and how to upload slides, video clips, and any other resources to avoid technical glitches.

Webinar Delivery Webinar presenters should log on at least 30 minutes before the start. A reminder slide can be posted at this time with details about the webinar topic, presenters, time, and how to get technical assistance or access resources. Presenters should close all other programs on their computer so extraneous background noise from email or social media notifications are not distracting. Sound and internet connections should be checked. Recording should be started and confirmed before the moderator and presenters start speaking. The webinar should begin on time and proceed as planned and rehearsed. Bates and Chiba[28] report that it is typical for only 30% to 60% of those who registered to participate, so there is no need to delay the start time. The backstage buddy should watch the time and may send private chat messages to presenters to help with this. Presenters should be aware of these techniques for communicating during the conference. The webinar should conclude with the moderator summing up key points in a few sentences, thanking presenters, and informing the audience how to obtain resources. If applicable, questions or discussion can follow with the assistance of the backstage buddy.

After the Webinar Recorded webinars may be edited, with technical assistance, to remove extraneous noise or distracting comments (like "ums"). Depending on the content, audio files without the slides may also be produced for listening while doing other activities. These edited files should also be announced and made available. Finally, an evaluation survey should be sent right after the webinar when participants are still thinking about their experience and suggestions.

Troubleshooting a Webinar Events that are unexpected should be anticipated. Plan B should be outlined and distributed to the team. For example, a remote presenter who loses internet connection may be able to call in via speaker phone while the backstage buddy advances slides. This may not be ideal, but it is better than completely losing the presenter. If part of the session includes using functions on internet sites, but this does not work as planned, having backup screenshots would be handy. Everyone has experienced technical glitches. Having a sense of humor and a plan B will help with delivering the webinar and prevent disaster.

Disseminating research findings using web conferences enables researchers to reach a wide audience. Though presenters will need to learn about and use technology resources beyond the traditional routes, it is well worth the effort.

Novel Approaches

An online community of practice is a new approach to building a robust partnership between the academic research world and the practice world. The National Cancer Institute, for example, launched Research to Reality in 2011 with the goal of enhancing cancer control practices by disseminating research and translating it into practice.[29] The program developers, including Margaret Farrell, MPH, RD, note that building trust through authentic community partnership is key. An online community of practice was established to develop ongoing (as opposed to one-time) knowledge transfer that would transcend varied work schedules and locations. Initially, interactive features included an online discussion forum, webinars, and partnerships. The program has evolved to include mentorship and a "virtual crosswalk" to other National Cancer Institute resources. This project has established ongoing research dissemination and dialogue between researchers and practitioners. In 2013, the website (https://researchtoreality.cancer.gov) had 80,000 views. The average webinar is viewed by 11,000. Research to Reality continues to grow annually. This virtual approach has a broad reach, can target those interested in very specific conditions, and fosters ongoing engagement.[29]

Another novel approach is the Philadelphia Collaborative Violence Prevention Center's use of digital animation to disseminate research findings related to evidence-based strategies for violence prevention with adolescents. Initially, the project planned to use cartoon characters and print media, but feedback from the community of interest, adoles-

cents, indicated that this would not be effective. The messages were reformulated, emphasizing humor and realism and delivered through texts, emails, and social media (namely, YouTube and Facebook).[26]

CONCLUSION

Researchers have an obligation to share their findings with communities of interest. Professional journal publications and conference presentations continue to be key strategies for research dissemination within the scientific community. Technological advances provide newer, creative methods to meet this goal, such as webinars. Researchers also have a responsibility to share their findings with consumers and stakeholder communities. These efforts are often less formal but nonetheless important so that findings can increase community awareness and inspire collective action toward problem solving and ultimately healthier individuals, families, and communities.

REFERENCES

1. World Health Organization. Module 5. Disseminating the research findings. In: *Implementation Research Toolkit.* Geneva, Switzerland: WHO; 2014. www.who.int/tdr /publications/year/2014/participant-workbook5_030414 .pdf?ua=1. Accessed January 26, 2017.

2. US National Library of Medicine. ClinicalTrials.gov Background. https://clinicaltrials.gov/ct2/about-site /background. Accessed October 15, 2017.

3. Ware M, Mabe M. *The STM report: An Overview of Scientific and Scholarly Journal Publishing.* 4th ed. The Hague, Netherlands: International Association of Scientific, Technical and Medical Publishers; 2015. www.zbw -mediatalk.eu/wp-content/uploads/2017/07/STM-Report .pdf. Accessed October 15, 2017.

4. *Journal of the Academy of Nutrition and Dietetics.* Information for Authors. www.andjrnl.org/content /authorinfo. Accessed January 12, 2017.

5. Switt J. What does the *Journal's* impact factor mean to you? *J Am Diet Assoc.* 2011;111(1):41-44.

6. International Scientific Institute. Impact Factor List. www .scijournal.org/about-us.shtml. Accessed February 9, 2017.

7. Elsevier. Journal of the Academy of Nutrition and Dietetics.: The official journal of the Academy of Nutrition and Dietetics. www.elsevier.com/journals/personal/journal-of -the-academy-of-nutrition-and-dietetics/2212-2672. Accessed February 12, 2019.

8. Elsevier. *Your Guide to Publishing Open Access with Elsevier.* August 2015. www.elsevier.com/__data/assets/pdf_file/0003 /78492/openaccessbooklet.pdf. Accessed February 23, 2017.

9. *American Journal of Clinical Nutrition.* Instructions to Authors. http://ajcn.nutrition.org/site/misc/ifa.xhtml. Accessed March 1, 2017.

10. Sheean P, Huifang L, Schiffer L, Arroyo C, Troy K, Solley M. Assessing the prevalence of compromised bone health among overweight and obese African-American breast cancer survivors: a case-control study. *J Cancer Surviv.* 2016; 10(1):21-30

11. von Elm E, Altman DG, Egger M, Pocock SJ, Gøtzsche PC, Vandenbroucke JP; STROBE Initiative. The Strengthening the Reporting of Observational Studies in Epidemiology (STROBE) statement: guidelines for reporting observational studies. *J Clin Epidemiol.* 2008;61(4):344-349.

12. Schulz KF, Altman DG, Moher D, for the CONSORT Group. CONSORT 2010 statement: updated guidelines for reporting parallel group randomised trials. *Ann Intern Med.* 2010;152(11):726-732

13. Academy of Nutrition and Dietetics. Dietetic practice groups list. www.eatrightpro.org/resource/membership/academy -groups/dietetic-practice-groups/list-of-dietetic-practice -groups. Accessed March 1, 2017.

14. Fisher Z. Maintaining a balanced diet poses a unique challenge in communities with limited food access. *Loyola Magazine.* www.luc.edu/loyolamagazine/stories/features /archive/fooddeserts.shtml. Accessed February 13, 2019.

15. Doerfler B, Allen T, Southwood C, Brenner D, Hirano I, Sheean P. Medical nutrition therapy for patients with advance system sclerosis (MNT PASS). Poster presented at Clinical Nutrition Week; January 16-19, 2016; Austin, TX.

16. Rowe N, Ilic D. What impact do posters have on academic knowledge transfer? A pilot survey on author attitudes and experiences. *BMC Med Educ.* 2009;9:71.

17. Saperstein AK, Lennon RP, Olsen C, Womble L, Saguil A. Infor-mation retention among attendees at a traditional poster presentation session. *Acta Med Acad.* 2016:45(2): 180-181.

18. Beamish AJ, Ansell J, Foster JJ, Foster KA, Egan RJ. Poster exhibitions at conferences: are we doing it properly? *J Surg Educ.* 2015:72(2):278-282.

19. McCleod KS, Stover KR. Tips for successful poster presenta-tion. *Am J Health Syst Pharm.* 2014;71:449-451.

20. Rowe N, Dragan, I. Poster presentation: a visual medium for academic and scientific meetings. *Paediatr Respir Rev.* 2011; 12:208-213.

21. Food and Nutrition Conference and Exhibition. Posters and abstract presenters. http://eatrightfnce.org/program /posters-abstract-presenters. Accessed March 18, 2017.

22. American Public Health Association. Presenter information. www.apha.org/events-and-meetings/annual/presenter -information. Accessed March 18, 2017.

23. Society for Nutrition Education and Behavior. SNEB annual conference call for abstracts. www.sneb.org/abstracts. Accessed March 18, 2017.

24. Wax JR, Cartin A, Pinette MG. Preparing a research presen-tation: a guide for investigators. *Am J Obstet Gynecol.* 2011; 205(1):28.e1-28.e5.

25. Fullilove M, Green LL, Hernández-Cordero LJ, Fullilove RE. Obvious and not-so-obvious strategies to disseminate research. *Health Promot Pract.* 2006;7(3):306-311.

26. Vaughn NA, Jacoby SF, Williams T, Guerra T, Thomas NA, Richmond TS. Digital animation as a method to disseminate research findings to the community using a community-based participatory approach. *Am J Community Psychol.* 2013;51(1-2):30-42.

27. Milat AJ, Bauman A, Redman S. Narrative review of models and success factors for scaling up public health interventions. *Implement Sci.* 2015;10:113.

28. Bates ME, Chiba C. Secrets of successful webinars. *Online Searcher.* 2015;39(5):10-15.

29. Farrell MM, LaPorta M, Gallagher A., Vinson C, Bernal SB. Research to Reality: moving evidence into practice through an online community of practice. *Prev Chronic Dis.* 2014;11: E78.

Chapter 27

Illustrating the Results of Research

Shortie McKinney, PhD, RD, FADA | *Kelsey M. Mangano, PhD, RD*

LEARNING OBJECTIVES

1. Describe the purpose of conveying research results through illustrations across various research designs in nutrition.

2. Outline guidelines for preparing and reading tables in nutrition research.

3. Identify current resources for aiding in the development of tables and figures for nutrition research.

4. Identify graph types that best convey research results across various research designs in nutrition.

Just as research becomes valuable when shared through scientific dissemination channels, research gains power and influence when conveyed in ways that are easy to understand. The combination of an understandable text and a clear presentation of the data helps the author make a stronger connection with consumers of research.

Transforming data into meaningful formats is an important skill for researchers to develop. Careful review of peer-reviewed, scientific journals can help point to effective examples of ways to present data. In addition, researchers can learn effective techniques of scientific dissemination from their colleagues at highly regarded scientific meetings by observing oral and poster presentations of research.

Effective presentation of research results can make the most complex study understandable. Achieving this goal poses a challenge to even the most experienced investigator. This chapter addresses the use of illustrations—tables, graphs, distribution maps, photographs, algorithms, and flowcharts—to enhance communication of research results. The basic methods of conveying research outcomes involve tables and graphs. Researchers need to use the basics well but should also be knowledgeable about other graphic methods that may more effectively communicate the findings.

This chapter emphasizes the most widely used types of illustrations—tables and graphs—as they are used in published works. In addition, less frequently used methods will be discussed as well as concepts to consider when developing illustrations.

The usefulness of illustrations in enhancing text (especially for textbooks) has been the subject of considerable study[1-4]; however, an extensive search of the literature reveals that relatively little research has been directed toward the types of illustrations used in reporting research results. In addition to the published references listed in this chapter, you are encouraged to use the internet to find online sources that show examples of various types of illustrations and resources to develop professional-looking illustrations.

PURPOSES OF ILLUSTRATIONS

Illustrations are used to make information more understandable, depict relationships, add needed emphasis, or present important data in a clear and compact form. Types of illustrations and their functions are listed here:

● **Table:** Represents exact data in compact form

● **Graph:** Displays trends or relationships in a quickly interpretable form
● **Distribution map:** Displays the location of data
● **Photograph:** Accurately represents the appearance of a subject (eg, a clinically observable disorder, microorganisms, newly developed equipment)
● **Algorithm, flowchart:** Displays the steps in a procedure that leads to one or more outcomes
● **Other diagrams:** Represent the subject in a simplified way

In their guidelines for reporting numbers and descriptive statistics, Lang and Altman[5] state, "Display data in tables or figures. Tables present exact values, and figures provide an overall assessment of the data." At the same time, authors need to consider the role of graphics in enticing the casual reader to look more closely at the text. The type of illustration selected should contain enough information to stand alone without referring to the text.

Illustrations will vary depending on the intended purpose. Published works, posters, slides, or transparencies should be prepared differently to support the method of viewing. Although all types of illustrations are generally suitable to include in research articles, some are unsuitable to display in a poster or on a screen where the goal is to share the message quickly. For these purposes, research results must be greatly simplified. Guidelines for preparing materials for posters[6-8] and slides[9-11] focus on simplicity and clarity.

CLEARLY CONVEY A MESSAGE THROUGH ILLUSTRATIONS

In deciding on illustrations for research articles, investigators should focus on the messages they wish to convey concerning the data, both in general and illustration by illustration. Different kinds of illustrations send different messages and serve different functions. Varying the methods used to illustrate similar data sets simply to introduce variety in an article is inappropriate. Extreme complexity in illustrations should also be avoided. Authors should strive to simplify as much as possible. Consider the audience and design the illustrations to match the knowledge base of the audience. Too many speakers in professional meetings apologize for the complexity of their data slides; generally, this is because they have used a published table or figure without considering the intended audience. Revising illustrations to match the mode of presentation is a better choice than using inappropriate graphs and charts that were designed for a different purpose. Authors and presenters who skip this step risk losing the interest of their audience.

ILLUSTRATIONS AS A SET

The number of illustrations included in a research article should be kept to a minimum so that the reader can easily comprehend the article's overall message and the data that support it. In fact, most journals echo this advice for authors, and reviewers frequently recommend that some illustrations be deleted or condensed. In contrast, more extensive illustration may be appropriate for monographs, technical reports, and some types of scientific books.

Consistency adds clarity. Scientific journals, therefore, require a specific style for tables. However, many journals do not have rigid specifications for graphs and other figures and typically reproduce the figures as they are submitted with the manuscript. Thus, authors should give special attention to consistency, accuracy, and scale when preparing a set of figures. In addition, authors should use consistent symbols throughout and similar proportions and style. For example, a series of graphs comparing food use by different ethnic groups should represent these groups using consistent symbols in line graphs or types of fill in bar graphs.

In contrast, when deciding the order in which comparisons are presented, as in tables or bar graphs, consistency from one manuscript to another is often *undesirable*. Instead, the order of presentation should ordinarily be determined by the message to be conveyed, as illustrated in Figure 27.1 on page 544. The preferred order appears in Figure 27.1B, because this approach places the groups in rank order for ease of comparison. (The category "Other" remains at the end because it includes many different groups with low individual rankings.)

GUIDELINES FOR PREPARING USEFUL TABLES

Many style manuals, such as the *Chicago Manual of Style*[12] and the *AMA Manual of Style,*[13] provide extensive guidelines for preparing tables. However, these manuals tend to deal only superficially with substantive issues in handling data. Gastel and Day[14] provide a number of examples of poorly designed and well-executed tables. Kellar and Kelvin,[15] Ehrenberg,[16] and Clark[17] (a noted editor) present complementary suggestions for making the data in tables more understandable. Many of their suggestions are listed in Box 27.1 on page 545.

Essential Categories of Information

Clark[17] specifies the categories of information that should be included in a table to provide a complete picture of the data. She recommends organizing information before actually preparing a table by producing a descriptor set using the categories listed in column 1 of Table 27.1 on page 546, which includes examples of Clark's approach using a hypothetical data set.

Stages of Table Reading

Table reading is an important skill to aid the reader in quickly interpreting data. Clark[17] identifies three stages of table reading: (1) scanning, (2) reading and making primary comparisons, and (3) making second-level comparisons. In the scanning stage, the reader looks across the column heads and down the stub (descriptive labels in first column on left side of table). More experienced readers will scan more intently. Clark asserts that, in the reading stage, readers glance across the rows of data and assume that the column heads are the categories being presented for comparison, even if that was not the author's intent. Ehrenberg[16] advises authors to present the numbers to be compared in columns rather than in rows. No scientific basis has been found for choosing one approach over the other, but if authors are formatting data in columns and readers are expecting to compare rows, misinterpretations will likely result. Authors should carefully consider the best ap-

A. Original graph (not recommended)

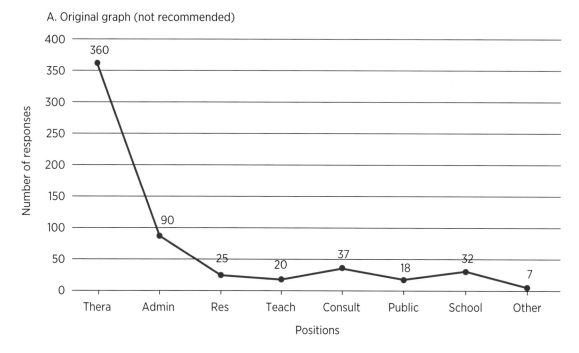

B. Revised bar graph (recommended)

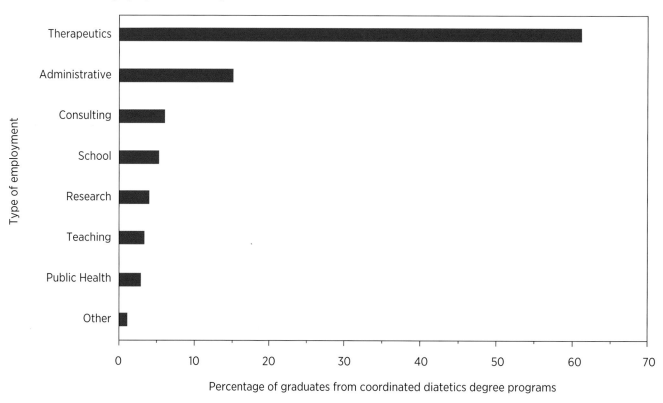

Figure 27.1 Examples of original and improved methods of depicting the same data

Example A is not recommended for several reasons: the implication of being a frequency polygon is misleading; the abbreviations are not standard and may not be clear to all readers; the data are not arranged in a logical order; and the actual frequencies are given on the graph. Further, the axis titles are nondescriptive, where a reader could not understand what the data are depicting by glancing at the figure. Additional descriptive text is needed, yet not desired. Example B is an improved version of the same graph. The type of bar graph has been changed to that of a vertical bar graph, which can aid in clear labeling; the order of the variables was changed so that the positions (type of employment) appear in descending order of frequency; the vertical axis displays the percentage of graduates in each type of position, rather than absolute numbers; the axis labels are descriptive so the reader can decipher the meaning of the figure, text, and axes simply at a glance and does not need supportive text; and use of simple grid marks declutters the graph.

Provide complete information in the table:

- Label clearly, making sure to include a label for the stub (the far left-hand column of the table) and the column heads. Difficulty in identifying a suitable label is likely to indicate a problem in the organization of the data.[17]
- Clearly indicate units of measurement.[15]
- Indicate totals, where applicable, to summarize the data in the table and to help reconcile the data with that in other tables and with material in the text.[15]
- Show in which direction the percentages add to 100% in order to inform the reader how the percentages were derived.[15]
- Use tables when they promote a clearer summary of results than would prose.
- Avoid complex tables.

Carefully consider table layout and organization[16]:

- Provide a visual focus by giving averages for the rows and columns. (Often this is not possible for the types of data displayed in dietetics journals.)
- Arrange the columns and rows in a logical order, and facilitate comparisons when relevant.
- Round appropriately to reflect the precision of the data collection instrument (ie, round the mean to no more than one decimal place beyond the data it summarizes and the standard deviation to no more than two decimal places).[18]
- Use the text to lead the reader to important patterns and exceptions.

Box 27.1 Tips for Creating Research Data Tables That Are Easy to Read and Understand

proach to organizing rows and columns for their particular data. Depending on the type and complexity of data, transposing columns and rows may be more or less difficult.

A major advantage of placing the data to be compared in columns is to facilitate labeling. Consistent units of measure for all items in a column is preferable. Nutrient comparisons generally do not follow this guideline, however, and nutrients are listed down the stub, which keeps nutrient data tables from becoming excessively wide and favors comparisons across the rows.

Strategies for Making Tables Stand Alone and Independent from Text Results

Readers often scan and review tables within an article or book before they turn their attention to the body of the text. Therefore, tables need to be self-explanatory without the support of text. Creating stand-alone tables that are concise, yet fully describe the data, can be challenging. To create self-explanatory tables that adequately convey the purpose and meaning behind data, use the following tips:

- Provide a clear and informative title. Titles of tables should not be vague but should clearly state the purpose of the table and provide any additional detail that may be pertinent to the interpretation of results. For example, a description of the study population, number of participants, and research purpose should be in one succinct statement.
- Ensure that column and row headings are detailed and contain units of measure or state briefly how measurements were captured and expressed.
- Provide footnotes to further explain methods, statistical comparisons, variable measurements, and abbreviations in more detail. For example, if numbers are expressed as xx±yy, a footnote could explain that the table shows means±standard errors. If categories are being presented, a footnote should denote what each category represents and/or the direction of ranking.

Further, results reported in text must not overlap with results presented in tables and figures. In other words, information in the results section of a manuscript should not duplicate data presented in tables or figures. Careful thought must be given as to which results should be reported via text and which

Category	Definition	Example (Comment)
Current source of the table	Author, publication date	From Smith and colleagues, 2017 (necessary only for data taken from sources apart from an original research effort; especially necessary in review articles)
Source of the data	Data collector and period of data collection	Statewide Preschool Nutrition Survey, 2015–2016
Observer	Respondents: Who reported the values?	Food intakes by preschoolers as reported by their mothers and day care providers
Matter	Entities involved in the event covered in the table	Preschoolers aged 3–5 years; milk consumption
Function	Nature of the event covered and factors that may influence it	Milk intake; race; income
Space	Location of the event	Large state; United States
Time	Period when the event occurred	2015–2016 (in studies examining past events—or exposures, as in case-control studies—this time may be much earlier than the time given by the period of data collection)
Aspect	What was measured and to what topic does this point?	Mean intake in grams in a single 24-hour period; points to weight of all forms of fluid milk
Domain	Range of values	0, . . . , 790 g
Sample size	Number of participants (total and in subgroups)	n = 100; men = 60, women = 40

Table 27.1 Categories of Information Necessary for a Complete Representation of Data in Tables[17]

are best represented by a table, figure, or a combination of the two. Figure 27.2 gives an example of how to make data in a table format stand alone from a text description of the same results.[19]

USE OF GRAPHS
Use of Computer Graphics Software

Computer graphics programs have been tremendously beneficial to researchers because they have made it easier for authors to enter data into a simple spreadsheet program and then graph it in a variety of ways. This ease of graphing data has likely reduced the need for highly skilled (and often expensive) illustrators to manually plot data and has increased the volume of illustrations in reports written by individuals of varying education levels, from elementary school students to academic researchers.[20] With graphics software, researchers can quickly flip through a series of illustration methods with the click of the mouse. Unfortunately, though the results of these programs are visually attractive, they do not always convey an appropriate message.

Researchers may need to experiment with a variety of software programs to find one that produces the desired graphics outcomes. The best of these software packages are relatively expensive, so be sure to evaluate several before a purchase. Although most spreadsheet programs have a graphing capability, they typically have more limitations than a program designed specifically for developing illustrations. Try out software to determine if the program offers the variety of illustrations required and sufficient flexibility to customize images. Graphing programs have changed a great deal in the past several years. Be sure to check on current versions, and be sure that the software matches the type of data and illustrations you seek. No one program will work for all researchers.

Following are examples of commonly used graphics software:

- GIMP; The GIMP Development Team
- GraphPad Prism; GraphPad Software, Inc.
- INKSCAPE; Free Software Foundation, Inc.
- MATLAB; MathWorks, Inc.
- Origin; OriginLab Corporation
- SigmaPlot; Systat Software Inc.

Text Describing Table 4 from the Results Section

Results on the comparisons of BMD across protein food clusters are presented in Table 4. After adjustment for relevant confounders and covariates, femoral neck BMD was significantly lower among participants in the processed foods cluster ($P = 0.02$) and red meat cluster ($P = 0.049$) compared with the low-fat milk cluster. BMD at other hip sites, but not the lumbar spine, showed similar trends, where BMD was lowest among participants in the processed foods and red meat clusters compared with the low-fat milk cluster; however, these associations did not reach statistical significance. Adjustment for physical activity did not change the least squares mean estimates at the femoral neck, although the P-value attenuated slightly for the difference between red meat and low-fat milk protein food clusters from $P = 0.049$ to $P = 0.056$ (see Table 4 for unchanged least squares mean estimates). Similarly, upon adjustment for physical activity, the least squares mean estimates for femoral neck did not change for the test of difference between processed foods protein food cluster and the low-fat milk protein food cluster (Table 4) (P-value unchanged at 0.02).

Table 4 Provides Complementary but Not Duplicated Information

Table 4. Association of dietary protein food clusters with bone mineral density (BMD) (in grams per centimeter^2) in 2,721 men and women from the Framingham Offspring Study

| Variable | n | Least Squares Mean ± Standard Error[a] for BMD by Protein Food Group | | | | |
		Cluster 1 Chicken	Cluster 2 Fish	Cluster 3 Processed foods	Cluster 4 Red meat	Cluster 5 Low-fat milk
Model 1[b]						
Femoral neck	2,720	0.909±0.005	0.910±0.007	0.897±0.004y	0.898±0.005y	0.919±0.007z
Trochanter	2,720	0.772±0.005	0.773±0.007	0.765±0.004	0.765±0.005	0.778±0.007
Total femur	2,720	0.956±0.006	0.956±0.007	0.948±0.005	0.948±0.005	0.964±0.007
Lumbar spine	2,721	1.224±0.009	1.208±0.011	1.208±0.008	1.212±0.009	1.226±0.011
Model 2[c]						
Femoral neck	2,689	0.908±0.006	0.911±0.007	0.897±0.005y	0.899±0.006	0.920±0.007z
Trochanter	2,689	0.771±0.005	0.774±0.007	0.766±0.004	0.765±0.005	0.777±0.007
Total femur	2,689	0.956±0.006	0.957±0.007	0.949±0.005	0.949±0.005	0.965±0.007
Lumbar spine	2,690	1.223±0.009	1.209±0.011	1.208±0.008	1.212±0.009	1.223±0.011

[a] The analyses were adjusted for multiple comparisons using Tukey's test (different superscripts [y, z] represent statistically significant differences at $P < 0.05$).
[b] Adjusted for age, sex, estrogen status, body mass index, height, total energy intake, current smoking status, energy-adjusted alcohol intake, calcium supplement use, and vitamin D supplement use.
[c] Further adjusted for physical activity (measured by Physical Activity Scale for the Elderly).

Figure 27.2 Example of how the information presented in a data table should complement but not duplicate the information presented in the text of the research article of which it is a part

Adapted with permission from: Mangano KM, Sahni S, Kiel DP, Tucker KL, Dufour AB, Hannan MT. Bone mineral density and protein-derived food clusters from the Framingham Offspring Study. *J Acad Nutr Diet.* 2015;115(10):1605.e1–1613.e1.[19]

Increased computer capabilities have resulted in rapid developments in the graphic display of results from multidimensional modeling. Suggestions for avoiding unintentional misrepresentation of data or other common problems that may be associated with the routine use of graphics software are incorporated in the sections that follow.

Guidelines for Preparing Useful Graphs

When adding text to graphs, use initial capital letters only, rather than all uppercase letters. Words written in lowercase letters are easier to read.[12,13,21,22] Avoid using boldface, italic, and underlined text in graphs unless the emphasis helps the reader understand the graph. Unless data are three-dimensional, do not use multidimensional computer graphs, which imply a z axis though the data are plotted only along the x- and y-axes.

Choosing a Graph Type

Standard graph types include line graphs, scatter graphs, histograms, frequency polygons, bar graphs, stacker bar graphs, and pie charts. Texts such as *Illustrating Science: Standards for Publication*[23] are good sources of information on the appropriate use of each type of graph. Authors should determine the message they want to convey and select graphs that will support that goal.

Graphs serve two general purposes: to examine data and to communicate data to others. Stem and leaf diagrams and scatterplots are types of graphs that are useful for finding out if a few data points are strongly influencing measures of effect. Such graphs are useful for data interpretation, but they are seldom used in communicating the results of studies. Box plots illustrate the spread and differences of samples.[24] (See articles by Hebert and Waternaux[25] and by Worthington-Roberts and associates[26] for examples of the use of a box plot graph for reporting the results of nutrition research.)

Important Characteristics of Graphs

According to Tufte,[22] "graphical excellence is the well-designed presentation of interesting data—a matter of substance, of *statistics,* and of *design.*" Tufte demonstrates ways to achieve clear, precise, and efficient communication of complex ideas and emphasizes displaying truthful messages with the data. He objects to graphs that have a small ratio of data to ink—as is the case with many bar graphs, for example. (See Figure 27.3 for a superior alternative to such bar graphs.[27]) Tufte compiled a useful list of suggestions for enhancing the visual display of statistical information:

● Choose the proper format and design.
● Use words, numbers, and drawing together (eg, short messages that help explain the data).
● Produce a balanced, well-proportioned graph with a relevant scale.
● Display complex detail (the data) in a simple manner (avoiding abbreviations and elaborate codes).
● Tell a story with the data, if appropriate.
● Draw the graph in a professional manner.
● Avoid decorations and moire effects (such as hatched lines).

Three important characteristics of graphs are as follows:

● Graphs should help the reader comprehend the material. A large number of variables are generally confusing, even with ingenious graph design.
● The axes of graphs should be clearly and concisely labeled and include the units of measure. More complete labeling (eg, Percentage of Calcium Absorbed) helps convey the message, whereas cryptic labeling of the vertical axis of graphs (eg, only the word "Percentage") does not quickly alert the reader to its content.
● Graphs should be scaled to represent the data and their importance accurately. Avoid using a small portion of the scale, which may exaggerate the difference between groups.

Improper or misleading scaling often occurs unintentionally, especially when using graphics programs. Computer default settings are designed to be user friendly by providing the user with standard preset elements. For graphics programs, default

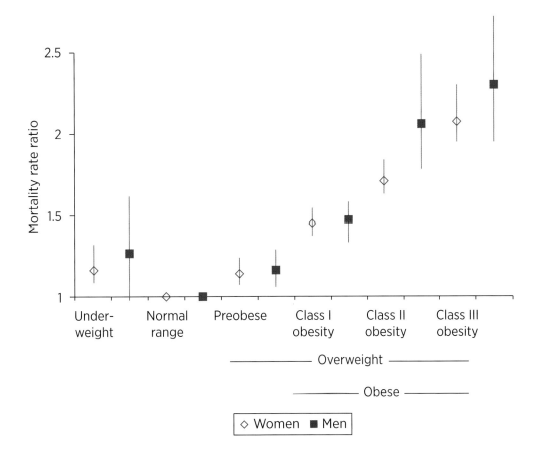

Figure 27.3 Rate ratios for death from all causes in white men (n = 57,073) and women (n = 240,158) by World Health Organization body mass index categories (underweight = 18.4 or less; normal range = 18.5 to 24.9; preobese = 25.0 to 29.9; class I obese = 30.0 to 34.9; class II obese = 35.0 to 39.9; class III obese = 40+)

Values were adjusted for age, education, and physical activity. All values were significantly different from normal range at *P*<.001.

This point graph illustrates the display of comparisons of means along with standard error (SE) among different categories of a factor. This graph is superior to bar graphs in displaying parameters of continuous variables, such as means, medians, and the accompanying standard error, standard deviation, or percentiles. Note that the parameters of interest are clearly shown, as is the range of values within the error bars, and that the graph does not distort the size of the differences between categories; a maximum ratio of data to ink is used, as recommended by Tufte.[22] A bar graph, in contrast, uses a small ratio of data to ink; the bars do not represent data points or any specific parameter from the data, and the relative size of the bars is not proportional to the difference among the categories compared. A bar graph is useful for frequency data (i.e., number or proportion of a discrete scale variable). A point graph more clearly shows the parameters of interest (here, the rate ratios along with SE).[28]

Adapted with permission from Stevens J, Cai J, Juhaeri, Thun MJ, Wood JL. Evaluation of WHO and NHANES II standards for overweight using mortality rates. *J Am Diet Assoc.* 2000;100(7):825-827.[27]

settings for the range, the scales of the *x*-axis and *y*-axis, the typeface, and so forth are intended to make it easy to produce standard graphs that look good (at least to the casual observer). Default settings for the range of the vertical axis are based on the range of the data being displayed. Therefore, they minimize unused space, which is generally a desirable outcome. However, the net result is that they often use an inappropriately high scale that makes minor differences appear major, as illustrated by Figure 27.4 on page 550. The researcher should make sure that the reader can easily tell if a scale does not start at zero and if the scales represent arithmetic or mathematical (eg, logarithmic) change; the investigator should also make sure that scales correspond exactly if graphs are to be compared. In all cases, authors must inspect all graphs visually for completeness, clarity, and accuracy before using them.

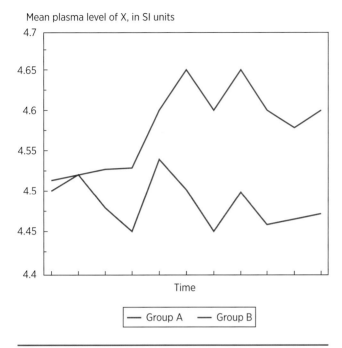

Mean plasma level of X, in SI units

Figure 27.4 Inappropriate graph overemphasizes the importance of data

This graph was produced using default settings in a graphics program. The scaling of the *y*-axis is inappropriate; the scale does not start at zero and no break in the *y*-axis is provided to shows this.

Achieving Consistency in Graphs

To achieve visual consistency, the same computer software should be used to prepare all the graphs for a given report. If two or more programs must be used, special steps may be required to achieve consistency in the use of symbols, fill, and lettering. Use of the same software to prepare all the graphs in a set does not ensure consistency of scale for graphs that are likely to be compared. For example, the linear distance in millimeters between tick marks on graph A should be identical to that on graph B. To achieve this consistency, the preparer of the graphs must avoid the use of default settings for the vertical axis and should be sure to specify the same range for all graphs to be compared (eg, "0% to 100%" or "2.0 mmol to 6.0 mmol"). Some graphics software allows the user to change the size of the graph. If this feature is used, identical changes in size should be made in all graphs that are to be compared. Furthermore, the authors must specify that identical reductions be made in preparing the art for printing.

Illustrating Science: Standards for Publication[23] contains an outstanding set of guidelines for preparing graphs, including detailed methods for improving visual clarity. The book advises researchers to choose symbols for data points that reproduce clearly and are easily discernable. The recommended symbols are ● ▲ and ■. The actual choice of symbols depends on what they represent and where they will appear in the graph. When only two symbols are required, black (filled) and white (open) circles are preferred. Similarly, white (open) symbols could be used to represent two groups before interventions and black symbols to represent them after the interventions (in this case, circles and triangles would be preferred). Although all of these symbols are acceptable, some shapes, such as circles and squares, should not be used next to each other because they are difficult to distinguish, especially if a graph is reduced in size. If only one symbol is needed, black circles are recommended because they are prominent and most like data points.

Graphical Perception

Graphical perception involves the way graphical information is interpreted and visually decoded by the reader; differences in line lengths, size of pie chart segments and color saturation can be used to quickly convey information.[28] According to the seminal work by Cleveland and McGill,[28] the elementary tasks in graphical perception can be ranked from most to least accurate, as shown in Box 27.2. Because a graph is successful only if it is accurately and efficiently decoded, researchers should keep abreast of new developments in the development of graphing techniques. The internet has accelerated the expansion of visual media. As society moves to more graphical information sharing, researchers will need to incorporate graphic techniques that resonate with the more visual nature of readers.

Other recommendations for creating an interpretable graphic include the use of sans serif typefaces, such as Arial or Helvetica; simplified imagery to delete unnecessary details; open spaces to guide the eye; and consistency of design, including reliance on a grid of implied lines. In addition, visual systems should be kept consistent by using the same colors,

Elementary Estimation Task	Examples
Position along a common scale	Height or length of a bar that is part of a bar graph
Position along nonaligned scales	Heights of segments in identical closed rectangles
Length, direction, angle	Comparison of line lengths without any point of reference; relative sizes of segments in a pie chart
Area	Difference in size of two charts
Volume, curvature	Difference in volume of two or more spheres
Shading, color saturation	Differences in shading on distribution maps

Box 27.2 Elementary Tasks in Graphical Perception in Decreasing Order of Accuracy[28]

axes, labels, and so on across multiple charts. Keep graphics simple using no more than six colors in one graph and avoid use of three-dimensional effects that make it hard to compare elements and judge areas.

Cleveland and McGill[28] provide qualitative evidence from experimental trials that specific graph types are interpreted more accurately than other types. In particular, they recommend dot charts (charts using dots to represent a particular number of individuals or data elements) or bar charts in place of pie charts, and dot or bar charts with grouping in place of stacked or divided bars. In perceptual experiments by Cleveland and McGill,[28] component (stacked) bar charts were inferior to bar charts (simple, either vertical or horizontal) because they require viewers to estimate length along nonaligned scales. Pie charts also require similar subjectivity in extracting numerical data by estimating angle and arc lengths of the pie. Due to the subjectivity and difficulty in interpreting data from pie charts and stacked bar charts, experts recommend conveying data through bar charts and dot charts. See Figure 27.5 on page 552.

Cleveland and McGill[28] further recommend the direct display of the differences between two curves in place of the curves themselves. Messages conveyed by curve-difference graphs are very different from those conveyed by graphs that depict the two curves separately. If the object is to show that one treatment consistently produces better results than another, a graph showing the two curves is more appropriate to use. If the difference between values at various time points is important, then curve-difference graphs or a table of differences would be superior. See Figure 27.6 on page 553.

Determine whether the difference between the curves warrants emphasis. Some readers who compare graphs in which the curves are close together suspect an error because of the great difficulty of visually perceiving absolute differences between two adjacent curves.

OTHER FORMS OF ILLUSTRATIONS
Histograms

Histograms display frequency distributions; the area of the rectangles in the histogram represents the frequency of the data. Accurate scaling of the horizontal axis must be maintained. Thus, if intervals are unequal—for example, they represent different time periods—the width of the rectangle should reflect this inequality. As shown earlier in Figure 27.1 (see page 544), graphics programs allow researchers to choose from many graph variations, not all of which are acceptable. A better alternative might be to use horizontal bar graphs (Figure 27.1) so that complete labels can be used rather than abbreviations.

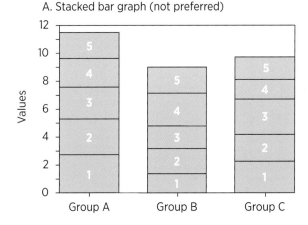

A. Stacked bar graph (not preferred)

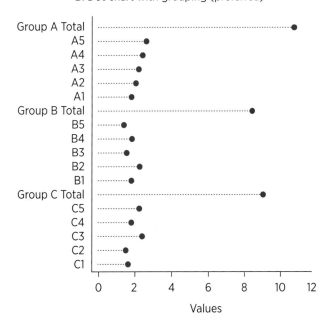

B. Dot chart with grouping (preferred)

Figure 27.5 Stacked bar graph (A) compared with dot chart with grouping (B)

Using Part B it is easier to estimate the relative frequencies of the items within groups. The program used to produce the stacked bar graph used differnet kinds of hatching to denote the different groups; the hatching was deleted to avoid a cluttered graph with moire (shimmering or wave-like) effects.

Adapted with permission from Cleveland WS, McGill R. Graphical perception: theory, experimentation, and application to the development of graphical methods. *J Am Stat Assoc.* 1984; 79:531–554.[28]

Distribution Maps

Distribution maps focus on the location of data and can be useful in depicting differences in rates, ratios, total amounts, or percentages by area. For example, a map of the United States in which states are grouped by census regions can be used to depict differences in breastfeeding rates in different parts of the country. A state map can be used to identify counties with an unusually high or low prevalence of obesity, and a city map can be used to identify census tracts where members of an ethnic minority reside in large numbers. Shades from light to dark are often used to depict numerical values from low to high. This practice has some drawbacks: regardless of the numerical value, large areas tend to appear more important, and differences in the shades of gray may be overestimated implying larger differences in the numerical values.[13] If such maps are used, seven intervals for the data should be the maximum number.

Cleveland and McGill[28] suggest using framed rectangle (blocked rectangle) charts as replacements for distribution maps in which shading denotes quantitative information. Framed rectangles show the level of a variable within a particular population group or region. They can be overlaid on a map to show how a variable varies geographically. See Figure 27.7 on page 554 for an example.

Photographs

Photographs bring the element of reality to the reader. A photograph showing clinical signs of a rarely seen nutrient deficiency reinforces the importance of nutrition intervention by showing how a specific treatment can lead to serious nutrition problems. *Illustrating Science: Standards for Publication*[23] and Melhuis[29] present contain detailed information on photography and points to consider when reproducing photographs. Staged photographs need to be used with care to avoid being misleading. Authors should ensure that a photograph conveys the correct message. Differing cultural perceptions need to be considered, too.

Images of gel electrophoresis are an example of a specialized use of photography entering the nutrition literature. Genetic researchers use these techniques to investigate how different tissues respond to a stimulus. If a gene is present or activated, a dark band is present at a particular point on the gel. Photographs of these gels are used to show results of an experiment.

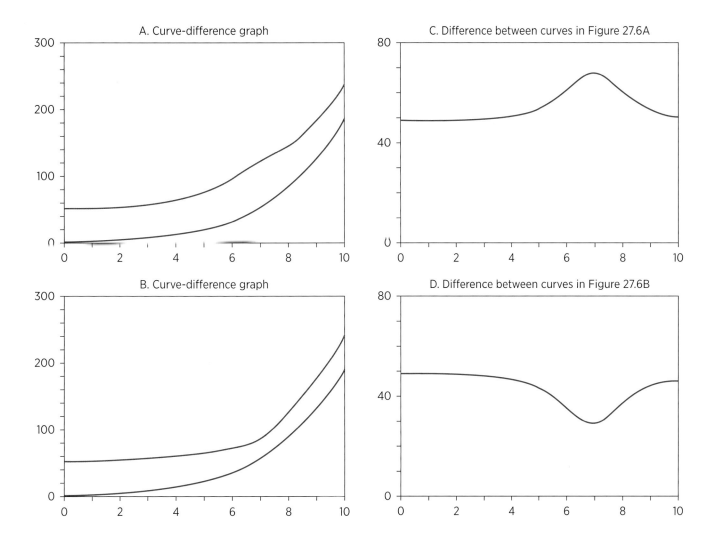

Figure 27.6 Curve-difference graphs

A and B depict data for each treatment over time, whereas C and D depict the absolute differences between the treatments over time. Note the difference in message; the author should determine whether the difference between the curves warrants emphasis. Some readers who compare the two types of graphs suspect an error because of the great difficulty of visually perceiving absolute differences between two adjacent curves.

Adapted with permission from Cleveland WS, McGill R. Graphical perception: theory, experimentation, and application to the development of graphical methods. *J Am Stat Assoc.* 1984; 79:531–554.[28]

Algorithms and Flowcharts

Increasing numbers of algorithms and flowcharts are appearing in dietetics literature. Algorithms are used to clarify complex decision-making processes by listing each step in a process and indicating points where various actions occur. Flowcharts are graphic representations of algorithms and make it easier for the reader to visualize steps in a process. Figure 27.8 on page 554 illustrates some features of a flowchart designed to show the total number of participants enrolled in the study population and the final number of participants included in analyses.[30] The major tasks involved are placed within carefully selected shapes and arranged logically. The shapes used are informative for those familiar with standard conventions, but knowledge of these conventions is not required to understand the diagram. In Figure 27.8, the alignment of the steps makes it easy to identify where in the study analysis participants were removed from the data due to missing or invalid data. To make the diagram easy to read, use active verbs and short, simple sentences. The number of participants is depicted in each box

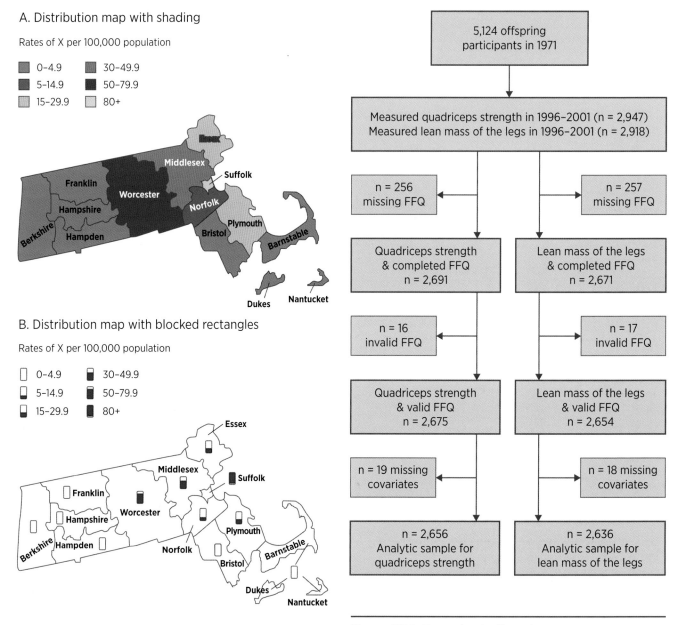

A. Distribution map with shading

Rates of X per 100,000 population

- 0–4.9
- 5–14.9
- 15–29.9
- 30–49.9
- 50–79.9
- 80+

B. Distribution map with blocked rectangles

Rates of X per 100,000 population

- 0–4.9
- 5–14.9
- 15–29.9
- 30–49.9
- 50–79.9
- 80+

Figure 27.7 Distribution maps

Map A (not recommended) depicts the conventional approach of using difference intensities of shading to denote different rates of X in various counties. Map B (recommended) depicts the framed (blocked) rectangle approach. In this approach, the area of the county has little or no effect on interpretation of the extent of the problem.

Figure 27.8 Example of a flow chart

FFQ = food frequency questionnaire

Adapted with permission from Sahni S, Mangano KM, Hannan MT, Kiel DP, McLean RR. Higher protein intake is associated with higher lean mass and quadriceps muscle strength in adult men and women. *J Nutr.* 2015;145(7):1569–1575.[30]

of the flow diagram so that the reader can calculate and verify how many particpants were included in final analyses and why.

The same symbol should not be used to represent two different variables. For example, if *N* is used in the legend to denote the number of participants, a different symbol, such as *T*, should be used to denote the time required for the activity. In Figure 27.8, only one symbol (n) was used. Both symbols and abbreviations should be denoted in the footnotes section.

Visualizing Big Data

In health care, the term *big data* refers to electronic health data sets so large and complex that they are difficult (or impossible) to manage with traditional software or hardware, nor can they be easily managed with traditional or common data management tools and methods.[31] Examples of big data include clinical data (such as health insurance, the Human Microbiome Project, or the Human Genome Project), patient data in electronic patient records, and social media posts. Discovering associations and understanding patterns and trends within big data have the potential to provide insights and solutions that cannot be discerned when viewing a smaller subset. This is particularly challenging when data are so large that they are difficult to analyze using traditional data-processing applications. Once the data are analyzed, an equally challenging problem is to determine how to adequately visualize and convey the data.

Data visualization techniques used for traditional data, as described earlier for histograms, distribution maps, flowcharts, and algorithms, also apply to big data; however, visualizing big data presents unique challenges because of what is known as the three *V*'s of big data: volume, velocity, and variety.[31] Large amounts of data (volume) are acquired at unprecedented rates (velocity) and therefore need to be analyzed in motion across multiple specialties (variety). Advanced interfaces and analytic tools have been developed to accommodate the challenges presented by the three *V*'s of big data. However, these new analytic tools are complex, programming intensive, and generally not user friendly. Methods have been developed to combat these challenges. Drawing from fields such as statistics, computer science, applied mathematics, and economics, a wide variety of techniques and technologies has been developed and adapted to aggregate, manipulate, analyze, and visualize big data in health care. A practical hands-on description of some methodologies that can be used in the health care setting are described by Raghupathi and Raghupathi.[31] Although visualizing big data is difficult, mastering techniques to properly analyze and convey results from big data in health care is of public health importance because of their potential to improve the health care system and our understanding of disease and health.

Areas of nutrition research utilizing big data include nutrigenomics, diet-microbiome interactions, and the use of social media apps in diet tracking. Keeping up to date with evolving technology to visualize and interpret big data is imperative for the field of nutrition to grow in an evolving health care research system.

PREPARING ILLUSTRATIONS FOR PUBLICATION

Illustrations require formatting before they are published in abstracts and manuscripts. Formatting is specific to the society or journal in which the authors are attempting to publish. Formatting requirements can generally be found on the society or journal website. For example, on the *Journal of the Academy of Nutrition and Dietetics* home page (https://jandonline.org), there is a link to "Information for Authors" from the "For Authors" dropdown menu. Within this section, readers can locate the "Tables and Figures" link for illustration requirements. In brief, tables must (1) be double spaced, (2) be consecutively numbered with Arabic numbers, (3) be detailed enough to stand alone (directions outlined above), (4) use footnotes with superscript letters to describe abbreviations and other statistical measures, and (5) cite the original source of data if it is published by permission from another source. Tables are submitted to the *Journal of the Academy of Nutrition and Dietetics* embedded at the end of the manuscript text. This is in contrast to figures, which must be submitted to the submission system in a separate file. Suggested figures include bar graphs, line graphs, and three-dimensional figures when appropriate. Figures must also be numbered consecutively using Arabic numbers and each must have a brief legend. Figures can be color or gray scale and should have a resolution of 300 dpi. Again, figures should stand on their own from the text and have an appropriate title and footnotes.

An abstract is a brief, written summary of the specific ideas or concepts to be presented, and a statement of their relevance to practice or research. Inclusion of graphs and figures in abstracts submitted to scientific meetings depends on the submission guidelines of that society. Some societies do not allow tables and graphs to be submitted with the abstract text. However, many societies are now accepting these components to support an abstract presentation. Pay particular attention to whether a table or figure is included in the required word count of the abstract. For more detailed step-by-step instructions in how to prepare an abstract for success, see the article by Manore.[32]

CONCLUSION

Researchers preparing illustrations to accompany their publication should select the proper type to serve specific functions, identify the messages to be conveyed, and develop the illustrations as a compatible set. They should pay particular attention to conveying important messages with clarity, simplicity, consistency, and accuracy. Once the illustrations are prepared, the investigator should examine the visual effect of those illustrations, both individually and as a set, and adjust as needed. Peer review of illustrations can be extremely helpful in identifying potential areas for misinterpretation and to determine if key points are accurately conveyed.

REFERENCES

1. Carney RN, Levin JR. Pictoral illustrations still improve students' learning from text. *Educ Psychol Rev.* 2002;14(1): 5-26.

2. Butcher K. Learning from text with diagrams: promoting mental model development and inference generation. *J Educ Psychol.* 2006;98(1):182-197.

3. Mayer RE. The promise of multimedia learning: using the same instructional design methods across different media. *Learn Instr.* 2003;13(2):125-139.

4. Mayer RE. Using illustrations to promote constructivist learning from science text. In: Otero J, ed. *The Psychology of Science Text Comprehension.* New York, NY: Routledge; 2013:333-356.

5. Lang TA, Altman DG. Basic statistical reporting for articles published in biomedical journals: the "Statistical Analyses and Methods in the Published Literature" or "The SAMPL Guidelines." *Int J Nurs Stud.* 2015;52(1):5-9.

6. Briggs DJ. A practical guide to designing a poster for presentation. *Nurs Stand.* 2009;23(34):35-39.

7. Boullata JI, Mancuso CE. A "how-to" guide in preparing abstracts and poster presentations. *Nutr Clin Pract.* 2007; 22(6):641-646.

8. Miller JE. Preparing and presenting effective research posters. *Health Serv Res.* 2007;42(1 part 1):311-328.

9. Alley M, Neeley KA. Rethinking the design of presentation slides: a case for sentence headlines and visual evidence. *Tech Commun.* 2005;52(4):417-426.

10. Strauss J, Corrigan H, Hofacker CF. Optimizing student learning: examining the use of presentation slides. *Mark Educ Rev.* 2011;21(2):151-162.

11. Alley M, Schreiber M, Ramsdell K, Muffo J. How the design of headlines in presentation slides affects audience retention. *Tech Commun.* 2006;53(2):225-234.

12. *The Chicago Manual of Style.* 17th ed. Chicago, IL: University of Chicago Press; 2017.

13. *AMA Manual of Style: A Guide for Authors and Editors.* 10th ed. New York, NY: Oxford University Press; 2007.

14. Gastel B, Day RA. *How to Write and Publish a Scientific Paper.* 8th ed. Santa Barbara, CA: Greenwood; 2016.

15. Kellar SP, Kelvin E. *Munro's Statistical Methods for Health Care Research.* 6th ed. Philadelphia, PA: Wolters Kluwer Health | Lippincott Williams & Wilkins; 2013.

16. Ehrenberg AC. The problem of numeracy. *Am Stat.* 1981;35: 67-71.

17. Clark N. Tables and graphs as a form of exposition. *Sch Pub.* 1987;19:24-42.

18. Lang TA, Secic M. *How to Report Statistics in Medicine: Annotated Guidelines for Authors, Editors, and Reviewers.* 2nd ed. Philadelphia, PA: American College of Physicians; 2006.

19. Mangano KM, Sahni S, Kiel DP, Tucker KL, Dufour AB, Hannan MT. Bone mineral density and protein-derived food clusters from the Framingham Offspring Study. *J Acad Nutr Diet.* 2015;115(10):1605.e1-1613.e1.

20. Fuhrmann S, MacEachren A, DeBerry M, et al. MapStats for kids: making geographic statistical facts available to children. *J Geog.* 2005:104(6):233-241.

21. Hartley J. Planning the typographical structure of instructional text. *Educ Psychol.* 1986;21:315-332.

22. Tufte ER. *The Visual Display of Quantitative Information.* 2nd ed. Cheshire, CT: Graphics Press; 2001.

23. Scientific Illustration Committee of the Council of Biology Editors. *Illustrating Science: Standards for Publication.* Bethesda, MD: Council of Biology Editors; 1988.

24. Krzywinski M, Altman N. Points of significance: visualizing samples with box plots. *Nature Meth.* 2014;11(2):119-120.

25. Hebert JR, Waternaux C. Graphical displays of growth data. *Am J Clin Nutr.* 1983;38(1):145-147.

26. Worthington-Roberts BS, Breskin MW, Monsen ER. Iron status of premenopausal women in a university community and its relationship to habitual dietary sources of protein. *Am J Clin Nutr.* 1988;47(2):275-279.

27. Stevens J, Cai J, Juhaeri, Thun MJ, Wood JL. Evaluation of WHO and NHANES II standards for overweight using mortality rates. *J Am Diet Assoc.* 2000;100(7):825-827.

28. Cleveland WS, McGill R. Graphical perception: theory, experimentation, and application to the development of graphical methods. *J Am Stat Assoc.* 1984;79(387):531-554.

29. Melhuish J. Know how. A guide to medical photography. *Nurs Times.* 1997;93(7):64-65.

30. Sahni S, Mangano KM, Hannan MT, Kiel DP, McLean RR. Higher protein intake is associated with higher lean mass and quadriceps muscle strength in adult men and women. *J Nutr.* 2015;145(7):1569-1575.

31. Raghupathi W, Raghupathi V. Big data analytics in healthcare: promise and potential. *Health Inf Sci Syst.* 2014;2:3.

32. Manore MM. Getting your abstract accepted: the key to success. *J Am Diet Assoc.* 2001;101(12):1410-1411.

Chapter 8

Research Publications: Perspectives of the Writer, Reviewer, and Reader

Jeffrey Harris, DrPH, MPH, RDN, LDN, FAND

LEARNING OBJECTIVES

1. Describe the publication process from the author's perspective, including the criteria used for authorship.

2. Identify the general questions a reviewer considers when reviewing a manuscript.

3. Discuss the role of literature from the reader's perspective to support evidence-based practice and knowledge.

4. Explain the processes of writing, reviewing, and reading nutrition research literature.

The writer, the reviewer, and the reader have different perspectives as they approach research publications. The writer might say, "I'm an expert in my area of research. I have something of value to contribute to the scientific community that advances knowledge, and I want it published as soon as possible. In addition, I want to present tentative answers to the research questions I have explored so that others may benefit." The reviewer might say, "I assist the writer, the reader, and the editor. I volunteer my time to help ensure the quality and clarity of research in the literature, and I do this in as timely a fashion as possible. I want to ensure that the scientific community publishes manuscripts that best add to the knowledge base, are consistent with the focus of the journal, and improve the practice of our discipline." The reader has still another point of view and might say: "I read in part to learn. I am not as familiar with some areas of research and have limited time to read. I want to engage in evidence-based practice, and I want to read articles that will improve my ability to do my job. Therefore, I expect articles to represent quality research and to be communicated in simple, logical terms that I can understand and apply."

A registered dietitian nutritionist (RDN) may assume the roles of writer, reviewer, and reader of research publications. Meaningful research that is original; is designed to answer specific research questions; and is current, well organized, meticulously conducted, and effectively communicated is the ideal from the perspectives of all three roles. Guidelines have been developed to help writers, reviewers, and readers implement, interpret, and communicate research. Furthermore, a statistical working group of the Board of Editors published a series of articles related to nutrition research in the *Journal of the Academy of Nutrition and Dietetics* to provide guidance in research design, data analysis, and manuscript preparation and evaluation.[1-10] Web-based literature archives and databases, online manuscript management systems, and online publishing provide writers with enhanced access, reduced costs, flexible formats, and faster turnaround for publishing articles. Open access publishing has increased the speed at which published information is available. Also, dietetics practitioners today have much easier access to journal articles and systematic reviews to study various subjects. Literature searches are easy to conduct, and tools are available to evaluate peer-reviewed journal articles. Current issues related to publishing include the subjectivity of the peer-review process, evaluation of journal quality, reviewer fatigue, difficulty finding reviewers, open access, and predatory publishing.[11-20] This chapter touches on those issues while addressing the three different roles an RDN can play in research and manuscript publishing.

THE WRITER'S PERSPECTIVE
Conducting the Research

The writer is responsible for demonstrating ethical and informed behavior when designing and completing research studies, intellectual honesty, and fair relational conduct with collaborators. The writer, as a scientist, has an idea that emerges from an area of interest, from professional experience, or from the literature; develops this idea into a research protocol; and fosters it through the stages of implementation, data collection, and data interpretation. Much of this book addresses these issues. The author has an ethical obligation to society to design research that furthers the advancement of the science and to submit research protocols and truthful results for peer review.

Consulting a statistician during the design phase and when results are analyzed is essential to prevent the collection of potentially worthless data and spurious analytic results. Researchers find it helpful to establish a network within their institution and work with individuals who have statistical expertise. Identifying a statistician who can assist in the specific domain of the researcher, whether it be foodservice management, clinical nutrition, dietetics education, or community nutrition, is important. Chapters 2, 25, 26, and 27 of this book review methods for design, data analysis, and presentation of research methods in nutrition and dietetics and provide a statistics review and update for researchers. In addition to the *Journal of the Academy of Nutrition and Dietetics* series on statistics,[1-10] a basic statistics text can provide helpful guidance.[21]

Preparing the Manuscript

The 2016 edition of the *Recommendations for the Conduct, Reporting, Editing and Publication of Scholarly Work in Medical Journals,*[22] formerly called the Uniform Requirements for Manuscripts Submitted to Biomedical Journals, should be familiar to authors. This comprehensive document, created by the International Committee of Medical Journal Editors, describes all aspects of conducting research as well as writing and submitting manuscripts for publication. The Academy of Nutrition and Dietetics also has guidelines for preparing manuscripts, which align with these recommendations.[23] The *Journal of the Academy of Nutrition and Dietetics* website has helpful documents, including manuscript preparation tips for getting a manuscript noticed and published. The recommendations and journal style documents are extremely helpful for all aspects of the publication endeavor. Authors can consult the "Journal Info" tab and find the Information for Authors page, which is a good example of comprehensive guidelines for preparing and submitting manuscripts.[23] The Information for Authors page also provides links to checklists from various sources that may be used as guides for writing and evaluating manuscripts.

The writer, as a communicator, needs to be logical, clear, and accurate in describing the research and should report negative and positive results. Discussion and conclusion sections need to be expressed in a fair and balanced way, reporting strengths and weaknesses of the research. Conclusions must not be overstated. Use restraint in the last paragraph of the manuscript; do not make naive policy recommendations or generic calls for more research. Also, do not overstate conclusions, such as making cause-effect deductions from a research design that does not warrant such conclusions.

Tailoring the format of the manuscript to suit the chosen journal and following that journal's guidelines for authors can expedite the reviewing process. For instance, the *Journal of the Academy of Nutrition and Dietetics* format is different from that of the *American Journal of Clinical Nutrition* or the *Journal of Foodservice Management and Education*. It is imperative to consult the specific journal website to access its guidelines for authors. In addition to following the author guidelines, authors can facilitate the review process by including page and line numbers throughout the manuscript to make it easier to link reviewer comments to the relevant place in the manuscript.

Choosing a Journal

The writer should consult the literature and learn which journals would be most appropriate for publishing a specific manuscript. One choice is whether to submit to a traditional or open access journal.[12,18,24,25] Traditional journals often publish articles in print and online formats, but many times access must be purchased through subscription or a per-article fee. The time from submission to publication is often longer than for open access journals. The publisher frequently retains strict copyright rules, including limitations in copying and disseminating the articles. Traditional journals generally have higher prestige than open access journals, however, and a more rigorous peer-review process.

In contrast, open access journals publish articles faster and have more liberal copyright rules. Often these types of journals allow free dissemination and use of articles if properly cited. Credible open access journals have the same manuscript peer-review process as traditional publishers, but it is often faster. Open access journals may charge authors a fee for publication. Access to the article is free and is usually only available online. Open access journals are growing in availability and status.[25] Authors should consider submitting manuscripts to open access journals as a viable option. The *Journal of the Academy of Nutrition and Dietetics* offers the option of traditional or open access publication.[23]

Authors must be careful to avoid predatory journals, which scam authors by collecting publishing fees without providing the quality publication services that are expected.[14,18,26] Be wary of solicitations that promise fast publishing for a fee. The motive of these journals is profit, not advancing knowledge. Not only do these journals lack peer review but they may also misinform authors about their connections with database services such as MEDLINE. Authors should avoid these at all costs, making sure to thoroughly vet open access journals before deciding to submit a manuscript. Signs of a predatory journal are presented in Box 28.1.

Publishes research on a larger number of topics than legitimate journals

Extremely low article processing charges—below $150 (vs $2,500 in charges for a legitimate journal)

Poorly maintained websites rife with spelling errors and distorted images

Article submission by email—often to non-professional or nonacademic email addresses—rather than via a submission system

No policies about retractions, corrections, errata, and plagiarism

Editorial board members with questionable credentials or unverifiable membership

Promised peer-review services are not provided

Bombards authors with emails encouraging submissions with promises that will go unfulfilled

Nonbiomedical interests

Website home page that speaks directly to authors

Use of Index Copernicus Value as index factor rather than more legitimate index factor services

No description of publishing process

Promises quick and unreasonable turnaround and publication processes

No information on how content will be preserved

Lack of copyright clarity

Publisher/journal email is generic (eg, Gmail)

Box 28.1 Signs of a Predatory Journal

Submitting the Manuscript

Submitting a manuscript for peer review can be an invaluable educational experience for an author.[27] Authors are entitled to expect a consistent response from the editor and prompt and courteous treatment

Consider and respond to all editor and reviewer comments and suggestions. Do not be defensive. Criticism is a normal part of the process.

Do not resubmit a manuscript to the same journal if it is refused for publication; instead, consider the reviewers' and editor's comments and submit to another journal.

Do not call the editor directly, unless invited to do so.

Do not approach the editor personally to discuss your manuscript at an annual meeting or elsewhere.

Box 28.2 Tips for Improving Communication Between Author and Editor

of their articles. They should feel free to question why an article was turned down. Authors frequently complain that the months of time spent reviewing and fine-tuning an article delays the transmission of knowledge. The time spent refining a manuscript, however, is well spent and relatively minor compared with the time spent completing the research and writing. Still, this is why some authors attempt to publish their manuscripts in open access journals, where publication may be quicker and peer review is more widespread and occurs directly online.

Many journals have online systems for manuscript submission and review. For instance, the *Journal of the Academy of Nutrition and Dietetics* has an online editorial manager that authors, reviewers, and editor use to process manuscripts. Anyone interested in publishing in the *Journal of the Academy of Nutrition and Dietetics* should become familiar with this website.[23]

An author can best interpret and respond to reviewers' and editors' comments by putting emotions aside. Constructive criticism should be taken as an opportunity to learn, not as rejection. Adhering to some suggestions can facilitate communication between the author and editor about current and future manuscripts (see Box 28.2).[28,29]

Irresponsible Authorship

In scientific publishing, irresponsible authorship and wasteful publication are considered offensive and perhaps far more damaging than fraud or plagiarism.[30] Irresponsible authorship is including, as authors, individuals who made little or no contribution to the work reported or omitting individuals who made major contributions. The responsible writer, as collaborator, acknowledges the complexity of modern dietetics research, which may require a variety of skills and techniques available only from the joint efforts of several individuals. Principles that can be used to justify multiple authorship are included in the *Recommendations for the Conduct, Reporting, Editing and Publication of Scholarly Work in Medical Journals*.[22] Authorship credit should be limited to those who made substantial contributions to (1) the conception and design or the analysis and interpretation of the data, (2) drafting the article or revising it critically for important intellectual content, and (3) achieving final approval of the version to be published. All three conditions must be met. Participation solely in acquiring funding or collecting data does not justify authorship, nor does general supervision of the research group. Individuals participating in these activities can be mentioned in the acknowledgments section of an article. Any part of an article critical to its main conclusions must be the responsibility of at least one author.

The order of authorship should be a joint decision of the coauthors. Because the order may be assigned in different ways, its meaning cannot be inferred accurately unless it is stated by the authors. Authors may wish to explain the order of authorship in a footnote. In deciding on the order, authors should be aware that many journals limit the number of authors listed in the table of contents and that the US National Library of Medicine lists only the first 24 plus the last author in MEDLINE when there are more than 25 authors. Many peer-reviewed journals provide clear guidelines for authorship.

Authors should avoid wasteful publication, which includes reporting the results of a single study in two or more papers or republishing the same material in successive papers that differ only in format and how the content is discussed. Wasteful publication also includes blending data from one study with additional data that are insufficient to stand on their own to create another paper, often called "meat extending."[30] The author is required to sign a copyright form stating that the article being submitted is exclusive and has not been published elsewhere. This procedure is designed to prevent repetitive publication.[30]

Electronic databases such as MEDLINE have made literature review easier and far less time-consuming for authors. With the many sources a literature search can generate, the author is responsible for finding, assessing the quality, and referencing the primary source of the information upon which the submitted work is based. This can ensure accurate referencing of the manuscript.

Technology advances during the past decades have created controversy around the issue of copyright control between authors and publishers involved in scholarly communication. Academic authors have historically viewed their work as having barter value only—that is, value in achieving tenure, obtaining time and money for research, and building and maintaining a reputation.[31] Academic authors are beginning to seek copyright control over scholarly communication in five areas. The first area is electronic prepublication, which allows anyone to see preprinted work and work that has not yet been peer reviewed. The second area is emerging knowledge environments in which the literature of an entire discipline or subdiscipline is brought together digitally for convenience. Authors in these environments are interested in securing the greatest possible flexibility in publishing. The third area is personal or laboratory websites, where authors can post original writing for teaching purposes. The fourth area is open access publication, which often allows free access, copying, and dissemination of journal articles. The final area is distance education, which requires printed material, video technology, and internet access in lieu of the traditional verbal classroom lecture. Advancements in technology and the changing marketplace for education will likely increase the need for authors to negotiate copyright agreements that allow the widest possible dissemination of their work and ensure that authors, rather than the publishers, have control over, and barrier-free access to, the accumulating body of scholarship on which future teaching and research will build.[31]

With the explosion of new journals, dietetics practitioners and academics should feel free to publish research related to their work. Practice-related manuscripts, narrative reviews, and systematic reviews are welcomed for submission because they add to the wealth of study-based publications.

THE REVIEWER'S PERSPECTIVE

Peer review is the critical, judicious evaluation of a manuscript performed by the authors' equals.[32] Peer review plays a critical role in determining a manuscript's value for publication. Many resources are available to assist reviewers in the specifics of the reviewing process.[29,32-36] The evaluating checklists provided by the Critical Appraisal Skills Programme UK are particularly helpful because they include evaluation lists for each type of manuscript from qualitative papers to randomized clinical trials.[33] General questions to ask when reviewing any manuscript are presented in Box 28.3.

Peer review is a positive, usually constructive, critical process that allows the author to enhance the publication. In comments to the author, the reviewer should present criticism dispassionately and avoid abrasive remarks.[29] These comments should be presented in a practical fashion so the author understands the issues and can respond accordingly. The reviewer assesses organization, originality, scientific reliability, clinical importance, clarity, correct and current referencing, and suitability for publication. For most journals the reviewer submits comments through an editorial management system, which is true of the *Journal of the Academy of Nutrition and Dietetics*. The author submits the manuscript through the same system. Note that a manuscript will generally have two or three reviewers to ensure thorough evaluation.

At the end of the process, the reviewer recommends whether to accept the paper for publication, accept it for publication after modification, or reject it. The reviewer may recommend that the manuscript be submitted to another journal, particularly if the manuscript is not a good fit; for example, an animal study would not be a good fit for the *Journal of the Academy of Nutrition and Dietetics*. Specific statements about the acceptability of a paper are directed to the editor in a confidential cover letter or on a form

Is the abstract clearly written?

Is the purpose stated clearly and specifically?

Are references current and from peer-reviewed journals in the literature review?

Are the methods and research design appropriate for effectively implementing the study?

Are the measuring techniques valid, reliable, and applied effectively?

Are the data analysis procedures appropriate and implemented effectively?

Are the results presented in an understandable format?

Does the discussion of the results connect with the review of literature?

Are the conclusions stated appropriately?

Are the study's strengths and weaknesses stated?

Are areas for future research described effectively?

Box 28.3 Questions Reviewers Should Ask When Reviewing a Manuscript

provided for that purpose. Editorial decisions are usually based on evaluations derived from several sources, however, and therefore a reviewer should not expect the editor to honor every recommendation. Keep in mind the subjectivity of peer review due to the lack of formal training of reviewers.[29,32,37] Very few journals offer their reviewers formal training in manuscript review. At times, reviews can lack ideal objectivity and a systematic application of guidelines for review. Short-term training workshops have been minimally effective in increasing review quality.[38]

Peer review not only influences the content of dietetics literature but also directly affects dietetics education in the classroom and workplace. The process influences the use or rejection of various dietetics-related interventions, educational models, preventive activities, behavior change strategies, or processes. Peer review also benefits readers by reducing the number of gross errors that appear in the literature, enforces some set of standards for practice, exerts a mechanism for quality control, and stimulates efforts to produce better work and better writing. Potential risks of peer review include delay in the transmission of helpful information and the exclusion of new ideas or approaches that conflict with orthodoxy, which can retard progress.

Even though the current referee system may fail from time to time, it represents today's single greatest protection of scientific integrity and excellence.[15,16] If the reviewer accepts the role of teacher by giving constructive criticism and remains open to feedback from the investigator, as in the case of a rebuttal, both investigator and reviewer gain an educational experience. Effective communication within the editorial review process makes a good paper better and an excellent paper superb.

Challenges with Peer Review

Several challenges are associated with peer review. As mentioned before, the lack and ineffectiveness of training can affect the quality and consistency of reviews. With open access publishing some manuscripts are posted without any peer review, and some will be reviewed while posted. This approach has positives and negatives. An article that receives a number of quality reviews may yield higher-quality criticism. If few reviews are done, then evaluation is limited. In addition, open access peer review is often conducted unblinded. Therefore, bias could be introduced into the process if the authors and reviewers know one another. Reviewers lacking statistical expertise might not vet the statistical procedures cited with the rigor needed to properly evaluate the article. Very few journals provide opportunities for a reviewer with statistical expertise to be placed on the team of reviewers for manuscripts.[13,15,16,17,19,20,32,37-40] An exception is the *Journal of the Academy of Nutrition and Dietetics*. Recruiting qualified reviewers can be difficult considering that services are offered for free and that the number of journals is growing. Also, reviewer fatigue can occur when reviewers are overloaded with reviews. Therefore, efforts must be made to improve peer review.

THE READER'S PERSPECTIVE

People read reports of research in the literature to keep abreast of current findings in their profession and areas of specialty and to improve their job performance and practice. The field of dietetics now emphasizes evidence-based practice, which is a model of decision-making that uses a systematic process to integrate the best research evidence with actual practice and patient or consumer values to optimize outcomes.[41] Dietetics practitioners must be effective miners of research evidence from the existing scientific literature so they can engage in effective evidence-based practice.

In recent years, university dietetics programs accredited by the Accreditation Council for Education in Nutrition and Dietetics have added a stronger emphasis on research and interpretation of research articles in their curricula. In fact, Drummond and Murphy-Reyes[42] recently wrote an excellent nutrition research book that will be a valuable resource for dietetics research courses. Dietetics graduates today are likely to have more competency in research literature evaluation than graduates in the past. However, it is imperative that graduates not rely solely on their university dietetics training, which in time will become outdated. Still, their training in research criticism and evaluation can be continually used to stay abreast of the dietetics field.

Reading and Evaluating the Literature

To access peer-reviewed dietetics-related literature, the reader must be familiar with databases to conduct computer searches. The most common databases used in the profession are EBSCO, CINAHL, MEDLINE, and PubMed. In addition, individual journals, such as the *Journal of the Academy of Nutrition and Dietetics* and *American Journal of Clinical Nutrition*, have options for searching past issues for relevant articles. Garrard[43] wrote an outstanding book on conducting literature searches. After identifying references from the literature review, full-text articles need to be obtained. With open access publishing, acquiring full-text articles has gotten much easier. Sometimes occupational institutions will buy subscriptions to provide employees with access to full-text articles. Some journals offer free access to full-text articles from back issues, but getting the full-text article can sometimes be a challenge.

The reader must follow certain guidelines for reading and evaluating the selected articles. The *Journal of the Academy of Nutrition and Dietetics* statistical series can provide a refresher on all aspects of nutrition research.[1-10] Though it dates from 1997, Greenhalgh's "how to read a paper" series in the *British Medical Journal* provides valuable information on interpreting statistics and reading scientific papers.[44] In a way, readers should think of themselves essentially as reviewers and consult references previously mentioned in order to critically evaluate articles.[33-36] The Critical Appraisal Skills Programme checklists are also extremely helpful.[33] The reader must approach the literature with a critical and evaluative mind. Just because an article is from a peer-reviewed journal does not mean it is necessarily of high quality or has valid results and conclusions. Box 28.4 lists questions a reader can ask to critically review a scientific article. The questions can serve as an evaluative checklist when reading the article.

Keeping Current

Strategies for keeping current with the literature include starting a journal club at work where professional colleagues and students may share and discuss research articles. Also, subscribers can establish PubMed email alerts to receive notifications about new articles. In addition, practitioners can subscribe to electronic table of content services from key nutrition journals. Another strategy is to read only articles specific to one's interest or area of expertise. Also, receiving daily emails from the *Journal of the Academy of Nutrition and Dietetics* about the most recently published research can be helpful.

In keeping current, dietetics practitioners may put too much faith in the results of a single publication. Every individual research study has weaknesses and limitations that reduce the validity and reliability of the results. Thus, conclusions from scientific evidence are best made from multiple studies. In the past, writers would compile review articles to summarize the research findings of several studies. The

Were the research questions clearly stated?

Was the selection of participants free of bias?

Were study groups comparable?

Was blinding used?

Were intervention procedures well described and strong enough for effect?

Were sample sizes large enough?

Were outcomes clearly defined?

Was the statistical analysis appropriate?

Was the literature review thorough enough?

Were the conclusions supported by the results?

Was there any potential bias due to funding source or sponsorship?

Was the project approved by an institutional review board?

Was the subject interesting, current, and relevant?

Could the intervention be applied effectively beyond the experimental situation?

Were the references current?

Box 28.4 Questions a Reader Should Ask to Critically Evaluate a Research Article

problem was that these reviews lacked standardized criteria for including articles, evaluating articles, and making conclusions. Currently, systematic reviews are being published at an ever-increasing rate on a variety of topics in which investigators are using standard procedures and criteria for analyzing evidence (see Chapter 10 on systematic reviews). Readers of systematic reviews get a concise summary of results for a particular topic. One well-known source for systematic reviews is the Cochrane Collaboration and its Cochrane Library.[45] The Cochrane Collaboration uses a consistent system of evidence analysis to review existing studies on various health care–related topics. These systematic reviews are published and posted at the Cochrane website. Dietetics practitioners will find it enlightening to become familiar with this website.

The Academy of Nutrition and Dietetics was progressive in establishing its Evidence Analysis Library.[46] Groups working on topics of interest to RDNs use a well-defined evidence analysis process to compile systematic reviews and evidence-based guidelines for practice. The four steps in the process of analysis are (1) identify the problem (or the specific question to be answered), (2) conduct an evidence search, (3) critique and grade the evidence by defined criteria, and (4) summarize the findings. Various groups have been recruited and convened to study specific topics, such as type 1 and type 2 diabetes, lipid disorders, and celiac disease. Many systematic reviews have been published and are currently being conducted. RDNs should become familiar with this rich source of information. Being familiar with systematic reviews and the associated original research articles could change the way RDNs practice.

CONCLUSION

RDNs are the expert resources for nutrition knowledge and the primary communicators of that knowledge to their scientific and administrative colleagues as well as to the lay public. The tools needed to fulfill these challenging roles lie in the development of a critical readership, a responsible authorship, and an invested group of peer reviewers. Critical readers will become critical reviewers of noteworthy information. Responsible authors will continue to be stimulated to research worthwhile ideas and effectively communicate the findings. Peer reviewers, through their efforts and expertise, guarantee high-quality, valid, published knowledge. Journals are, and will continue to be, the most current source of nutrition knowledge; therefore, personal commitment to develop and maintain skills in all aspects of the periodical arena is necessary for RDNs to become the readers, writers, and reviewers they are called on to be.

REFERENCES

1. Bruemmer B, Harris J, Gleason P, et al. Publishing nutrition research: a review of epidemiologic methods. *J Am Diet Assoc.* 2009;109(10):1728-1737.

2. Boushey C, Harris J, Bruemmer B, Archer SL, Van Horn L. Publishing nutrition research: a review of study design, statistical analyses, and other key elements of manuscript preparation, part 1. *J Acad Nutr Diet.* 2006;106(1):89-96.

3. Boushey CJ, Harris J, Bruemmer B, Archer SL. Publishing nutrition research: a review of sampling, sample size, statistical analysis, and other key elements of manuscript preparation, part 2. *J Am Diet Assoc.* 2008;108(4):679-688.

4. Gleason PM, Boushey CJ, Harris JE, Zoellner J. Publishing nutrition research: a review of multivariate techniques–part 3: data reduction methods. *J Acad Nutr Diet.* 2015;115(7): 1072-1082.

5. Harris JE, Boushey C, Bruemmer B, Archer SL. Publishing nutrition research: a review of nonparametric methods, part 3. *J Am Diet Assoc.* 2008;108(9):1488-1496.

6. Harris JE, Sheean PM, Gleason PM, Bruemmer B, Boushey C. Publishing nutrition research: a review of multivariate techniques—part 2: analysis of variance. *J Acad Nutr Diet.* 2012;112(1):90-98.

7. Harris JE, Gleason PM, Sheean PM, Boushey C, Beto JA, Bruemmer B. An introduction to qualitative research for food and nutrition professionals. *J Am Diet Assoc.* 2009; 109(1):80-90.

8. Sheean PM, Bruemmer B, Gleason P, Harris J, Boushey C, Van Horn L. Publishing nutrition research: a review of multivariate techniques—part 1. *J Am Diet Assoc.* 2011;111(1): 103-110.

9. Gleason PM, Harris J, Sheean PM, Boushey CJ, Bruemmer B. Publishing nutrition research: validity, reliability, and diagnostic test assessment in nutrition-related research. *J Am Diet Assoc.* 2010;110(3):409-419.

10. Zoellner J, Van Horn L, Gleason PM, Boushey CJ. What is translational research? Concepts and applications in nutrition and dietetics. *J Acad Nutr Diet.* 2015;115(7):1057- 1071.

11. EQUATOR Network. Enhancing the Quality and Transparency of Health Research. 2017. www.equator-network.org. Accessed February 19, 2017.

12. Björk BC. Open access to scientific articles: a review of benefits and challenges. *Intern Emerg Med.* 2017;12(2):247-253.

13. Breuning M, Backstrom J, Brannon J, Gross BI, Widmeier M. Reviewer fatigue? Why scholars decline to review their peers' work. *PS Polit Sci Polit.* 2015;48(04): 595-600.

14. Moher D, Moher E. Stop predatory publishers now: act collaboratively. *Ann Intern Med.* 2016;164(9):616-617.

15. García JA, Rodriguez-Sánchez R, Fdez-Valdivia J. Bias and effort in peer-review. *J Assoc Inf Sci Technol.* 2015;66(10): 2020-2030.

16. Leopold SS. Editorial: CORR will change to double-blind peer review—what took us so long to get there? *Clin Orthop Relat Res.* 2017;475(2):297-299.

17. Levis AW, Leentjens AFG, Levenson JL, Lumley MA, Thombs BD. Comparison of self-citation by peer-reviewers in a journal with single-blind peer-review versus a journal with open peer-review. *J Psychosom Res.* 2015;79(6):561-565.

18. McNaught K. The changing publication practices in academia: inherent uses and issues in open access and online publishing and the rise of fraudulent publications. *J Electron Publ.* 2015;18(3): On Access. doi:10.3998 /3336451.0018.308.

19. Missimer T. Journal paper peer-review: a broken system? *Ground Water.* 2015:53(3): 347.

20. Vercellini P, Buggio L, Viganò P, Somigliana E. Peer-review in medical journals: beyond quality of reports towards transparency and public scrutiny of the process. *Eur J Intern Med.* 2016;31:15-19.

21. Rosner B. *Fundamentals of Biostatistics.* 7th ed. Boston, MA: Brooks/Cole; 2011.

22. International Committee of Medical Journal Editors. *Recommendations for the Conduct, Reporting, Editing and Publication of Scholarly Work in Medical Journals.* 2016. www.icmje.org/about-icmje/faqs/icmje-recommendations. Accessed February 21, 2017.

23. Information for Authors. *Journal of the Academy of Nutrition and Dietetics.* 2017. www.andjrnl.org/content /authorinfo. Accessed February 19, 2017.

24. Hua F, Walsh T, Worthington H, Glenny AM. "Predatory" publishing and open access in dentistry. *J Am Dent Assoc.* 2016;147(8):600-601.

25. Lone MI, Khan NJ. Open access journal publishing: a DOAJ perspective with reference to environmental sciences. *Int J Inf Dissem Technol.* 2016;6(4):242-246.

26. Oermann MH, Conklin JL, Nicoll LH, et al. Study of predatory open access nursing journals. *J Nurs Scholarsh.* 2016;48(6):624-632.

27. Turale S. So you want to publish in *International Nursing Review*? A few words of advice for authors. *Int Nurs Rev.* 2016;63(4):519.

28. Awati M. How to respond to comments by peer-reviewers. *Editage Insights.* 2013; www.editage.com/insights/how-to -respond-to-comments-by-peer-reviewers. Accessed February 25, 2017.

29. Bagchi R, Block L, Hamilton RW, Ozanne JL. A field guide for the review process: writing and responding to peer-reviews. *J Consum Res.* 2017;43(5):860-872.

30. Kumar S, Sartaj A. Medical research misconduct: a review study on duplicate publications. *Int J Contemp Microbiol.* 2016;2(2):25-29.

31. Laakso M, Lindman J. Journal copyright restrictions and actual open access availability: a study of articles published in eight top information systems journals (2010–2014). *Scientometrics.* 2016;109(2):1167-1189.

32. Akers KG. Being critical and constructive: a guide to peer-reviewing for librarians. *J Med Libr Assoc.* 2017;105(1):1-3.

33. Critical Appraisal Skills Programme UK (CASP). CASP Appraisal Checklists. 2017. www.casp-uk.net/casp-tools -checklists. Accessed February 19, 2017.

34. Quality Assessment Tool for Quantitative Studies. 2017. www.ephpp.ca/tools.html. Accessed February 19, 2017.

35. Mar CD, Hoffmann TC. A guide to performing a peer-review of randomised controlled trials. *BMC Med.* 2015;13(1):248.

36. Moher D. Optimal strategies to consider when peer-reviewing a systematic review and meta-analysis. *BMC Med.* 2015;13:1-4.

37. Derraik J. The principles of fair allocation of peer-review: how much should a researcher be expected to contribute? *Sci Eng Ethics.* 2015;21(4):825.

38. Bruce R, Chauvin A, Trinquart L, Ravaud P, Boutron I. Impact of interventions to improve the quality of peer-review of biomedical journals: a systematic review and meta-analysis. *BMC Med.* 2016;14(1):85.

39. Heinze G. Statistical reviewing: constructive criticism towards reproducible research. *Transpl Int.* 2016;29(4): 388-389.

40. Stahel PF, Moore EE. Peer-review for biomedical publications: we can improve the system. *BMC Med.* 2014;12:179.

41. Byham-Gray LD, Gilbride JA, Dixon B, Stage FK. Evidence-based practice: what are dietitians' perceptions, attitudes, and knowledge? *J Am Diet Assoc.* 2005;105(10):1574-1581.

42. Drummond K, Murphy-Reyes A. *Nutrition Research: Concepts and Applications.* Burlington, MA: Jones and Bartlett Learning; 2018.

43. Garrard J. *Health Sciences Literature Review Made Easy.* 5th ed. Burlington, MA: Jones and Bartlett Learning; 2017.

44. Greenhalgh T. How to read a paper. statistics for the nonstatistician. I: different types of data need different statistical tests. *BMJ.* 1997;315(7104):364-366.

45. The Cochrane Library. The Cochrane Collaboration website. http://www.cochrane.org. Accessed February 26, 2017.

46. The Academy of Nutrition and Dietetics Evidence Analysis Library website. www.eatrightpro.org/resources/research /applied-practice/evidence-analysis-library. Accessed February 26, 2017.

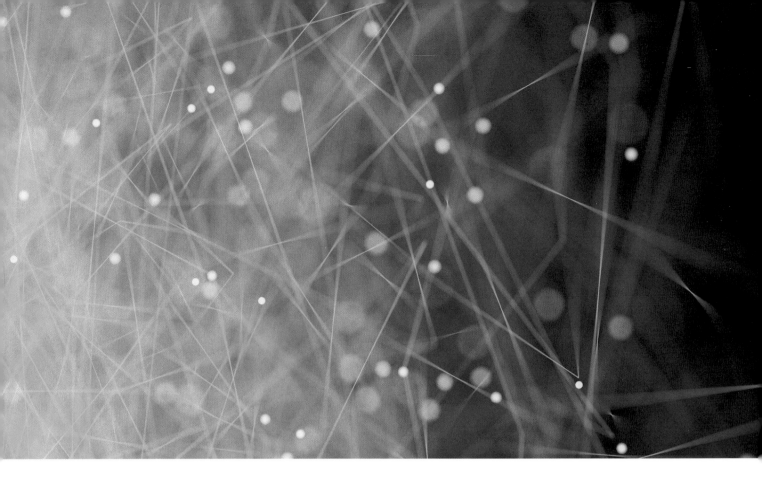

Applications of Research to Practice

Chapter 29

Bridging Research into Practice

Judith A. Gilbride, PhD, RDN, FAND | *Laura D. Byham-Gray,* PhD, RDN, FNKF

LEARNING OBJECTIVES

1. Describe the important role of research in nutrition and dietetics practice.

2. Explain the steps in the research process to document or modify practice.

3. Identify ways to build research effectiveness in any dietetics practice setting.

The nutrition and dietetics profession integrates several disciplines, so it requires a broad theoretical and applied research base. Since the evolution of the profession, research and its application to practice have been valued and sought after. In fact, research has been described as the "body" and the "backbone" for the dietetics profession—research drives practice and practice drives research.[1] The involvement of registered dietitian nutritionists (RDNs) has changed in the past decade, supported by revised dietetics education standards and practice-based research initiatives of the Academy of Nutrition and Dietetics. Practicing RDNs are applying evidence-based resources that advance the profession.[2] Theoretical and applied research courses and projects have increased in undergraduate and graduate dietetics programs,[3] and clinical doctoral degrees have emerged in dietetics, similar to the other health professions. For example, Rutgers University–Biomedical and Health Sciences, Department of Nutritional Sciences and the University of North Florida, Department of Nutrition and Dietetics, both offer a doctorate in clinical nutrition.

Long recognized as the backbone and foundation of the profession, research plays a major role in what all practitioners should do. A call for stronger links between research and practice began in the mid-1980s with the belief that research is driven by the practice of nutrition and dietetics.[4] This linkage is advanced by a conscientious commitment to identifying and solving scientific problems, ensuring sound methods, and interpreting research outcomes. As research is the basis of dietetics profession, today RDNs are building on the work of predecessors and forging ahead by involving more practitioners in the process of analyzing, implementing, and evaluating how research affects practice. RDNs should continue to lead and answer the research practice questions that contribute to the research foundation of the profession. This chapter provides the background of research advancing the profession, examples of how research contributes to practice, and information that will increase the investigative opportunities for RDNs.

IMPORTANCE OF RESEARCH IN NUTRITION AND DIETETICS PRACTICE

The discovery of new knowledge is the foundation and framework of the dietetics profession.[1,2-5] Research helps RDNs develop professionally and allows them to integrate findings into their work. Nutrition practitioners who work with the public must be able to interpret food and nutrition studies accurately and correct any misinformation for consumers.[5] Moreover, in all practice settings, generating and interpreting scientific data keep RDNs up to date and give credibility to what they say.[1,6]

To integrate research into practice, resources must be skillfully organized and managed. Collecting and analyzing data help practitioners solve some problems that they observe and face every day. A research perspective is useful in monitoring ongoing activities in all areas of nutrition and dietetics and provides the feedback necessary for changing program or departmental policies, standard protocols, or patient care guidelines to improve the general health of individuals. Well-designed studies can also generate data to expand food and nutrition services, ensure quality and cost savings, evaluate systems, determine effectiveness of medical nutrition therapy, and substantiate clinical and cost outcomes from dietetics interventions.[7] In an early commentary on research opportunities in the profession, Wylie-Rosett and colleagues[8] identified four categories or levels in a continuum: (1) using a scientific approach in practice, (2) collaborating to translate research into practice or for publication, (3) participating in research studies, and (4) leading a research initiative. According to Wylie-Rosett,(EdD) "evidence-based care should be informed by a reciprocal relationship between research and practice" (personal email communication, March 13, 2007). A delicate balance should exist to ensure that the best possible evidence is available and accessible for the care of patients and clients.

READING THE PROFESSIONAL LITERATURE

The proliferation of nutrition articles in health and medical journals and the explosion of information on the internet make targeted reading of research critical for today's busy practitioners. Although evidence analysis summaries, daily scientific updates, and abstracts help in making decisions at the bedside, a reflective approach is important to consider the body of existing evidence and to determine any knowledge gaps that might affect practice. RDNs who want to improve their analytic skills and better understand statistical tests and interpretation of significance should adopt a disciplined approach to reading the literature (see Box 29.1 on page 572).

Acquiring the ability to judge the value, methods, and clinical and practical significance of research studies can ultimately enhance the care of patients and clients. An RDN should ask: What do the study results really mean? Is it relevant to my

Set up PubMed and Ovid alerts to receive emails listing articles of interest.

Sign up for electronic table of contents for key journals (eg, *Journal of the Academy of Nutrition and Dietetics, Journal of Nutrition, American Journal of Clinical Nutrition*).

Read the *Journal of the Academy of Nutrition and Dietetics* monthly and scan the brief article reviews at the back of each issue.

Organize a monthly journal club at work or school.

Monitor tables of content from one's specialty practice area journals.

Expand research network to relevant interdisciplinary journals.

Box 29.1 Practical Tips for Keeping Up with the Research Literature

patients? Following are some suggestions to consider when deciphering an article:

- Avoid the abstract, introduction, and discussion unless the intent is to simply scan the literature or gain an overall perspective.
- Concentrate on the design and methods section first and determine how the study was planned and executed.
- Analyze what the statistical significance means as well as the clinical (impact on patient care) and practical (relevant to altering practice) significance. Gain confidence in interpreting tables and graphs because they usually summarize the primary and secondary study outcomes.
- Reflect on the soundness and reliability of the methods, the strengths and limitations of the design and implementation, and the clinical relevance and practical significance of the study before analyzing other references from the bibliography and designing a research project.[9]

Although many questions can be answered from research, job demands, limited resources, and time constraints may hamper the efforts of investigators to solve practice problems. Practitioners are often so busy concentrating on meeting their routine responsibilities that they have little time to begin a research project or even become engaged in an ongoing study. Collaborating with faculty in academic settings, pursuing a graduate degree or advanced training, and finding research mentors are helpful strategies for practicing RDNs to increase participation in research.[10]

RESEARCH PRIORITIES AND OPPORTUNITIES IN THE PROFESSION

For practitioners, there are some positive aspects to becoming more involved in research. King and colleagues[11] explored the topic of research outcome expectations when they surveyed members of the Nutrition Research Network (NRN) and members of the Academy of Nutrition and Dietetics who identified research as their primary area of practice. Besides leadership opportunities and career advancement, respondents identified an increased sense of self-worth, personal satisfaction, financial opportunities, expansion of knowledge, and respect from others.

As is evident from its professional website (www.eatrightPRO.org), the Academy of Nutrition and Dietetics strongly supports research.[12] Nutrition research benefits the profession by improving patient outcomes and increasing reimbursement, collaborative relationships, and recognition for nutrition science. Personal satisfaction is often enhanced by job advancement, the acquisition of new skills and professional knowledge, as well as internal and external visibility.[12] For many researchers, helping patients and others is the most satisfying outcome, along with mentoring practitioners and contributing to the growing body of literature on the value of food and nutrition for preventing and treating disease.

Box 29.2 provides a list of questions practitioners can use to determine if they are prepared to become a practitioner-researcher. These questions may help practitioners explore their potential and

What activities are important to my profession and to my personal career development?

Do I search databases for answers to practice questions?

Do I evaluate research studies critically?

Do I apply research findings in my practice setting?

Do I use evidence-based practice guidelines and/or science-based findings?

Do I help colleagues and students interpret nutrition and dietetics research?

Do I review research proposals, projects, and manuscripts for publication?

Do I develop policies or protocols based on evidence-based practice?

Do I demonstrate evidence-based practice as a mentor or team member?

Do I present findings of quality improvement projects?

Do I design applied research studies or systems to measure outcomes?

Do I participate in quality improvement methods or translational research studies?

Do I help colleagues develop and design research?

Do I initiate or participate in narrative or systematic reviews?

Do I apply for grant funding?

Do I author or coauthor peer-reviewed research articles?

Do I serve as a principal investigator or key investigator on a grant?

Do I advocate for research opportunities at work or in my profession?

Do I advocate for research opportunities at a national or global level?

Box 29.2 Self-Assessment Questions for Determining Potential for Increasing Research Involvement in Nutrition and Dietetics Practice

Adapted with permission from Byham-Gray LD. *Dietitians' Perceptions, Attitudes, and Knowledge of Evidence-Based Practice and Involvement in Research Activities* [dissertation]. New York, NY: New York University; 2004.[13]

determine the level of research involvement they may want to achieve.

The role of research in the dietetics and nutrition profession has been an ongoing theme for the past 15 years. Over this time, practitioners have seen an increase in member resources from the Academy of Nutrition and Dietetics. Major revisions, initiated and approved by the House of Delegates in 2002 (with broad input from members and external experts), strengthened the Academy of Nutrition and Dietetics infrastructure to expand resources for members and to increase research opportunities in all practice settings. The House of Delegates endorsed practice-based research to measure outcomes that may affect reimbursement, legislation, and policy decisions. Delegates supported wide dissemination and implementation of research findings to add value for patients who receive dietetics services and to enhance the overall quality of care.[14] Valuable contributions for members have been generated through the online Evidence Analysis Library (EAL) and posted on their website (www.andeal.org) and the formation of the NRN (known at that time as the Dietetics Practice-Based Research Network).[15,16] Other fundamental resources developed and sustained within the Academy of Nutrition and Dietetics by the Research, International and Scientific Affairs team include the adoption of the Nutrition Care Process and Terminology, tools for collecting data, and the Academy of Nutrition and Dietetics Health Informatics Infrastructure (ANDHII) in 2013.[2,14]

The Council on Research provides direction for Academy of Nutrition and Dietetics research activities, in alignment with public policy and advocacy priority areas. The Academy of Nutrition and Dietetics has evolved its role in leading research within the profession and has made great strides in helping practitioners. It is committed to a foundational model that supports practice, education, and policy decisions for the Academy of Nutrition and Dietetics. Six areas of research were categorized in 2009: Dietetics Research (dietetics services, nutrition care process, outcomes of nutrition intervention); Nutrition Research (nutrition functions and biomarkers); Behavioral and Social Sciences Research (behavior from social and psychological perspectives and applied to community and public health nutrition); Management Research (systems, finance, and operations); Basic Science Research (biochemistry, cellular and molecular biology, physiology, genomics, pharmacology); and Food Science Research (chemistry, physical structure, effects of processing and food preparation).[2]

Dietetics research is used to demonstrate the application of knowledge in the field to help individuals choose a healthy diet and lifestyle. The Academy of Nutrition and Dietetics set a goal to increase member involvement in dietetics research in 1993 in four practice areas: disease prevention and health promotion, acute and long-term care, food service, and consumer education.[14] Research topics and priorities are established by the Academy of Nutrition and Dietetics Council on Research and reexamined periodically. In a 2011 survey of the Research Dietetic Practice Group,[15] the Council on Research compiled the following Academy of Nutrition and Dietetics research priorities:

● Nutrition and lifestyle change intervention to prevent obesity and chronic diseases
● Nutrition care process and health outcome measures
● Safe, secure, and sustainable food supply
● Nutrients and systems biology (nutrigenetics and nutrigenomics)

Six roles were also identified as critical to advancing the Academy of Nutrition and Dietetics research agenda in the profession and to promote collabora-

tion with other scientists and organizations: advocate, facilitator, convener, educator, funder, and disseminator.[14] The Academy of Nutrition and Dietetics advocates for work to be done with federal and nongovernmental agencies. As a facilitator, the Academy of Nutrition and Dietetics devises key questions for the profession. As a convener of scientists and practitioners, the Academy of Nutrition and Dietetics brings professionals together and leads discussions of the key research issues, such as preventing and treating childhood obesity and maintaining a safe, sustainable food supply. As an educator, the Academy of Nutrition and Dietetics teaches members and the public about key nutrition and dietetics findings and the impact on diet and health. The Academy of Nutrition and Dietetics may also fund selected research projects to conduct relevant studies that help and educate members. As a disseminator, the Academy of Nutrition and Dietetics publishes and distributes practice-based nutrition and dietetics research to professionals and to the public in various media outlets.

According to the spring 2014 House of Delegates Backgrounder, *Engaging Members in Research*, the breadth of Academy of Nutrition and Dietetics research relies on varied methods. A conceptual model for the Academy of Nutrition and Dietetics has five primary foci, including translational, epidemiologic, practice-based, quality improvement, and evidence analysis.[14,16] All affect the interpretation and implementation of nutrition and dietetics practice.

Translational research is considered the most traditional focus and has been emphasized by the National Institutes of Health (NIH) as foundational for advancing health and clinical care. Translational research originates in academia and progresses from the lab to animal and clinical trials before it is applied in medical centers and other small health facilities.[17] Translational research begins with facts discovered from animal studies, theoretical methods, and laboratory experiments. Through new findings and implementation research, translational research encourages adoption of evidence-based clinical practice into nutrition and dietetics.[18] For example, new roles for RDNs are warranted in nutritional genomics. With a strong knowledge base in nutritional genetics and nutritional genomics, RDNs can be the connection for converting new findings into applied nutrition practice.[19]

The NRN has been successful in involving more practicing clinical RDNs into the research process. Its purpose is to "conduct, support, promote, and advocate research in practice-based settings."[18] This collaborative model exemplifies how practitioners can become involved in research and add to the body of the dietetics literature while being mentored simultaneously.

The NRN surveyed Academy of Nutrition and Dietetics members on their perceptions of research, their extent of participation, and any barriers or resources needed to initiate research. Of the 4,134 respondents, 71% reported involvement in at least one research project throughout their careers. Almost unanimously, 99.5% of participants, thought research was important to the profession, but they perceived greater value in applying research than participating in the research process. Evidence-based practice (EBP) and guidelines were deemed important by 84.4% of the sample. The barriers reported were structural rather than disinterest; the most frequent barrier was lack of time followed by funding, importance of other work, administrative support, lack of employer interest, and regulatory requirements. Resources they identified that have been instrumental in guiding them are tools like the EBP guidelines and the health informatics initiatives.[20]

The Academy of Nutrition and Dietetics commitment to help practitioners conduct meaningful research is supported with many online tools. ANDHII is a platform that allows expanded use of the Nutrition Care Process And Terminology for Academy of Nutrition and Dietetics members to apply in research with human participants. ANDHII has three facets: a Dietetics Outcome Registry, Smart Visits, and Nutrition Research Information. All facilitate data collection and management. Moreover, the Dietetics Outcome Registry deidentifies data for nutrition research and quality improvement projects.[2] Thus, the online platform assists RDNs with procedures to track patient outcomes of care and helps researchers and practitioners summarize data from electronic health records. As an approach for research that applies privacy rules by deidentifying patient data, it allows users to evaluate data for effectiveness and outcome studies.[21]

More than three quarters of the respondents in another survey indicated that they have searched and critiqued the scientific literature, focusing on dietetics research that encompasses nutrition intervention of specific disorders and nutrition support, dietetics education, medical nutrition therapy, outcomes research, and a variety of miscellaneous areas. Other categories identified were nutrition research, behavioral and social science research, management research, basic science research, food science research, and general research methods.[2]

Both practitioners and educators seem to be interested in research. The Academy of Nutrition and Dietetics promotes the confluence of academia and dietetics practice to advance the research agenda for members. Dalton[22] documents several examples of this convergence where RDNs were able to translate research into practice and make positive improvements in the health of individuals and communities. The breadth of research by Dalton's doctoral students ranged from testing tuberous vegetables in the laboratory to reduce the amount of available potassium for patients on hemodialysis to evaluating how a weight-management strategy of two vs eight meals affects weight, insulin levels, and hunger. Another doctoral candidate focused on state school wellness policies and used qualitative and quantitative methods (termed a *mixed-methods study*) to implement school policies effectively in one school district.[22]

Practice-based studies can document nutrition interventions and assess the effectiveness of nutrition protocols and dietary treatment. After effectiveness is determined, researchers may evaluate the costs of intervention procedures and measure them against the efficacy of outcomes. Outcome evaluation and quality improvement projects keep nutrition and dietetics competitive as a profession. The NIH has also addressed the need for more nutrition science through increased support of randomized controlled nutrition trials, the National Nutrition Research Agenda, and the creation of the Nutrition Section of the National Institute of Diabetes and Digestive and Kidney Diseases. In this era of financial accountability in health care, providing EBP in nutrition and dietetics can further demonstrate the value of RDNs in preventing and treating complex diseases.[23,24]

Scholarly activities begin with a strong background in research and the curriculum enhancements proposed in the Academy of Nutrition and Dietetics 2017 Standards of Education.[25,26] Similar to the 2012 standards[27] for didactic programs, dietetics internships, and coordinated programs, the 2017 version supports research skills and knowledge and EBP for students in accredited programs. The final draft of the 2017 standards includes core knowledge and competencies for integrating scientific information and translating research into practice. The didactic portion delineates basic knowledge about research methods, needs assessments, and outcomes research and in-depth knowledge of the scientific method and quality improvement methods.[26]

Educators have already increased the research content in dietetics curriculums and have initiated novel approaches to applied research skills, heeding the call for increasing research content in curricula. Adding research to undergraduate, practice, and graduate programs has enhanced the focus on critical thinking and how to conduct rigorous studies, interpret the research literature, and apply evidence in nutrition care practice. One program director created a master's degree in nutrition with a research focus.[28] In addition to collecting and analyzing data and presenting findings at meetings, the program is designed to have students write a grant proposal and develop literature reviews and research manuscripts.

The criteria for evaluating dietetics education programs rely on the ability of graduates to interpret current research and basic statistics. Harris and colleagues[29] reported on an online survey of 269 supervised practice programs and the status of research education in their programs. The program directors who responded (51%; n = 152) confirmed that in 76% of programs, interns have research content in their supervised practice. Furthermore, 69% of the programs required interns to use the EAL, 45% required at least one research project to be completed during the program, and 30% required interns to do more than one project.[29]

APPLYING RESEARCH TO PRACTICE

Research studies do not always have immediate, practical application but rather may build on what was learned in prior studies. The application of sound research principles can confirm impressions or observations about patient care. Research is a systematic process of deductive-inductive reasoning to provide answers to questions and to develop theories. Such answers may be abstract and general in qualitative studies and concrete and specific in clinical trials. In both descriptive and analytic research, the investigator uncovers facts and then formulates a generalization based on the exploration, description, and explanation of those facts.[30]

Applying research to practice is the central element of evidence-based medicine (now more broadly known as EBP). Evidence-based medicine is a model of clinical decision-making that uses a "systematic process to integrate the best [research] evidence with clinical expertise and patient values to answer a question about one patient's plan of care in order to optimize outcomes."[30] This model incorporates a five-step process for making appropriate patient care decisions: (1) writing an answerable clinical question, (2) effectively searching the literature, (3) critically appraising the literature, (4) applying research findings to practice, and (5) evaluating patient and practitioner outcomes. Such methods let RDNs link the best research evidence to clinical decisions and practice. Investigations by Byham-Gray and colleagues[31] and Vogt and colleagues[32] indicated that EBP is the bridge across the theory-practice gap in dietetics; in other words, the higher the knowledge of EBP among RDNs, the greater their level of research involvement. The NRN website also provides many resources for conducting practice-based research, from study design to data analysis to manuscript assistance (www.eatrightpro.org/research /projects-tools-and-initiatives/nutrition-research -network/academy-research-toolkit-2011).[16]

What Is the Health Insurance Portability and Accountability Act

The Health Insurance Portability and Accountability Act (HIPPA), enacted in 1996, affects all health professionals, including RDNs, and ensures the security and privacy of all forms of patient personal health data. Protected health information (PHI) has certain common identifiers (name, address, date of birth, Social Security number, and payer identification) that must be deidentified for conducting research. Other information in electronic health records includes health record data on past, present, and future physical and mental health and provision of health care services. In nutrition and dietetics, PHI includes medical nutrition therapy services and counseling in health care institutions and private practice and is essential for billing and reimbursement.[21]

Before any research project begins, all administrators and supervisors should be informed of the design and any specific protocols for the study that will affect the patients or study participants. Besides gaining approval to conduct a research project by an institutional review board (IRB), HIPAA regulations and informed consent procedures must be followed and addressed in the protocol. The amount of patient information has increased considerably with electronic records, and information must be de-identified for research purposes.

Security and confidentiality of data are protected in HIPAA by safeguarding electronic PHI for individuals maintained by a covered entity as defined in the rules. HIPAA defines covered entities as a health plan, a health care provider, or a health care clearinghouse. RDNs are considered a covered entity if even one patient is billed electronically in their practice or institution. If an RDN is a covered entity, HIPAA rules apply to all services, and patient health data must be protected. It is important to know institutional procedures and payer agreements that may also require HIPAA compliance. Moreover, in addition to following the HIPAA rules, RDNs must comply with state laws, which may exceed or be less rigid than federal requirements. HIPAA is often cited as and considered a best practice for securing patient or client data.[21]

THE CYCLE OF RESEARCH IN PRACTICE

The application of research techniques to practice focuses on everyday operations and problem solving. Data collection and interpretation can provide insight and direction for collaborative projects with other colleagues and health care professionals. The cycle of practice-based research begins with questions generated by practice; a workable research question is clarified through an extensive literature search, and the research methods are refined. The design and implementation of the research project seeks to answer unresolved problems in practice. Conducting the project produces new facts that necessitate careful analysis. However, integrating that new information into practice requires determining its practical relevance to current procedures. The final steps are disseminating findings to colleagues and other practitioners and applying the new knowledge to improve practice. Thus, a cycle is completed and starts again as other practice questions are raised and solutions to new, perplexing problems are sought.

Case Example

A nutrition intervention study can illustrate the cycle of research as in the following case study based on the trial on the effects of medical nutrition therapy by practitioners on patients with prediabetes who participated in a randomized controlled study by Parker and colleagues.[33]

The Problem

One of the investigators is an RDN in a freestanding research clinic. In addition to coordinating clinical research trials for diabetes, she provides dietary counseling for patients with prediabetes. She wondered about the impact of medical nutrition therapy among patients with prediabetes. A research question was formulated to study the problem: Among patients with prediabetes in a free-standing research clinic, how does medical nutrition therapy vs usual care affect fasting plasma glucose values, hemoglobin A1c (HbA1c) levels, lipid levels, and diabetes risk score, given demographic characteristics, clinical characteristics, and comorbidities, from baseline to the end of a 12-week intervention?[33]

Clarifying the Question

The investigators conducted a review of the scientific literature to find and examine studies regarding dietary intervention in patients with prediabetes. The research question was further refined to study a gap in knowledge. The investigators developed a protocol to explore how medical nutrition therapy affects fasting plasma glucose values, HbA1c levels, lipid levels, and diabetes risk score from baseline to the end of a 12-week intervention in patients with prediabetes who received usual care vs medical nutrition therapy. The protocol included four visits with the RDN, including an initial assessment visit of 60 minutes, and three follow-up visits of 30 to 45 minutes each to determine the following questions:

● What are the demographic characteristics (sex, age, race, ethnicity, family history of diabetes, exercise habits), clinical characteristics (body mass index and waist circumference), and comorbidities (hypertension, dyslipidemia, and obesity)?

● At baseline, what are the fasting plasma glucose values, HbA1c levels, lipid levels, and diabetes risk score?

● After the 12-week intervention, what are the fasting plasma glucose values, HbA1c levels, lipid levels, and diabetes risk score?

● Given demographic characteristics, clinical characteristics, and comorbidities, how does medical nutrition therapy vs usual care affect fasting plasma glucose values, HbA1c levels, lipid levels, and diabetes risk score from baseline to end point after a 12-week intervention?

Conducting the Study

The investigators enrolled 120 participants; 39 individuals did not meet the inclusion criteria and were excluded. The remaining 81 participants were assigned to either the treatment or usual care group. The inclusion criteria for the study specified age 18 years or older; no previous history or treatment for type 2 diabetes; impaired fasting glucose, which was as defined as >100 mg/dL and <126 mg/dL or an HbA1c of 5.7% to 6.4%; body mass index ≥25; and not already regularly active (defined as >30 min-

utes each day of moderate-intensity activity for 5 days). Exclusion criteria included a history of type 2 diabetes or use of antidiabetic medications; concomitant medication known to interfere with glucose metabolism, such as systemic corticosteroids; use of weight loss drugs; pregnancy or breastfeeding; refusal or inability to give informed consent to participate in the study; hospitalization for heart disease, stroke, or transient ischemic attack in the previous 6 months; and mental incapacity, unwillingness, or language barrier precluding adequate understanding or cooperation.[33]

At the second visit, participants who met the criteria were randomized into the study to receive medical nutrition therapy or usual care. Participants in the usual care group returned after 12 weeks to complete a final visit. They did not receive medical nutrition therapy.

Intervention

The treatment group received medical nutrition therapy provided by the RDN based on the American Diabetes Association Standards of Medical Care in Diabetes–2017 providing EBP recommendations for preventing diabetes.[34] Recommendations included education to promote moderate weight loss of 5% to 7% of starting weight, regular physical activity (150 min/week), and strategies to reduce energy and dietary fat intake.[34] Individualized goals included risk factors associated with type 2 diabetes and appropriate weight loss goals. Macronutrient distribution was individually modified for the participant, but all were encouraged to consume foods containing whole grains. Alcohol was limited to moderate consumption (one drink per day or less for adult women and two drinks per day or less for adult men).[35] The RDN calculated caloric goals for each participant using the Mifflin-St. Jeor equation as recommended by the Academy of Nutrition and Dietetics EAL for calculating resting metabolic rate for individuals who are overweight or obese.[36] The carbohydrate content of meals and snacks was kept consistent.

Interpreting and Determining Relevance to Practice

The medical nutrition therapy group achieved a greater magnitude of change from baseline in HbA1c levels compared with the usual care group. Mean HbA1c in the medical nutrition therapy group decreased from 5.99% to 5.79%, while HbA1c in the usual care group increased to 6.01%.

Dissemination of Findings and Application to Practice

The authors had the following conclusion: "With the increasing prevalence of prediabetes, the role of MNT [medical nutrition therapy] following practice guidelines can lead to improvement in metabolic control. Preliminary results indicate MNT by a RDN was associated with improved clinical outcomes, specifically HbA1c and Diabetes Risk Score. In addition, changes in behavior were cited in the MNT group due to increased fruit and vegetable consumption as well as physical activity. It seems reasonable to conclude that the beneficial medical outcomes from MNT may prevent or delay the onset of [type 2 diabetes]. With the economic burden resulting from diabetes, MNT should be considered for reimbursement in the treatment of prediabetes to reduce diabetes risk."[33]

New research questions were developed from this study, including the following:

- Would a longer intervention period with multiple sites show similar results?
- Does a longer period of intervention result in a further decrease in HbA1C levels?
- What are the optimal number and frequency of intervention visits to RDNs to decrease HbA1C levels?

Thus, new research questions are devised and the practice-research-practice cycle continues with related or follow-up studies. For example, in another study, the intensive lifestyle intervention group in the Diabetes Prevention Program had a greater effect on HbA1c levels than the metformin group and the standard lifestyle recommendation group.[36]

USING RESEARCH TO HELP SOLVE PROBLEMS: CASE EXAMPLES

As RDNs read research studies in the literature, they should look for ways to integrate findings into prac-

tice and carefully weigh the scientific evidence. When reading and examining reports, key questions should come to mind: Are there practical applications for these investigative findings? How does this study affect patients or the setting? How can I apply this information to my setting? Such questions are the basic tenets of EBP, and evidence analysis databases should be consulted for additional insight and applicable studies.

Knowledge of research methods is required to understand articles in the scientific literature. Critical analysis is useful when reading investigative reports and articles to determine if the purpose and need of the study are supported, the methods are appropriate, the findings indicate accurate interpretation of the data, conclusions are sound, strengths and limitations are presented, and references are well chosen and up to date. Some published research studies may contain inconsistencies or gaps in knowledge. Practitioners should evaluate the quality of each report and determine if the study has weaknesses that limit its application to a particular health care setting. After a thorough literature search from a myriad of information sources, including narrative and systematic reviews, the clinical question can be further refined to include the patient or problem; intervention (cause, prognostic factors, and treatment); comparison intervention, if appropriate; and outcomes to be measured. The Academy of Nutrition and Dietetics uses a Quality Criteria Checklist: Primary Research, available at the EAL, which can assist practitioners with the appropriate questions for guiding the critical appraisal of the study's relevance and validity to practice.[37]

To develop a framework for investigating a nutrition intervention, various research theories and methods can be used to collect data about the patient population, institution, and community.[17] This information is vital in planning and testing the most efficient and effective delivery of nutrition services. An instrument can be developed to collect pertinent information for a pilot study, or an instrument that incorporates the nutrition care process can be pretested and adapted to a specific setting. Questions such as the following can be asked:

- What population is served by this institution or agency (numbers, age, gender, economic status)?

- What are the poulation's nutritional needs (diagnosis, health status, mobility)?
- What resources are available to help deliver nutrition services (infrastructure, time, funds, personnel, other health care professionals)?

The past two decades have seen an increase in randomized clinical trials that include nutrition. Research sponsored by the NIH, other governmental agencies, and food and pharmaceutical companies have broadened the responsibilities of RDNs as study managers and clinical coordinators, investigators in clinical and translational research centers, and employees in independent research organizations. For RDNs who are entering these positions or embarking on research in clinical settings, perusing the Academy of Nutrition and Dietetics EAL or other systematic databases helps the investigator review the published research to determine the extent of practical and clinical relevance before changing or testing treatment protocols. Data should be carefully scrutinized to determine the validity of the study and the importance to clinical and patient outcomes for an individual setting, as shown in the earlier cycle of research example.[34]

EPB that measures outcomes is the standard the medical and nutrition professions expect to have a positive effect on delivering patient care, evaluating economic factors, and controlling clinical and functional outcomes in intervention trials. Outcomes research tests the effectiveness of an intervention under ordinary or usual circumstances.[21] Research on outcomes (clinical, patient, or cost) helps determine what is effective and what is not effective in health care. For example, the cost-effectiveness of a new nutrition intervention can be tested by comparing it with the usual treatment option or by analyzing medical nutrition therapy outcomes for a subset of patients with diabetes. The purpose is to help patients, providers, payers, and administrators make the appropriate choices regarding medical treatment options and health care policy. Outcomes research builds evidence for nutrition practice.[21]Applying an evidence-based approach has created a model to show the effectiveness of medical nutrition therapy for the profession along with guidelines and tool kits for practitioners to apply during their daily responsibilities.[36]

Research to Observe and Alter Practice

Documenting and measuring practice standards can provide evidence of the effectiveness of nutrition care being delivered. Standards of professional practice and evidence-based guidelines are intended to help RDNs decide how various food and nutrients are delivered.[38] If the practitioner cannot demonstrate effectiveness, the research findings can lead to further investigation to alter practice and produce more positive outcomes.

EXAMPLE
Research to Observe Practice

Portion control and appropriate portion sizes are a continuing topic for RDNs in private practice, outpatient clinics, inpatient facilities, and community settings. A recent qualitative study provides an example of how to address visual estimates of dietary intakes of hospital patients. In Japan, 10 nurses and 10 dietitians were interviewed to assess their perceptions of accuracy of patient intakes using visual estimation methods. Three methods were discussed: self-reports, visual estimates, and the weighed method as the gold standard for measuring hospital food intake. Their observations of how food is served and evaluation of plate waste were recorded and analyzed. Based on grounded theory, three themes emerged: measurement, data input, and training for raters. The researchers found that no standard procedures were set for recording estimates of individual food intake. Dietitians and nurses differed in how they evaluated meals consumed. Nurses and nursing assistants always recorded plate waste, but portion sizes were difficult to assess because they did not see the food when it was served. Dietitians reported that they understood portion sizes but had less access to measuring plate waste. They visited patients selectively based on nutritional status, special interventions, need of feeding assistance, poor appetite, and postsurgery or tube feedings. The authors concluded that the project provided data to support better training of staff and refinement of practices to improve accuracy of measuring dietary intake of hospital patients.[39]

Research to Change Practice

Research is useful to monitor activities or procedures, solve problems, and change practice by finding a better way to deliver food and nutrition services. According to Zoellner and colleagues,[17] dissemination and implementation models can be applied to change practice in translational research.

EXAMPLE
Research to Change Practice

With the publication of the Chronic Kidney Disease-Mineral and Bone Disorder Clinical Practice Guidelines of the National Kidney Foundation [40] and guidelines of the Kidney Disease-Improving Global Outcomes group,[41] as well as the increased implementation of treatment algorithms,[42] registered dietitian nutritionists (RDNs) are noticing new demands to change their current practice and assume the role of bone mineral managers within their respective institutions. As integral members of the heath care team, RDNs are especially suited to take an active role in managing their patients' bone mineral algorithms, as they have the requisite didactic knowledge and experiential training. This 18-month retrospective study of adult patients undergoing maintenance hemodialysis (n=252) examined the effectiveness of an RDN-managed bone metabolism algorithm compared with one managed by non-RDNs (a registered nurse and a nephrologist) for addressing serum phosphorus levels and related clinical outcomes (corrected serum calcium level, intact parathyroid hormone level, incidence of parathyroidectomy) before and after the change in management of a comprehensive bone metabolism treatment algorithm. On average, serum phosphorus, parathyroid hormone, and serum calcium levels were equivalent during both the RDN-managed and non–RDN-managed time points, thereby indicating that RDNs may be as equally effective as non-RDNs in bone metabolism management. Further research is needed to prospectively examine the impact of RDN management on these specific bone disease outcomes or parameters. Nonetheless, this study provides convincing evidence for a potentially expanding role for RDNs practicing in chronic kidney disease setting, and identifies areas to change clinical care within these settings.[43]

EXAMPLE
Research to Change Practice

A retrospective chart review was done before and after implementation of nutrition support guidelines to determine how the guidelines affected energy and protein intake for critically ill children. The sample included 520 admissions to a pediatric intensive care unit (PICU). A PICU regisetered dietitian nutritionist (RDN) conducted a 45-minute introductory training session and clarified the clinical care guidelines to the interdisciplinary pediatric team on rounds over a 2-month period. One month after the training period, enteral, parenteral, and intravenous feeding data were collected over an 8-day period. Energy and protein needs were calculated, along with anthropometrics, severity of illness, and malnutrition parameters. The nutrition support team found higher intakes of energy and protein after the guidelines were instituted. These findings suggest that communications and training by the RDN and other team members are required to support continuous quality improvements. By implementing the nutrition support guidelines, this project demonstrated a positive effect on clinical outcomes and the potential to achieve optimal feeding for critically ill children in a PICU.[44]

Research to Document Effectiveness

More and more research studies and projects document patient and cost outcomes with medical nutrition therapy provided by RDNs. The advent of EBP has made a difference in assessing the effectiveness of RDNs who deliver medical nutrition therapy for chronic diseases. Early intervention and monitoring of patients can help reduce the incidence of diabetes, cardiovascular disease, and cancer.[36,45] Besides EBP, adoption of the nutrition care process in dietetics helps to solidify a strong foundation for research in the profession. Use of the nutrition care process encourages RDNs and dietetics students to increase the body of dietetics research through the measurement of outcomes.[46]

EXAMPLE
Effectiveness in Practice

A partial feeding study assessed the adoption of a Mediterranean-style diet for postmenopausal women based on selected cardiovascular health outcomes. Over a 6-month period, 16 participants entered a control and intervention phase. The intervention included diet counseling by an RDN that emphasized increased fruits, vegetables, fiber, and n-3 polyunsaturated fatty acids and reduced saturated fat, n-6 polyunsaturated fatty acids, and simple sugars. The participants met four times with RDNs for dietary guidance, learned principles of the Mediterranean-style diet, and were given selected foods (olive oil, walnuts, and fatty fish) at 3-week intervals during the intervention. The investigators measured 3-day food records and serum fatty acid and lipid profiles. The RDN counseling resulted in patients following the Mediterranean-style diet regimen as indicated from food records and improvements in their lipid profiles. Triglycerides showed a clinically meaningful decline, and high-density lipoprotein cholesterol increased. This pilot study primarily focused on postmenopausal women with age as the primary risk factor and the adoption of a dietary pattern. A larger intervention study with diet counseling by RDNs could document the effectiveness of medical nutrition therapy and nutrition education for cardiovascular disease in a similar population.[45]

EXAMPLE
Effectiveness in Practice

The systematic accumulation of a body of scientific evidence can be used to incorporate new approaches into clinical practice and to influence nutrition policy. A systematic review and meta-analysis were conducted to address the effectiveness, cost, and cost-effectiveness for diabetes prevention. The effects of instituting lifestyle interventions by RDNs compared with non-RDNs and by mode of delivery were the primary measures (in person vs technology). Six databases were accessed for relevant articles, and 69 articles met the inclusion criteria for the analysis and synthesis of study findings. Although only 4 of the 69 studies reported costs, the investigators found that lifestyle interventions were effective in reducing weight and glucose-related outcomes. Although RDN interventions, including nutrition education, accomplished greater weight loss than interventions by other personnel, the in-person vs technology-delivered interventions were comparable and showed a similar trend across different delivery channels.[47]

The systematic collection of a body of scientific evidence can be used to incorporate new approaches into dietetics practice. Systematic reviews, which typically take 18 months or more, summarize the scientific literature on a particular topic or research question, following a rigid methodology to conduct a thorough search and weighing the quality, strength, and significance of each study or publication. The summary of evidence should be balanced and unbiased. Often, a meta-analysis accompanies a systematic review and is done to combine studies into one result that estimates the statistical strength of the evidence.[21]

Research Reports to Solve Practice Problems

An examination of resources and guidelines to explain and augment practice projects helps to clarify and justify the process of incorporating new inquiries into practice-based research. When confronting a practice problem, some steps may facilitate planning the project and moving it along. These steps include appointing a committee or work group, defining the problem and specific aims, making assignments to committee members, setting a time frame, and organizing ongoing meetings or periodic contacts to discuss progress, refocusing if necessary, and keeping the project on target to completion. Close collaboration and agreement on each step break down the project to small units according to each hypothesis, type of analysis, or step in the investigative process.

EXAMPLE
Collaborative Study

An inpatient staffing study, conducted through the Clinical Nutrition Management dietetic practice group and the Nutrition Research Network of the Academy of Nutrition and Dietetics, helped to answer a long-standing question: What is the appropriate RDN staffing ratio in acute care settings? Investigators collected data at three levels: facility, RDN, and patient. A total of 353 RDNs in 78 facilities across the United States participated and tracked their time caring for each inpatient. All RDNs were trained on how to collect and document patient encounters to obtain consistent and accurate data. The project represented a wide range of bed sizes and complex patient cases. Based on data from 47,000 adult and pediatric patient encounters, the investigators were able to create an equation that clinical nutrition managers could use to predict staff time needed based on the number of patients and complexity of cases. The project did not collect patient outcomes, so it cannot be considered a gold standard model, but it helped to answer a question that was important to clinical nutrition managers. As a collaboration between research experts (Nutrition Research Network staff and statisticians) and clinical nutrition managers who were experts in the practice area, the project was designed to be feasible for the participating RDNs to contribute data.[46] Data were gathered in 3 months and then compared, analyzed, and shared with an oversight committee for further interpretation. When the project was completed, the clinical nutrition managers disseminated the results to their colleagues at meetings and to other health care providers in their institutions through a similar format.

Research to Improve Quality of Patient-Centered Care

Quality improvement (QI) is one important way to apply research techniques to measure practice and "to design and test interventions to change pro-cesses and systems of care."[48] RDNs are qualified to lead these efforts, and well-planned studies combine aspects of EBP and QI. Quality management is the area where there is overlap for applying qualitative and quantitative measures to collect structural, procedural, or outcome data and to improve daily patient care.

QI has been aligned with nutrition and dietetics practice since the 1990s. Much of the original efforts to ensure its adoption in the profession came from the Quality Management Committee of the Academy of Nutrition and Dietetics.[2] Emphasis on QI has persisted, and the Institute of Medicine has called for the delivery of patient-centered care and respect for all patients.[48] The focus for QI is to "identify errors and hazards in care and measure quality of care (structures, process, and outcomes) for patients."[49] For RDNs, quality care means listening to patients, giving clear food and nutrition information, and being an advocate for prevention and health.[21]

Renewed interest in QI has occurred with an emphasis on food and nutrition quality services. The Institute of Medicine report *Health Professions Education: A Bridge to Quality* spurred health care providers to refocus their efforts on improving practice. The report encouraged five educational priorities to prepare health care professionals for future practice: patient-centered care, EBP, QI, interdisciplinary teamwork, and health informatics.[48] Various health professional organizations have examined their adherence to these priorities. In 2015, an online survey was sent to 535 directors of accredited dietetics education programs to determine the extent to which the Institute of Medicine recommendations were implemented in their programs. The directors (response rate=35%) reported inclusion of EBP and patient-centered care most frequently, at 92% and 84%, respectively, followed by interdisciplinary teams and health informatics. QI was included the least at 42%. Respondents noted barriers to incorporating all of the education priorities (lack of faculty, inadequate time in the curriculum, and few university structures for implementation).[49]

EXAMPLE
Research to Improve Quality Practices for Patient-Centered Care

The clinical nutrition literature supports the need for adequate enteral nutrition in intensive care unit patients, but underfeeding still exists. A quality improvement (QI) project was instituted to determine the effect of volume-based feeding on adequacy of enteral nutrition delivery and provision of energy and protein in a surgical/trauma intensive care unit (STICU) compared with usual practice (prescribed hourly rate). Based on a prior QI audit indicating that only 37% of enteral nutrition was being supplied to patients on the unit, the STICU team, led by an RDN, instituted a feeding protocol (Feed Early Enteral Diet Adequately for Maximum Effect or FEED ME). Several steps were taken to begin the project:

- gaining approval of the institutional review board and QI committee,
- addressing the concerns of the medical staff,
- establishing a clear protocol for calculating new feeding rates, and
- launching a 10-week educational campaign with physicians and nurses.

Electronic health records of 111 mechanically ventilated STICU patients, fed at least 72 hours after achieving their target goal of enteral nutrition during their first week of admission, were reviewed retrospectively. Data were obtained before (n=54) and after (n=56) initiation of a volume-based feeding protocol. The two groups were similar in patient demographics, clinical characteristics, and nutrition practices. The proportion of enteral nutrition volume and energy delivered increased significantly (rate based, 63%; FEED ME, 89%), as did grams of protein per kilogram body weight using the FEED ME protocol. Only slightly more diarrhea was noted in gastric-fed patients, and the incidence of gastric residual volume and emesis was similar. Success of FEED ME depended on nursing compliance (90% during the QI review and 82% after an 11-month reaudit). A change in the standard of practice was achieved by an enteral nutrition volume-based feeding approach in a STICU based on a significant improvement in the adequacy of energy and protein delivered, with only a slight increase in diarrhea.[50]

DEFINING THE PROBLEM: EMPHASIS ON THE BEGINNING TO GET TO THE END

A research project should begin with a clearly written and definitive practice question that is specific to what should be measured. When using the EBP framework, the practice question may contain four critical components: statement of the patient or problem of interest (P), the intervention (I), the comparison with a control group (C), and the measured outcomes (O). An example of a practice-based question related to nutrition and chronic kidney disease might be the following: Does a modular supplement (I) increase serum albumin levels (O) higher than a nutritionally complete product (C) does in patients on maintenance dialysis (P)? Practice-based questions may also arise from the results of a QI study in an institution or through online dietetic practice group forums and practitioner-focused webinars. The inquiry begins with a problem or question: what one wants to know about one's practice that would be useful. The question should be clearly defined at the outset with an answer that is measurable. After putting the question in writing, the practitioner should work on refining and clarifying it. With further thought, the question usually expands and evolves into a broader statement; however, an effort should be made to tighten and focus the problem and allow measurement of very specific variables. Coulston[51] proposes the following format for research questions in clinical dietetics practice:

- What is the nutritional status of patients with, or at risk of developing, specific diseases?
- What are the nutrient requirements of patients with specific diseases, and how do they differ from the requirements of the healthy population?
- What is the efficacy of nutrition intervention: in the prevention of disease, as adjunctive therapy, as primary treatment for specific diseases?

An extensive review of the literature provides ideas for methodology and shows how other researchers have handled similar questions. A review can disclose sources of information, including unpublished work that may not be known. The review can help the investigator evaluate the proposed project and allows comparisons with other studies. For RDNs embarking on new ventures, scientific databases and systematic reviews (Cochrane Database of Systematic Reviews, EAL, Evidence-Based Medicine Reviews) have expanded access to investigations and researchers worldwide (see Chapter 10). A comprehensive search can give information on descriptions of participants, sample selections, inclusion and exclusion criteria for participants, outcomes or end points used, validated instruments or researcher-designed tools, reported results and significance, and gaps and limitations of previous studies. The investigator should locate the strongest available evidence and then determine the following:

● What is the unique contribution of the proposed study?
● Will the proposed study contribute to expanding knowledge or will it verify previous investigations?
● Does the proposed study validate outcomes of a nutrition intervention or improve patient care?

In appraising the clinical nutrition literature, it may be wise to begin with the EAL to determine what questions have been asked and to discern gaps in the research related to nutrition and dietetics practice. It may help pose questions to clarify the problem and the study design. Can new information or additional qualitative and quantitative data help solve the problem? An exhaustive search sometimes provides the information that answers the question without the need for further study.

It can also be useful to explore whether an existing theoretical model can be used to tackle the problem. Some studies may provide such a model and eliminate some steps in the research process or identify key investigators to contact for more explanation of study designs and their analysis. Discussions with peers—especially peers with research experience—often help refine the details of the study plan or protocol. Collaborative partnerships like the NRN also offer an opportunity for joining professionals in educational institutions, research centers, and practice settings to conduct projects

that benefit the community or a specific patient population.

After developing the question and conducting the literature search, a design for the study is selected. Preparing a proposal or research protocol is necessary to clearly delineate the procedures and processes for data collection and IRB approval. A pilot study is useful to test for any problems in the methodology and provides an opportunity to make adaptations before undertaking a larger investigation or applying for internal or external funding.

The data analysis procedures should be planned at the beginning of the study, not after the data are collected. In conducting research in the practice setting, resources for collecting, analyzing, and interpreting data may be limited. The process may need to be simplified to complete the project with the resources available. Assistance may be obtained from a senior staff member, a statistician, or an academician interested in practice-based research.

Finally, investigators must remember to disseminate findings within and outside their own institution or agency. If the study or project was conducted according to the plan approved by the IRB or the investigators sought guidance from colleagues and internal committees, results should be shared broadly (see Box 29.3).

Present a poster session at a regional or national meeting.

Give a lecture or demonstration to a local, regional, or national meeting.

Represent your specialty on an interdisciplinary team or community committee.

Provide periodic research updates to colleagues.

Publish findings in a scientific or practice-focused journal.

Contribute regularly to an affiliate or dietetic practice group newsletter or blog about new research findings in nutrition and dietetics.

Box 29.3 Ways to Disseminate Practice-Based Research

OVERCOMING BARRIERS TO QUALITY RESEARCH: WHERE DO WE GO FROM HERE?

Despite the concerted effort to enhance and increase research involvement, RDNs still have limited activity in the research process.[52-55] Some of the factors that affect RDNs' research involvement are related to their level of education or academic training; research knowledge and skills; areas of practice; and perceptions, attitudes, and knowledge of EBP. A number of barriers to conducting research are described as individual or organizational factors.[56] Individual factors relate to the extent of research experience, level of confidence, and content knowledge and skills. Organizational factors concern time, staffing, money, institutional and administrative support, and other resources.[57]

Getting started with research in the practice setting is the first giant step. Assessing the needs and resources available to implement investigations is crucial to productive planning. Although not technically a research method, a QI project could be the first attempt at doing research in the workplace. QI is a technique to study a complex institutional process or system and to solve ongoing problems in caring for patients.[21] Sometimes QI projects precede a fully developed research study that examines patient outcomes of care and establishes an RDN-led team of researchers in an institution.[50]

Knowledge Constraints

Many investigators have examined ways to overcome barriers and widen the practitioner-researcher base in the dietetics profession. Lack of knowledge and skills is the principal barrier to involvement in RDN surveys. Knowledge of research methods is facilitated with practice-based studies. Studies have shown that EBP has a positive effect on increasing research activity.[53,54] Overall, knowledge can be improved by taking courses or pursuing an advanced degree or training. Participating in actual projects and developing strong organizational skills to manage data and research team members or volunteers also build confidence.

Continuing professional education (CPE) is often mentioned as the key to improving knowledge and skills. The 2011 Academy of Nutrition and Dietetics member survey identified not only CPE but also adding more skills in undergraduate education and actual participation in research projects.[15] Sometimes CPE is better received in a group format or a collaborative project reinforced by colleagues. Another recommendation for increasing skills has been to get involved with EBP as a consumer, reviewer, evidence analyst, NRN member, or mentor.

Learning how to conduct research is essential for success. Many individuals are afraid to initiate investigations, but involvement usually builds confidence. Following are some ideas for building research knowledge and skills[52-56]:

- Obtain an advanced degree with a research-focused curriculum.
- Take a research design, methods, or statistics course.
- Critique the research literature and talk with researchers.
- Test protocols and validated practice guidelines.
- Learn about experiences in conducting research projects to avoid pitfalls.
- Join a practice-based network to reach out to other investigators for practical advice.
- Contact local universities for research guidance and mentoring.
- Use tools like ANDHII to access anonymous data for large collaborations.
- Participate in webinars and elearning about how to conduct investigations.
- Establish research affiliations within and outside the workplace.
- Learn how to do systematic reviews and write grants and proposals.
- Join an interdisciplinary research group as the RDN researcher.
- Become a peer reviewer for clinical manuscripts.
- Guide students and interns in conducting a QI project or research study.

Time and Other Constraints

Sufficient time, another concern of dietetics practitioners, must be found to conduct practice-related research. Lack of time is the second most frequent reason for not becoming involved in research.[10] Time for research needs to be carved out of an already full schedule within the daily or weekly routine. Finding support from a supervisor to set a certain amount of time aside for research may occur if QI or cost-effectiveness studies or other topics benefit the organization.[57]

Responsibilities could be augmented to devote time to do research. An evaluation of existing responsibilities as part of the clinician's annual goal setting may help reset priorities for research time. Consulting evidence-based resources, where the content is already critically reviewed, helps practitioners stay abreast of emerging research and new findings, an especially helpful technique when time is limited. Structuring professional reading time or journal clubs into daily activities also keeps practitioners current. Despite these suggestions, a willingness to devote some personal time to early development of any research investigation is usually necessary. However, time commitment for research was less of a concern in a recent examination of research outcome expectations.[58]

Staff members may not be available or interested in assisting the principal investigator when a research project is in the planning stages. Enlisting department staff members to collaborate in at least some part of the project is vital. It may be easier to motivate staff (representatives from QI, HIPAA or research compliance, medical records, informatics) if the investigation has the potential to make their jobs easier or more efficient and if the focus is a QI project or a research initiative of the larger organization. Other health professionals (physicians, nurses, therapists, pharmacists) within an institution may be interested in the project and provide essential content expertise that is integral to the project's success. Study coordinators in a research office may help with patient recruitment, the IRB process, and institutional requirements, and statisticians can assist with study design, data analysis, and interpretation of results. Undergraduate and graduate students are another valuable resource. Students are often eager to participate in projects that expose them to the research process and opportunities to interact with other professionals.[28,29]

Dietetics practitioners must recognize that funds generally are not allocated for their first efforts at research. Selecting data that are readily available is desirable; for example: What laboratory values are already collected that could be used for end points? Are data analysis systems in place in the institution? Working through a pilot study may be an excellent method of learning how to utilize an existing data analysis program. The project should be planned to keep within the resources available. If the investigator must input data manually, the study design should be in keeping with this limitation. Even though new investigator funds are limited, occasionally institutions or dietetic practice groups contribute funds for projects that can advance practice or improve systems of care. Discussing potential research projects with administrative leadership may uncover foundations or intramural sources of funding that have shared interests in the research concept.

Implementing any research necessitates permission from supervisors or superiors. Reorganization of duties or staffing must be authorized. Cooperation and permission are needed to make use of equipment and facilities, such as space and computer time. Permission from physicians, patients, and IRBs is necessary for human participant research. HIPAA and state regulations that protect patient privacy must also be adhered to. Practitioners must go through the appropriate channels to organize a project. Explaining the possible benefits of the study or the potential for higher productivity often encourages cooperation from the institution or agency.

Turning Barriers into Opportunities

Barriers can become opportunities by adopting new behaviors and attitudes toward research in practice. Supports identified in the literature include education, especially CPE on evidence-based research, teamwork, and building research capacity and interprofessional networks.[58,59] Mentoring and finding research guidance are identified as important to increasing confidence and a sense of accomplishment.[58] Mentors encourage ingenuity, collaboration, and persistence for managing the barriers that may impede implementation of practice-related research projects.

Several investigators have examined ways to overcome barriers and enlarge the practitioner-researcher base in the nutrition and dietetics profession.[53-59] A personal interest in research has been a chief motivator for becoming involved in research.[14] The more RDNs are interested in research activities, the more likely they are to be become involved. Studies found early experience with research stimulated more interest and predicted involvement.[32,34,53] Other predictors of research involvement include level of education, attitudes and knowledge about EBP, number of prior research courses, frequency and continuity of reading research, and keeping professionally up to date and active.[32,34,53,54] Early educational experiences in research have also been recommended by the Institute of Medicine. The report calls for undergraduate exposure to research and research-focused curriculum with an emphasis on EBP for all health practitioners.[48]

Barriers can be offset by the rewards of engaging in research and new discovery. Some supports for increasing research engagement by RDNs have been suggested: engaging in organized and self-directed CPE, participating in interprofessional collaborations and team projects, joining a professional network, and gaining administrative support and recognition.[58,59] In a study of research outcome expectations by King and colleagues,[59] the most frequently identified research outcome expectations were professional development and respect from others. They also noted personal satisfaction; self-worth; financial, job, and professional opportunities; and associations with others as benefits. Discussion forums in the qualitative arm of the study revealed three additional categories important to RDNs: impact on patient care, confidence, and communication with the health care team. King and colleagues suggest interventions to help RDNs achieve research knowledge and skills as shown in their education intervention study.

An array of topics could be studied by researcher-practitioners to improve practice and open up new vistas for the dietetics profession. The following research topics might be addressed to expand the body of research literature in nutrition and dietetics:

- Document clinical practice and assess the effectiveness of medical nutrition therapy in selected nutrition-related diseases.
- Investigate the team approach to determine what RDN-provided aspect of care (eg, EBP guidelines, education, counseling) contributed to improved patient or client outcomes.
- Measure patient outcomes based on RDN staffing in health care facilities.
- Compare different prevention and treatment models of nutrition intervention and outcomes for patients over time.
- Evaluate the achievement of QI methods of food and nutrition services in various settings.
- Participate in joint projects across institutions as a contributor to the NRN.

CONCLUSION

By incorporating research, the opportunities to refine and change dietetics practice are endless. Important to making research a part of every RDN's responsibilities are good analytic skills and a commitment to building the evidence base for ethical and scientific nutrition and dietetics practice. RDNs should contribute to the advancement of the profession by reading critically, designing and executing studies carefully, and disseminating findings broadly.

REFERENCES

1. Smitherman AL, Wyse BW. The backbone of our profession. *J Am Diet Assoc.* 1987; 87:1394-1396.

2. Stein K. Propelling the profession with outcomes and evidence: building a robust research agenda at the Academy. *J Acad Nutr Diet.* 2016;116(6):1014-1030.

3. Tatum C, Touger-Decker R, Brody R, Byham-Gray L, O'Sullivan-Maillet J. Perceived needs for graduate level clinical nutrition education for registered dietitians. *Top Clin Nutr.* 2008;23(4):320-332.

4. Sims LS, Simko MD. Applying research methods in nutrition and dietetics: embodiment of the profession's backbone. *J Am Diet Assoc.* 1988;88:1045-1046.

5. Byham-Gray LD. A review of the "body" and the "backbone"for the dietetics profession. *Top Clin Nutr.* 2005;20(1):2008-2015.

6. Dwyer JT. Scientific underpinnings for the profession: dietitians in research. In: *Challenging the Future of Dietetic Education and Credentialing: Dialogue, Discovery, Directions.* Proceedings of the Consensus Conference held June 12–14, 1994, Itasca, IL. Chicago, IL: American Dietetic Association; 1993.

7. Monsen ER, ed. *Research: Successful Approaches.* 2nd ed. Chicago, Ill: American Dietetic Association; 2003.

8. Wylie-Rosett J, Wheeler M, Krueger K, Halford B. Opportunities for research-oriented dietitians. *J Am Diet Assoc.* 1990;90(11):1531-1534.

9. Gehlbach SH. *Interpreting the Medical Literature.* 6th ed. New York, NY: McGraw-Hill; 2009.

10. Byham-Gray LD. Gilbride JA, Dixon LB, Stage FK. Predictors for research involvement among dietitians. *J Am Diet Assoc.* 2006;106(12): 2008-2015.

11. King C, Parrott JS, Hand R. A cross-sectional exploration of research outcome expectations. *Top Clin Nutr.* 2016; 31(2):147-167.

12. Making the case for research. Academy of Nutrition and Dietetics website. www.eatrightpro.org/research /philosophy-and-structure/making-the-case-for-research. Accessed May 4, 2018.

13. Byham-Gray LD. *Dietitians' Perceptions, Attitudes, and Knowledge of Evidence-Based Practice and Involvement in Research Activities* [dissertation]. New York, NY: New York University; 2004.

14. Academy of Nutrition and Dietetics House of Delegates. *Engaging Members in Research.* HOD Backgrounder. Chicago, IL: Academy of Nutrition and Dietetics; 2014.

15. Hand RK. Research in nutrition and dietetics–what can the Academy do for you? *J Acad Nutr Diet.* 2014;114(1): 131-135.

16. Anchondo IM, Campbell C, Zoellner J. Academy of Nutrition and Dietetics 2011 survey on member research activities, needs and perceptions. *J Acad Nutr Diet.* 2014; 114(5):803-810.

17. Zoellner J, Van Horn L, Gleason PM, Boushey CJ. What is translational research? Concepts and applications in Nutrition and Dietetics. *J Acad Nutr Diet.* 2015;115(7): 1057-1071.

18. Dougherty CM, Burrowes JD, Hand RK. Why registered dietitian nutritionists are not doing research—perceptions, barriers, and participation in research from the Academy's Dietetics Practice-Based Research Network Needs Assessment Survey. *J Acad Nutr Diet.* 2015;115(6): 1001-1007.

19. Camp K, Trijullo E. Position of the Academy of Nutrition and Dietetics: nutritional genomics. *J Acad Nutr Diet.* 2014;114(2):299-312.

20. Molinar LS, Childers AF, Hoggle L, Kent S, Porter H, Rusnak S. Informatics initiatives at the Academy of Nutrition and Dietetics. *J Acad Nutr Diet.* 2017;117(8): 1293-1301.

21. Drummond KE, Murphy-Reyes A. *Nutrition Research: Concepts and Applications.* Burlington, MA: Jones & Bartlett Learning; 2018.

22. Dalton S. The confluence of research and practice. *Top Clin Nutr.* 2009;24;(1):3-5.

23. Cohen DA, Byham-Gray L, Denmark RM. Impact of two pulmonary enteral formulations on nutritional indices and outcomes. *J Hum Nutr Diet.* 2013;26(3):286-293.

24. Byham-Gray LD, Drasher T, Deckman K, et al. Effect of aggressive osteodystrophy management on clinical outcomes in stage 5 chronic kidney disease. *J Ren Nutr.* 2009;19(4):321-333.

25. Accreditation Council for Education in Nutrition and Dietetics (ACEND). ACEND Accreditation Standards for Nutrition and Dietetics Internship Programs (DI). Academy of Nutrition and Dietetics website. www.eatrightpro .org/-/media/eatrightpro-files/acend/about-program -accreditation/accreditation-standards/2017 -standardsfordiprograms.pdf?la=en&hash=B1F08833AAB C0FA8A6EBB7B76778A09BE7EDB667. Updated January 26, 2018. Accessed May 4, 2018.

26. Accreditation Council for Education in Nutrition and Dietetics (ACEND) ACEND Accreditation Standards for Nutrition and Dietetics Didactic Programs (DPD). Academy of Nutrition and Dietetics website. www.eatrightpro .org/-/media/eatrightpro-files/acend/about-program -accreditation/accreditation-standards/2017 -standardsfordpdprograms.pdf?la=en&hash=18A1A38F32 363415418B9E72E055AC98DD0438C0. Updated January 26, 2018. Accessed May 4, 2018.

27. 2012 ACEND Accreditation Standards in Nutrition and Dietetics. Didactic Programs, Internship and Coordinated Programs. www.eatrightpro.org. Last update March 2015.

28. AbuSabha R. Developing research knowledge and competence in master's students: individualizing group research projects. *J Acad Nutr Diet.* 2016;116(3): 389-394.

29. Harris J, Bruemmer B, Boushey C. Integrating research into dietetics education. Paper presented at the Dietitian Education Program Meeting, Areas 6 and 7. March 25, 2010.

30. Strauss SE, Richardson WS, Glasziou P, Haynes RB. *Evidence-Based Medicine: How to Practice and Teach EBM.* 3rd ed. Edinburgh; New York: Elsevier/Churchill Livingstone; 2005.

31. Byham-Gray LD, Gilbride JA, Dixon LB, Stage FK. Evidence-based practice: what are dietitians' perceptions, attitudes, and knowledge? *J Am Diet Assoc.* 2005;105: 1574-1581.

32. Vogt EA, Byham-Gray L, Touger-Decker R. Perceptions, attitudes, knowledge, and clinical use of evidence-based practice among US registered dietitians: a prospective descriptive pilot study. *Top Clin Nutr.* 2013;28(3):283-294.

33. Parker A, Byham-Gray L, Denmark R, Winkle PJ. The effect of medical nutrition therapy by a registered dietitian nutritionist in patients with prediabetes participating in a randomized controlled clinical research trial. *J Acad Nutr Diet.* 2014;114(11):1739-1748.

34. American Diabetes Association. Standards of Medical Care in Diabetes—2017. *Diabetes Care.* 2017;40 (1):S1-S132.

35. American Diabetes Association. Nutrition recommendations and interventions for diabetes. *Diabetes Care.* 2008;31(suppl 1):S61-S78.

36. Diabetes Prevention Program Research Group. Reduction in the incidence of type 2 diabetes with lifestyle intervention or metformin. *N Engl J Med.* 2002;346(6): 393-403.

37. Academy of Nutrition and Dietetics. *Evidence Analysis Manual: Steps in the Academy Evidence Analysis Process.* Appendix 8: Quality Criteria Checklist: Primary Research, p. 91. www.andeal.org/vault/2440/web/files/2016_April _EA_Manual.pdf. Published April 2016. Accessed March 1, 2017.

38. Academy Quality Management Committee and Scope of Practice Subcommittee of the Quality Management Committee. Academy of Nutrition and Dietetics: revised 2012 Standards of Practice in Nutrition Care and Standards of Professional Performance for Registered Dietitians. *J Acad Nutr Diet.*2013;113(6 suppl):S29-S45.

39. Kawasaki Y, Kijima Y, Akamatsu R. Measuring patient dietary intake using visual estimation methods in Japanese hospitals. *Top Clin Nutr.* 2016; 31(4):335-345.

40. National Kidney Foundation. K/DOQI clinical practice guidelines for bone metabolism and disease in chronic kidney disease. *Am J Kidney Dis.* 2003;42(4 suppl 3): S1-S201.

41. Kidney Disease: Improving Global Outcomes (KDIGO) CKD–MBD Work Group. KDIGO clinical practice guideline for the diagnosis, evaluation, prevention, and treatment of chronic kidney disease–mineral and bone disorder (CKD–MBD). *Kidney Int.* 2009;76(suppl 113): S1-S130.

42. Blair D, Byham-Gray LD, Sweet SJ, et al. Effect of a dietitian-managed bone algorithm on serum phosphorus level in maintenance hemodialysis patients. *J Ren Nutr.* 2013;23(2):98-105.

43. Thompson KL, Davidson P, Swan WI, et al. Nutrition care process chains: the "missing link" between research and evidence-based practice. *J Acad Nutr Diet.* 2015;115(9): 1491-1497.

44. Kyle UG, Lucas L, Mackey G, et al. Implementation of nutrition support guidelines may affect energy and protein intake in the pediatric intensive care unit. *J Acad Nutr Diet.* 2016;116(5):844-851.

45. Bihuniak JD, Ramos A, Huedo-Medina T, et al. Adherence to a Mediterranean-style diet and its influence on cardiovascular risk factors in postmenopausal women. *J Acad Nutr Diet.* 2016;116(11):1767-1775.

46. Hand RK, Jordan B, DeHoog S, Pavlinac J, Abram JK, Parrott JS. Inpatient staffing needs for registered dietitian nutritionist in 21st century acute care facilities. *J Acad Nutr Diet.* 2015;115(6):985-1000.

47. Yu S, You W, Almeida F, Estabrooks P, Davy B. The effectiveness and cost of lifestyle interventions including nutrition education for diabetes prevention: a systematic review and meta-analysis. *J Acad Nutr Diet.* 2017;117(3): 404-421.

48. Institute of Medicine. *Health Professions Education: A Bridge to Quality.* Washington DC: National Academy Press; 2003.

49. Turner P, Eliot K, Kent S, Rusnak S, Landers P. Level of implementation of the Institute of Medicine recommended core competencies among dietetics education programs. *J Acad Nutr Diet.* 2017;117(11): 1709-1716.

50. Taylor B, Brody R, Denmark R, Southard R, Byham-Gray L. Improving enteral delivery through the adoption of the "Feed Early Enteral Diet adequately for Maximum Effect (FEED ME)" protocol in a surgical trauma ICU: a quality improvement review. *Nutr Clin Pract.* 2014; 29(5):639-648.

51. Coulston AM. Make a career of clinical nutrition research. *Top Clin Nutr.* 1995;10(3):29-33.

52. Murphy WJ, Steiber AL. A new breed of evidence and the tools to generate it: introducing ANDHII. *J Acad Nutr Diet.* 2015; 115(1):19-22.

53. Boyd M, Byham-Gray L, Touger-Decker R, Marcus AF, King C. Research interest and research involvement among United States registered dietitians. *Top Clin Nutr.* 2016; 31(3):267-277.

54. Plant MK, Marcus AF, Ziegler J, Byham-Gray L. Testing of a tool to measure practice-based research involvement for registered dietitian nutritionists in clinical practice. *Top Clin Nutr.* 2017;32(1):47-59.

55. King C, Byham-Gray L, Parrott JS, Maillet JOS, Roberts MM, Splett P. Applying social cognitive career theory to registered dietitian research involvement: a randomized controlled trial. *J Allied Health.* 2014;43(4):201-211.

56. Howard A, Ferguson M, Wilkinson P, Campbell K. Involvement in research activities and factors influencing research capacity among dietitians. *J Hum Nutr Diet.* 2013; 26(suppl 1):180-187.

57. King C, Byham-Gray L, Maillet JO, Parrott JS, Splett P, Roberts MM. Dietitians and facilitating research involvement *Top Clin Nutr.* 2014;29(3):227-238.

58. King C, Byham-Gray L, Parrott JS, Maillet JO. Registered dietitians research outcomes expectations: a mixed methods study for content validation. *Digest (Wash D C).* 2015;50(4): 1-8.

59. King C, Byham-Gray L, Parrott JS, Maillet JO, Roberts MM, Splett P. Research self-efficacy in clinical registered dietitians: outcomes of continuing professional education. *Digest (Wash D C).* 2015;50(2):1-12.

Chapter 30

Community-Based Research with a Focus on Diet

Linda Snetselaar, PhD, RDN, LD, FAND | *Angela Odoms-Young, PhD* | *Maria O. Scott, MPH*

LEARNING OBJECTIVES

1. Describe community-based research designs that are used in nutrition and dietetics.

2. Distinguish between qualitative and quantitative outcome measures of community-based research and how they can be used to determine the success of a community intervention.

3. Recognize the importance of community partnerships in community-based research.

Community-based research became an important area of emphasis with the advent of translational research, which follows the path from the biological basis of health and disease to interventions that improve the health of individuals and the public.[1] As one of the pillars of translating research findings into meaningful health outcomes, community-based research provides insights that cannot be achieved in a laboratory or with clinical trials. These insights inform the improvement of interventions and the development of new research questions. The National Center for Advancing Translational Research developed a graphic to show the stages

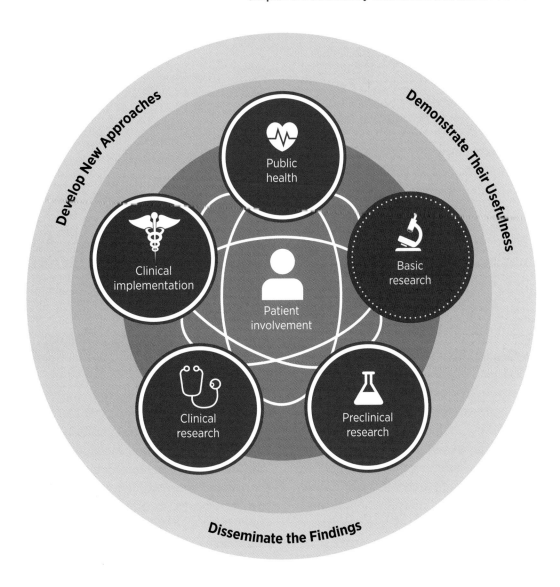

Figure 30.1 The translational science spectrum

Adapted with permission from the National Center for Advancing Translational Sciences.[1]

of research and the way they interact in translational research (see Figure 30.1).[1] Box 30.1 on page 594 explains the types of research included in each stage of the translational research spectrum. The spectrum is not linear as each stage builds on and informs the others.[1,2]

Specific to dietary change, community-based studies give researchers a picture of how successful recommendations can be when not all factors (eg, food availability, social environment) can be controlled. This chapter provides information about the types of community-based research designs and methods used in nutrition and dietetics as well as the importance of community engagement in implementing this work.

COMMUNITY-BASED RESEARCH DESIGN

Consistent with approaches used in health and medicine research, more broadly, community-based study designs in nutrition and dietetics include observational (epidemiologic), quasi-experimental, and experimental methods. Observational studies in community nutrition primarily focus on identifying or understanding risk factors and explaining the

T0: Basic Research	Preclinical and animal studies
T1: Translation to Humans	Proof-of-concept studies and phase 1 clinical trials (highly controlled settings)
T2: Translation to Patients	Phase 2 and 3 clinical trials (clinical application)
T3: Translation to Practice	Comparative effectiveness and clinical outcomes research; dissemination and implementation research
T4: Translation to Communities	Population-level outcomes research

Adapted with permission from The Institute for Clinical and Translational Research, supported by the Clinical and Translational Science Award (CTSA) program, the National Center for Advancing Translational Sciences (NCATS), grant 1UL1TR002373.[1]

Box 30.1 Institute of Medicine Classification System Showing Where Research Sits on the Translational Research Spectrum

patterns of disease associated with dietary behaviors. Quasi-experimental and experimental studies (or community trials)[3] examine the impact of an intervention at the individual/family, organization, community, policy level, or some combination of these to improve dietary behaviors.[4,5]

While not specific to community nutrition research, observational studies examining nutrition-related behaviors can be conducted in a community and typically use a cohort or cross-sectional design to establish links between diet-related risk factors and health outcomes. For example, in prospective cohort studies, a segment or subset of the population is followed over time to determine if a certain exposure or behavior (eg, poor dietary quality) is associated with a specific health outcome (eg, cardiovascular disease).[4-6] Retrospective cohorts are less common and use previously collected data to determine the exposure/disease relationship. Case-control designs are also retrospective but start by identifying individuals with the outcome of interest and then comparing differences in exposure. Observational data can help researchers understand the exposure/outcome relationship as well as the prevalence of the exposure and outcome in a community to help determine an intervention approach. Figure 30.2 outlines various observational study designs and examples of what each can contribute to a specific research question. See Chapter 7 for an explanation of the advantages and disadvantages of various observational and experimental designs.

In community trials, individuals, families, or communities that receive an intervention (eg, nutrition education related to behavioral change) are compared with a control group that has not been exposed to the intervention. Studies that test individual/group interventions commonly use behavioral (eg, dietary behaviors, food purchasing practices, food insecurity) or physiological (eg, body mass index, blood pressure, blood lipids) changes at the population level as outcome measures.[7] When the assignment to intervention or control is random, this design is a randomized controlled trial. Allocation can occur at the individual level or in clusters/groups (cluster-randomized controlled trial). When assignment to the intervention or control group is not random, this design is quasi-experimental. Randomized controlled trials have the most power to detect differences between intervention and control groups. Outcomes are compared using the two groups. Pre/post single group or crossover design, a type of quasi-experimental design where a before and after comparison is made within a single group, has less power than randomized controlled trials. A positive element of pre/post design is that confounding characteristics, such as gender, race, and genetic predisposition, are controlled; a disadvantage is the confounder of time, where external elements like advertising for a new fad diet or a downturn in the economy that causes a population to eat in a different way may confound the study results. Figure 30.3 outlines various experimental

Research Question: Are Cardiovascular Disease (CVD) Risk Factors Associated with Diet Quality?		
Experimental Design	**Approach**	**Findings**
Prospective cohort	Follow a group of children into young adulthood and measure diet quality (exposure) and CVD risk factors (outcome)	Incidence of CVD risk factors in exposed (low diet quality) persons
		Incidence of CVD risk factors in nonexposed (high diet quality) persons
		Association between diet quality and CVD risk factors
		Measures include relative risk, odds ratio, and attributable risk
Cross-sectional	Survey of young adults, including CVD diagnosis and recall of diet quality in childhood	Association between diet quality and CVD risk factors
		Prevalence of CVD factors
		Overall diet quality
Case-control	Compare the childhood diet quality of cases (young adults with CVD) to that of controls (young adults without CVD)	Odds ratio for having CVD risk factors with a specific level of diet quality
		Estimate of attributable risk of CVD risk factors associated with diet quality

Figure 30.2 Sample observational study designs and potential findings

Research Question: Does a Nutrition Education Intervention Improve Diet Quality and Reduce Cardiovascular Disease (CVD) Risk Factors?		
Experimental Design	**Approach**	**Findings**
Randomized controlled trial	Nutrition education intervention to improve diet quality and reduce CVD risk factors; control group receives regular care	Add to evidence base for dietary recommendations
		Measure impact of dietary change in practice compared with more controlled settings (clinical trials)
		Demonstrate causality
Cluster/group randomized controlled trial	Participants are randomized by community to receive either a nutrition education intervention to improve diet quality and reduce CVD risk factors or regular care; environmental changes in intervention communities will also be a part of the intervention (eg, increased availability of healthy options at school and work cafeterias, sales on fruits and vegetables at the supermarket)	Add to evidence base for dietary recommendations
		Measure impact of dietary change in practice compared to more controlled settings (clinical trials)
		Measure impact of community changes
		Demonstrate causality
Quasi-Experimental Design	**Approach**	**Findings**
Pre/post single group	Participants receive nutrition education intervention to improve diet quality and reduce CVD risk factors; preintervention and postintervention measures are compared	Measure impact of dietary change in practice
		Demonstrate causality

Figure 30.3 Sample experimental/quasi-experimental designs and potential findings

study designs and examples of what each can contribute to a specific research question. See Chapter 8 for a discussion of the many factors that must be considered in experimental designs.

Another study design that focuses on communities and behavioral change is the natural experiment, where a real-world community event allows researchers to compare levels of exposure. An example is the building of a full-service supermarket in a disadvantaged neighborhood. The naturally occurring event will allow one community to be compared with another where a full-service supermarket is not available. This type of study allows for a situation that resembles a planned experiment.

QUANTITATIVE AND QUALITATIVE DATA: IDENTIFYING COMMUNITY NEEDS AND EVALUATING COMMUNITY-BASED RESEARCH

Successful community-based research starts with understanding the population. A community needs assessment can be part of the community research process to best meet the needs of the population. This process involves various approaches to gathering information, including, but not limited to, surveys, interviews, focus groups, and checklists of available resources. It can also include data from observational studies. Statistics from surveys, checklists, and observational studies provide quantitative data (ie, results expressed in numbers). Methods such as focus groups and interviews provide qualitative data, which give researchers insight into motives, opinions, feelings, relationships—"the subtleties behind the numbers."[8]

While traditionally quantitative methods alone have been used to identify community needs and evaluate the efficacy of community-based dietary interventions (using measures such as dietary intake assessment), an emerging body of research emphasizes the importance of qualitative methods.[5,9,10] Qualitative research methods are particularly useful for designing a new intervention to ensure that it will meet the needs of a particular target population (eg, low-income pregnant women, college students) and for evaluating satisfaction and effectiveness after a pilot intervention.[11] Both quantitative and

qualitative methods have strengths and weaknesses, and, used together, they can provide a clearer picture of a community's needs and the success of an intervention than they would alone.[12] Often, the most accurate information is found with a mixed-methods approach, that is, using a variety of methods.[10,12]

Qualitative Aspects of Community-Based Research

Recognition is growing of the importance of using qualitative research approaches in understanding dietary behaviors and determining related health and social consequences. Qualitative research includes a collection of naturalistic methodologies and techniques. Qualitative researchers study individuals in their natural settings and attempt to make sense of, or interpret, phenomena in terms of the meanings, concepts, definitions, and characteristics individuals bring to them.[11,13] They acknowledge that experience is subjective—that is, filtered through the perceptions and world views of the individuals undergoing it—and that it is important to understand those perceptions and world views.[8,11,13,14] In community-based research with a focus on diet, qualitative methods can be used in a variety of ways: to provide an in-depth understanding of factors that influence food choice behaviors, as well as the contexts in which these decisions are made; to inform the development or identification of effective intervention strategies for supporting and sustaining dietary behavior; to help evaluate program outcomes; to generate a hypothesis or validate a theory; and to serve as a complement to quantitative research approaches, such as surveys in mixed-methods research, to help better understand quantitative findings.[9,10,14] See Box 30.2.

Consistent with assumptions and designs in qualitative research, sampling approaches and data collection methods center on gaining in-depth perspectives and narratives from the individuals participating in the study. In contrast to most quantitative research designs, qualitative research samples are not intended to be statistically representative. Thus, a type of nonprobability sampling known as *purposive sampling* is commonly used to identify participants, settings, or other sampling

Ethnography: description or interpretation of a population and its culture

Phenomenology: emphasizes individuals' subjective or lived experience and their interpretations of the world around them

Grounded theory: an inductive approach where data are collected and analyzed to generate a theory reflecting the phenomena of interest

Case study: detailed information about a particular participant or small group

Box 30.2 Qualitative Research Strategies[11]

units that reflect the specific characteristics or features needed to support detailed exploration and understanding of the phenomenon under study.[14] Data collection methods—including in-depth unstructured (eg, using a topic list) or semistructured (eg, guides including required or recommended questions and probes) interviews, focus groups, observation, visual methodologies (eg, photovoice and photo elicitation)—are iterative and provide the flexibility for participants to share their conceptualizations and values while allowing researchers to avoid imposing their predetermined definitions or view of the issue. For example, in one study researchers conducted focus groups with families who completed a community-based, family-oriented obesity treatment program to better understand intervention outcomes.[15] To help inform potential recommendations for changes in food assistance policy, another study used in-depth, semistructured interviews to explore experts' opinions about the factors that influence the eating patterns and dietary behaviors of Supplemental Nutrition Assistance Program (SNAP) recipients and elicited strategies to improve nutrition in SNAP.[16] As is common in qualitative research, data in these studies were audiorecorded, transcribed verbatim, and coded and analyzed for thematic content related to settings, contexts, actions, and meanings. While many studies conducted before 2000 coded transcripts and other types of qualitative data manually, most studies now use qualitative management software to organize and maintain data, (eg, Atlas.ti from Berlin Scientific or NVivo from QSR International).

As expected, the criteria for evaluating the quality of community-based qualitative research differs from the standard approaches to validity and reliability traditionally used in quantitative investigations. Lincoln and Guba[17] proposed the following "trustworthiness criteria" for evaluating the quality of qualitative research:

- Credibility: confidence in the truth of the findings
- Transferability: demonstrating that the findings are applicable in other contexts
- Dependability: showing that the findings are consistent and could be repeated
- Confirmability: the degree of neutrality or the extent to which the findings of a study are shaped by the respondents and not researcher bias, motivation, or interest

Techniques for establishing trustworthiness include prolonged engagement (ie, spending adequate time in the field), checking with members (ie, testing and sharing interpretations and conclusions with members of the target population), and triangulation (ie, using multiple data sources to produce a comprehensive understanding of the phenomena under study).[17,18] The observer's long-term involvement in the research setting increases participant trust and the likelihood that real behaviors, perceptions, and attitudes will be observed.[10] Observers can check with members by conducting interviews until response saturation is reached or no new information is provided (often after 25 to 30 interviews in a target population).[12] Conducting interviews and then confirming findings with a focus group is an example of triangulation and increases dependability.[11] Comparing findings with similar qualitative studies, confirming findings with a few experts in the field, and having more than one person analyze the data are techniques to increase confirmability.[12,13]

Quantitative Aspects of Community-Based Research

Qualitative aspects of community-based research provide a guide for selecting quantitative measures of impact in community settings. Quantitative measures may include impact factor models for evaluating the success of an intervention in a community as well as more traditional measures, such as dietary intake assessment and body weight, blood pressure, or biospecimen collection.

Impact Factor Models: Quantifying Success in Community Settings

One way to quantify the impact of an intervention in a community is to build a model for an impact factor. Identifying the factors to consider for this model often starts with looking at community projects that community partners have identified as successful, less successful, or unsuccessful. The division between successful and unsuccessful will be the dividing point for quantifying impact. For a dietary intervention in a community setting, the following factors might be of value:

● **Number of hours faculty, staff, students, and community partners work collaboratively to develop and implement projects:** The time spent to develop and implement a project allows external groups and community partners to bond. This close working relationship results in a more successful end result and impact on the community.

● **Number of community partners involved in project development and decision-making:** Identify the percent of actively participating key partners identified in the community who will extend the reach of the intervention.

● **Number of citizens the project touched through open houses, survey work, and so on:** Participation of community members is a measure of success of the intervention within a community. Tracking participation in every aspect of the intervention puts a pulse on overall reach.

● **Number of years the project continued in the community:** The sustainability of a project once a team of nutrition experts leaves a community is a mark of how the project or intervention effected community change.

● **Number of additional projects or initiatives that were spun off from original project:** Within a community, one project or intervention may

lead to other spin-off projects that continue to have a lasting effect on improving the quality of health within a community.

● **Economic impact of a project in the community (assessed on a sliding scale of 1 to 10 chosen by community partners):** When a community partner equates research work in a community with dollar amounts, the project and its potential savings become a return on investment that has new meaning for a community.

● **Safety (assessed on a sliding scale of 1 to 10 chosen by community partners):** In the book *Methods for Community-Based Participatory Research,*[9] the authors posit that in order to achieve an impact in a community, community partners must feel a level of safety. They must believe their needs are of the highest priority and the outcomes or interventions are upheld throughout the project.

● **Humility (assessed on a sliding scale of 1 to 10 chosen by community partners):** It is vital that the community partners' ideas and input are the most important factors in designing and implementing a community intervention. Many projects have been unsuccessful because the researchers' demands overshadowed those of the community partner.

While researchers working in each community setting may have different ideas on what constitutes impact, once a model is established for a community, projects within that community can then be compared using a single impact factor. Both community partners and researchers should provide input on the factors to consider and, within each of those, what constitutes success. Assigning numbers to each factor provides a numeric dividing point to identify the impact in each of the community interventions.

Dietary Intake Assessment and Biospecimen Data Collection

Other more traditional means of measuring the success of a nutrition-focused community intervention include a variety of quantitative methods to assess dietary intake. The data collection method used to do this will depend on both the population being studied and the resources available to the researchers. The major quantitative self-report measure for diet is the standard 3-day, 24-hour dietary recall. Trained staff should conduct the interviews using the US Department of Agriculture's Automated Multiple-Pass Method[19] and record data using such software as the Nutrition Data System-Research software (Minneapolis, Minn) or the National Cancer Institute's Automated Self-Administered 24-Hour Dietary Assessment Tool, ASA24. Recalls in nutrition studies may be completed by telephone.[20-22] When collecting data on children, this process can be facilitated by sending each child home with a serving-size book to use during the 24-hour dietary recall telephone calls as a reference for amounts of foods eaten. This proved useful in the Diet Intervention Study in Children.[23-25]

Often in large community-based trials, 24-hour recalls are too labor and resource intensive, so food frequency questionnaires[26] or brief scanners[27] can be used to assess dietary intake. These methods are often lower in cost and less burdensome for participants. The study outcomes and resources available should guide the choice of dietary intake assessment.

Health assessment methods are also important pieces of quantitative data in community-based research. In a dietary intervention these measures would likely include: body weight, height, body mass index, blood pressure, and waist circumference. Relevant diagnoses (eg, hypertension, diabetes) should also be recorded.

Biospecimen data collection may also be included as a quantitative measure of the diet intervention outcome. The choice of outcome assessment depends on the setting, feasibility, and resources available. For example, bioelectrical impedance analysis or a fingerstick lipid panel may be more feasible in a community research setting than some of the very accurate methods used in clinical research to measure impact of dietary change (eg, dual-energy x-ray absorptiomety or a blood lipid panel). Another biomarker used to assess adherence to the dietary intervention is urine sodium, an important biomarker of dietary sodium intake.[28,29] Unlike blood draws, urine sample collections are noninvasive and have proved to be feasible in community research.[29]

IMPORTANCE OF COMMUNITY PARTNER INVOLVEMENT

Most community-based research approaches involve some collaboration between community members, community-based organizations, and academic researchers.[9] The level of community engagement is an important consideration in community-based studies[2]; it can range from researchers maintaining exclusive control over the research process, with the community having no or minimal engagement (eg, research participants, outreach, community advisory boards), to fully collaborative partnerships (eg, identifying research questions, deciding about research design).[30] Goodman and colleagues[30] proposed that higher levels of community engagement help facilitate a deeper understanding of the complexities associated with poor health outcomes and a better translation of findings to practice and policy.

In nutrition and dietetics, community-based participatory research (CBPR) is one of the most frequently used community-engaged approaches. CBPR "equitably involves all partners in the research process, recognizes the unique strengths that each brings, and begins with a research topic of importance to the community with the aim of combining knowledge and action for social change."[31,32] To engage in this process, the community has to initially be recognized as a unit of identity, which is frequently defined based on its shared geography, cultural interests, values, and norms. Informed by Brazilian educator Paulo Freire's concept of popular education, a common aspect of CBPR (and other community-engaged paradigms) is to empower individuals who have traditionally been marginalized by research to take an active role.[33,34] Goodman and colleagues[30] developed a quantitative measure to assess levels of community engagement that could subsequently be correlated with research outcomes. Because CBPR is an approach and not a research design, various research designs can be used, including any of the community-based approaches previously discussed.

Community-Based Research Sample

The following example of CBPR uses existing relationships between an academic institution and community resource development centers across a state. Researchers used a cluster-randomized controlled trial design to examine the impact of a culturally tailored diet intervention to reduce blood pressure in Hispanic/Latino middle school students. The importance of community partner involvement for recruitment, randomization, and adherence in this example is detailed in the next section.

Recruitment in Community-Based Research

Having an initial partnership within communities before developing a community-based research project is vital. The project involving a nutrition intervention in middle schools, for example, is more achievable when community partners who have already worked with the schools approach the school administrators first. With these community partners paving the way with an introduction, the researcher's work takes several steps forward that might not have been possible without the community partner's involvement.

Seasoned researchers are aware of the importance of having specific scenarios for recruitment that fit the community and know that even with tailored approaches, recruitment does not always go as planned. Several recruitment strategies that varied according to the communities involved were proposed for the example study. Offering financial incentives for completing data collection procedures was a primary strategy. Other strategies included having information available at back-to-school nights, at school orientation, and during school physicals, which enabled the researchers to obtain consent or assent on the spot (see Box 30.3). Group presentations during physical education classes or study halls could also be used to garner interest in the study. Identifying a teacher at each school to act as a liaison between project coordinators and students is another avenue to recruit through the school. In the community, flyers could be posted at various locations, including the local YMCA, community health centers, and grocery stores; information booths could also be set up periodically at these locations during the recruitment phase. Similarly, a booth at the county and state fairs could aid recruitment. Having a familiar and trusted local person and local organizations

When is parental consent required?

If a child is younger than 18 years old, parents must provide consent for the child's participation. The child's agreement to participate is called assent.

See Chapter 3 for more on ethical issues in conducting research.

Box 30.3 Parental Consent for Children Participating in Research

endorse the project is another way to gain community support. If recruitment lags (or attrition is eventually reached), researchers could identify additional communities with populations similar to those targeted for the study and make sure those that have expressed a desire to participate are ready for screening.

Having a simple screening tool and process can also make recruitment easier. Figure 30.4 shows a form used in screening participants in a study that used blood pressure measurements as a quantitative outcome.

Randomization of Clusters Spanning Several Communities

Randomization also requires community involvement. Ensuring that each community understands that randomization could mean participants in their community are the control group and may not receive the intervention is just as important as ensuring that they understand how to implement the intervention. Figure 30.5 on page 602 provides an example of a plan for screening and eventually randomizing clusters into the arms of the community-based intervention study. The study design also includes the intervention and data collection points.

A plan for screening and study entry for community-based research should include a staggered recruitment plan followed by the nutrition intervention. For most community-based studies, recruitment will occur over several years in a stag-

Date: _____/_____/_____

Full Name: _____

Address: _____

Phone: (_____) - _____- _____

Sex: M / F   Birthdate: _____/_____/_____   Age: _____   Grade in school: _____

Race (circle one): Hispanic/Latino / non-Hispanic/Latino

Have you ever been told by a physician that you have diabetes? Yes / No

Do you have or have you had cancer in the past 5 years? Yes / No

Have you ever been told by a physician that you have kidney disease? Yes / No

Have you ever been told by a physician that you have high blood pressure/hypertension? Yes / No

        If yes, are you being treated for high blood pressure now? Yes / No

        If yes, what type of treatment? Diet / Medication / Other _____

Are you taking any medication? Yes / No

        If yes, which one(s)*? _____

        _____
        *study staff will ask participants to bring current medications with them at screening

---

FOR STUDY STAFF:

Measure	Height (cm)	Weight (kg)	Waist Circumference (cm)	Blood Pressure (mm Hg)		
				SBP / DBP	L / R	Time
1st				_____/_____	L / R	:
2nd				_____/_____	L / R	:
3rd	**	**	**	_____/_____	L / R	:

**only necessary when 1st and 2nd measurements differ by more than 1.0 cm or more than 0.3 kg.

Average of 2nd and 3rd BP measures: _____/_____mm Hg   Percentile for height: _____

REFER TO PROVIDER IF BLOOD PRESSURE IS GREATER THAN 98th PERCENTILE FOR HEIGHT.

PCP signature required if blood pressure falls between 95th-98th percentile for height.

Staff signature: _____   Date: _____

Participants excluded if they are not Hispanic/Latino, answer yes to any of the first three screening questions, or have a blood pressure >98th percentile for height.

Figure 30.4 Sample screening form for participants in a study on blood pressure management
Abbreviations: PCP = primary care physician; BP = blood pressure

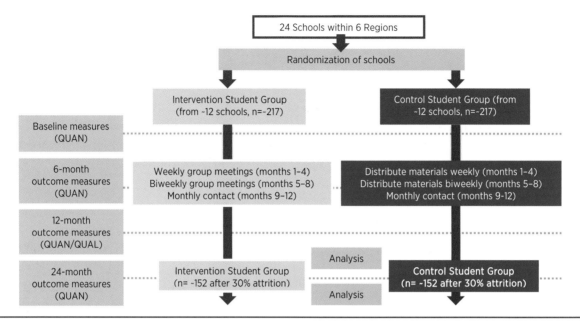

Figure 30.5 Sample community-based study design

Abbreviations: QUAN = Quantitative (height, weight, waist circumference, blood pressure, 24-hour diet recall, urine sodium, questionnaires regarding skills confidence and barriers to adherence); QUAL = Qualitative (exit interviews).

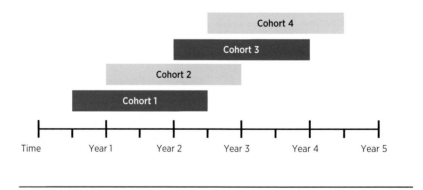

Figure 30.6 Staggered recruitment and intervention strategy

gered fashion. This will allow for slower recruitment in some communities and will help the researchers eventually achieve the numbers needed to show statistical significance. Additionally, this recruitment schedule allows study staff to be involved in each stage in each community. Figure 30.6 provides an example of a staggered recruitment and implementation schedule.

Maintaining Adherence in a Community-Based Intervention

Tracking attendance at group sessions and participant monitoring related to dietary behaviors are essential elements in a community-based intervention. For example, if students in the example study have difficulty meeting their fruit and vegetable intake goals, researchers trained in motivational interviewing could have brief sessions to help uncover barriers that prevent participants from meeting goals. Solutions to these barriers to adherence will come from the students through use of reflections and affirmations that lead to lasting dietary changes. Makeup sessions can also be offered to ensure that session content and motivation to follow the dietary and physical activity regimens are sustained.

While the incentives offered with recruitment (for completing data collection) also help with the goal to enhance adherence, researchers can provide additional incentives during group sessions. The incentives should be specific to each of the group sessions and might include healthy snacks and similar items that have the potential to increase adherence to the dietary regimen. Grocery store vouchers can also serve as an incentive. Staggering the monetary incentives throughout the study, providing small incentives for completing each data collection point, and awarding an additional bonus at the end of the data collection period for those completing all data collection points can also maintain adherence. This gives participants more reasons to stay committed to the study until the end.

Figure 30.7 on page 604 provides a sample form used in maintaining quality control, fostering adherence, and identifying problems as the study moves through the screening and implementation phases. This form also allows for consistent data collection and follow-up to identify and solve problem situations before they become detrimental to the study.

STUDY RESULTS AND THE COMMUNITY FOCUS

Community-based research approaches have been used to examine a variety of nutrition topics, including managing obesity and weight control, promoting diabetes self-management, implementing community-wide sodium reduction, lowering risk of cardiovascular disease, assessing dietary quality in children, improving the foods served in restaurants and schools, and examining the impact of opening new grocery stores and other food retail establishments.[35-43] In each case, outcomes should be closely tied to the original study hypotheses. Observational studies might aim to assess overall diet quality in a community. Policy changes as part of an intervention could aim to improve food served in restaurants or schools. Determining the study hypotheses before designing the study and using them to direct each aspect of the intervention and implementation ensures that appropriate measures are used and essential data are collected. Maintaining quality control throughout the study is also essential to ensure that the results are valid. As outlined earlier, both qualitative and quantitative measures are important to provide the complete picture of the success of the intervention.

CONCLUSION

Community-based studies are an important component of the body of knowledge related to diet and nutrition research. In the spectrum of translational research, community-based research helps investigators understand how dietary behavior change affects related health outcomes and informs directions for future research across the spectrum. Not only can community-based research add to the understanding of risk factors and the success of interventions but the results can also inform decision-making by allowing researchers to justify the choice of outcome measures based on feasibility and validity.

Both qualitative and quantitative research methods are important in measuring the success of community interventions. Used together, they can provide a more complete understanding of the factors influencing dietary behaviors and intervention success and whether these factors are specific to the community being studied or applicable to the larger population. Community partnerships and engagement are important measures of success in community research design and implementation.

DASH Study Status Update

Recruitment and Participation as of TIME, DATE

Study Staff Training

Session	Region 1	Region 2	Region 3	Region 4	Region 5	Region 6
Training Date						
Attendees						

Screening/Enrollment

	Screened (last week)	Eligible* (last week)	Enrolled (last week)	Total Enrolled/ Total Eligible	Total Enrollment Rate
Region 1					
Region 2					
Region 3					
Region 4					
Region 5					
Region 6					
TOTAL					

*Eligible = n Enrolled + n Refused + n Missed

<u>Reasons for Not Enrolling (Not mutually exclusive):</u>

- Refusal (n)
- Missed Recruit (n)
- Unable to provide PCP signature (n)
- BP >98th percentile (n)

- Diabetic (n)
- Chronic Disease (n)
- Significant psych history (n)
- Unable to complete study procedures (n)

Drop out notes:

Group Session Attendance (attendees/enrolled)

Session	Region 1	Region 2	Region 3	Region 4	Region 5	Region 6
1						
2						
3						
4						
5						
6						
7						
8						
9						
10						

Data Collection

Region	Baseline Eligible	Baseline Complete	6 month Eligible	6 month Complete	12 month Eligible	12 month Complete	24 month Eligible	24 month Complete
1								
2								
3								
4								
5								
6								

Figure 30.7 Study status update form

REFERENCES

1. Translational Science Spectrum. National Center for Advancing Translational Sciences website. https://ncats .nih.gov/translation/spectrum#public-health. August 21, 2017. Accessed October 2, 2017.

2. What are the T0 to T4 Research Classifications? University of Wisconsin Institute for Clinical and Translational Research website. https://ictr.wisc.edu /what-are-the-t0-to-t4-research-classifications. Accessed October 2, 2017.

3. Merrill RM. Experimental studies in epidemiology. In: Merrill RM. *Introduction to Epidemiology*. 7th ed. Burlington, MA: Jones & Bartlett Learning; 2017: 160-161.

4. Atienza A, King A. Community-based health intervention trials: an overview of methodological issues. *Epidemiol Rev*. 2002;24(1):72-79.

5. Blumenthal DS, DiClemente RJ. *Community-Based Health Research: Issues and Methods*. New York, NY: Springer; 2004.

6. Willett W. *Nutritional Epidemiology*. 3rd ed. New York, NY: Oxford University Press; 2012.

7. Remler DK, Van Ryzin GG. *Research Methods in Practice: Strategies for Description and Causation*. Thousand Oaks, CA: Sage Publications; 2011.

8. Assessing community needs and resources. University of Kansas Center for Community Health and Development Community Tool Box website. http://ctb.ku.edu/en/table -of-contents/assessment/assessing-community-needs -and-resources. Accessed September 25, 2017.

9. Israel BA, Eng E, Schulz AJ, Parker EA. *Methods in Community-Based Participatory Research for Health*. San Francisco, CA: Jossey-Bass; 2005.

10. Harris JE, Gleason PM, Sheean PM, Boushey D, Beto JA, Bruemmer B. An introduction to qualitative research for food and nutrition professionals. *J Am Diet Assoc*. 2009; 109(1):80-90.

11. Creswell JW. *Qualitative Inquiry and Research Design: Choosing Among Five Approaches*. 2nd ed. Thousand Oaks, CA: Sage; 2007.

12. Zoellner J, Harris JE. Mixed-methods research in nutrition and dietetics. *J Acad Nutr Diet*. 2017;117(5):683-697.

13. Denzin NK, Lincoln YS. *Handbook of Qualitative Research*. 2nd ed. London, United Kingdom: Sage Publications; 2000.

14. Ritchie J, Lewis J, eds. *Qualitative Research Practice: A Guide for Social Science Students and Researchers*. London, United Kingdom: Sage Publications; 2003.

15. Cason-Wilkerson R, Goldberg S, Albright K, Allison M, Haemer M. Factors influencing healthy lifestyle changes: a qualitative look at low-income families engaged in treatment for overweight children. *Child Obes*. 2015;11(2): 170-176.

16. Leung CW, Hoffnagle EE, Lindsay AC, et al. A qualitative study of diverse experts' views about barriers and strategies to improve the diets and health of Supplemental Nutrition Assistance Program (SNAP) beneficiaries. *J Acad Nutr Diet*. 2013;113(1):70-76.

17. Lincoln YS, Guba EG. Establishing trustworthiness. In: Lincoln YS, Guba EG. *Naturalistic Inquiry*. Newbury Park, CA: Sage Publications; 1985:289-331.

18. Schwandt TA, Lincoln YS, Guba EG. Judging interpretations: but is it rigorous? Trustworthiness and authenticity in naturalistic evaluation. *New Dir Eval*. 2007; 114:11-25.

19. Moshfegh AJ, Rhodes DG, Baer DJ, et al. The US Department of Agriculture Automated Multiple-Pass Method reduces bias in the collection of energy intakes. *Am J Clin Nutr*. 2008;88(2):324-332.

20. Rocha-Goldberg M, Corsino L, Batch B, et al. Hypertension Improvement Project (HIP) Latino: results of a pilot study of lifestyle intervention for lowering blood pressure in Latino adults. *Ethn Health*. 2010;15(3):269-282.

21. Ard JD, Coffman CJ, Lin PH, Svetkey LP. One year follow-up study of blood pressure and dietary patterns in Dietary Approaches to Stop Hypertension (DASH-Sodium) participants. *Am J Hypertens*. 2004;17(122):1156-1162.

22. Funk KL, Elmer PJ, Stevens VJ, et al. PREMIER—a trial of lifestyle interventions for blood pressure control: intervention design and rationale. *Health Promot Pract*. 2008;9(3):271-280.

23. Hartmuller VW, Snetselaar L, Van Horn L, et al. Creative approaches to cholesterol-lowering used in the Dietary Intervention Study In Children (DISC). *Top Clin Nutr*. 1994;10:71-78.

24. Snetselaar L, Lauer R. Children and cholesterol: potential prevention for future good health. *Bol Asoc Med PR*. 1991; 83(11):505-507.

25. Van Horn L, Stumbo P, Moag-Stahlberg A, et al. The Dietary Intervention Study In Children (DISC): dietary assessment methods for 8- to 10-year-olds. *J Am Diet Assoc*. 1993;93(12):1396-1403.

26. Shim J-S, Oh K, Kim HC. Dietary assessment methods in epidemiologic studies. *Epidemiol Health*. 2014;36: e2014009.

27. Yaroch AL, Tooze J, Thompson FE, et al. Evaluation of three short dietary instruments to assess fruit and vegetable intake: the National Cancer Institute's Food Attitudes and Behaviors (FAB) Survey. *J Acad Nutr Diet.* 2012;112(10):1570-1577.

28. Brown IJ, Dyer AR, Chan Q, et al. Estimating 24-hour urinary sodium excretion from casual urinary sodium concentrations in Western populations: the INTERSALT study. *Am J Epidemiol.* 2013;177(11):1180-1192.

29. *National Health and Nutrition Examination Survey (NHANES): Home Urine Collection.* Rockville, MD: NHANES, Centers for Disease Control and Prevention; 2013.

30. Goodman MS, Thompson VLS, Arroyo Johnson C, et al. Evaluating community engagement in research: quantitative measurement development. *J Community Psychol.* 2017;45(1):17-32.

31. Minkler M, Wallerstein N, eds. *Community Based Participatory Research in Health.* San Francisco: Jossey-Bass; 2003.

32. Wallerstein N, Duran B. Community-based participatory research contributions to intervention research: the intersection of science and practice to improve health equity. *Am J Public Health.* 2010; 100(suppl 1):S40-S46.

33. Strand KJ. Community-based research as pedagogy. *Mich J Community Serv Learn.* 2000;7:85-96.

34. Strand K, Marullo S, Cutforth N, Stoecker R, Donohue P. *Community-Based Research and Higher Education: Principles and Practices.* San Francisco CA: Jossey Bass; 2003.

35. Carson JA, Michalsky L, Latson B, et al. The cardiovascular health of urban African Americans: diet-related results from the Genes, Nutrition, Exercise, Wellness, and Spiritual Growth (GoodNEWS) trial. *J Acad Nutr Diet.* 2012;112(11):1852-1858.

36. Cohen JF, Kraak VI, Choumenkovitch SF, Hyatt RR, Economos CD. The CHANGE study: a healthy-lifestyles intervention to improve rural children's diet quality. *J Acad Nutr Diet.* 2014;114(1):48-53.

37. Gittelsohn J, Lee-Kwan SH, Batorsky B. Community-based interventions in prepared-food sources: a systematic review. *Prev Chronic Dis.* 2013;10:E180.

38. Gittelsohn J, Rowan M, Gadhoke P. Interventions in small food stores to change the food environment, improve diet, and reduce risk of chronic disease. *Prev Chronic Dis.* 2012; 9:E59.

39. Kane H, Strazza K, Losby JL, et al. Lessons learned from community-based approaches to sodium reduction. *Am J Health Promot.* 2015;29(4):255-258.

40. Rosas LG, Thiyagarajan S, Goldstein BA, et al. The effectiveness of two community-based weight loss strategies among obese, low-income US Latinos. *J Acad Nutr Diet.* 2015;115(4):537-550.e2

41. Roy R, Kelly B, Rangan A, Allman-Farinelli M. Food environment interventions to improve the dietary behavior of young adults in tertiary education settings: a systematic literature review. *J Acad Nutr Diet.* 2015; 115(10):1647-1681.

42. Seidu S, Walker NS, Bodicoat DH, Davies MJ, Khunti K. A systematic review of interventions targeting primary care or community based professionals on cardio-metabolic risk factor control in people with diabetes. *Diabetes Res Clin Pract.* 2016;113:1-13.

43. Silveira JA, Taddei JA, Guerra PH, Nobre MR. The effect of participation in school-based nutrition education interventions on body mass index: a meta-analysis of randomized controlled community trials. *Prev Med.* 2013; 56(3-4):237-243.

Index

608 • *Research: Successful A*

American Oil Chemist
American Society fo
Group, I
American Tim
amino acids
assemb
gen
G

Page numbers followed by *b*, *f*, or *t* refer to boxes, figures or tables.

E

H

HACCP. *See* Hazard Analysis and Critical Control Point
Handbook for Guideline Development (World Health
    Organization), 214*b*
Harris-Benedict equation, 146
Harvard Food Frequency Questionnaire, 256
Harvard School of Public Health, 47
Hawthorne effect, 111
Hazard Analysis and Critical Control Point (HACCP), 446
HBM. *See* health belief model
HBSC. *See* Health Behavior in School Aged Children
HDL-C. *See* high-density lipoprotein cholesterol
Health and Diet Survey, 162*t*, 173
health assessment methods, 599
Health Behavior in School Aged Children (HBSC), 164*t*
health belief model (HBM), 406, 407, 407*t*, 408–409
Health Information Index, 176*b*
Health Information National Trends Survey, 173
Health Insurance Portability and Accountability Act
    (HIPAA), 41, 576–577
Health Professions Education: A Bridge to Quality
    (Institute of Medicine), 583
Healthy Eating Index (HEI), 231, 258
Healthy Eating Index-2015, 109
Healthy People 2020, 9, 156*b*, 528
HEI. *See* Healthy Eating Index
heptadecanoic acid, 318
Herb Research Foundation, 431*b*
HHS. *See* Department of Health and Human Services
high-density lipoprotein cholesterol (HDL-C), 353–354,
    354*f*, 354*t*
high-performance liquid chromatography (HPLC), 314,
    318
    quality assurance and, 326
HIPAA. *See* Health Insurance Portability and
    Accountability Act
Hispanic Community Health Study/Study of
    Latinos, 320, 321
histidine, 386*t*
histograms, 490, 492*f*, 493*f*, 544*f*, 551
Homescan, 164*t*
homogenous sampling, 91*b*
hormone therapy, 3
HPLC. *See* high-performance liquid chromatography
HuGENet™ Handbook of Systematic Reviews, 213*b*
human error, 35–36
human genetics, 381–383
    diet exposure and response and, 384, 385*t*–389*t*, 389
Human Genome Project, 555
Human Microbiome Project, 555
Human Nutrition Research Information Management
    system, 425
human subjects
    institutional review board role in protecting, 37–38
    training resources for protection of, 38*t*
hunger, meal size and, 337
hydrocinnamte, 388*t*
hyperkalemia, 351
HyperRESEARCH, 95*b*
hypertension, 115, 140
    defining, 122
hypoglycemia, 24
hypothesis
    alternative, 469–470, 484–485
    defining, 10, 129, 130*f*
    examples for nutrition studies, 130*f*

null, 469–470, 484–486
primary, 129
secondary, 129
hypothesis testing
    assumption of normality, 487–488
    courtroom analogy, 486, 487*b*
    errors in, 486
    logic of, 486
    one-sided, 485–486
    statistical significance in, 497–498
    study design and statistical analysis, 484–486
    two-sided, 485–486

I

IBD. *See* inflammatory bowel disease
Icahn School of Medicine, Mount Sinai, 430*t*
IFPS. *See* Infant Feeding Practices Survey
IJCME. *See* International Committee for Medical
    Journal Editors
Illinois Transdisciplinary Obesity Program (I-TOPP), 224
Illustrating Science: Standards for Publication, 548, 550
illustrations. *See also* research, illustrating results
    algorithms and flowcharts, 553–554
    distribution maps, 552
    graphs, 546–551
    histograms, 490, 492*f*, 493*f*, 544*f*, 551
    message conveyed through, 542–543
    photographs, 542, 552
    preparing for publication, 555–556
    purposes, 542
    tables, 543, 544*f*, 545–546, 545*b*
    visualizing big data, 554–555
immunoassay, 318
impact evaluation measures, 61*t*
impact factor models, 598
incentives
    in clinical nutrition studies, 143
    training impacts of, 21
incidence
    calculating, 76*b*
    defining, 77*b*
    measurement of, 75–76
incidence-prevalence bias, 110
incidence rate, 75–76
incidence ratio, 24
inconsistent findings among nutrition studies, 121–122
indels. *See* insertion-deletion variants
independent groups
    with continuous data, 472–473
    proportions and sample size, 474
    three or more, 473
independent samples, study design and statistical
    analysis, 483
indirect benefits, 372
indirect calorimetry, 318–319
industry, funding from, 56
Infant Feeding Practices Survey (IFPS), 164*t*
inflammatory bowel disease (IBD), 12
INFOODS. *See* International Network of Food Data
    Systems
informatics, 361
information bias, 110
informed consent
    components of form for, 40*b*
    equipoise and, 45
    processes for, 38, 40–41